Stroke Therapy

Stroke Therapy

Second Edition

Edited by
Marc Fisher, M.D.

Professor and Vice Chairman, Department of Neurology, University of Massachusetts
Medical School, Worcester; Department of Neurology, UMASS/Memorial Health
Care, Worcester

with 38 contributing authors

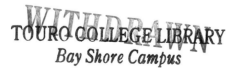
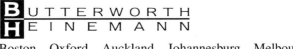

BUTTERWORTH
HEINEMANN

Boston   Oxford   Auckland   Johannesburg   Melbourne   New Delhi

Library of Congress Cataloging-in-Publication Data

Stroke therapy/ edited by Marc Fisher, with 38 contributing authors.—2nd ed.
    p. ; cm.
  Includes bibliographical references and index.
  ISBN 0-7506-7236-6 (alk. paper)
   1. Cerebrovascular disease—Treatment. I. Fisher, Marc, 1948–
  [DNLM: 1. Cerebrovascular Accident—therapy. 2. Brain Ischemia—therapy. WL 355
S9213736 2001]
  RC388.5 .S8568 2001
  616.8'1— dc21

                                                   00-066745

British Library Cataloguing-in-Publication Data
A catalogue record for this book is available from the British Library.

Contents

Contributing Authors

Alex Abou-Chebl, M.D.
Cerebrovascular Fellow, Department of Neurology, Cleveland Clinic Foundation

S. Hinan Ahmed, M.D.
Department of Neurology, Washington University School of Medicine, St. Louis

Gregory W. Albers, M.D.
Professor, Department of Neurology and Neurological Sciences, Stanford University School of Medicine, Stanford, California; Director, Stanford Stroke Center, Palo Alto, California

Andrei V. Alexandrov, M.D.
Assistant Professor of Neurology and Radiology, Stroke Treatment Team, University of Texas—Houston Medical School

Ursula E. Anwer, M.D.
Assistant Professor, Department of Neurology, University of Massachusetts Medical School, Worcester; Department of Neurology, UMASS/Memorial Health Care, Worcester

Viken L. Babikian, M.D.
Professor of Neurology, Boston University School of Medicine; Associate Visiting Neurologist, Boston University Medical Center; Associate Chief of Neurology, Boston Veterans Affairs Medical Center

Alison E. Baird, M.D., Ph.D.
Visiting Scientist, National Institute of Neurological Disorders and Stroke, National Institutes of Health, Bethesda, Maryland

Markus Bertram, M.D.
Medical Assistant, Department of Neurology, Ruprecht-Karls Universität, Heidelberg, Germany

Serge A. Blecic, M.D.
Associate Professor, Stroke Unit, Department of Neurology, Erasme Hospital, Free University of Brussels, Belgium

Bernadette Boden-Albala, M.P.H.
Project Manager, The Northern Manhattan Stroke Study, Department of Neurology and Division of Socio-Medical Science, Columbia University College of Physicians and Surgeons, New York

Natan M. Bornstein, M.D.
Professor of Neurology, Tel Aviv University Sackler School of Medicine, Tel Aviv, Israel; Chief of Stroke Unit, Department of Neurology, Tel Aviv Sourasky Medical Center, Tel Aviv

Lawrence M. Brass, M.D.
Professor of Neurology and Epidemiology and Public Health, Department of Neurology, Yale University School of Medicine, New Haven, Connecticut; Attending Neurologist, Department of Neurology, Yale-New Haven Hospital, New Haven

Stephen M. Davis, M.D., F.R.A.C.P.
Professor of Neurology, Department of Medicine, University of Melbourne, Victoria, Australia; Director, Department of Neurology, Royal Melbourne Hospital, Victoria

Gregory J. del Zoppo, M.D.
Associate Professor, Department of Molecular and Experimental Medicine, The Scripps Research Institute, La Jolla, California; Member, Department of Medicine, Division of Hematology/Medical Oncology, Scripps Clinic, La Jolla

Gérald Devuyst, M.D.
Associate Doctor, Department of Neurology, CHUV, Lausanne, Switzerland

Marc Fisher, M.D.
Professor and Vice Chairman, Department of Neurology, University of Massachusetts Medical School, Worcester; Department of Neurology, UMASS/Memorial Health Care, Worcester

Alejandro M. Forteza, M.D.
Director of Cerebrovascular Division, Assistant Professor of Neurology, University of Miami School of Medicine; Division Chief of Stroke Service, Department of Neurology, Jackson Memorial Hospital, Miami

Anthony J. Furlan, M.D.
Head, Section of Stroke and Neurological Intensive Care, Department of Neurology, Cleveland Clinic Foundation

Larry Bruce Goldstein, M.D.
Associate Professor of Medicine, Division of Neurology, Duke University School of Medicine, Durham, North Carolina; Director, Duke Center for Cerebrovascular Disease, Duke University Medical Center, Durham; Head, Stroke Policy Program, Center for Clinical Health Policy Research, Duke University; Attending Neurologist, Durham Veterans Affairs Medical Center

Camilo R. Gomez, M.D.
Professor, Department of Neurology, University of Alabama School of Medicine, Birmingham; Director, Comprehensive Stroke Center, Department of Neurology, University of Alabama at Birmingham

Werner Hacke, M.D.
Professor and Chairman, Department of Neurology, University of Heidelberg, Heidelberg, Germany

Gerhard Hamann, M.D.
Neurologische Klinik, Klinikum Grosshadern, Ludwig-Maximilians-Universität, Munich, Germany

Naoshia Hosomi, M.D.
Second Department of Internal Medicine, Kagawa Medical University, Kagawa, Japan

Chung Y. Hsu, M.D., Ph.D.
Professor and Head of Cerebrovascular Disease Section, Department of Neurology, Washington University School of Medicine, St. Louis; Professor and Director of Stroke Center, Department of Neurology, Barnes-Jewish Hospital, St. Louis

Chaur-Jong Hu, M.D.
Staff Neurologist, Department of Neurology, Taipei Municipal Jcn-Ai Hospital, Taipei, Taiwan

Markku Kaste, M.D., Ph.D.
Professor, Department of Neurology, University of Helsinki, Helsinki, Finland; Chairman, Department of Neurology, Helsinki University Central Hospital, Helsinki

Fuhai Li, M.D.
Research Instructor, Department of Neurology, University of Massachusetts Medical School, Worcester; Research Associate, Department of Neurology, UMASS/Memorial Health Care, Worcester

Kazuo Minematsu, M.D.
Director of Cerebrovascular Division, Department of Medicine, National Cardiovascular Center, Osaka, Japan

Fenwick T. Nichols III, M.D.
Professor, Department of Neurology, Medical College of Georgia School of Medicine, Augusta; Department of Neurology, Medical College of Georgia, Augusta

Richard Paczynski, M.D.
Department of Neurology, Washington University School of Medicine, St. Louis

James Paskavitz, M.D.
Assistant Professor, Department of Neurology, University of Massachusetts Medical School, Worcester; Department of Neurology, UMASS/Memorial Health Care, Worcester

Peter A. Rasmussen, M.D.
Assistant Staff, Department of Neurosurgery, Cleveland Clinic Foundation

Ralph L. Sacco, M.D., M.S.
Associate Chair of Neurology and Associate Professor of Neurology and Public Health (Epidemiology), Columbia University College of Physicians and Surgeons, New York; Associate Director of Stroke Service, Department of Neurology, New York Presbyterian Hospital

Wolf-Rüdiger Schäbitz, M.D.
Resident, Department of Neurology, University of Heidelberg, Heidelberg, Germany

Stefan Schwab, M.D.
Assistant Professor, Department of Neurology, University of Heidelberg, Heidelberg, Germany

David C. Tong, M.D.
Assistant Professor, Department of Neurology and Neurological Sciences, Stanford University School of Medicine, Stanford, California; Associate Director, Stanford Stroke Center, Palo Alto, California

Steven Warach, M.D., Ph.D.
Chief of Section on Stroke Diagnostics and Therapeutics, National Institutes of Health, National Institute of Neurological Disorders and Stroke, Bethesda, Maryland

John P. Weaver, M.D.
Associate Professor, Division of Neurosurgery, University of Massachusetts Medical School, Worcester; Director, Cerebrovascular Program, Division of Neurosurgery, UMASS/Memorial Health Care, Worcester

Takenori Yamaguchi, M.D.
President, National Cardiovascular Center, Osaka, Japan

Preface

Many important advances have occurred in the treatment of cerebrovascular disease since the first edition of this book was published in 1994. This revision represents an update of the inaugural edition with the addition of several new topics. Understanding the scope and pathophysiology of cerebrovascular disorders leads to an enhanced comprehension of which patients to treat with the most rational therapies. Advances in diagnostic capability enables clinicians to better target therapies to the most appropriate patients. The appropriate evaluation of new therapies in animal models and well-designed clinical trials is critical for the development of new stroke therapies. Since the mid-1990s, much effort has been focused on prevention strategies to reduce the incidence of acute stroke. An increasing variety of medical, surgical, and interventional procedures are available to reduce stroke risk. Acute stroke therapy has lagged in comparison; however, one therapy, recombinant tissue-type plasminogen activator administered within 3 hours of stroke onset, is of established value. Many other acute therapies have been evaluated, and valuable lessons for the future have been derived. The management of hemorrhagic cerebrovascular disorders has also advanced slowly. The promise of restorative therapies to enhance stroke recovery is beginning to be explored. All of these topics are reviewed in-depth by the contributions of acknowledged experts in the cerebrovascular disease field.

The compilation of a book on stroke therapy must be viewed as a work in progress that lends itself to periodic updates as this burgeoning and important field moves forward. It is my distinct honor and pleasure to assemble the information provided by the distinguished and dedicated group of contributing authors into this volume. I anticipate many further advances in the coming years and hope that future editions provide evidence of further advances to reduce the frequency and improve the outcome of cerebrovascular disorders.

Marc Fisher, M.D.

Acknowledgments

I dedicate this volume to my grandmother, Ella, who lived for several years with the devastating effects of a major, dominant-hemisphere ischemic stroke. I greatly appreciate the support and encouragement of my wife, Deborah, without whom my professional and personal development would not have been possible. I appreciate the help and encouragement of Susan Pioli and her staff at Butterworth–Heinemann, the best publisher and support staff that any editor could envision. Finally, I salute the chapter authors for their expertise, valuable contributions, and exhaustive efforts. Without them and their invaluable knowledge, this work would not have become a reality.

Stroke Therapy

Chapter 1

Stroke Risk Factors: Identification and Modification

Ralph L. Sacco and Bernadette Boden-Albala

Stroke is one of the top three causes of death in the United States, as well as in many countries throughout the world.[1] However, mortality rates alone do not represent the true impact of stroke, as stroke morbidity is frequently followed with functional dependence (Table 1-1). An understanding of the epidemiology of stroke is necessary to plan effective strategies for reducing the morbidity and mortality of this major public health problem. Although epidemiology allows the provider to recognize important risk factors for stroke, such identification alone only aids the provider in identifying individuals at greater risk for an event. Only when complemented with an understanding of the effects of modifying these risk factors can one attempt to reduce the impact of stroke morbidity and mortality in the community. In the United States, the 50% decline in stroke mortality since the 1980s indicates that many causes of stroke may be modifiable.[2] Prospective studies of stroke have identified many factors considered to carry a strong risk for stroke. Clearly, many of the strongest risk factors are beyond modification, including age, gender, race or ethnicity, and genetic causes. Many other factors are potentially modifiable and require early identification and treatment (Table 1-2).

Nonmodifiable Risk Factors

Age

The strongest determinant of stroke is age. Stroke incidence rises exponentially with age, with the majority of strokes occurring in persons older than 65 years of age. The age-specific incidence rates in Taiwan, for example, rose 10-fold over a 25-year span, from nearly 100 per 100,000 at 38 years of age to 1,000 per 100,000 at 63 years of age.[3] In Rochester, Minnesota, the incidence rate increased 10% per year of age.[4] As the population ages, the burden of stroke becomes even more apparent.

Gender

Gender differences in stroke incidence and mortality have been consistently demonstrated and indicate a greater risk of stroke among men. The male to female ratio has been estimated to be 1.3 to 1.0 and differs by stroke subtype. In Rochester, the stroke incidence rate was 70% higher in men for both lacunar and nonlacunar stroke.[4] In Sweden and Taiwan, stroke incidence was respectively 66% and 16% greater in men than in women.[3,5] Because women are more likely to survive a stroke, the prevalence and mortality rates among women are greater than men.[6,7]

Table 1-1. Estimated Public Health Impact of Stroke in the United States

Incidence	Prevalence	Mortality	Cost (billions)
731,000 new strokes/yr	4,000,000 survivors of stroke	160,000 stroke deaths/yr; third leading cause of death	$19.7 for stroke-related care: Hospital/nursing home: $14.7 Lost productivity: $2.8 Physician/nurse services: $1.9 Medication: $0.3

Race and Ethnicity

A decline in stroke mortality has occurred in each race and gender group, but the relative difference between the races has remained fairly uniform, with nearly twofold increased stroke mortality in blacks.[8] Few studies have the appropriate race and ethnic mixture to compare stroke incidence in multiethnic groups in the same region. Prior studies in Alabama and the Lehigh Valley of Pennsylvania have found that blacks have a greater incidence of stroke than whites of comparable age, sex, and residence.[9–11] In the National Health and Nutrition Survey, the relative risk of stroke for blacks was higher than for whites even after adjustment for age, hypertension, and diabe-

Table 1-2. Potential Stroke Risk Factors: Nonmodifiable and Modifiable

Nonmodifiable	Modifiable / Modification
Age	Hypertension/antihypertensives, diet
Gender	Heart disease/antiplatelets, anticoagulants, antiarrhythmics
Race and ethnicity	Atrial fibrillation/anticoagulants
Heredity	Diabetes mellitus/glucose control
	Hypercholesterolemia/lipid-lowering medication, diet
	Asymptomatic carotid stenosis/antiplatelets, endarterectomy
	Smoking/cessation
	Heavy alcohol intake/quantity reduction
	Physical inactivity/moderate exercise routine
	Recent TIA or stroke/antiplatelets, anticoagulants

TIA = transient ischemic attack.

tes.[12,13] In northern Manhattan, the overall age-adjusted 1-year stroke incidence rate for blacks was 2.4 times that of whites in a population-based stroke incidence study among white, black, and Hispanic residents (Figure 1-1).[14] In England and Wales, mortality from cerebrovascular disease was highest in Caribbeans, followed by Africans and Indians.[15] Moreover, physical and functional impairments after stroke were significantly more severe in blacks compared with whites in Durham County, North Carolina.[16] In Cincinnati, there was an increased risk of subarachnoid and intracerebral hemorrhages in blacks.[17] Blacks had 2.1 times the risk of subarachnoid hemorrhage of whites and 1.4 times the risk of intracerebral hemorrhage. The excess risk of hemorrhage for blacks was greatest for those of younger age in Cincinnati, whereas the increased incidence of intracerebral hemorrhage among blacks in northern Manhattan persisted even in the oldest population.

In contrast with blacks, Hispanics have rarely been identified separately in epidemiologic studies of stroke.[18–20] In northern Manhattan, Hispanics, predominately from the Dominican Republic, had an overall age-adjusted 1-year stroke incidence rate 2 times that of whites.[14] Finally, in other studies, Asians, particularly Chinese and Japanese, have exceedingly high stroke incidence rates, which seem to be decreased among those who have migrated to Hawaii and California.[21]

One explanation for the increased mortality from stroke in blacks, Hispanics, and Asians is that increased mortality is directly related to increased incidence. Others have shown that different groups have a unique burden of stroke risk factors after controlling for differences in socioeconomic status and other demographic variables.[22] By calculating the attributable risk or

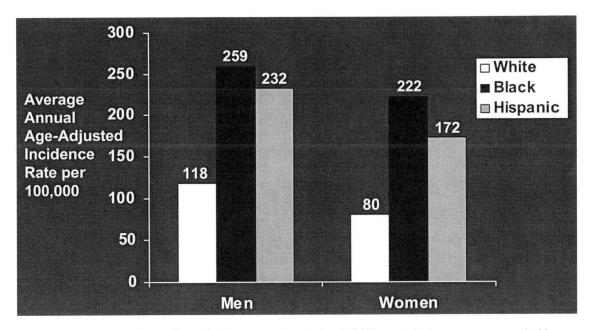

Figure 1-1. Average annual age-adjusted incidence rates of stroke (per 100,000 population) among persons aged ≥20 years in northern Manhattan by sex and race/ethnicity, July 1, 1993–June 30, 1996. (Modified from RL Sacco, B Boden-Albala, R Gan, et al. Stroke incidence among white, black and Hispanic residents of an urban community. The Northern Manhattan Stroke Study. Am J Epidemiol 1998:147:259–268.)

etiologic fraction of the risk factor, one can gauge the differential burdens in stroke risk across different groups. Identification of differences in risk factor profiles across racial and ethnic groups allows more targeted and better-justified therapeutic or preventive interventions.

Heredity

The hereditability or genetic risk of cerebrovascular disease has been underemphasized. Stroke is predominantly a complex disease, influenced by both genetic and environmental factors. Although there are more than 50 monogenic disorders associated with stroke, most are rare and account for a small proportion of stroke cases. It is thought that stroke is caused by several different genes whose individual effects are determined by certain environmental triggers in a complex gene-environmental interaction causal model.

Studies in different populations have demonstrated familial aggregation of stroke. A family history of stroke among first-degree relatives was a determinant of stroke mortality in women in south-

ern California, even after adjusting for other stroke risk factors.[23] Among Swedish men, a maternal history of death from stroke was an independent predictor of stroke.[24] Based on analyses from the Twin Registry crossed with the master index file of the Veterans Affairs Administration, the proband concordance rate for stroke was 17.7% for monozygotic pairs and only 3.6% for dizygotic pairs, yielding a significant relative risk of 4.3%.[25] Data from the Framingham Study indicated that both paternal and maternal history of stroke was associated with an increased stroke risk among the offspring cohort.[26]

Relatives of people with ischemic stroke often share the same risk factors, making it difficult to separate genetic factors from shared environment. The familial effect is thought to represent indirect genetic influences that operate through well-documented risk factors such as hypertension, diabetes mellitus (DM), cardiac diseases, and abnormal lipid states. Each of these risk factors remains under genetic influences that may or may not interact with environmental factors, and this observation argues against the notion that any single gene is a sufficient or necessary cause of stroke. Knowledge of these possible indirect genetic causes of stroke is incomplete. Potential genetic stroke risk factors include apolipoprotein E, lipoprotein(a), and genetic markers of thrombosis such as factor V Leiden and fibrinogen. At present, genetic screening is not available for atherosclerosis and stroke. The identification of genetic determinants for stroke would allow early identification of persons with increased risk of stroke through genetic screening and lead to more intensive environmental risk factor modification.

Modifiable Stroke Risk Factors

Besides the reported differences in stroke occurrence by age, gender, and race, numerous stroke risk factors have been identified in asymptomatic populations that are potentially modifiable. Stroke morbidity and mortality are more likely to be significantly reduced by identification and control of environmental factors in the stroke-prone individual. Modifiable stroke risk factors, as determined by prospective cohort and case-control studies, include hypertension, diabetes, cardiac disease (particularly atrial fibrillation [AF]), hypercholesterolemia, cigarette use, and alcohol use.

Hypertension

Hypertension and Stroke Risk

Hypertension, after age, is the most powerful stroke risk factor. It is prevalent in the U.S. population in both men and women and is of even greater significance in blacks. The risk of stroke rises proportionately with increasing blood pressure. In the Framingham Study, the age-adjusted relative risk of stroke among those with definite hypertension (blood pressure >160/95) was 3.1 for men and 2.9 for women.[27] Even among borderline hypertensives, the relative risk was 1.5 compared to normotensives. Isolated systolic hypertension is increasingly prevalent with age and increases the risk of stroke two- to fourfold, even after controlling for age and diastolic blood pressure. In the British Regional Heart Study, men with systolic blood pressures (SBPs) between 160 and 180 had approximately

four times the risk of stroke compared with men with SBPs below 160.[28] Those with SBPs above 180 had a sixfold greater stroke risk. A risk factor profile based on the Framingham cohort was developed that included SBP and the use of antihypertensive treatment, as well as other stroke risk factors (Figure 1-2).[29] The relative risk of stroke for a 10-mm Hg increase in SBP was 1.9 for men and 1.7 for women after controlling for other known stroke risk factors.

Hypertension Control

Data from Rochester, Minnesota, show a decline in stroke incidence between 1950 to 1959 and 1970 to 1979.[30] A corresponding analysis of hypertension during this period revealed an almost linear inverse relationship between hypertension control and stroke incidence in women. Men were found to have delayed management of hypertension, with a corresponding delayed decline in stroke incidence. Estimates from New Zealand attribute 10% of the observed reduction in stroke during 1973–1982 to hypertension management.[2] Other researchers emphasize that stroke incidence was decreasing as early as the 1950s, predating the widespread use of antihypertensive therapy and indicating that hypertensive management is not solely responsible for the decline.[31]

Prospective studies and clinical trials have consistently shown a decreased risk of stroke with control of mild, moderate, and severe hypertension in all age groups. A meta-analysis of nine prospective studies, including 420,000 individuals followed for 10 years, found that stroke risk increased by 46% for every 7.5-mm Hg increase in diastolic blood pressure (DBP) (Figure 1-3).[32] This analysis disclosed a graded relationship with no low threshold. A subsequent meta-analysis of 14 treatment trials, including 37,000 unconfounded randomized individuals followed for a mean of 5 years, confirmed the expected reduced stroke risk (Figure 1-4).[33,34] The analysis showed a mean diastolic reduction of 5–6 mm Hg with a corresponding 35–40% reduction in stroke incidence. This reduced risk was identified regardless of the level of the index DBP. Other meta-analyses have documented benefits among various subgroups.[35] The authors here concluded that antihypertensive therapy should be prescribed for all moderate hypertensives with

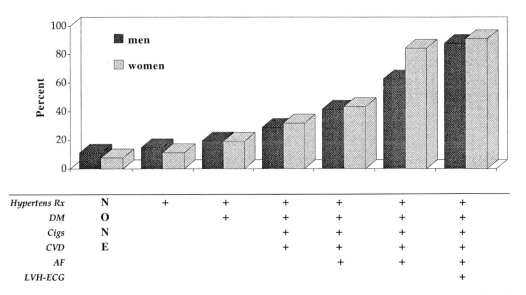

Hypertens Rx	N	+	+	+	+	+	+
DM	O		+	+	+	+	+
Cigs	N			+	+	+	+
CVD	E			+	+	+	+
AF					+	+	+
LVH-ECG							+

Figure 1-2. Probability of stroke within 10 years for men and women free of previous stroke: Framingham stroke risk profile. Bar graph of probability of stroke during 10 years in 70-year-old men and women at systolic blood pressure of 160 mm Hg: Impact of other risk factors. (AF = atrial fibrillation; Cigs = cigarette smoking; CVD = previously diagnosed coronary heart disease, cardiac failure, or intermittent claudication; DM = diabetes mellitus; Hypertens Rx = antihypertensive therapy; LVH-ECG = left ventricular hypertrophy by electrocardiogram.) (Modified from PA Wolf, RB D'Agostino, AJ Belanger, et al. Probability of stroke: a risk profile from the Framingham Study. Stroke 1991;22:312–318.)

high stroke risk. Also, as no low threshold for risk was found with DBP, antihypertensive therapy may also be considered for "normotensive" high-risk patients.[36]

In addition to the preceding meta-analysis, individual trials have also made significant contributions to the knowledge of the relationship between hypertension control and stroke risk. The STOP-Hypertension program (Swedish Trial in Old Patients with Hypertension) followed 1,627 randomized hypertensive patients aged 70–84 years for an average of 25 months.[37] This study indicated the benefit of managing hypertension in the elderly, finding a significant decline in stroke morbidity and mortality, as well as in total mortality. The SHEP (Systolic Hypertension in the Elderly Program) trial randomized 4,736 individuals older than 60 years of age with isolated systolic hypertension (SBP >160 mm Hg with DBP <90 mm Hg) and followed for 4.5 years.[38] The resulting 36% reduction in total stroke incidence confirmed the significance of managing isolated systolic hypertension, a condition affecting two-thirds of elderly hypertensives.[36] The Syst-Eur trial demonstrated that treatment of older patients

with isolated systolic hypertension led to a 42% reduction in stroke risk with no significant decline in overall mortality.[39] In absolute terms, these trials indicated that treating only 10–20 patients for 5 years prevents one major cardiovascular event.[40]

Current guidelines for treatment of hypertension have been published by the Joint National Committee on prevention, detection, evaluation, and treatment of high blood pressure.[41] Definitions of hypertension have been broadened to include individuals who were once considered "borderline hypertensive." Because the attributable stroke risk for hypertension (proportion of strokes explained by hypertension) ranges from 35% to 50% depending on age, even a slight improvement in the control of hypertension could translate into a substantial reduction in stroke frequency.[42] The National Stroke Association (NSA) recommends that to help decrease the risk for a first stroke, the three following things should be done: (1) blood pressure should be controlled in patients with hypertension who are most likely to develop stroke, (2) physicians should check the blood pressure of all their patients at every visit, and

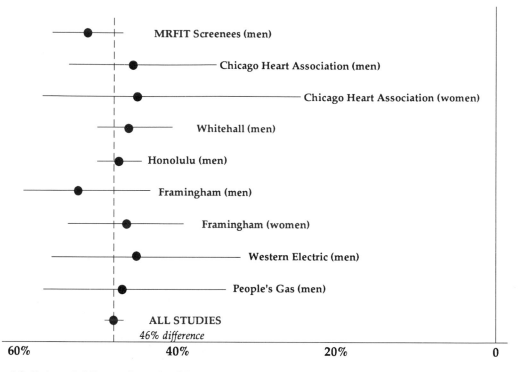

Figure 1-3. Estimated difference in stroke risk associated with a 7.5-mm Hg reduction in usual diastolic blood pressure. The horizontal lines represent the 95% confidence intervals for the estimated difference in risk. The broken vertical line represents a 46% difference in risk—the weighted mean difference in risk for all studies combined. (MRFIT = Multiple Risk Factor Intervention Trial.) (Modified from S MacMahon, R Peto, J Cutler, et al. Blood pressure, stroke, and coronary heart disease. Part 1. Prolonged differences in blood pressure: prospective observational studies corrected for the regression dilution bias. Lancet 1990;335:765–774.)

(3) patients with hypertension should monitor their blood pressure at home.[43]

Cardiac Disease

Cardiac Disease and Stroke Risk

Cardiac disease has been clearly associated with increasing the risk of ischemic stroke, particularly AF, valvular heart disease, myocardial infarction, coronary artery disease, congestive heart failure, electrocardiographic evidence of left ventricular hypertrophy, and perhaps mitral valve prolapse. Because certain stroke risk factors, like hypertension, may also be determinants of cardiac disease, some cardiac conditions may be viewed as intervening events in the causal chain for stroke.

Chronic AF affects more than 1 million Americans and becomes more frequent with age. AF accounts for 7–30% of all strokes in patients older than 60 years of age and more than 75,000 cases of stroke per year. In the Framingham Study, AF was a strong predictor of stroke, with nearly a fivefold increased risk of stroke.[44] In those with coronary heart disease (CHD) or cardiac failure, AF doubled the stroke risk in men and tripled the risk in women. The attributable risk of stroke from AF (percentage of strokes that could be attributed to AF) increased significantly with age, approaching that of hypertension in the oldest age group (Figures 1-5 and 1-6). In contrast, the attributable risk of stroke from hypertension remains relatively constant, with a slight decline in the oldest age group. When there is coexisting valvular disease, AF has an even greater impact on the relative risk of stroke. In the Stroke Prevention in Atrial Fibrillation study,[45] recent congestive heart failure, hypertension, and prior thromboembolism were found to

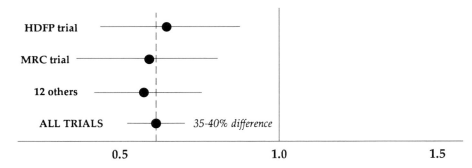

Figure 1-4. Reduction in odds of stroke with mean diastolic blood pressure difference of 5–6 mm Hg for 5 years in the Hypertension Detection Follow-Up Program (HDFP) trial, the Medical Research Council (MRC) trial, and 12 other smaller, unconfounded randomized trials of antihypertensive therapy. (Modified from R Collins, R Peto, S MacMahon, et al. Blood pressure, stroke, and coronary heart disease. Part 2. Short-term reductions in blood pressure: overview of randomised drug trials in their epidemiological context. Lancet 1990;335:827–838.)

identify high-risk groups for arterial thromboembolism among patients with nonvalvular AF. Left ventricular dysfunction and increased left atrial size by echocardiography were also predictors of increased thromboembolic risk.[45,46]

Stroke risk nearly doubles in those with antecedent coronary artery disease and nearly quadru-

ples in subjects with cardiac failure.[44] Relative risk significantly declined with advanced age. Acute myocardial infarction has also been associated with stroke, particularly when it is transmural and when the anterior wall is involved.[47] The attributable risk of stroke for CHD was approximately 12% and ranged from 2.3% to 6.0% for cardiac

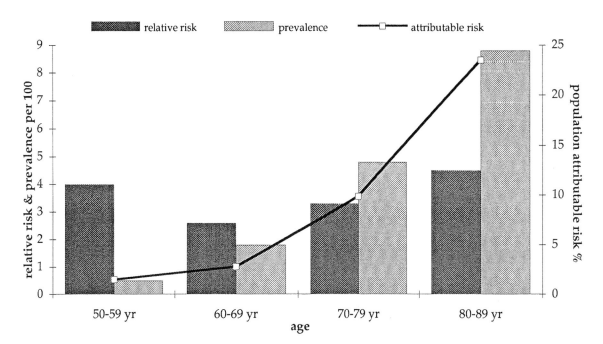

Figure 1-5. Prevalence, relative risk, and population attributable risk for atrial fibrillation by age. Relative risk adjusted for coronary heart disease, cardiac failure, and hypertension. Prevalence rate per 100. (Data from PA Wolf, RD Abbott, WB Kannel. Atrial fibrillation as an independent risk factor for stroke. Stroke 1991;22:983–988.)

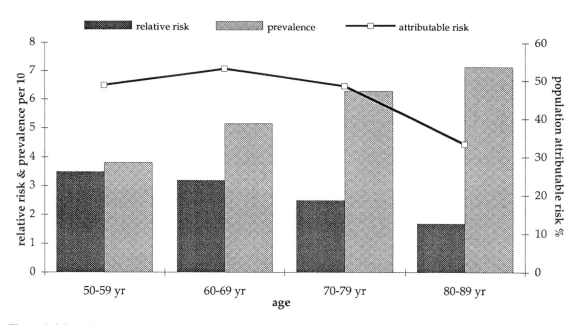

Figure 1-6. Prevalence, relative risk, and population attributable risk for hypertension by age. Relative risk adjusted for coronary heart disease, cardiac failure, and atrial fibrillation. Prevalence rate per 10. (Data from PA Wolf, RD Abbott, WB Kannel. Atrial fibrillation as an independent risk factor for stroke. Stroke 1991;22:983–988.)

failure. In British men with definite evidence of myocardial infarction, there was a fourfold increase in risk of stroke compared with men with no prior ischemic heart disease.[28]

Electrocardiographic evidence of left ventricular hypertrophy is more prevalent with advancing age and elevated blood pressure and has been found to increase the risk of stroke. Even after adjusting for the presence of other risk factors, such as hypertension, left ventricular hypertrophy increased the risk of stroke by 2.3% in both men and women.[29] Left ventricular hypertrophy is markedly influenced by the degree of obesity.[48] In British men, the effect of left ventricular hypertrophy was observed only in those with pre-existing ischemic heart disease.[28]

Improved cardiac imaging has led to the increased detection of potential stroke risk factors: mitral valve prolapse,[49–51] mitral annular calcification,[52] spontaneous echo contrast (a smokelike appearance in the left cardiac chambers visualized on transesophageal echocardiography),[53] left atrial enlargement,[54] atrial septal aneurysms,[55,56] patent foramen ovale,[57–59] and aortic arch atherosclerotic disease.[60,61]

Treatments for Cardiac Conditions

Numerous medications have been tested for various cardiac conditions. Measures effective in reducing the incidence of cardiac disease could lead to a reduction in stroke incidence. Antiplatelet agents have proven efficacy in the reduction of nonfatal myocardial infarction in primary prevention studies. Beta blockers have been shown to reduce the risk of myocardial infarction. Warfarin appears beneficial in the prevention of cardiogenic embolism among patients with acute anterior wall myocardial infarction, left atrial or ventricular thrombus, and prosthetic valvular replacements.

Numerous randomized clinical trials have demonstrated the superior therapeutic effect of warfarin compared to placebo in the prevention of thromboembolic events among patients with nonvalvular AF.[62–68] The relative risk reduction of stroke ranged from 42% to 86%. Warfarin use was relatively safe, with major bleeding rates ranging from 0.8% to 2.1%. Aspirin may also have some efficacy among lower risk groups or those who have relative contraindications to anticoagulation. The Stroke Prevention in Atrial Fibrillation III study demonstrated that warfarin with an international normalized ratio (INR) of 2–3 was far superior to aspirin and mini-dose warfarin with an INR <1.5 in the prevention of stroke among high-risk patients with nonvalvular AF.[69] The recommendation from the fifth American College of Chest Physicians Consensus Conference on Antithrombotic Therapy was that long-term oral warfarin therapy (INR 2.0–3.0, target 2.5) be used in patients with AF who are eligible for anticoagulation, except in patients younger than 60 years of age who have no associated cardiovascular disease.[70]

Diabetes Mellitus

Diabetes has also been associated with an increased stroke risk. Relative risks range from 1.5 to 3.0, depending on the type and severity. Death from cerebrovascular disease is greatly increased among subjects with elevated blood glucose values.[71] In British men, the mean serum glucose level was significantly higher in those who developed stroke but lacked significance after adjusting for age and hypertension.[28] In the Framingham Study, the impact of diabetes was much clearer. The study found the stroke risk from diabetes in both men and women did not diminish with age, and was independent of hypertension.[27] In the Copenhagen City Heart Study, diabetes had a marked independent effect on stroke risk.[72] Diabetes was associated with a twofold increased adjusted risk of thromboembolic stroke among Japanese men living in Hawaii[73] and in men and women in Rancho Bernardo, California.[74]

Worldwide there seems to be an extraordinary increase in type 2 diabetes, from an estimated 124 million cases in 2000 to a predicted 221 million cases by 2010, with only 3% of all patients with type 1 diabetes.[75] Based on preliminary data from the Northern Manhattan Stroke Study, the prevalence of diabetes may be as high as 22% among elderly blacks and 20% among elderly Hispanics, with the corresponding attributable risks of stroke estimated at 13% and 20%, respectively.[22]

Intensive treatment of both type 1 and type 2 diabetes aimed at maintaining near normal levels of blood glucose can substantially reduce the risk of microvascular complications such as retinopathy, nephropathy, and neuropathy, but has not been conclusively shown to reduce macrovascular complications, including stroke.[76–78] The UK Prospective Diabetes Study group, however, reported that aggressive treatment of high blood pressure (<150/85 mm Hg) among type 2 diabetics helped significantly reduce the risk of stroke by 44%.[79] Guidelines for management of diabetes have been published by the American Diabetes Association and have lowered the target fasting blood glucose level to 126 mg/dl.[80] The NSA recommends rigorous comprehensive control of blood sugar levels for adherent patients with type 1 DM and type 2 DM to prevent microvascular complications.[43]

Lipids

Lipid Level and Stroke Risk

Abnormalities in the levels of serum lipids, triglycerides, cholesterol, low-density lipoprotein (LDL) and high-density lipoprotein (HDL) are regarded as risk factors, more for coronary artery disease than cerebrovascular disease.[81] Cholesterol and LDL have a direct relationship with the incidence of heart disease, whereas HDL has an inverse relationship. In prior studies from Framingham, a quadratic or U-shaped relationship was described between serum total cholesterol level and stroke incidence. In the Multiple Risk Factor Intervention Trial, mortality from ischemic stroke was greater among men with high cholesterol levels.[82] In the Honolulu Heart Program, there was a continuous and progressive increase in both CHD and thromboembolic stroke rates with increasing levels of cholesterol, with a relative risk of 1.4 comparing highest and lowest quartiles.[83] Meta-analyses among prospective studies have either found no or only a minimally increased relative risk of stroke due to elevated total cholesterol.[84,85] The absence of a consistent significant relationship between cholesterol and stroke may be partially explained by the recognition that there are multiple stroke subtypes that are not all attributed to atherosclerosis. Additionally, most prospective studies were done among younger populations and focused on cardiac outcomes, and lipoprotein fractions were not always evaluated separately from total cholesterol.

When lipid subfractions have been measured, some studies have documented a protective association between HDL and ischemic stroke.[71] In the Oxfordshire Community study, a dose-dependent, inverse relationship was demonstrated between HDL and transient ischemic attacks (TIAs) or minor stroke risk, with nearly one-third the stroke risk found in those with higher HDL levels.[86] In northern Manhattan, a significant protective dose-response relationship was found between HDL and ischemic stroke.[87] Degree and progression of carotid atherosclerosis have been found to be directly related to cholesterol and LDL levels and inversely related to HDL levels.[88,89] Other lipid markers, such as a high serum lipoprotein(a), have been found to be a risk factor in a group of patients with early onset of cerebral infarction.[90]

Control of Hyperlipidemia

Before the introduction of statins, clinical trials analyzing the relationship between lipid-lowering strategies and stroke found no benefits.[91] The Multiple Risk Factor Intervention Trial study showed a paradoxical increase in hemorrhagic stroke risk with low cholesterol levels.[92] Modern clinical trials analyzing the efficacy of statins in lowering lipid levels have demonstrated impressive reductions in stroke risk in various high-risk populations with cardiac disease. In these studies, stroke was either a secondary endpoint, or a nonspecified endpoint determined by post-hoc analyses.[93] Two

large trials in which stroke was prespecified as a secondary endpoint have also shown significant reductions with pravastatin among subjects with coronary artery disease and normal to modest cholesterol elevations.[94,95] Meta-analyses of some of these trials have found significant reductions in stroke risk, with a 29% overall reduced risk of stroke and a 22% reduction in overall mortality.[96,97] Secondary prevention trials showed a 32% stroke risk reduction, and primary trials demonstrated a 20% reduction. Using serial carotid ultrasound measurements, some clinical trials have also demonstrated carotid plaque regression with statins.[98–102]

The mounting evidence from observational and clinical trial data provides support for the role of lipoproteins as precursors of carotid atherosclerosis and ischemic stroke, and the benefits of cholesterol lowering in stroke reduction. Individuals with cholesterol levels above 200 mg/dl and cardiovascular risk factors should have a complete lipid analysis (total cholesterol, LDL, HDL, triglycerides) and most likely would benefit from cholesterol-lowering regimens, including statins (Table 1-3).[43]

Asymptomatic Carotid Artery Disease

Asymptomatic carotid artery disease, which includes nonstenosing plaque or carotid stenosis, is common and increases with age, occurring in 53.6% of subjects 65–94 years of age.[103] Among individuals with asymptomatic carotid disease, the annual stroke risk was 1.3% in those with stenosis of 75% or less and 3.3% in those with stenosis of more than 75%, with an ipsilateral stroke risk of 2.5%.[104] The combined TIA and stroke risk was 10.5% per year in individuals with more than 75% carotid stenosis. Cardiac event rates also were greater in the severe carotid stenosis group (8.3% per year). Moreover, silent (subclinical) strokes on computed tomography scans have been found in 19% of individuals with asymptomatic carotid stenosis.[105] The occurrence of symptoms may depend on the severity and progression of the stenosis, the adequacy of collateral circulation, the character of the atherosclerotic plaque, and the propensity to form thrombus at the site of the stenosis. The benefits of interventions for asymptomatic

Table 1-3. Stroke Reduction with Statin Agents

Treatment	N	No. of Stroke Events	Percent Reduction
4S trial[93]			
Simvastatin[93]	2,221	61	
Placebo	2,223	95	30 (P = .024)
CARE trial[94]			
Pravastatin	2,081	54	
Placebo	2,078	78	31 (P = .03)
Lipid study[95]			
Pravastatin	4,512	169	
Placebo	4,502	201	19 (P = .048)

CARE = Cholesterol and Recurrent Events trial.

carotid disease are discussed in subsequent chapters on surgical therapies.

Cigarette Smoking

Cigarette Smoking and Increased Stroke Risk

Cigarette smoking has been clearly established as a biologically plausible, independent determinant of increased stroke risk.[106] In case-control studies, the effect of cigarette smoking remained significant after adjustment for other factors, and a dose-response relationship was apparent.[107,108] In cohort studies, such as the Honolulu Heart Study[109] and the Nurses' Health Study,[110] cigarette smoking was an independent predictor of ischemic stroke, with adjusted relative risks of 2.5 for men and 3.1 for women, respectively. In the Framingham Study, cigarette smoking accounted for an adjusted relative risk of brain infarction of 1.7 after controlling for other cardiovascular risk factors.[29] Stroke risk was increased twofold in heavy smokers (>40 cigarettes per day) compared to light smokers (<10 cigarettes per day).[111] In middle-aged British men, stroke incidence rose with increasing number of cigarettes smoked, and among hypertensive smokers the relative risk of stroke was 12.2.[28]

In a meta-analysis of 32 separate studies, the overall pooled relative risk of stroke was 1.5 (95%; CI, 1.4–1.6) among cigarette smokers.[112] A dose-response relationship was observed. The risk decreased with age, and a small increased risk was noted in women compared to men. The stroke risk attributed to cigarette smoking was greatest for subarachnoid hemorrhage,[113,114] intermediate for cerebral infarction, and lowest for cerebral hemorrhage.

The mode of action of cigarette smoking in causing stroke is not entirely clear, but acceleration of atherosclerosis is one possibility. Cigarette smoking was found to be an independent determinant of carotid artery plaque thickness[115,116] and the strongest predictor of severe extracranial carotid artery atherosclerosis.[117,118] The relationship between cigarettes and atherosclerosis suggests that the effect of smoking may vary by ischemic stroke subtype. This observation may help explain the lack of an association between stroke and smoking in some studies, particularly Japanese cohorts in which cholesterol levels are lower and stroke subtypes are different.[119] Other potential biological mechanisms that can induce stroke include increased blood viscosity, hypercoagulability, elevated fibrinogen levels, enhanced platelet aggregation, and elevation of blood pressure.[120]

Cigarette Smoking Cessation

Although no randomized clinical trial has been performed to support the benefits of cigarette smoking cessation, there is ample evidence from observational epidemiologic studies that smoking cessation leads to a reduction in stroke risk. In a prospective study of 177,006 female registered nurses, the excess risk of ischemic stroke for former smokers disappeared after 2 years of cessation.[121] This reduction was found regardless of the number of cigarettes smoked, age at starting, and other stroke risk factors. Data from the Framingham Study confirm that the risk of stroke for former smokers approaches the risk for those who never smoked within 5 years of cessation.[122] An intervention program randomizing 1,445 British men found that at 10 years, the intervention group was smoking 53% less than the controls.[123] Although stroke mortality was not measured, the reduction was associated with an 18% reduction in CHD mortality.

Despite the absence of confirmatory clinical trials, the data from prospective cohort studies have demonstrated convincingly that cessation of cigarette smoking can reduce the risk of stroke. The methods to encourage smoking cessation include education, biofeedback, behavioral conditioning, hypnosis, financial disincentives, and nicotine patches. It has been estimated that if cigarette smoking could be eliminated in the United States, the number of strokes occurring each year could be reduced by 61,500, saving $3.08 billion in stroke-related health care.[124] The NSA recommends the cessation of smoking as a stroke prevention measure, in accordance with guidelines by the Agency for Healthcare Research and Quality that address various topics, including tobacco screening, smoking cessation advice and motivation, interventions, smoking cessation pharmacotherapy, and relapse prevention.[43]

Alcohol

Alcohol Consumption and Stroke Risk

The role of alcohol as a stroke risk factor is controversial.[125] Study results range from a definite independent effect in both men and women, an effect only in men, and no effect after controlling for other confounding risk factors such as cigarette smoking. As with other studies regarding stroke risk factors, discrepancies in the results are in part explained by the definition of the exposure variables, choice of comparison groups, and the subtype composition of the stroke group. The various mechanisms through which alcohol may increase the risk of stroke include hypertension, hypercoagulable states, cardiac arrhythmia, and cerebral blood flow reduction. However, there is also evidence that light to moderate drinking can increase HDL-cholesterol, reduce the risk of coronary artery disease, and increase endogenous tissue plasminogen activator. These variable mechanisms complicate the interpretation of alcohol as a stroke risk factor.

The biological effects of alcohol are consistent with the epidemiological observation of a J-shaped relationship between alcohol and stroke, with an elevated stroke risk for moderate to heavy alcohol consumption and a protective effect in light drinkers compared to nondrinkers.[126] A significant effect of heavy ethanol use (odds ratio = 4.0 for 300 g per week or more) was found for men in Birmingham, England, whereas light drinkers (odds ratio = 0.5 for 10–90 g per week) were relatively protected from stroke.[127] Heavy alcohol intake increased the risk of stroke twofold in middle-aged British men without previously diagnosed cardiovascular disease.[28] In northern Manhattan, a J-shaped relationship between alcohol and stroke was found with an elevated stroke risk for heavy alcohol consumption and a protective effect in light to moderate drinkers (two or fewer drinks per day) when compared to nondrinkers.[128] Among nurses, moderate alcohol consumption led to a 30% reduction in stroke risk.[129] In the Framingham Study, moderate to heavy alcohol consumption was associated with an increased relative risk of stroke, whereas light drinking was associated with reduced relative risk when compared to nondrinkers. However, the effect was only significant in men.[130] Other studies

have corroborated the protective effects of mild to moderate alcohol intake against stroke.[131,132]

Alcohol Reduction

No trials of the relationship between alcohol use modification and stroke risk have been performed. Such studies will be difficult because of the nonlinear dose-response relationship between alcohol and stroke, as well as the ethical concerns. Elimination of heavy drinking can undoubtedly reduce the incidence of stroke. Because some ingestion of alcohol, perhaps up to two drinks per day, may actually help reduce the risk of stroke, drinking in moderation should not be discouraged for most of the public.[43]

Physical Activity

The vascular benefits of physical activity have been emphasized by numerous public health organizations.[133,134] Previous studies evaluating the association between physical activity and stroke have found beneficial effects predominately among white populations, more apparent for men than women, and generally described for younger rather than older adults.[135–143] The Honolulu Heart Program, which investigated older men of Japanese ancestry, showed a protective effect of habitual physical activity from thromboembolic stroke only among nonsmokers.[135] The Framingham Study demonstrated the benefits of combined leisure- and work-time physical activities for men, but not for women.[136] In the Oslo Study, increased leisure-time physical activity was related to a reduced stroke incidence among men aged 40–49.[137] Among women aged 40 to 65 years old, the Nurses' Health Study showed an inverse association between the level of physical activity and the incidence of any stroke.[139] In the Northern Manhattan Stroke Study, the benefits of leisure-time physical activity were noted for all age, gender, racial and ethnic subgroups.[140] The protective effect of physical activity may be partly mediated through its role in controlling various risk factors such as hypertension, diabetes, and obesity. Other than control of risk factors, biological mechanisms, such as increased HDL and reduced homocysteine levels, may also be responsible for the effect of physical activity.[143–145]

Physical activity is a modifiable behavior that requires greater emphasis in stroke prevention campaigns. The 1994 Behavioral Risk Factor Surveillance Survey found that 60% of adults did not achieve the recommended amount of physical activity, and people with the lowest incomes and less than a twelfth grade education were more likely to be sedentary.[146] Moreover, 70% to 80% of older women surveyed reported levels less than the recommended amount of physical activity.[146] Public health goals are to increase the proportion of people who engage in regular physical activity and reduce the proportion of those who engage in no leisure-time physical activity, particularly among people aged 65 and older.[147] Leisure-time physical activity could translate into a cost-effective means of decreasing the public health burden of stroke and other cardiovascular diseases among the United States' rapidly aging population.[43]

Dietary Factors

Few studies have been able to clarify the relationship of diet to stroke because of the complex issues associated with dietary intake and nutritional status. Early large ecological studies have suggested that excess fat intake associated with migration may lead to increased risk of both CHD and stroke.[148] High daily dietary intake of fat is associated with obesity and may act as an independent risk factor or may affect other stroke risk factors such as hypertension, diabetes, hyperlipidemia, and cardiac disease. Results from the Framingham Study, however, have suggested conflicting findings, with an inverse association between dietary fat and ischemic stroke.[149] Dietary sodium may also be associated with increased stroke risk. Specifically, increased sodium intake is involved with an increased risk of hypertension.[150]

Another important dietary component is homocysteine. Case-control studies have demonstrated an association between moderately elevated homocysteine and vascular disease, including stroke.[151,152] Genetic and environmental causes of increased serum homocysteine have been implicated as a modifiable determinant of cardiovascular

and cerebrovascular events.[153,154] The Framingham Study found that deficiencies in folate, vitamin B_{12}, and pyridoxine accounted for the majority of elevated homocysteine levels in the study cohort.[155] Additionally, evidence from case-control studies has suggested that increased dietary and supplemental intake of vitamin B_6 may decrease stroke risk.[156] Large studies, such as the Vitamin in Stroke Protection Trial, are currently investigating the protective effects of vitamins B_6 and B_{12} and folate against recurrent stroke.

Dietary intake of fruits and vegetables may reduce the risk of stroke. These foods may contribute to stroke protection through antioxidant mechanisms or through elevation of potassium levels.[157–160] Dietary antioxidants, including vitamin C, vitamin E, and beta-carotene, belong to a group of antioxidants called *flavonoids* that are found in fruits and vegetables. These scavengers of free radicals are thought to be associated with stroke risk reduction through the free-radical oxidation of LDL, which inhibits formation of atherosclerotic plaques.[161] The large Western Electric cohort found a moderate decrease in stroke risk associated with a higher intake of both beta-carotene and vitamin C.[162] Other dietary factors associated with a reduced risk of stroke include milk, calcium,[134] and fish oils.[163–165]

Other Potential Stroke Risk Factors

Other potential stroke risk factors have been identified in some studies but need confirmation and clarification through further epidemiologic investigations (Table 1-4). Migraine-associated stroke has been observed. However, there are few conclusive epidemiologic studies on migraine-associated stroke. In a case-control study of young women with stroke, migraine had a significant odds ratio of 1.7 when compared to neighborhood controls but failed to be significant when compared to hospitalized controls.[166] In Rochester, Minnesota, the incidence of migraine-associated stroke was 1.7 per 100,000 population[167] and in Oxfordshire, England, the incidence rate was 3.4 per 100,000 population, but this association accounted for only 3% of ischemic infarcts.[168]

Oral contraceptive use has been associated with a higher stroke risk, particularly in women older

Table 1-4. Potential Stroke Risk Factors Under Further Epidemiologic Investigations

Genetic markers and lipids
    Lipoprotein fractions (Lp[a])
    Apolipoprotein E
Hormone use/replacement
Cardiac disease
    Patent foramen ovale
    Atrial septal aneurysm
    Spontaneous echo contrast
    Aortic arch plaque
    Valve strands
Migraine
Diet
    Hyper-homocystinemia
    Vitamin B_6, vitamin E
    Antioxidants
Hypercoagulable states
    Antiphospholipid antibodies
    Lupus anticoagulant
    Protein C, free protein S deficiencies
    Prothrombin fragment 1•2
    Factor V Leiden

than 35 years of age who smoke or have hypertension.[169,170] Former users were not found to be at increased risk of stroke.[171] The older formulations of contraceptive pills with a higher dose of estrogen were thought to impart a higher risk than the current low-dose pills. However, the relationship between amount of estrogen and stroke risk has not been adequately investigated.

There have been conflicting reports about snoring as a stroke risk factor. In one case-control study, habitual or frequent snoring was associated with a significant odds ratio of 2.1 for brain infarction,[172] whereas in a separate study, snoring was

not an independent risk factor for cardiovascular disease.[173]

Various laboratory abnormalities, often reflective of an underlying metabolic or hematologic disturbance, have been associated with stroke and identified as possible stroke precursors. These include hematocrit,[174] polycythemia, sickle cell anemia, white blood cell count, fibrinogen,[86,175,176] hypokalemia,[177] hyperuricemia,[54] hyper-homocystinemia,[178,179] protein C and free protein S deficiencies,[180,181] lupus anticoagulant, and anticardiolipin antibodies.[182] Some are clear stroke risk factors, whereas others require further epidemiologic investigations to verify a relationship. In particular, transient factors that may be acquired poststroke could lead to biases in case-control studies, and therefore prospective investigations are required to establish their role as risk factors.

Risk Factor Modification Programs

In general, risk factor modification efforts may take two forms: the *high-risk* approach and the *mass* approach (Table 1-5). The high-risk approach seeks to modify the degree of the factor in individuals identified as at an elevated risk of disease. The mass approach attempts to make a modest adjustment of the risk factor in the entire population. The secondary prevention involved in the high-risk method is already evident in the U.S. medical system, involving the detection and treatment of factors such as hypertension, typically through pharmacologic intervention. The primary prevention of the mass approach is less apparent in the United States' current health care system and more difficult to achieve without broad support to promote a screening program in the disease-free population (Figure 1-7).

Table 1-5. Comparison of the Mass and High-Risk Approaches to Stroke Prevention

	Mass Approach	High-Risk Approach
Prevention	Primary	Secondary
Target	Small effect in general population	Large effect in select population at risk
Benefit	Community	Individual
Emphasis	Behavior modification	Detection and treatment: behavior/pharmacologic
Example	Increased tax on cigarettes	Hypertension detection/treatment program

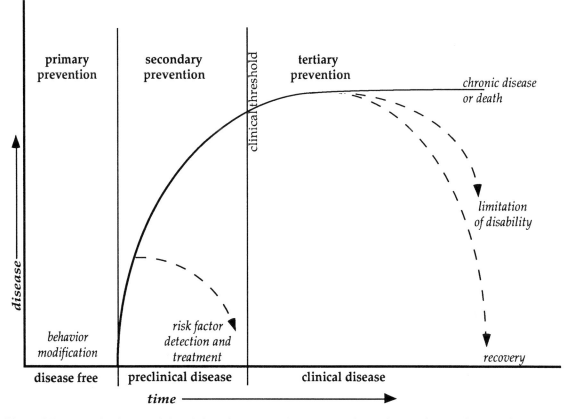

Figure 1-7. Schematic diagram of the relationship between disease progression and stage of prevention over time. Dashed lines represent potential benefit of preventive intervention.

The initial component of the high-risk approach involves identification of stroke risk factors. Various methods have been suggested for the identification of individuals at high risk for stroke. Analysis of the Framingham Study data has led to the development of a stroke risk profile based on physical examination, medical history, and electrocardiogram.[27] By screening for five stroke risk factors and identifying the 10% of individuals at highest risk, it is estimated that 50% of strokes may be avoided.[36] High-risk patients may also be identified by noninvasive screening of carotid artery plaque as a marker for patients at risk of systemic atherosclerotic disease or by detecting left ventricular hypertrophy by cardiac imaging.[183] One may base antihypertensive or antihyperlipidemic therapy on the presence of preclinical disease, which may involve a more direct association with stroke than the observation of risk factors alone (Figure 1-8). Additional factors in the identi-

fication of high-risk individuals may include recent TIA, recent-onset AF, recent myocardial infarction, or recent mild stroke.[27,184]

However, efforts in the detection of such high-risk individuals may not always be practical. Noninvasive screening of asymptomatic persons would be costly. In addition, by exclusively emphasizing those at highest risk for disease, a prevention program excludes a substantial percentage of the population at risk. Even if screening for five risk factors identified those at risk for 50% of strokes, the remaining one-half of all stroke patients would not have been reached for prevention. Although those with increased exposure to many factors have the highest risk for disease, much stroke mortality is found among those with normal cholesterol levels and those considered "normotensive."[35] In addition, the high-risk screening method typically involves the additional cost of pharmacologic intervention and the associated potential side effects.

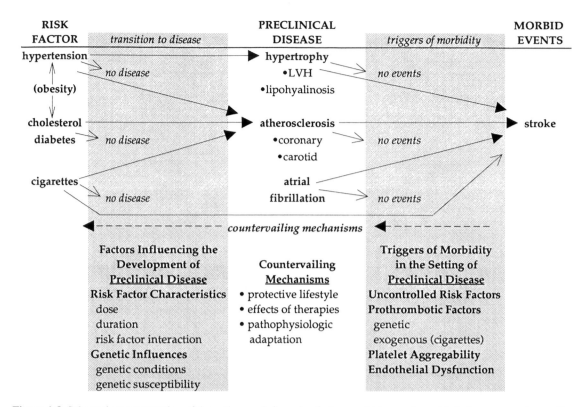

Figure 1-8. Schematic representation of the pathways, influencing factors, and triggers from risk factor exposure to preclinical disease and ultimate development of clinically morbid event. Note that at each step some individuals do not make the next transition. (LVH = left ventricular hypertrophy.) (Adapted from RB Devereux, MH Alderman. Role of preclinical cardiovascular disease in the evolution from risk factor exposure to development of morbid events. Circulation 1993;88[part 1]:1444–1445.)

Modification of risk factors through the high-risk approach may fail to reduce stroke risk. This phenomenon may be due to the fact that the development of precursor stroke conditions, such as atherosclerosis, is a chronic process in which the strong relationship between the risk factor and the disease reflects decades of exposure. In this case, stroke risk may be reduced by a modification of the exposure only if it occurs early enough. The timing of the intervention among high-risk individuals is critical to the success of the program.

The mass approach to risk factor modification is not applicable for all stroke risk factors. In general, a risk factor should be independently and strongly associated with a disease in a wide spectrum of the population at risk and be dose-dependent when applicable.[36] An important distinction to be made in assessing a factor's eligibility for modification is that of relative and absolute risk.

Although a large relative risk implies that the risk factor has a strong association with the disease, this measure does not correlate with the actual prevalence of the risk factor in the community. As an absolute measure, the attributable risk reflects the amount of disease that is attributable to a particular risk factor, reflecting the public health impact of the risk factor.[185] The population attributable risk takes into consideration both the attributable risk and the prevalence of the factor in the population (see Figures 1-5 and 1-6). Planning a mass strategy for a risk factor with a high relative risk but low prevalence confers a benefit applicable to few in the community. A large number of people exposed to a risk factor with a low relative risk is likely to produce more cases of disease than a small number of people exposed to a high risk.[186] Although the mass approach results in large benefit to the community as a whole, little benefit is offered to each participat-

Table 1-6. Estimated Savings (in Lives and Dollars) Attributable to Stroke Prevention*

Risk Factor	Estimated Percentage Exposed	Estimated Relative Risk (%)	Estimated Population Attributable Risk (%)	Estimated Strokes Prevented	Estimated Savings (billions)
Hypertension	56.20	2.73	49.3	246,500	$12.33
Cigarette smoking	27.00	1.52	12.3	61,500	$3.08
Atrial fibrillation	3.98	3.60	9.4	47,000	$2.35
Heavy alcohol	7.20	1.68	4.7	23,500	$1.18
Hypercholesterolemia	36.00	1.40	20.0	100,000	NA

NA = not available.
*Prevalence and relative risk based on averages from the Framingham data and other national data sources. Population attributable risk based on A/1 + A where A = prevalence multiplied by (relative risk − 1).
Source: Adapted from PB Gorelick. Stroke prevention: windows of opportunity and failed expectations? A discussion of modifiable cardiovascular risk factors and a prevention proposal. Neuroepidemiology 1997;16:163–173.

ing individual.[186] This paradox adds to the difficulty of implementing such a program community-wide.

In the high-risk model, hypertension modification may involve population screening to identify those considered to be borderline hypertensive. From this point, an effective treatment would be implemented, typically involving a pharmacologic intervention. Overall, this model involves the high cost of a population screen, as well as the cost and potential side effects of antihypertensive medication. Using the mass model, a modest decrease in blood pressure would be sought in the general population, typically through health education, social pressure, economics, convenience, and legislation. For example, the recommendation of salt intake restriction has been a simple and economical method for reducing blood pressure in the effort to reduce stroke.[187] It has been estimated that the reduction in risk by the high-risk strategy in the United Kingdom of treating all antihypertensives is equivalent to a mass decrease of only 2–3 mm Hg in the general population.[186] Such a decrease may be implemented by a decrease in sodium and alcohol use and an increase in potassium and polyunsaturated fatty acid intake.[36] A 6-month education program in Newfoundland encouraging decreased sodium, fat, and cholesterol intake resulted in a decrease in blood pressure, serum cholesterol, and body mass index.[188] With the end of the intervention program, however, levels seemed to rise again, approaching those before the program began. This implies that mass programs may need continual reinforcement to prevent return to prior levels of exposure.

Gorelick has estimated the potential savings, in lives and dollars, associated with a mass or high-risk prevention program (Table 1-6).[189] Based on the estimated prevalence of risk factors and their attributable risks for stroke in the United States, it is estimated that 246,500 strokes may be prevented from the control of hypertension alone, saving $12.33 billion. A prevention program aimed at cigarette smoking may prevent more than 61,000 strokes, with an associated cost of more than $3 billion. Even if these programs were only 25% successful in reducing hypertension and smoking, more than $3.8 billion may be saved in stroke-related care. Treatment of AF and modification of heavy alcohol use could eliminate 47,000 and 23,500 strokes, respectively. Clearly, there should be increased emphasis by all health care providers on the modification of risk factors before morbidity and mortality occur. An ideal prevention strategy requires implementation of aspects of both the high-risk and the mass approaches. Patients identified as at increased risk for stroke should be aggressively treated, with particular emphasis on the management of hypertension. Efforts to reduce the overall risk in the population should be applied concurrently to attempt a modest reduction in the risk for the general community. Further research is needed to identify new stroke risk factors and improve the ability to eliminate and control these exposures, with the goal of preventing stroke and reducing this great public health burden.

References

1. American Heart Association. Heart and Stroke Facts: 1994 Statistical Supplement. Dallas: American Heart Association, 1993.
2. Bonita R, Beaglehole R. Does treatment of hypertension explain the decline in mortality from stroke? BMJ 1986;292:191–192.
3. Hu H-H, Sheng W-Y, Chu F-L, et al. Incidence of stroke in Taiwan. Stroke 1992;23:1237–1241.
4. Sacco SE, Whisnant JP, Broderick JP, et al. Epidemiological characteristics of lacunar infarcts in a population. Stroke 1991;22:1236–1241.
5. Jerntorp P, Bergland G. Stroke registry in Malmo, Sweden. Stroke 1992;23:357–361.
6. Wolf PA, D'Agostino RB. Secular trends in stroke in the Framingham Study. Ann Epidemiol 1993;3:471–475.
7. Brown RD, Whisnant JP, Sicks JS, et al. Stroke incidence, prevalence and survival: secular trends in Rochester, Minnesota, through 1989. Stroke 1996;27:373–380.
8. Cooper R, Sempos C, Hsieh SC, Kovar MG. Slowdown in the decline of stroke mortality in the United States, 1978–1986. Stroke 1990;21:1274–1279.
9. Sacco RL. Ischemic Stroke. In PA Gorelick, MA Alter (eds), Handbook of Neuroepidemiology. New York: Marcel Dekker, 1994;77–122.
10. Gross CR, Kase CS, Mohr JP, et al. Stroke in south Alabama: incidence and diagnostic features—a population based study. Stroke 1984;15:249–255.
11. Friday G, Lai SM, Alter M, et al. Stroke in the Lehigh Valley: racial/ethnic differences. Neurology 1989;39: 1165–1168.
12. Kittner SJ, White LR, Losonczy K, et al. Black-white differences in stroke incidence in a national sample—the contribution of hypertension and diabetes mellitus. JAMA 1990;264:1267–1270.
13. Sacco RL, Hauser WA, Mohr JP. Hospitalized stroke incidence in blacks and Hispanics in Northern Manhattan. Stroke 1991;22:1491–1496.
14. Sacco RL, Boden-Albala B, Gan R, et al. Stroke incidence among white, black and Hispanic residents of an urban community. The Northern Manhattan Stroke Study. Am J Epidemiol 1998;147:259–268.
15. Balarajan R. Ethnic differences in mortality from ischemic heart disease and cerebrovascular disease in England and Wales. BMJ 1991;302:560–564.
16. Horner RD, Matchar DB, Divine GW, Feussner JR. Racial variations in ischemic stroke-related physical and functional impairments. Stroke 1991;22:1497–1501.
17. Broderick JP, Brott T, Tomsick T, et al. The risk of subarachnoid and intracerebral hemorrhages in blacks as compared with whites. N Engl J Med 1992;326:733–736.
18. Bruno A, Carter S, Qualls C, et al. Incidence of spontaneous intracerebral hemorrhage among Hispanics and non-Hispanic whites in New Mexico. Neurology 1996;47: 405–408.
19. Morgenstern LB, Spears WD. A triethnic comparison of intracerebral hemorrhage mortality in Texas. Ann Neurol 1997;42:919–923.
20. Kattapong VJ, Becker TM. Ethnic differences in mortality from cerebrovascular disease among New Mexico's His-panics, Native Americans, and non-Hispanic whites, 1958–1987. Ethn Dis 1993;3:471–475.
21. Reed DM. The paradox of high risk of stroke in populations with low risk of coronary heart disease. Am J Epidemiol 1990;131:579–588.
22. Abel GA, Sacco RL, Lin IF, et al. Race-ethnic variability in etiologic fraction for stroke risk factors. The Northern Manhattan Stroke Study. Stroke 1998;29(abstract):277.
23. Khaw K, Carrett-Connor EB. Family history of stroke as an independent predictor of ischemic heart disease in men and stroke in women. Am J Epidemiol 1986;123:59–66.
24. Welin L, Svardsudd K, Wilhelmsen L, et al. Analysis of risk factors for stroke in a cohort of men born in 1913. N Engl J Med 1987;317:521–526.
25. Brass LM, Isaacsohn JL, Merikangas KR, Robinette CD. A study of twins and stroke. Stroke 1992;23:221–223.
26. Kiely DK, Wolf PA, Cupples LA, et al. Familial aggregation of stroke: the Framingham Study. Stroke 1993;24: 1366–1371.
27. Wolf PA, Cobb JL, D'Agostino RB. Epidemiology of Stroke. In HJM Barnett, JP Mohr, BM Stein, FM Yatsu (eds), Stroke-Pathophysiology, Diagnosis, and Management. New York: Churchill Livingstone, 1992;3–27.
28. Shaper AG, Phillips AN, Pocock SJ, et al. Risk factors for stroke in middle aged British men. BMJ 1991;302:1111–1115.
29. Wolf PA, D'Agostino RB, Belanger AJ, Kannel WB. Probability of stroke: a risk profile from the Framingham Study. Stroke 1991;22:312–318.
30. Garraway WM, Whisnant JP. The changing pattern of hypertension and the declining incidence of stroke. JAMA 1987;258:214–217.
31. Fletcher AE, Bulpitt CJ. Epidemiological aspects cardiovascular disease in the elderly. J Hypertens 1992;10(Suppl 2):S51–S58.
32. MacMahon S, Peto R, Cutler J, et al. Blood pressure, stroke, and coronary heart disease. Part 1. Prolonged differences in blood pressure: prospective observational studies corrected for the regression dilution bias. Lancet 1990;335:765–774.
33. Collins R, Peto R, MacMahon S, et al. Blood pressure, stroke, and coronary heart disease. Part 2. Short-term reductions in blood pressure: overview of randomised drug trials in their epidemiological context. Lancet 1990;335:827–838.
34. MacMahon S, Peto R, Cutler J, Stamler J. Antihypertensive drug treatment: potential, expected, and observed effects on stroke and on coronary heart disease. Hypertension 1989;13(Suppl I):I45–I50.
35. Hebert PR, Moser M, Mayer J, et al. Recent evidence on drug therapy of mild to moderate hypertension and decreased risk of coronary heart disease. Arch Intern Med 1993;153:578–581.
36. Dunabibin DW, Sandercock PAG. Preventing stroke by the modification of risk factors. Stroke 1990;21(Suppl IV):IV36–IV39.
37. Dahlöf B, Linholm L, Hansson L, et al. Morbidity and morality in the Swedish Trial in Old Patients with Hypertension (STOP-Hypertension). Lancet 1991;338:1281–1285.
38. SHEP Cooperative Research Group. Prevention of stroke by antihypertensive drug treatment in older persons with

isolated systolic hypertension. Final results of the Systolic Hypertension in the Elderly Program (SHEP). JAMA 1991;265:3255–3264.

39. Staessen JA, Fagard R, Thijs L, et al. Randomized double-blind comparison of placebo and active treatment for older patients with isolated systolic hypertension. Lancet 1997;350:757–764.

40. Yusef S, Lessem J, Jha P, Lonn E. Primary and secondary prevention of myocardial infarction and strokes: an update of randomly allocated controlled trials. J Hypertens 1993;11(Suppl 4):S61–S73.

41. The Sixth Report of the Joint National Committee on prevention, detection, evaluation, and treatment of high blood pressure. Arch Intern Med 1997;157:2413–2446.

42. McMahon S, Rodgers A. The epidemiological association between blood pressure and stroke: implications for primary and secondary prevention. Hypertens Res 1994;17(Suppl 1):S23–S32.

43. Gorelick PB, Sacco RL, Smith DB, et al. Prevention of a first stroke: a review of guidelines and a multidisciplinary consensus statement from the National Stroke Association. JAMA 1999;281:1112–1120.

44. Wolf PA, Abbott RD, Kannel WB. Atrial fibrillation as an independent risk factor for stroke: the Framingham Study. Stroke 1991;22:983–988.

45. The Stroke Prevention in Atrial Fibrillation Investigators. Predictors of thromboembolism in atrial fibrillation: I. Clinical features of patients at risk. Ann Intern Med 1992;116:1–5.

46. The Stroke Prevention in Atrial Fibrillation Investigators. Predictors of thromboembolism in atrial fibrillation: II. Echocardiographic features of patients at risk. Ann Intern Med 1992;116:6–12.

47. Dexter DD, Whisnant JP, Connolly DC, O'Fallon WM. The association of stroke and coronary heart disease: a population study. Mayo Clin Proc 1987;62:1077–1083.

48. Kannel WB. Left ventricular hypertrophy as a risk factor: the Framingham experience. J Hypertens 1991;9(Suppl 2):S3–S9.

49. Barnett HJM, Boughner DR, Taylor DW, et al. Further evidence relating mitral valve prolapse to cerebral ischemic events. N Engl J Med 1980;302:139–144.

50. Gilon D, Buonanno FS, Joffe MM, et al. Lack of evidence of an association between mitral valve prolapse and stroke in young patients. N Engl J Med 1999;341:8–13.

51. Freed LA, Levy D, Levine RA, et al. Prevalence and clinical outcome of mitral-valve prolapse. N Engl J Med 1999;341:1–7.

52. Benjamin EJ, Plehn JF, D'Agostino RB, et al. Mitral annular calcification and the risk of stroke in all elderly cohort. N Engl J Med 1992;327:374–379.

53. Briley DP, Giraud G, Spear G, et al. Spontaneous echo contrast, ischemic stroke, and risk of recurrent stroke. Ann Neurol 1992;32(abstract):237.

54. Di Tullio MR, Sacco RL, Sciacca RR, et al. Left atrial size and the risk of ischemic stroke in an ethnically mixed population. Stroke 1999;30:2019–2024.

55. Pearson AC, Nagelhout D, Castello R, et al. Atrial septal aneurysm and stroke: a transesophageal echocardiographic study. J Am Coll Cardiol 1991;18:1223–1229.

56. Labovitz AJ, Camp A, Castello R, et al. Usefulness of transesophageal echocardiography in unexplained cerebral ischemia. Am J Cardiol 1993;72:1448–1452.

57. Gautier JC, Durr A, Koussa S, et al. Paradoxical cerebral embolism with a patent foramen ovale—a report of 29 patients. Cerebrovasc Dis 1991;1:193–202.

58. Jeanrenaud X, Kappenberger L. Patent foramen ovale and stroke of unknown origin. Cerebrovasc Dis 1991;1:184–192.

59. Di Tullio MR, Sacco RL, Gopal AS, et al. Patent foramen ovale as a risk factor for cryptogenic stroke. Ann Intern Med 1992;117:461–465.

60. Amarenco P, Duyckaerts C, Tzourio C, et al. The prevalence of ulcerated plaques in the aortic arch in patients with stroke. N Engl J Med 1992;326:221–225.

61. Amarenco P, Cohen A, Baudrimont M, Bousser MG. Transesophageal echocardiographic detection of aortic arch disease in patients with cerebral infarction. Stroke 1992;23:1005–1009.

62. Peterson P, Boysen G, Godfredsen J, et al. Placebo-controlled, randomised trial of warfarin and aspirin for prevention of thromboembolic complications in chronic atrial fibrillation. Lancet 1989;1:175–185.

63. Stroke Prevention in Atrial Fibrillation Investigators. Preliminary report of the Stroke Prevention in Atrial Fibrillation Study. N Engl J Med 1990;322:863–868.

64. Stroke Prevention in Atrial Fibrillation Investigators. Stroke Prevention in Atrial Fibrillation Study—final results. Circulation 1991;84:527–539.

65. The Boston Area Anticoagulation Trial for Atrial Fibrillation Investigators. The effect of low-dose warfarin on the risk of stroke in patients with nonrheumatic atrial fibrillation. N Engl J Med 1990;323:1505–1511.

66. Connolly SJ, Laupacis A, Gent M, et al. Canadian Atrial Fibrillation Anticoagulation (CAFA) study. J Am Coll Cardiol 1991;18:349–355.

67. Ezekowitz MD, Bridgers SL, James KE, et al. Warfarin in the prevention of stroke associated with nonrheumatic atrial fibrillation. N Engl J Med 1992;327:1406–1412.

68. Stroke Prevention in Atrial Fibrillation Investigators. Warfarin versus aspirin for prevention of thromboembolism in atrial fibrillation: Stroke Prevention in Atrial Fibrillation II Study. Lancet 1994;343:687–691.

69. Stroke Prevention in Atrial Fibrillation Investigators. Adjusted-dose warfarin versus low-intensity, fixed-dose warfarin plus aspirin for high-risk patients with atrial fibrillation: stroke prevention in atrial fibrillation III randomised clinical trial. Lancet 1996;348:633–638.

70. Laupacis A, Albers G, Dalen J, et al. Antithrombotic therapy in atrial fibrillation. Chest 1998;114(Suppl):579S–589S.

71. Balkau B, Shipley M, Jarrett RJ, et al. High blood glucose concentration is a risk factor for mortality in middle-aged nondiabetic men. 20-year follow-up in the Whitehall Study, the Paris Prospective Study, and the Helsinki Policemen Study. Diabetes Care 1998;21:360–367.

72. Boysen G, Nyboe J, Appleyard M, et al. Stroke incidence and risk factors for stroke in Copenhagen, Denmark. Stroke 1988;19:1345–1353.

73. Abbott RD, Donahue RP, MacMahon SW, et al. Diabetes and the risk of stroke: the Honolulu Heart Program. JAMA 1987;257:949–952.

74. Barrett-Connor E, Khaw K. Diabetes mellitus: an independent risk factor for stroke? Am J Epidemiol 1988;128:116–123.

75. Watkins PJ, Thomas PK. Diabetes mellitus and the nervous system. J Neurol Neurosurg Psychiatry 1998;65:620–632.

76. Effect of intensive diabetes management on macrovascular events and risk factors in the Diabetes Control and Complications Trial. Am J Cardiol 1995;75:894–903.

77. UK Prospective Diabetes Study Group. Intensive blood-glucose control with sulphonylureas or insulin compared with conventional treatment and risk of complications in patients with type 2 diabetes: UKPDS 33. Lancet 1998;352:837–853.

78. The effect of intensive treatment of diabetes on the development and progression of long-term complications in insulin-dependent diabetes mellitus. The Diabetes Control and Complications Trial Research Group. N Engl J Med 1993;329:977–986.

79. UK Prospective Diabetes Study Group. Tight blood pressure control and risk of macrovascular and microvascular complications in type 2 diabetes: UK PDS38. BMJ 1998;317:703–713.

80. American Diabetes Association. Clinical practice recommendations 1998. Diabetes Care 1998;21(Suppl 1):S1–S89.

81. Smith GD, Shipley MJ, Marmot MG, Rose G. Plasma cholesterol concentration and mortality. JAMA 1992;267:70–76.

82. Iso H, Jacobs DR, Wentworth D, et al. Serum cholesterol levels and six-year mortality from stroke in 350,977 men screened for the Multiple Risk Factor Intervention Trial. N Engl J Med 1989;320:904–910.

83. Benfante R, Yano K, Hwang LJ, et al. Elevated serum cholesterol is a risk factor for both coronary heart disease and thromboembolic stroke in Hawaiian Japanese men. Implications of shared risk. Stroke 1994;25:814–820.

84. Prospective Studies Collaboration. Cholesterol, diastolic blood pressure, and stroke: 13,000 strokes in 450,000 people in 45 prospective cohorts. Lancet 1995;346:1647–1653.

85. Qizilbash N, Duffy SW, Warlow C, Mann J. Lipids are risk factors for ischemic stroke—overview and review. Cerebrovasc Dis 1992;2:127–136.

86. Qizilbash N, Jones L, Warlow C, Mann J. Fibrinogen and lipid concentrations as risk factors for transient ischaemic attacks and minor ischaemic strokes. BMJ 1991;303:605–609.

87. Kargman DE, Berglund LF, Lin IF, et al. High density lipoprotein: a protective stroke risk factor. The Northern Manhattan Stroke Study. Ann Neurol 1997;42:491.

88. O'Leary DH, Anderson KM, Wolf PA, et al. Cholesterol and carotid atherosclerosis in older persons: the Framingham Study. Ann Epidemiol 1992;2:147–153.

89. Salonen R, Seppanen K, Rauramaa R, Salonen JT. Prevalence of carotid atherosclerosis and serum cholesterol levels in eastern Finland. Atherosclerosis 1988;8:788–792.

90. Shintani S, Kikuchi S, Hamaguchi H, Shiigai T. High serum lipoprotein(a) levels are an independent risk factor for cerebral infarction. Stroke 1993;24:965–969.

91. Atkins D, Pstay B, Koepsell T, et al. Cholesterol reduction and the risk factors for stroke in men. A meta analysis of randomized, controlled trials. Ann Intern Med 1993;119:136–145.

92. Hiroyasu I, Jacobs D, Wentworth D, et al. Serum cholesterol levels and six-years mortality from stroke in 350,977 men screened for the Multiple Risk Factor Intervention Trial. N Engl J Med 1989;320:904–910.

93. Scandinavian Simvastatin Survival Study Group. Randomized trial of cholesterol lowering in 4,444 patients with coronary heart disease: the Scandinavian Simvastatin Survival Study (4S). Lancet 1994;344:1383–1389.

94. Sacks FM, Pfeffer MA, Moye LA, et al. The effect of pravastatin on coronary events after myocardial infarction in patients with average cholesterol levels. N Engl J Med 1996;335:1001–1009.

95. The Long-Term Intervention with Pravastatin in Ischemic Disease (LIPID) Study Group. Prevention of cardiovascular events and death with pravastatin in patients with coronary heart disease and a broad range of initial cholesterol levels. N Engl J Med 1998;339:1349–1357.

96. Hebert PR, Gaziano JM, Chan KS, Hennekens CH. Cholesterol lowering with statin drugs, risk of stroke, and total mortality. An overview of randomized trials. JAMA 1997;278:313–321.

97. Blauw GJ, Lagaay AM, Smelt AHM, Westendorp RGJ. Stroke, statins, and cholesterol. A meta-analysis of randomized, placebo-controlled, double-blind trials with HMG-CoA reductase inhibitors. Stroke 1997;28:946–950.

98. Blakenhorn DH, Selzer RH, Crawford DW, et al. Beneficial effects of colestipol-niacin therapy on the common carotid artery. Two- and four-year reduction of intima-media thickness measured by ultrasound. Circulation 1993;88:20–28.

99. Furberg CD, Adams HP, Applegate WB, et al. Effect of lovastatin on early carotid atherosclerosis and cardiovascular events. The Asymptomatic Carotid Artery Progression Study (ACAPS) Research Group. Circulation 1994;90:1679–1687.

100. Crouse JR, Byington RP, Bond MA, et al. Pravastatin, Lipids, and Atherosclerosis in the Carotid Arteries (PLAC-II). Am J Cardiol 1995;75:455–459.

101. Solonen R, Nyyssonen K, Porkkala E, et al. Kuopio Atherosclerosis Prevention Study (KAPS): a population-based primary prevention trial of the effect of LDL lowering on atherosclerotic progression in carotid and femoral arteries. Circulation 1995;92:1758–1764.

102. Hodis HN, Mack WJ, LaBree L, et al. Reduction in carotid arterial wall thickness using lovastatin and dietary therapy: a randomized, controlled clinical trial. Ann Intern Med 1996;124:548–556.

103. Pujia A, Rubba P, Spencer MP. Prevalence of extracranial carotid artery disease detectable by echo-Doppler in an elderly population. Stroke 1992;23:818–822.

104. Norris JW, Zhu CZ, Bornstein NM, Chambers BR. Vascular risks of asymptomatic carotid stenosis. Stroke 1991;22:1485–1490.

105. Norris JW, Zhu CZ. Silent stroke and carotid stenosis. Stroke 1992;23:483–485.

106. Higa M, Davanipour Z. Smoking and stroke. Neuroepidemiol 1991;10:211–222.

107. Gorelick PB, Rodin MB, Langenberg P, et al. Weekly alcohol consumption, cigarette smoking, and the risk of

ischemic stroke: results of a case control study at three urban medical centers in Chicago, Illinois. Neurology 1989;39:339–343.

108. Bonita R, Scragg R, Stewart A, et al. Cigarette smoking and risk of premature stroke in men and women. BMJ 1986;293:6–8.

109. Abbott RD, Yin Y, Reed DM, Yano K. Risk of stroke in male cigarette smokers. N Engl J Med 1986;315:717–720.

110. Colditz GA, Bonita R, Stampfer MJ, et al. Cigarette smoking and risk of stroke in middle-aged women. N Engl J Med 1988;318:937–941.

111. Wolf PA, D'Agostino RB, Kannel WB, et al. Cigarette smoking as a risk factor for stroke: the Framingham Study. JAMA 1988;259:1025–1029.

112. Shinton R, Beevers G. Meta-analysis of relation between cigarette smoking and stroke. BMJ 1989;298:789–794.

113. Bonita R. Cigarette smoking, hypertension and the risk of subarachnoid hemorrhage: a population-based case control study. Stroke 1986;17:831–835.

114. Longstreth WT, Nelson LM, Doepsell TD, van Belle G. Cigarette smoking, alcohol use, and subarachnoid hemorrhage. Stroke 1992;23:1242–1249.

115. Howard G, Wagenknecht LE, Burke GL, et al. Cigarette smoking and progression of atherosclerosis: The Atherosclerosis Risk in Communities (ARIC) Study. JAMA 1998;279:119–124.

116. Sacco RL, Roberts JK, Boden-Albala B, et al. Race-ethnicity and determinants of carotid atherosclerosis in a multi-ethnic population. The Northern Manhattan Stroke Study. Stroke 1997;27:929–935.

117. Whisnant JP, Homer D, Ingall TJ, et al. Duration of cigarette smoking is the strongest predictor of severe extracranial carotid artery atherosclerosis. Stroke 1990;21:707–714.

118. Mast H, Thompson JLP, Lin IF, et al. Cigarette smoking as a determinant of high-grade carotid artery stenosis in Hispanic, black, and white patients with stroke or transient ischemic attack. Stroke 1998;29:908–912.

119. Fujishima M, Kiyohara Y, Ueda K, et al. Smoking as cardiovascular risk factor in low cholesterol population: the Hisayama Study. Clin Exp Hypertens 1992;A14:99–108.

120. Wolf PA. Cigarettes, alcohol and stroke. N Engl J Med 1986;315:1087–1089.

121. Kawachi I, Colditz G, Stampfer M, et al. Smoking cessation and decreased risk of stroke in women. JAMA 1993;269:232–236.

122. Wolf PA, Belanger AJ, D'Agostino RB. Management of risk factors. Neurol Clin 1992;10:177–191.

123. Rose G, Hamilton PJS, Colwell L, Shipley MJ. A randomised controlled trial of anti-smoking advice: 10 year results. J Epidemiol Community Health 1982;36:102–108.

124. Gorelick PB. Stroke prevention: windows of opportunity and failed expectations—a discussion of modifiable cardiovascular risk factors and a prevention proposal. Neuroepidemiology 1997;16:163–173.

125. Gorelick PB. The status of alcohol as a risk factor for stroke. Stroke 1989;20:1607–1610.

126. Camargo CA. Moderate alcohol consumption and stroke. The epidemiological evidence. Stroke 1989;20:1611–1626.

127. Gill JS, Zezulka AV, Shipley MJ, et al. Stroke and alcohol consumption. N Engl J Med 1986;315:1041–1046.

128. Sacco RL, Elkind M, Boden-Albala B, et al. The protective effect of moderate alcohol consumption on ischemic stroke. JAMA 1999;281:53–60.

129. Stampfer MJ, Colditz GA, Willett WC, et al. A prospective study of alcohol consumption and the risk of coronary disease and stroke in women. N Engl J Med 1988;319:267–273.

130. Wolf PA, D'Agostino RB, Odell P, et al. Alcohol consumption as a risk factor for stroke: the Framingham Study. Ann Neurol 1988;24:177.

131. Gaziano JM, Gaziano TA, Glynn RJ, et al. Light-to-moderate alcohol consumption and mortality in the Physicians' Health Study enrollment cohort. J Am Coll Cardiol 2000;35:96–105.

132. Truelsen T, Gronbaek M, Schnohr P, Boysen G. Intake of beer, wine, and spirits and risk of stroke—the Copenhagen City Heart Study. Stroke 1998;29:2467–2472.

133. NIH Consensus Development Panel on Physical Activity and Cardiovascular Health. Physical activity and cardiovascular health. JAMA 1996;276:241–246.

134. Fletcher GF. Exercise in the prevention of stroke. Health Rep 1994;6:106–110.

135. Abbott RD, Rodriguez BL, Burchfiel CM, Curb JD. Physical activity in older middle-aged men and reduced risk of stroke: The Honolulu Heart Program. Am J Epidemiol 1994;139:881–893.

136. Kiely DK, Wolf PA, Cupples LA, et al. Physical activity and stroke risk: the Framingham Study. Am J Epidemiol 1994;140:608–620.

137. Haheim LL, Holme I, Hjermann I, Leren P. Risk factors of stroke incidence and mortality. A 12-year follow-up of the Oslo Study. Stroke 1993;24:1484–1489.

138. Gillum RF, Mussolino ME, Ingram DD. Physical activity and stroke incidence in women and men—the NHANES I Epidemiologic Follow-up Study. Am J Epidemiol 1996;143:860–869.

139. Hu FB, Stampfer MJ, Colditz G, et al. Physical activity and risk of stroke in women. JAMA 2000;283:2961–2967.

140. Sacco RL, Gan R, Boden-Albala B, et al. Leisure-time physical activity and ischemic stroke risk. The Northern Manhattan Stroke Study. Stroke 1998;29:380–387.

141. Wannamethee G, Shaper AG. Physical activity and stroke in British middle aged men. BMJ 1992;304:597–601.

142. Manson JE, Stampfer MJ, Willett WC, et al. Physical activity and incidence of coronary heart disease and stroke in women. Circulation 1995;91(Suppl):5.

143. Lee IM, Hennekens CH, Berger K, et al. Exercise and risk of stroke in male physicians. Stroke 1999;30:1–6.

144. Williams PT. High-density lipoprotein cholesterol and other risk factors for coronary heart disease in female runners. N Engl J Med 1996;334:1298–1303.

145. Nygard O, Vollset SE, Refsum H, et al. Total plasma homocysteine and cardiovascular risk profile—the Hordaland Homocysteine Study. JAMA 1995;274:1526–1533.

146. U.S. Department of Health and Human Services. Physical Activity and Health: A Report of the Surgeon General. Atlanta: U.S. Department of Health and Human Services, Centers for Disease Control and Prevention, National Center Chronic Disease Prevention and Health Promotion; 1996.

147. U.S. Department of Health and Human Services. Healthy People 2000: National Health Promotion and Disease Pre-

vention Objectives. Washington: U.S. Department of Health and Human Services, 1991. DHHS publication no. (PHS) 91-50213.

148. Takeya Y, Popper JS, Schmimizu Y, et al. Epidemiologic studies of coronary heart disease and stroke in Japanese men living in Japan, Hawaii and California. Stroke 1984;15:15–23.

149. Gillman MW, Cupples A, Millen B, et al. Inverse association of dietary fat with development of ischemic stroke in men. JAMA 1997;278:2145–2150.

150. Stampfer J, Rose G, Stamler R, et al. INTERSALT study findings. Public health and medical care implications. Hypertension 1989;14:570–577.

151. Ueland PM, Refsum H, Brattstrom L. Plasma Homocysteine and Cardiovascular Disease. In Francis RB, Jr. (ed), Atherosclerotic Cardiovascular Disease, Hemostasis, and Endothelial Function. New York: Marcel Dekker, 1992:183–236.

152. Boushey CJ, Beresford SAA, Omenn GS, Motulsky AG. A quantitative assessment of plasma homocysteine as a risk factor for vascular disease. Probable benefits of increasing folic acid intakes. JAMA 1995;274:1049–1057.

153. Giles WH, Croft JB, Greenlund KJ, et al. Total homocyst(e)ine concentration and the likelihood of nonfatal stroke: results from the Third National Health and Nutrition Examination Survey, 1988–1994. Stroke 1998;29:2473–2477.

154. Sacco RL, Roberts JK, Jacobs BS. Homocysteine as a risk factor for ischemic stroke: an epidemiological story in evolution. Neuroepidemiology 1998;17:167–173.

155. Selhub J, Jaques PF, Bostom AG, et al. Association between plasma homocysteine concentration and extracranial carotid-artery stenosis. N Engl J Med 1995;332:286–291.

156. Jacobs BS, Sacco RL, Lui RC, et al. Low dietary intake of vitamin B6 is associated with an increased risk of ischemic stroke. Stroke 1999;30:252.

157. Gillman MW, Cupples LA, Posner B, et al. Protective effects of fruits and vegetables on development of stroke in men. JAMA 1995;273:1113–1117.

158. Gey KF, Stahelin HB, Eichholzer M. Poor plasma status of carotene and vitamin C is associated with higher mortality from ischemic heart disease and stroke. Clin Invest Med 1993;71:3–6.

159. Khaw KT, Barrett-Connor E. Dietary potassium and stroke-associated mortality. N Engl J Med 1987;316:235–240.

160. Benson RT, Jacobs B, Boden-Albala B, et al. Vitamin E intake: a primary preventive measure in stroke. Neurology 1999;52:A146.

161. Diaz MN, Frei B, Vita JA, Keaney JF. Antioxidants and atherosclerotic heart disease. N Engl J Med 1997;282:408–416.

162. Dietary vitamin C, beta-carotene and 30-year risk of stroke: results from the Western Electric Study. Neuroepidemiology 1997:16:69–77.

163. Abbott RD, Curb D, Rodriguez BL, et al. Effect of dietary calcium and milk consumption on risk of thromboembolic stroke in older middle-aged men. The Honolulu Heart Study. Stroke 1996;27:813–818.

164. Orenica AJ, Daviglus ML, Dyer AR, et al. Fish consumption and stroke in men. 30 year findings of the Chicago Western Electric Study. Stroke 1996;27:204–209.

165. Morris M, Manson J, Rosner B, Buring J, et al. Fish consumption and cardiovascular disease in the Physicians' Health Study: a prospective study. Am J Epidemiol 1995;142:166–175.

166. Collaborative Group for the Study of Stroke in Young Women. Oral contraceptives and stroke in young women. JAMA 1975;231:718–722.

167. Broderick JP, Swanson JW. Migraine-related strokes: clinical profile and prognosis in 20 patients. Arch Neurol 1987;868–871.

168. Henrich JB. The association between migraine and cerebral vascular events: an analytical review. J Chronic Dis 1987;44:868–871.

169. Stadel BV. Oral contraceptives and cardiovascular disease. N Engl J Med 1981;305:672–677.

170. Longstreth WT, Swanson PD. Oral contraceptives and stroke. Stroke 1984;15:747–750.

171. Stampfer MJ, Willett WC, Colditz GA, et al. A prospective study of past use of oral contraceptive agents and risk of cardiovascular diseases. N Engl J Med 1988;319:1313–1317.

172. Palomaki H. Snoring and the risk of ischemic brain infarction. Stroke 1991;22:1021–1025.

173. Zaninelli A, Fariello R, Boni E, et al. Snoring and the risk of cardiovascular disease. Int J Cardiol 1991;32:347–352.

174. Kannel WB, Gorden T, Wolf PA, et al. Hemoglobin and the risk of cerebral infarction: the Framingham Study. Stroke 1972;3:409–419.

175. Kannel WB, Wolf PA, Castelli WP, D'Agostino RB. Fibrinogen and risk of cardiovascular disease: the Framingham Study. JAMA 1987;258:1183–1186.

176. Wilhelmsen L, Svardsudd K, Korsan-Bengsten K, et al. Fibrinogen as a risk factor for stroke and myocardial infarction. N Engl J Med 1984;311:501–505.

177. Khaw K, Barrett-Connor E. Dietary potassium and stroke associated mortality: a 12-year prospective population study. N Engl J Med 1987;316:235–240.

178. Boushey CJ, Beresford SAA, Omenn GS, Motulsky AG. A quantitative assessment of plasma homocysteine as a risk factor for vascular disease: probable benefits of increasing folic acid intakes. JAMA 1995;274:1049–1057.

179. Bostom AG, Rosenberg IH, Silbershatz H, et al. Nonfasting plasma total homocysteine levels and stroke incidence in elderly persons: the Framingham Study. Ann Intern Med 1999;131:352–355.

180. Sacco RL, Owen J, Mohr JP, Tatemichi TK. Free protein S deficiency: a possible association with intracranial vascular occlusion. Stroke 1989;20:1657–1661.

181. Mayer SA, Sacco RL, Hurlet-Jensen A, et al. Free protein S deficiency in acute ischemic stroke: a case-control study. Stroke 1993;42:224–227.

182. Kittner SJ, Gorelick PB. Antiphospholipid antibodies and stroke: an epidemiologic perspective. Stroke 1992;23(Suppl 2):I19–I22.

183. Devereux RB, Alderman MH. Role of preclinical cardiovascular disease in the evolution from risk factor exposure

to development of morbid events. Circulation 1993;88: 1444–1455.

184. Fisher M, Jones S, Sacco RL. Prophylactic neuroprotection for cerebral ischemia. Stroke 1994;25:1075–1080.

185. Fisher M, Jones S, Sacco RL. Measures of Disease Frequency and Association. In CH Hennekens, JE Buring. Epidemiology in Medicine. Boston: Little, Brown, 1987;54–100.

186. Rose G. Strategy for prevention: lessons from cardiovascular disease. BMJ 1981;282:1847–1851.

187. Isles CG. Recent development in primary prevention of stroke. Scott Med J 1993;38(Suppl 3):S6–S7.

188. Chockalingam A, Fodor JG. Cardiovascular risk factors in Newfoundland population and modification of their level through nonpharmacological intervention. J Cardiovasc Pharmacol 1990;16(Suppl 8):S54–S56.

189. Gorelick PB. Stroke prevention: windows of opportunity and failed expectations? A discussion of modifiable cardiovascular risk factors and a prevention proposal. Neuroepidemiology 1997;16:163–173.

Chapter 2
Pathophysiology of Ischemic Injury

S. Hinan Ahmed, Chaur-Jong Hu, Richard Paczynski, and Chung Y. Hsu

The brain seems uniquely vulnerable to ischemic injury. While comprising only 2% of the human body's mass, the brain receives up to 20% of cardiac output to meet its tremendous metabolic requirements and depends on a continuous supply of oxygen and glucose. If perfusion of the cerebrum is suspended or critically reduced, there are limited capacities for compensation and minimal energy reserves.[1] Until recently, the recognition of this tenuous state of existence, together with the erroneous assumption that neurologic deficits detected during an ischemic event are synonymous with tissue death, had fostered a generally passive and pessimistic attitude toward management of acute stroke. Functional deficits and cell death are not equivalent,[2] however, and it has been known since the 1980s that central nervous system (CNS) tissues can remain viable under ischemic conditions for longer than had been traditionally believed.[3,4] Moreover, since 1990 there has been tremendous expansion in both the breadth and depth of the understanding of events on the cellular and molecular levels that accompany or mediate ischemic brain injury, with obvious implications for medical intervention. This has led to identification of various therapeutic agents that could potentially block these ischemia-induced cell death pathways.

This chapter begins with a review of hemodynamic factors pertinent to acute stroke. The discussion then turns to a more detailed consideration of developments in the understanding of cellular and biochemical events critical to the establishment and maturation of focal ischemic brain injury. The interactions between the unique metabolic environment of focal ischemia and the various physical and biochemical derangements possibly mediating brain damage are emphasized throughout.

Thresholds of Ischemia

Clinical studies and data from animal models of stroke suggest that ischemic brain injury can be conceived as a series of interlocking thresholds, each of which relates a decrement in regional cerebral blood flow (CBF) to key pathologic events. An introduction to these "ischemic thresholds" provides a framework for better understanding ischemic pathophysiology on the cellular and biochemical levels. First, the compensatory mechanisms that must be exhausted before hypoperfusion results in reduction of CBF and disturbed cerebral energy metabolism are discussed.

Autoregulation of Blood Flow and Increased Oxygen Extraction

Stroke is foremost a disturbance of brain perfusion. Not all disturbances of perfusion produce ischemia, however, and not all ischemia results in stroke.

Compensatory changes in cerebrovascular tone and the degree of extraction of circulating oxygen can maintain normal CBF and rates of aerobic metabolism when there is decreased brain perfusion. Autoregulation is still a poorly understood process whereby precapillary resistance vessels dilate or constrict in response to decreases and increases, respectively, in regional cerebral perfusion pressure (CPP)—the mean systemic arterial blood pressure minus the intracranial pressure (ICP)—to maintain a constant regional CBF.[5,6] CBF can be expressed simply as the ratio of CPP to cerebrovascular resistance (CVR), according to Ohm's law:

$$CBF = CPP/CVR$$

Patients with hemodynamically significant carotid stenoses and chronically hypoperfused brain regions can maintain normal CBF via autoregulatory decreases in CVR.[7] Similar compensatory mechanisms may be operative after acute reductions in CPP throughout the cerebrovasculature.[8,9] Autoregulatory decreases in CVR to maintain constant CBF in the face of declining CPP largely reflect increases in vessel diameter that are invariably accompanied by increases in cerebral blood volume. The mechanisms and consequences of autoregulation are complex and have been reviewed (Figure 2-1).[5]

Autoregulation maintains a nearly constant average resting CBF of approximately 50 ml of blood per 100 g of brain tissue per minute to the cerebral hemispheres of humans over a wide range of CPPs. This average value reflects the contribution of higher flows in the cortex and basal ganglionic structures and lower flows in white matter.[5,6] In adults, the lower limit of autoregulation—the perfusion pressure at which autoregulatory vasodilatation has reached a maximum and further decline of CPP will result in proportional decreases in CBF—is typically observed at approximately 60 mm Hg.[5,7] This lower limit is variable and can be altered under a number of conditions, however, most notably chronic arterial hypertension and prior ischemic insult[5,10] (see Figure 2-1). It is important to note that CBF is influenced by a number of other factors such as systemic arterial oxygen content, blood carbon dioxide tension, local pH, and degree of local functional activation of neurons.[11,12] Therefore,

although reduction in perfusion pressure is the major acute consequence of obstructive embolus, occlusive thrombus, or vasospasm, all of these interrelated factors must be taken into consideration when interpreting pathologic changes in CBF.

Beyond the limits of maximal dilatation of resistance vessels, CBF declines with further decreases in CPP. Extraction of oxygen from the blood then increases—expressed as an increasing oxygen extraction fraction (OEF)—to sustain aerobic metabolism from the remaining modicum of substrate. OEF may rise from an average resting value of 30–40% to more than 90% and can maintain normal rates of cerebral oxygen metabolism ($CMRO_2$).[6,7] It is important to note that, in contrast to the more profound degrees of perfusion failure to be described in the section Threshold for Ionic Failure and Calcium Overload (Severe Ischemia), there are data suggesting that "compensated" low flow states associated with high OEF, normal $CMRO_2$, and normal neurologic function—as can be observed in individuals with severe carotid artery stenoses—may be sustainable for years.[7,13] With little "reserve" flow left, however, the patients with symptomatic carotid occlusion and increased OEF arc at substantially greater risk of developing stroke.[14] Increases in OEF in the ischemic region of the brain after an acute ischemic event represent another pathologic state in which the similar compensatory mechanism may contribute to sustain the viability of the ischemic brain tissue (see Figure 2-1).[15,16]

Failure of Aerobic Metabolism (Mild Ischemia)

Under normal physiologic conditions, the human brain extracts and metabolizes more than five times as much oxygen (165 mmol/100 g/minute) as glucose (30 mmol/100 g/minute), indicating that the vast majority of the energy required for the brain's work is normally derived from oxidative metabolism.[1,6] This oxygen to glucose consumption ratio of approximately 5.5 (rather than 6 if oxidation of glucose was complete) indicates a modest basal production of lactate via glycolysis. When flow is further reduced in a brain region already sustaining a maximum OEF through a maximally dilatated vasculature, the $CMRO_2$ must fall.[7] Both primate

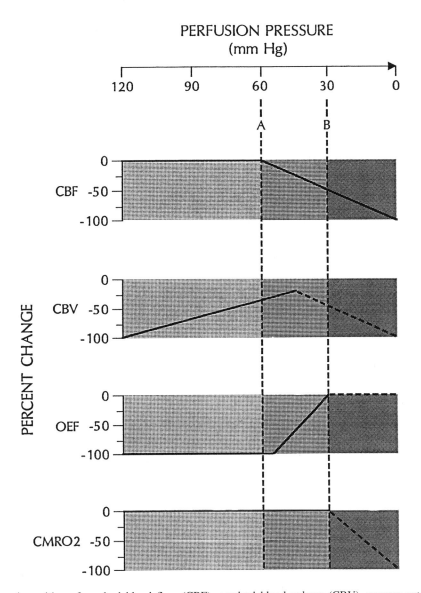

Figure 2-1. Superimposition of cerebral blood flow (CBF), cerebral blood volume (CBV), oxygen extraction fraction (OEF), and cerebral oxygen metabolism (CMRO$_2$) maps during graded reduction of cerebral perfusion pressure (CPP). When CPP declines, diminished CBF does not occur (A) until autoregulatory decreases in cerebrovascular resistance (reflected in increasing CBV) approaches a maximum; similarly, the CMRO$_2$ and related tissue functions do not deteriorate (B) until tissue metabolic demands exceed the maximum available oxygen supply (achieved through increasing OEF) from the remaining CBF. The CPP below which CBF declines (A) is typically approximately 60 mm Hg (the lower limit of cerebrovascular autoregulation), but can vary considerably. In chronic hypertension, for example, the autoregulatory curve is typically "shifted to the right" such that the lower limit of autoregulation—and CBF reduction—is met at considerably higher absolute values of systemic blood pressure. Because tissues surrounding a focus of recent ischemic injury typically fail to autoregulate, it is essential to avoid conditions that will result in reduction of "pressure-passive" flow to these regions. These considerations are particularly relevant in individuals with chronic hypertension, who may require considerably higher CPPs to maintain adequate CBF. In general, it is advisable to avoid therapeutic attempts at systemic blood pressure reduction during acute stroke unless clear-cut hypertensive end-organ damage (e.g., retinopathy, congestive heart failure) is occurring. Even relative hypotension can worsen existing ischemic neurologic deficits and the ultimate extent of tissue infarction.[7,10] (Adapted from WJ Powers. Cerebral hemodynamics in ischemic cerebrovascular disease. Ann Neurol 1991;29:231.)

and small-animal studies indicate that this metabolic threshold may be reached at approximately 50–65% of normal CBF.[17,18] At these flows—still compatible with cerebral electrical function—tissue lactate and hydrogen ion concentrations rise, indicating an increase in the rate of anaerobic glycolysis.[17,19,20] Energy charge is compromised, as reflected in declines in tissue phosphocreatinine and elevated inorganic phosphate levels, despite the capacity of tissues to temporarily maintain adenosine triphosphate (ATP) concentrations within or near normal limits.[21] In fact, an early decrease in intracellular pH and interstitial pH starts when the ATP levels are still high.[22] The interstitial pH begins to decrease within 15 seconds after the onset of ischemia, with the intracellular pH declining to 6.5–6.8.[23,24] Protein translation in general may be suppressed, but the products of specific gene families appear in abundance (especially the "immediate-early genes"; see Protein Metabolism and Gene Activation).[25] It is important to stress that mildly ischemic tissues have little energy reserve and limited capacity to respond to increases in metabolic demand and may therefore be vulnerable to secondary insults (inflammatory response, electrical spreading depression) (Figure 2-2).

The extent to which human cerebral tissues can sustain increases in the rate of anaerobic glycolysis or use of alternative fuels to maintain adequate high-energy phosphate supplies under mildly

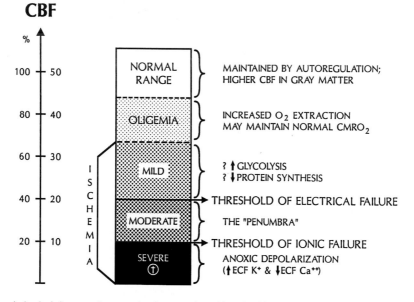

Figure 2-2. Ischemic brain injury can be conceived as a series of interlocking thresholds, each of which relates a decrement in cerebral blood flow (CBF) to key pathologic events. The normal range of CBF is maintained by cerebrovascular autoregulation. Modest reductions in CBF may produce no disturbances of tissue metabolism or function because increased oxygen extraction can maintain normal rates of cerebral oxygen metabolism (CMRO$_2$). More substantial reductions in CBF result in failure of CMRO$_2$ and progressive deterioration of various tissue functions—ischemia. Increases in the rate of tissue glycolysis and suppression of protein translation may be some of the earliest pathologic changes resulting from reduced CBF. However, there is very little available data from humans subjected to sustained "mild" ischemia. At a CBF of approximately 20 ml/100 g per minute (approximately 40% of resting flow), the threshold of electrical failure is met. At this threshold the electroencephalogram flattens, evoked potentials are attenuated, and neurologic deficits appear. Moderate ischemia can be defined as the range of CBF between this threshold for functional failure and the CBF threshold for ionic failure (approximately 20% of resting flow), below which cells rapidly become nonviable. Moderately ischemic tissues are presumed to contribute to the clinical deficit while being capable of responding to therapeutic intervention—the "ischemic penumbra." In severely ischemic tissues, normal ion gradients are reversed (anoxic depolarization), as reflected in increases in extracellular fluid (ECF) K$^+$ and movement of Ca^{2+} into cells (decreased ECF Ca^{2+}). (Adapted from K-A Hossmann. Pathophysiology of Cerebral Infarction. In PJ Viken, GW Bruyn, HL Klawans [eds], Handbook of Clinical Neurology. Vol. 53. New York: Elsevier, 1988;117.)

ischemic conditions is not known. Ischemia is traditionally defined in terms of CBF reduction of sufficient severity to produce symptomatic disruption of cerebral energy metabolism. It is controversial whether sustained modest reductions in CBF resulting in mildly decreased $CMRO_2$—yet above the traditionally defined CBF threshold for cerebral electrical failure—ultimately produce clinically significant changes in brain function. However, there is evidence from models of incomplete global ischemia and graded hypoxia that energy metabolism may deteriorate in a gradual, stepwise fashion, even in the presence of stable CBF.[26] The measured CBF threshold for energy failure—the CBF at which cell ATP levels are severely degraded—can actually increase over time in marginally perfused tissues.[27] This has led to the concept of preconditioning in cerebral ischemia. Animals undergoing non-lethal short exposures to ischemia were found to be more resistant to lethal ischemic insults. This ischemic tolerance usually requires 2–4 days to develop. Similar tolerance is observed after short periods of thermal stress,[28] mechanical stimulation,[29] cortical spreading depression,[30] and endotoxin pretreatment. The period required for tolerance to manifest is suggestive of the involvement of protein synthesis in this process. Various proteins that have been proposed are heat shock proteins (hsp), neurotrophins, or Bcl-2. There is also evidence showing that elevation of interleukin-1α (IL-1α), IL-1β, or tumor necrosis factor-α (TNF-α) may induce this ischemic tolerance.[31]

An exciting new field of stroke research has been the regulation of angiogenesis after cerebral ischemia. The severe reduction of blood supply and low oxygen tension in ischemia leads to compensatory neovascularization in the affected regions. Hypoxic stress leads to the induction of hypoxia-inducible factor-1 (HIF-1), a mediator of physiologic and pathologic responses to hypoxia.[31] HIF-1 regulates various hypoxia-inducible genes, including vascular endothelial growth factor (VEGF) and VEGF receptors.[32] In addition, glucose deprivation during ischemia may regulate VEGF in a manner independent of HIF-1.[33] Other factors that regulate VEGF include a whole range of growth factors and cytokines such as platelet-derived growth factor (PDGF), transforming growth factor β, TNF, or IL-1β. VEGF,[34,35] as well as the other angiogenic factors such as PDGF[36] and

basic fibroblast growth factor,[37] are upregulated after focal cerebral ischemia with a time course that parallels angiogenesis. Some data demonstrate that ischemia also regulates the expression genes encoding angiopoietin-1, angiopoietin-2, and receptor tyrosine kinases (Tie-1 and Tie-2).[38] The angiopoietin/Tie receptor system may contribute to angiogenesis and vascular remodeling by mediating interactions of endothelial cells with smooth muscle cells and pericytes. The temporal profile of the angiogenesis factors suggests that angiopoietin-2 interacts with VEGF in regulating vessel sprouting, whereas angiopoietin-1 may play a role in stabilizing the vasculature.[38]

Threshold for "Electrical Failure" and Disturbed Calcium Homeostasis (Moderate Ischemia)

Further decreases in cerebral perfusion herald the onset of so-called electrical failure: At 18–25 ml/100 g per minute or 40–50% of normal resting hemispheral CBF, the electroencephalogram slows, evoked potentials are attenuated,[39,40] and the generation of synaptic potentials by individual cortical neurons declines.[41] This functional threshold, similar in both global and focal ischemia, corresponds in essence to the appearance of neurologic deficits.[42] It must be emphasized that tissue ATP content may be normal or only slightly depressed at the threshold for functional failure.[21] The precise mechanisms of this reversible functional failure are unknown but likely reflect the exquisite vulnerability of certain neurotransmitter systems to even moderate hypoxia-ischemia and decreases in tissue pH.[43] The common occurrence of transient ischemic attacks suggests the paramount importance of duration as well as depth of ischemia in producing permanent tissue damage.

The CBF threshold for electrical failure lies in close relation to the experimentally determined CBF threshold for large-scale release of amino acids into the extracellular fluid (ECF) space from various cells (estimated at CBF <20 ml/100 g/minute), in particular the excitatory amino acids (EAAs) glutamate and aspartate.[44] This flow threshold for EAA release overlaps the CBF threshold for early tissue edema formation (approximately 20 ml/100 g/minute). When reductions of CBF below these levels are maintained for approximately one-half hour or more, astrocytes are thought to swell as a consequence of their removal of osmotically active lactate and EAA molecules from the ECF.[45–47] There is emerging awareness of the possibility that all these changes associated with moderate ischemia—cerebroelectric functional failure, EAA release, and early edema—can occur in tissues in which neither severe energy failure, gross disturbance of cellular ion homeostasis, or sustained disruption of blood-brain barrier integrity have developed.[12,17,44,45]

The extracellular Ca^{2+} content in neurons is much higher than the concentration $[Ca^{2+}]_i$, because much of the intracellular Ca^{2+} is sequestered in the organelles. Various factors that determine the net $[Ca^{2+}]_i$ include Ca^{2+} influx through voltage-gated Ca^{2+} channels (VGCCs) and ligand-gated Ca^{2+} channels (LGCCs), sequestration in internal storage organs such as mitochondria and endoplasmic reticulum, buffering by Ca^{2+}-binding proteins, and active Ca^{2+} extrusion.[48] The extrusion of Ca^{2+} occurs via a high affinity Ca^{2+}-activated adenosine triphosphatase (ATPase) and a low affinity Na^+/Ca^{2+} exchanger, driven by the plasma membrane Na^+ gradient. Ca^{2+} influx and the disturbance of Ca^{2+} homeostasis are the critical steps in initiating ischemic cell death. In moderately ischemic tissues subject to an increased release of EAAs, Ca^{2+} probably enters exposed neurons early through the EAA receptor–linked LGCCs. One of the most intensely studied LGCCs is the Ca^{2+} channel associated with the receptor for the glutamate analog N-methyl-D-aspartate (NMDA)[49] (see Pathways of Ischemic Injury for further discussion of excitotoxicity). There is strong indirect evidence from in vitro work that Ca^{2+} entry through the NMDA receptor–associated channels occurs at a magnitude of membrane depolarization substantially less than that required for Ca^{2+} entry through voltage-sensitive Ca^{2+} channels (VSCCs), indicating a possible rank order of different modes of Ca^{2+} mobilization in the pathogenesis of ischemic injury. The initial massive neuronal depolarization required for activation of NMDA receptors in energetically stable tissues may reflect an EAA-induced increase in conductances of ligand-operated sodium (Na^+) channels.[49,50] After a mild elevation of $[Ca^{2+}]_i$, the Na^+-Ca^{2+} exchanger uses the electrochemical gradient for Na^+ that is maintained by the Na^+-K^+ pump to exchange extracellular Na^+ for intracellular Ca^{2+}. If cellular energy reserves are adequate to manage the expulsion of Ca^{2+}, $[Ca^{2+}]_i$ remains stable, and there may be no dire consequences of LGCC-mediated Ca^{2+} entry. However, entry of Ca^{2+} through ligand-operated Ca^{2+} channels can be devastating if it is excessive and/or neurons lack the energy reserves necessary to contain elevation in $[Ca^{2+}]_i$[49] and rectify ionic derangement (see next section).

Threshold for Ionic Failure and Calcium Overload (Severe Ischemia)

Finally, still more profound ischemia—flows less than 10–12 ml/100 g per minute or approximately 20–30% of normal—results in the gross deterioration of transmembrane ionic gradients: the threshold of ionic failure. This depth of ischemia seems incompatible with tissue survival in small-animal models if sustained beyond approximately 1 hour.[12] Both severe substrate depletion and the negative feedback of hydrogen ions at the phosphofructokinase step will result in cessation of glycolysis, leading to complete degradation of high-energy phosphate.[19] Electrodes in the ECF space detect striking increases in the concentration of potassium ions (K^+) and marked declines in Ca^{2+}, indicating Ca^{2+} entry into cells—the characteristic features of so-called "anoxic depolarization."[17,18] Hypoxic-ischemic insults of more than 3–5 minutes' duration result in anoxic depolarization or rapid depolarization (–20 mV) of all neurons. The mechanism of this anoxic depolarization is not completely understood but may be secondary to the reduction of intracellular ATP, with the consequent inhibition of Na^+/K^+ ATPase activity and subsequent K^+ efflux. This is supported by the studies showing early increase in the extracellular K^+ concentration ($[K^+]_e$). These ion shifts reflect multifactorial changes in membrane permeability and the progressive failure of multiple energy-dependent membrane pumps and transport systems (e.g., Na^+-K^+-ATPase, Ca^{2+} ATPase, and the Na^+-Ca^{2+} antiporter) that normally maintain the steep electrochemical gradients essential for neuronal membrane polarization[51] (see Figure 2-2).

K^+ channels are the major contributors for maintaining the cells' resting membrane potential in a hyperpolarized state. The early increase in $[K^+]_e$ is due to the activation of ATP-sensitive K^+ channels. Astrocytes attempt to buffer this increase in $[K^+]_e$ by switching to anaerobic glycolysis and swelling up, but eventually are unable to cope. The increased $[K^+]_e$ concentration in severely ischemic brain regions may help sustain ischemic injury by a number of mechanisms. First, elevated $[K^+]_e$ creates an electrophysiologic environment that leads to the depolarization of neighboring neurons and may provide an important trigger for electrical spreading depression, a pathologic wave of depolarization that has been implicated in the extension of tissue injury beyond the region of severe ischemia in several animal models of stroke. Spreading depression may be harmful by promoting Ca^{2+} entry into neuronal populations rendered vulnerable to further Ca^{2+} loading secondary to ischemic energy depletion.[52] At the time of anoxic depolarization, the interstitial concentrations of other ions, such as Na^+, Cl^-, and Ca^{2+}, have been shown to decrease. Second, increased $[K^+]_e$ within the brain parenchyma may diffuse toward the cerebral microvasculature and stimulate the activity of Na^+-K^+-ATPase along the abluminal surface of endothelial cells, promoting movement of intravascular Na^+ and water into the ECF space. This may occur at a level of tissue oxygenation that alters parenchymal Na^+-K^+-ATPase activity, resulting in a net transfer of Na^+ and water from the vasculature into neurons and glia to maintain intracellular osmolarity. The consequence of such an ionic shift is "cytotoxic" edema.[53] To achieve an electric neutrality, there is a passive entry of Cl^- and water. Cl^- influx can also be enhanced with the activation of γ-aminobutyric acid[54] receptors, as an increase in γ-aminobutyric acid release also occurs after ischemia.[54] Furthermore, extremely high $[K^+]_e$ may promote vasoconstriction, compromising residual blood flow to severely ischemic regions.[55]

There is evidence that Ca^{2+} entry into neurons via VGCC begins abruptly and massively when $[K^+]_e$ rises to approximately 10–15 mmol.[17] Additional mechanisms to increase $[Ca^{2+}]_i$ include second messenger–mediated mobilization of Ca^{2+} from various high-capacity intracellular sites (e.g., phosphatidyl inositol activation), reversal of the neuronal membrane's Na^+-Ca^{2+} exchanger under conditions of cellular Na^+ overload, and passage of ions through nonspecific "leak" conductances that may develop across severely damaged cellular membranes. The resting membrane permeability to Ca^{2+} is very low, and transient physiologic elevations in $[Ca^{2+}]_i$ are usually rapidly reversed at the expense of metabolic energy by a number of regulatory mechanisms and intracellular buffers. At the point that massive Ca^{2+} entry through VGCC occurs with anoxic depolarization, however, the capacity of cells to normalize $[Ca^{2+}]_i$ may be severely compromised, and true Ca^{2+} overload is established.[49]

Elevations in $[Ca^{2+}]_i$ accompany and most likely mediate myriad pathologic processes, many of which are thought to be related to the irreversible damage to mitochondria, cellular membranes, and enzyme systems that best define cell necrosis.[56,57] First, attempted cellular reversal of Ca^{2+} overload challenges already scarce supplies of ATP, and Ca^{2+} ions may directly induce uncoupling of oxidative phosphorylation as they compete with hydrogen ions for sequestration sites on mitochondrial membranes (competition between Ca^{2+} and pH buffering systems).[55,56] Scarce oxygen supplies are then diverted from energy production into "futile cycling" of ions across the mitochondrial cristae. Second, sustained increases in $[Ca^{2+}]_i$ are associated with the disordered activation of a wide range of enzyme systems, including phospholipase A_2 and C, endonucleases, calpains, and various other proteases. These functional alterations have far-reaching consequences for the structural integrity of cell membranes, genetic material, neurofilaments, and other structural proteins.[49,56–58] In addition, Ca^{2+} entry into vascular smooth muscle promotes increases in CVR that may threaten residual blood flow.[59]

Specific pharmacologic antagonists of Ca^{2+} channels have been reported to improve CBF in marginally perfused tissues,[60] reverse disturbances of cellular energy metabolism,[61] and reduce the volume of tissue infarction in some animal models of stroke[62] but not others.[63] More consistent benefit is observed with pretreatment (before onset of ischemic insult), but it has been difficult to determine the specific mechanism of the therapeutic effect, given the multiple levels at which blockage of Ca^{2+} entry might alter lesion formation. However, there have been many substantial data supporting the role of the dihydropyridine VSCC antagonist nimodipine in preventing ischemic sequelae of cerebral vasospasm secondary to subarachnoid hemorrhage.[64] However, other studies offer no definite evidence to support the clinical benefit from postischemic administration of nimodipine in patients with acute ischemic stroke.[65,66]

Topography and Time Course of Focal Ischemia

A sudden, sharp decline in CPP, as after cardiac arrest, results in near immediate suspension of CBF, loss of consciousness within 10 seconds, loss of spontaneous and evoked electrical activity within 20 seconds,[67] and rapid depletion of high-energy phosphate. Collapse of normal tissue ion homeostasis occurs within minutes.[68] Episodes of severe global ischemia as brief as 5 minutes can result in the delayed deterioration and death of certain selectively vulnerable neurons in the CA1 region of the hippocampus, inner layers of the cerebral cortex, portions of the striatum, and Purkinje's cells in the cerebellum.[69] More sustained global ischemia results in patchy laminar necrosis of the cortical ribbon and strio-pallidum, but frank infarction—large-scale necrosis, including death of glia and endothelium—does not usually occur unless global ischemia is prolonged or produced under hyperthermic conditions.[12,19,70]

In the setting of focal ischemia more relevant to stroke, however, flow reduction is rarely total, even in the most severely hypoperfused regions. The flow is regionally heterogeneous, due to a variably efficient network of anatomic vascular collaterals.[71,72] In focal ischemia, CBF may differ substantially between contiguous brain regions, in a range from normal to severely reduced (below the threshold for ionic failure). "Flow gradients" can be defined both with respect to the surface of the cerebral hemispheres and the cross-sectional depth of the neuraxis (Figure 2-3).

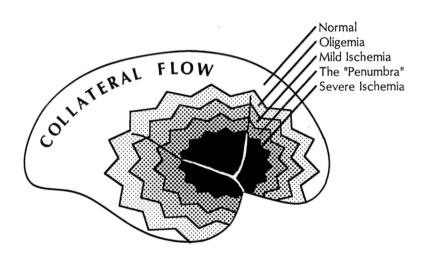

Figure 2-3. Depiction of hypothetical "flow gradient" over the convexity of a primate hemisphere subjected to acute proximal middle cerebral artery (MCA) occlusion. Collateral blood flow from adjacent vascular territories may maintain normal or only modestly reduced cerebral blood flow (CBF) to a large percentage of the hemispheral surface. Total arrest of CBF is not usually observed in focal ischemia. A roughly circumferential gradient of ischemic CBF suggests regional variation in vulnerability to infarction. Because it occupies the site most remote from leptomeningeal collateral flow, the sylvian operculum is frequently infarcted after proximal MCA occlusions. Similarly, less well-perfused structures within the depths of the hemisphere may be more vulnerable to ischemic injury than the richly collateralized cortex. The ultimate extent of tissue infarction is highly variable and reflects both the depth and duration of ischemia. (Adapted from J Astrup, BK Siesjo, L Symon. Thresholds in cerebral ischemia: the ischemic penumbra. Stroke 1981;12:723.)

These flow gradients provide a first order of approximate estimation of regional vulnerability to infarction. For example, critical reduction of CPP distal to an extracranial carotid stenosis may result in severe ischemia between the border zones of the ipsilateral major intracranial vascular territories, but normal or only mildly reduced flow over most of the cerebral convexity.[73,74] In contrast, after acute occlusion of the proximal portion of the middle cerebral artery in normotensive primates, CBF is reduced maximally—to approximately 20–25% of control—in the sylvian region (frontal, parietal, and temporal opercula), anterior basal ganglia, and supradjacent white matter. Circumscribing these densely ischemic regions are zones of less severe CBF reduction across a range from 40% to 80% of the normal level, depending on the distance from the ischemic core and local collateral supply[75,76] (see Figure 2-3). Distal occlusions of leptomeningeal branch arteries result in similarly demarcated cores of dense ischemia with halos of intermediate flow reduction.[77] Considerable heterogeneity of CBF may occur at the microvascular level as well.[78] Correlative histopathologic and radiographic data corroborate the relevance of these concepts to focal ischemic lesions in humans.[79]

The weight of available evidence suggests that tissue infarction—pan-necrosis of all tissue elements—is detectable in the regions of lowest blood flow after approximately 1 hour and then progressively expands in a radial fashion toward its maximum volume over 3–4 hours in rodents,[80] 6–8 hours in subhuman primates,[42] and over an uncertain time in humans.[15,81,82] Brain regions initially outside of the zones of severe ischemia are eventually recruited into the infarction if sufficient time elapses. It is increasingly clear that systemic hyperthermia greatly accelerates this process of infarct evolution and even moderate hypothermia dramatically retards it,[12] with important therapeutic implications. Elevated brain temperature increases the $CMRO_2$, promoting mismatch between demand and limited oxygen supply. In addition, hyperthermia may alter the integrity of the blood-brain barrier, promote "vasogenic edema," and bring the normally sequestered brain ECF space into contact with the potentially toxic contents of the plasma.

Furthermore, during the period of infarct evolution, marginally perfused tissues are vulnerable to further reductions in oxygen delivery because of the combination of widespread loss of normal cerebrovascular autoregulation (flow becomes "pressure passive")[10] and the not uncommon occurrence of systemic cardiopulmonary dysfunction that may decrease blood pressure and arterial oxygen content.[83,84] These considerations underscore the importance of vigilant supportive care, including avoidance of iatrogenic reduction of systemic blood pressure during acute stroke. Even under stable systemic conditions, however, marginal cerebral tissues frequently deteriorate toward infarction unless rapidly reperfused.[42,80] Understanding this process of "spontaneous" deterioration remains one of the central goals of research into the pathophysiology of stroke.

Ischemic Penumbra: Why Does It Deteriorate?

As described previously in the section Topography and Time Course of Focal Ischemia, in acute focal cerebral ischemia there are corridors of tissue interposed between normal and densely ischemic regions that contain cells that are nonfunctioning electrically but potentially viable. This "ischemic penumbra"—likened to the shadow region that surrounds a complete solar eclipse—was originally defined as a state of moderate CBF reduction between the thresholds for electrical and ionic failure.[4] Cells in this state are presumed to contribute to the clinical deficit while being capable of responding to therapeutic intervention. The proper definition, pathophysiology, and degree of stability of the ischemic penumbra as it pertains to acute stroke in humans remain areas of intense controversy.[85–87]

Perfusion Pressure and the Penumbra

It is established that even under stable systemic conditions, initially viable tissues are recruited into evolving cerebral infarctions. There are numerous factors intrinsic to the brain and its vasculature that may contribute to the deterioration of an ischemic penumbra. The anatomic extent of any one region receiving a stable rate of penumbral CBF is variable and depends on the tone, number, and proximity of collateral channels, the blood viscosity, and the CPP.[12,85] The latter factor is of particular importance because it may be readily subject to therapeutic manipulation. CPP is the difference between arterial inflow and venous back pressures; however, CPP is usually expressed as a function of mean arterial blood pressure (MABP) and ICP, because changes in the pressure of cerebral tissues or the cerebrospinal fluid spaces they freely communicate with are effectively and rapidly transmitted to the thin-walled cerebral veins:

$$CPP = MABP - ICP$$

It is possible then that even under stable systemic MABP, global increases in ICP or compartmentalized increases in local tissue pressure could reduce CPP to the penumbra level by impeding outflow.[88] CBF might then be brought below the threshold for ionic failure with loss of tissue viability. Despite considerable experimental effort, however, the difficult problem of the role of progressive flow failure in infarct evolution remains unresolved. Substantial local tissue pressure gradients—on the order of 10–20 mm Hg—have been recorded in association with acute experimental ischemic stroke, but they have had no measurable effect on regional CBF.[89] Other investigators have reported declines in CBF in edematous tissues, but the relationships are complex, and they may reflect the reflex alterations in cerebrovascular reactivity and tone but are unrelated to tissue pressure per se.[90,91] Experimental efforts are hampered by the inherent difficulty of measuring CBF and oxygen delivery to the tissues at the microvascular level.

The balance of available evidence suggests that the mechanical aspects of edema (effects on perfusion pressure and CBF) are unlikely to contribute substantially to primary ischemic brain damage under conditions most commonly encountered in ischemic stroke.[12] *Primary damage* can be defined as the destruction of neurons and the capacity for integrated neurologic function, which traditionally was assumed to precede the breakdown of glia and endothelium, leukocyte invasion, vascular sludging, and other "secondary" processes.[70,92] Tissue-pressure gradients evolve over time and may be more relevant to secondary tissue injury. Although these secondary processes are important, there is evidence that they may be late events, occurring "after the fact" of primary neuronal injury.[89,93] The clinical significance of secondary injury processes is usually thought to derive from their contribution to edema formation, increases in ICP, cerebral herniations, impaired microcirculation, and inflammation[88,94] (Table 2-1). The sec-

Table 2-1. Categorization of Ischemic Brain Injury

	Primary (Early)	Secondary (Late)
Gross changes	Pyknosis and eosinophilia of dying neurons	Necrosis of glia and endothelium; leukocyte accumulation; hemorrhage
	Cerebral electrical failure	Re-expansion of ECF space ("vasogenic edema")
	Shrinkage of ECF space as glia swell ("cytotoxic edema")	Distortion of tissues/cerebral herniations
Mechanisms	Depletion of neuronal high-energy phosphates	Release of cytokines from activated leukocytes
	Impaired protein synthesis	Changes in permeability of blood-brain barrier secondary to prostaglandin accumulation, build-up of leukotrienes, leukocyte invasion, contraction of endothelium, free radicals, tissue acidosis, etc.
	Exposure to toxic compounds released from ischemic cells (e.g., glutamate, lactate)	Increased blood viscosity
	Accumulation of Ca^{2+} within cells (many consequences)	Brain hyperemia
	Alterations in structure/expression of genetic material	

ECF = extracellular fluid.

ondary injury processes are discussed in the section Postischemic Inflammatory Reaction.

However, contemporary data on the early breakdown of endothelial components of the blood-brain barrier, leukocyte infiltration of tissues, and rapid development of vasogenic edema under specific (and likely clinically relevant) circumstances, such as hyperthermic ischemia,[95] dense ischemia with reperfusion,[96] and microembolism,[97] have suggested a causal link between early edema formation and primary ischemic brain damage. Indeed, the traditional distinction between "primary" pathology occurring in neurons and "secondary" pathology involving other cerebral tissue elements is somewhat artificial and may be overly restrictive (see Table 2-1).

Beyond Blood Flow

A more intriguing possibility is that deterioration of the penumbra occurs independently of further reductions in CBF. Over the time course, most likely relevant to infarct evolution, CBF is stable or changes only very gradually in many animal models of stroke. However, progression of stable hypoperfused tissues toward infarction as reflected in changes in tissue pH, glycolytic metabolites, ATP concentration, and histology is regularly observed.[42,77,89,98] It is as if the effectiveness of residual flow declines in a time-dependent fashion once a critical reduction in brain perfusion is established. For example, the measured CBF threshold for energy failure—the level of flow at which tissue high-energy phosphate levels become severely degraded—increases with time.[27] Stated another way, the CBF threshold for histologic lesions in primates with permanent ischemia (no reperfusion) is 17–18 ml/100 g per minute. If the duration of ischemia is limited to only 1 hour, however, only tissues with CBF reduced to 5–6 ml/100 g per minute or less go on to infarct.[42]

Specific hypotheses that may explain these time-dependent changes in viability of stable, hypo-perfused tissues include interference with residual aerobic metabolism by calcium overload or byproducts of glycolysis, or both[1,49]; exposure of marginal tissues to potentially damaging plasma constituents in the setting of early blood-brain barrier damage[95]; diffusion of toxic mediators that alter ion homeostasis from ischemic neurons[49,99]; and the invasion of the penumbra by waves of electrical spreading depression originating from the regions of dense ischemia.[52] The critical determinant of deterioration of the penumbra, then, may not be the spontaneous decline of marginal flow but the proximity of vulnerable tissues to specific threats emanating from core ischemic regions. There is little information about the anatomic extent or biochemical status of the focal ischemic penumbra in humans.[82] Data on the time course and relative roles of ischemic versus "toxic" processes during truly acute ischemia—within a few hours of symptom onset—are sorely needed. Advances in imaging technology in correlative clinical studies are beginning to fill this void (see Chapter 3).

Pathways of Ischemic Injury

Beyond Energy Failure

Although some degree of tissue energy depletion is a constant feature of all ischemic insults,[100] under many circumstances complete energy failure—degradation of ATP and related high-energy phosphate compounds—is neither necessary nor sufficient to produce irreversible neuronal injury. Evidence to support this perhaps surprising statement comes from several different perspectives. First, the degree of ATP depletion may correlate better with initial neurologic deficits[101] than ultimate outcome[102] after ischemic insult. Second, it is well documented that cerebral protein synthesis—vital for cell survival—may be abnormal at degrees of CBF reduction well above the threshold for cerebral energy failure.[25] Furthermore, certain vulnerable neuronal populations may undergo delayed necrosis after even brief periods of sufficiently severe ischemia, long after restoration of energy charge,[103,104] whereas many brain cells are capable of surviving for periods of severe hypoxia-ischemia lasting as long as 1 hour that result in total energy failure.[105] Finally, neuronal susceptibility to ischemic injury is non-uniform and reflects the regional and developmental variation in cellular expression of receptors for certain neurotransmitters[106] and other dynamic aspects of neuronal connectivity.[107]

Therefore, additional factors, brought into play in relation to the reduction of cellular energy supplies but not necessarily dependent on frank energy failure for their continuing adverse influence, must be invoked to explain these experimental observations (Figure 2-4). The remainder of this chapter provides a more detailed account of several of the better-characterized mediators of primary and secondary ischemic injury and closes with a brief introduction to the consequences of reperfusion.

Excitotoxicity

There are abundant data from diverse sources indicating a pivotal role for the EAA neurotransmitters, especially glutamate, in both the initiation and elaboration of ischemic brain injury. A consistent pattern of structural damage is obtained when neurons are exposed to high concentrations of EAAs in vitro, and the vulnerability of both hippocampal and cortical neurons to anoxia and hypoglycemia in vivo has been related to glutamate release from presynaptic terminals.[108–110] Neurons in culture exposed to glutamate even briefly rapidly swell—a reflection of increased permeability to Na^+ ions and passive influx of chloride and water—and later accumulate Ca^{2+} subsequent to massive entry through both ligand-operated Ca^{2+} channels and VSCCs.[111,112] The aggregate effects of this rapid osmotic disturbance and more delayed Ca^{2+} loading comprise *excitotoxicity*, a term first coined by Olney, who described glutamate toxicity in relation to its capacity to excite or depolarize neurons.[113] However, it is now well appreciated that glutamate toxicity is far more complex than the induction of cation flux, and that the toxic potential of glutamate analogs may not correlate well with excitatory potential per se.[114] In particular, glutamate and other EAAs may stimulate the production of the potentially toxic compound nitric oxide (NO), generate other free radicals (FRs), and induce changes in gene structure and expression.[115–117]

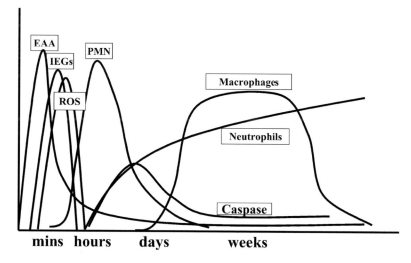

Figure 2-4. Ischemic neuronal injury is initiated by many mediators. Very early after the onset of the ischemic injury, excitatory amino acids (EAAs) induce Ca^{2+} influx by activating the *N*-methyl-D-aspartate receptor and then damage neurons and glia. A number of immediate early genes (IEGs) express, such as c-fos, c-jun, within 30 minutes. Reactive oxygen species (ROSs) are free radicals, which are products from aerobic metabolism, cascades arachidonic acid, lipid peroxidation, or activated phagocytes. ROSs damage virtually all of the cellular components, including the DNA. Pro-inflammatory gene expression indicates the synthesis of inflammatory mediators. Consequently, the expression of adhesion molecules on endothelial cell surface would interact with polymorphonuclear neutrophils (PMNs), which migrate into the ischemic brain tissue. Macrophages and monocytes follow neutrophils and enter the brain parenchyma. Caspase-dependent cell death (apoptosis) appears in the more delayed stage and demises the ischemic tissue. Increases in messenger RNA for neurotrophins also occur in the more delayed stage. The x-axis reflects the evolution of the major events of time, whereas the y-axis illustrates an arbitrary unit.

The importance of excitotoxicity to the understanding and potential treatment of ischemic brain injury can be considered from several distinct perspectives. First, pathologic glutamate release into the ECF space of ischemic cerebral tissues (where it may access a broad spectrum of cellular receptors) appears to occur temporally "upstream" from more severe postischemic insults to ion homeostasis, cellular membranes, and enzyme systems (Table 2-2). Work using brain microdialysis techniques indicates that when regional CBF is reduced to below approximately 20 ml/100 g per minute (35–40% of normal), massive release of glutamate into the ECF space begins[44,118]; these levels of flow reduction are above the CBF threshold for ATP depletion, ionic failure, and tissue autocatalysis. Glutamate release into the extracellular space is caused by a decline in cellular energy reserves and disturbed Na^+ gradients. Impairment in glutamate uptake mechanism due to metabolic derangement of glial element further accentuates the extracellular

elevation of glutamate levels.[119] Therefore, excitotoxins may be viewed as "early" mediators of ischemic injury. Second, by various mechanisms, glutamate may influence the status of neural tissues remote from the site of its release. For example, elevated ECF glutamate may, like pathologic increases in extracellular K^+, incite potentially harmful waves of spreading depression in cortical tissues.[52,120]

Third, compelling evidence from animal models of focal and, to a lesser extent, global ischemic injury indicates that specific pharmacologic antagonists of the various glutamate receptor subtypes can significantly reduce neuronal necrosis or volume of tissue infarction, or both.[121–125] Among the three major subtypes of neuronal glutamate receptor so far identified, the NMDA receptor has generally been assumed to play the most important role in excitotoxicity by inducing the influx of Ca^{2+} via a LGCC, triggering a host of Ca^{2+}-mediated or accelerated pathologies[126] (see Table 2-2). Ca^{2+} entry into neurons occurs rapidly in the presence of

Table 2-2. Excitatory Amino Acid (EAA) Receptors

	Physiologic Properties	Functional/Pathologic Effects
NMDA receptor	Present on dendritic (postsynaptic) membranes throughout CNS Receptor activation triggers entry of both Na^+ and Ca^{2+} into neurons Ca^{2+} entry causes activation of many second-messenger systems, including phospholipase C, protein kinase C, nitric oxide synthetase, phosphatases, and various proteases May be expressed by endothelium	Mediates long-term potentiation/ depression of neuronal networks and so is essential for neuronal plasticity Likely mediator of both acute and chronic neuronal degeneration after ischemic insult via Ca^{2+}-linked events
AMPA/kainate receptor	Widely distributed throughout CNS on postsynaptic (and possibly presynaptic) membranes Receptor activation triggers entry of Na^+ (and possibly Ca^{2+}) into neurons May provide initial depolarizing effect in regions of moderate ischemia	Critical in fast excitatory neurotransmission and cell signaling throughout CNS Increasingly recognized as playing a key role in ischemic cellular injury
Quisqualate	"Metabotropic" receptor: unlike NMDA and AMPA/kainate receptors, the major effect is to activate a G protein and in turn multiple neuronal enzyme systems Modulates activity of ion channels linked to other EAA receptor subtypes	Recognized role in central control of nociception and basal ganglia function Role in ischemic injury uncertain

NMDA = *N*-methyl-D-aspartate; AMPA = alpha-amino-3-hydroxy-5-methyl-4-isoxazole propionic acid; CNS = central nervous system.

NMDA receptor agonists, in contrast to the delayed and less massive Ca^{2+} loading that follows isolated application of specific agonists of the alpha-amino-3-hydroxy-5-methyl-4-isoxazole propionic acid (AMPA) and kainate receptors[127] (Figure 2-5). Furthermore, specific pharmacologic antagonists of the NMDA receptor efficiently protect cultured neuronal populations from otherwise lethal hypoxic and ischemic insults.[128] However, in vivo data suggest that NMDA antagonists may be of limited value under conditions of severe ischemia (complete global or severe focal ischemia), due in part to down-modulation of these receptors by the local decreases in pH and energy charge characteristic of densely ischemic tissues.[124] These and other reasons could explain the fact that clinical trials of several NMDA receptor

blockers, such as dextrorphan, selfotel (CGS 19755), and aptiganel (Cerestat, CNS 1102), ended in failure.[129] Adverse effects that were found common to NMDA antagonists include psychotic, phencyclidine (PCP)-like reactions and cardiosuppressive effects, formation of neuronal vacuoles, and neuronal necrosis.[130] Therefore, the doses of NMDA antagonists that are safe for stroke patients might not reach the therapeutic levels that are neuroprotective in animal stroke models. Some studies on NMDA antagonism have been directed to NMDA receptor subtype antagonists that may be devoid of undesirable side effects. GV150526, a selective inhibitor of the glycine site of the NMDA receptor, is free of hemodynamic CNS adverse effects and has gone through extensive clinical trials.[131,132] However, results from two phase III trials

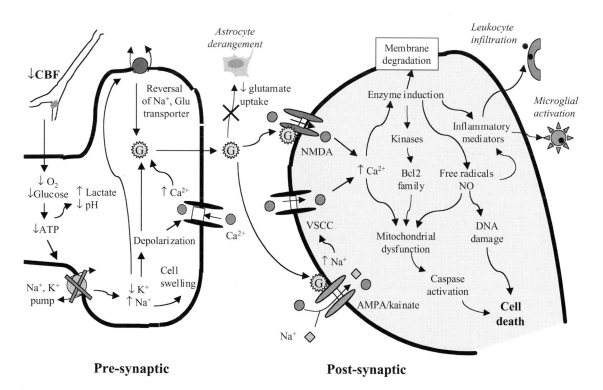

Pre-synaptic   **Post-synaptic**

Figure 2-5. Decrease of cerebral blood flow (CBF) induces hypoxic depolarization, intracellular acidosis, increase of $[Na^+]_i$, $[Ca^{2+}]_i$, decrease of $[K^+]_i$ and cell swelling in pre-synaptic neurons. Glutamate (G) is released, and it further activates the glutamate receptors (N-methyl-D-aspartate [NMDA], alpha-amino-3-hydroxy-5-methyl-4-isoxazole propionic acid [AMPA]/kainate) in post-synaptic neurons. By-standing, deranged astrocytes cannot uptake glutamate as in a normal situation. Large amounts of Ca^{2+} entering into the post-synaptic neurons increases the activity of enzymes and kinase. Elevation of $[Ca^{2+}]_i$ is accompanied by activation of pro-inflammatory mediators, free radicals formation, and mitochondrial dysfunction. All of the preceding demise neurons by the pathways of necrosis (membrane degradation) or apoptosis. (ATP = adenosine triphosphate; Glu = glutamate; VSCC = voltage-sensitive Ca^{2+} channels; NO = nitric oxide.)

showed that GV150526 was without any therapeutic benefit in stroke patients (unpublished observations). A new class of antagonists of the AMPA/kainate subtype receptors may, however, exert neuroprotective effects even in regions of severe focal or global ischemia,[133] possibly via both Ca^{2+}-dependent and Ca^{2+}-independent mechanisms.[134] PNQX (quinoxalinedione PD 152247), a selective AMPA receptor antagonist, was shown to reduce stroke lesion volume by 51% in a rat model of temporary focal ischemia.[135] Although some AMPA antagonists are associated with serious side effects and precluded from entering large-scale trials, others with excellent safety profiles are entering the early stage of clinical studies.

A potentially important advantage of AMPA antagonists is that they also exert neuroprotective effects on white matter. The conventional view that white matter is less vulnerable to ischemic injury than gray matter is being questioned. Increasing in vivo evidence indicates functional deficit after ischemic insults may be due primarily to damage in white matter in the spinal cord[136] and the brain.[137] Although excitotoxins play a major role in the pathogenesis of ischemic gray matter injury,[110] the role of glutamate receptor action in ischemic white matter lesion is less clear. Glial elements and axons have traditionally been considered resistant to injury caused by excitotoxin exposure.[138] However, activation of the AMPA/kainate glutamate receptor has been shown to cause oligodendrocyte death in vitro and in vivo.[139,140] AMPA/kainate receptor antagonism also has been found selectively in salvaging white, but not gray, matter after ischemic spinal cord injury in rats.[141]

In addition to Na and Ca, another ion, namely zinc, has also been implicated in ischemic neuronal death. Zinc is a divalent cation that physiologically serves as a neurotransmitter in addition to being an integral element of metalloenzymes and transcription factors. During ischemia, zinc may be released with glutamate to exert cytotoxic effects.[142] The role of zinc in selective neuronal death after ischemia has been demonstrated in a global ischemia model.[143] In contrast to zinc, magnesium, another endogenous ion abundant within cells, could be neuroprotective in the setting of cerebral ischemia. Magnesium ions may act at multiple points in the ischemic cascade. Magnesium blocks the NMDA-associated ion channel in a voltage-dependent manner.[144] In addition, magnesium may act as a neuroprotective agent through vascular effects, such as increasing regional CBF to the ischemic tissue and providing protection against oxygen FR production.[144]

Hyperthermia greatly facilitates edema formation and primary neuronal injury due to excitotoxic mechanisms.[145] This has prompted the exploration of hypothermia as a neuroprotective strategy in both global and focal ischemia.[146] In this regard, the brain temperature rather than the rectal temperature is a more reliable indicator in determining the hypothermic effects on ischemic brain injury.[147] Whereas very low temperature (<25°C) offers nearly complete protection against ischemic injury, it is associated with severe adverse effects. Mild to moderate temperature reductions of 1–3°C may still confer substantial neuroprotection in animal stroke models without serious side effects.[148] The protective effect of intraischemic hypothermia can be explained by a number of mechanisms, including reduced metabolic demand, improved local glucose utilization, reversal of protein synthesis inhibition, suppression of glutamate release, and decreased generation of FRs, NO, and other deleterious substances.[149] One prospective study showed that ischemic stroke patients with mild hypothermia on admission had a lower mortality rate and improved outcome as compared to hyperthermic patients.[150] However, prospective study of the efficacy of hypothermic interventions in reducing brain damage after stroke remains to be done.

Anaerobic Metabolism and Tissue Acidosis

As a form of incomplete CBF reduction, focal ischemia is unique in that hypoperfused tissues beyond the limits of maximum oxygen extraction continue to receive a modicum of glucose-bearing flow. Under mild to moderately ischemic conditions, neural tissues appear to accelerate glycolysis, and cellular elements are exposed to its byproducts.[17,19,20] Hyperglycemia can exacerbate ischemic brain damage: "Pretreatment" of animals with glucose in models of both global and focal ischemic injury leads to worsened histologic, electrophysiologic, and behavioral outcome.[151,152] There is some evidence that intraischemic—but probably not postischemic—hyperglycemia may be similarly deleterious.[153] Although rigorous proof is lacking, it is widely accepted that tissue lactic acidosis is the major factor underlying these observations. Lactate and hydrogen ion concentrations measured in the ischemic brain are proportionately related to brain glucose and glycogen stores.[154] In 1983, Plum and colleagues theorized that acidosis of glia was the key factor distinguishing selective neuronal necrosis—isolated "dropping out" of vulnerable populations of neurons as classically seen after brief, severe global ischemia—from tissue infarction.[155] The still emerging picture of tissue acidosis in brain infarction is considerably more complicated, however, than a matter of selective glial acidosis under ischemic conditions.[156] It is debated whether acidosis per se or some other aspect of glycolysis and lactate production are responsible for the worsened outcomes that can be observed in hyperglycemic ischemia. For example, in addition to the direct denaturing effects of low pH on enzyme function and structural proteins, lactate causes cellular swelling. In particular, glia take up large quantities of newly formed osmoles that accumulate in the brain ECF space and increase in volume. Although this early "cytotoxic" edema may be an epiphenomenon of a desirable compensation (removing lactate from the ECF), encroachment of engorged glial end-feet along their associated capillary walls could impede CBF at the microvascular level.[116] Furthermore, depletion of tissue bicarbonate levels in the setting of lactic acidosis may facilitate iron-catalyzed FR reactions, which, in turn, may increase secondary tissue injury[156–158] (see Free Radicals and Nitric Oxide).

In contrast to the wealth of evidence suggesting that severe tissue acidosis and lactate accumulation increase the likelihood of tissue infarction, a growing body of in vitro data supports the possibility that low pH has a protective effect on cultured neurons exposed to excitotoxins[99]; pH reduction to less than 6.8 in vitro (compatible with pathophysiologic conditions in vivo) virtually abolishes Ca^{2+} entry via the NMDA receptor.[159] These observations are not necessarily contradictory. Although exaggerated lactic acid production may contribute to the gross destruction of glia and endothelial cells in areas of dense ischemia, it may offset events leading to selective neuronal necrosis in less severely ischemic brain regions. The complexity of the relationships between plasma glucose concentration, brain energy metabolism, and tissue acidosis under ischemic conditions precludes universal recommendations, although there is a growing consensus that euglycemia should be pursued as a goal of acute stroke management.

Kinases

Sustained elevation in intracellular Ca^{2+} initiates "cytotoxic cascades" that involve activation of catalytic enzymes such as protein kinases, proteases, phospholipases, endonucleases, and others. The activity of kinases, a large family of signaling enzymes involved in cell proliferation, differentiation, and death, is altered after both focal and global ischemia. They participate in the major signaling pathways that are important for cell growth and survival. The protein tyrosine and serine/threonine kinases, such as protein kinase A, the Ca^{2+}/phospholipid-dependent kinase C (PKC) and the Ca^{2+}/calmodulin-dependent kinase II, are activated rapidly after ischemia and may contribute to the development of ischemic neuronal damage. Conflicting results suggesting both neuroprotective and deleterious roles for PKC have been obtained using the PKC inhibitor staurosporine.[160,161] However, one study using mutant mice knocked out for the γ isoforms of PKC showed that γPKC has a neuroprotective role in focal cerebral ischemia.[162] Other kinases that have also been reported to be modulated by cerebral ischemia include cyclin-dependent protein kinase 5, c-Jun NH2-terminal kinase, stress-activated protein kinase (SAPK), SAPK/extracellularly regulated kinase (ERK) kinase, and the mitogen-activated protein kinase (Figure 2-6).

Prote

One of the key events after increased [Ca^{2+}] is the activation of proteolytic enzymes, including the two families of cysteine proteases called *calpains* and *caspases*. Calpains play an important role in the proteolytic degradation of cellular proteins, a

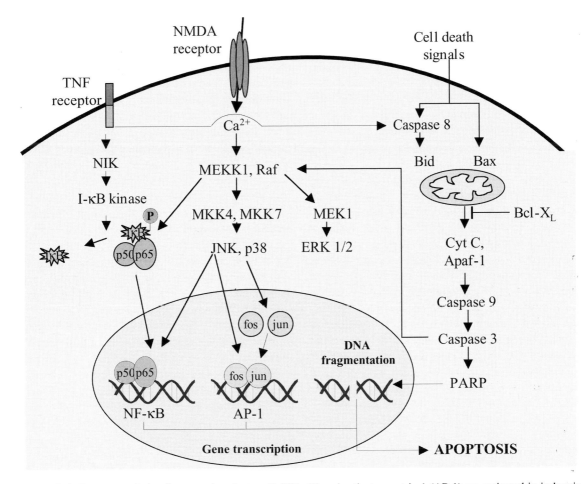

Figure 2-6. Gene transcription factor nuclear factor-κB (NF-κB) and activator protein-1 (AP-1) are activated in ischemic injury. AP-1 is an immediate early gene. NF-κB and AP-1 affect the expression of a number of downstream genes. Mitochondrial dysfunction causes cytochrome c (Cyt C) to be released from the intermembrane space. Cyt C and apoptosis protease-activating factor 1 (Apaf-1) in cytoplasm initiate the caspase cascade and finally induce DNA fragmentation and poly-ADP ribose polymerase (PARP) cleavage. Bcl-2 family, including Bid, Bax, and Bcl-X$_L$, involve the mechanism for stability of mitochondrial outer membrane, which regulates release of Cyt C from mitochondria. (TNF = tumor necrosis factor; NMDA = N-methyl-D-aspartate; NIK = NF-κB–inducing kinase; I-κB = inhibitory protein of NF-κB; P = phosphorylation; MEKK = MAP-ERK kinase kinase kinase; MKK = MAP kinase kinase.)

feature of neurodegeneration. Calpain is ubiquitously present in the proenzyme heterodimer (m- and μ-calpain) form in resting brain cells and is activated by $[Ca^{2+}]_i$ and autolytic processing.[163] Calpain activity is also regulated by the endogenous protein inhibitor calpastatin. The substrates of activated calpain include cytoskeletal proteins (spectrin, microtubule-associated protein 2 [MAP2], actin, tubulin, tau, microtubules, neurofilaments), plasma-membrane associated proteins (epidermal growth factor receptor, PDGF receptor, glutamate receptors), signal transduction (protein kinase C, G-proteins, calcineurin, calpain, calmodulin-dependent proteins), and transcription factors. It leads to cleavage of various cytoskeletal proteins, breakdown of microtubules, and probably mitochondrial dysfunction.[164] Inhibitors of calpain activity, such as leupeptin,[165] AK-275,[166] and MDL-28170,[167] are neuroprotective in both global and focal ischemia models. In addition to the necrotic cell death paradigm, calpain activation may also play a role in apoptotic cell death after ischemia. This is supported by studies showing calpain activation in apoptotic cell death, which is inhibited by calpain inhibitors. The role of another protease family, caspases, is discussed later under Role of Apoptosis.

Lipid Catabolism and the Arachidonic Acid Cascade

High concentrations of complex, lipid-rich compounds in cellular membranes underscore another of the brain's particular vulnerabilities. With a decrease in energy charge, the usual balance between anabolic and degradative processes in cell membranes is overturned, leading to a number of specific derangements. The critical link is the accumulation of diglycerides in tissues subsequent to the shutdown of the ATP-dependent glycerophospholipid synthetic pathways and the acceleration of membrane lipid catabolism via Ca^{2+}-dependent phospholipase A_2 and C as the intracellular Ca^{2+} concentration rises.[168] Diglycerides are hydrolyzed by several Ca^{2+}-dependent lipolytic enzymes, resulting in a 10- to 20-fold increase in tissue free fatty acid (FFA) concentrations in densely ischemic tissues.[169] Under catabolic conditions, not only are normal phospholipid structures degraded, but accumulated FFAs also tend to further disrupt cell membranes, affecting permeability to various ions.[170,171] Furthermore, FFAs and their metabolites contribute to regional declines in pH and increasing tissue osmolality.[55]

Arachidonic acid (AA) is the preeminent FFA released because of lipolysis. This polyunsaturated fatty acid may contribute to the evolution of ischemic brain damage in several distinct ways. In the presence of tissue reperfusion, AA metabolism results in the production of an important class of compounds: eicosanoids, which act as mediators of inflammation. Eicosanoids are produced through the cyclooxygenase and the oxygen-sensitive lipoxygenase pathways. These molecules exert complex effects on vascular reactivity, platelet aggregation, leukocyte adhesion, and blood-brain barrier permeability.[171] Cyclooxygenase isozymes (COX-1 and COX-2) are constitutively expressed in the brain, with neuronal expression of COX-2 also being rapidly inducible after cerebral ischemia.[172] Transient COX-2 expression occurs

after ischemic insult, most prominently in cortical neurons that are at high risk of dying after focal brain ischemia[173] and in the vulnerable hippocampal neurons in global ischemia models.[174] COX-2 activation leads to increased prostaglandin synthesis and generation of oxygen FRs.[175] After ischemia, the prostaglandin levels in the brain increase rapidly from their low basal levels.[175] One study has demonstrated that induced COX-2 directly contributes to the pathogenesis of NMDA receptor–mediated neurotoxicity in mixed cortical cell culture.[176] The activation of COX-2 is most likely due to the postischemic activation of nuclear factor-κB (NF-κB), cytokines, and inducible nitric oxide synthase (iNOS) expression.[174,177] The lipooxygenase pathway of AA metabolism leads to the production of leukotrienes. Leukotriene production has been demonstrated in the brain[175] and increases after ischemia-reperfusion,[170,178,179] inducing broad changes in the permeability of microvascular endothelium and facilitating edema formation.[171]

Reactive oxygen species or FRs, in particular the superoxide anion, are produced as byproducts of arachidonate metabolism at several enzymatic loci.[169] It is of particular relevance that in the setting of rapid AA metabolism and FR formation (which occurs during reperfusion/reoxygenation), the usual balance between the production of prostacyclin (vasodilating, platelet antiaggregant) and thromboxane (vasoconstricting, platelet proaggregant) may be overturned in favor of the latter.[171] This biochemical shift may lead to increases in CVR and has been implicated in the decrease of CBF that may occur after reperfusion (see Consequences of Reperfusion). Both AA metabolites and platelet-activating factor, a glycerophosphocholine also produced in large quantities during ischemia-induced breakdown of cellular membranes, can modulate trophic reactions of leukocytes in ischemic tissues. Activated leukocytes release degradative enzymes, generate FRs, and have been implicated in secondary tissue injury.[180]

Despite an accepted role of therapeutic strategies that manipulate AA metabolism in ischemic stroke prevention (e.g., aspirin), evidence supporting this approach in acute stroke is quite limited. Dietary regimens that aim to reduce AA metabolite production during ischemia by incorporating alternative fatty acids into cell membranes are probably of limited effectiveness and benefit.[181] Pharmacologic inhibitors of cyclooxygenase have been reported to improve blood flow in some stroke models,[182] but relationships to outcome have not been established yet. Despite early promise, two randomized clinical trials of the potent vasodilator prostacyclin produced no significant benefit in acute stroke, but the results were tempered by the delayed entry of subjects and the compound's tendency to produce systemic hypotension at the doses used.[183,184] Manipulation of AA metabolite-triggered leukocyte and endothelial cell activations, particularly as it relates to reperfusion injury, remains an area of active research.

Free Radicals and Nitric Oxide

Reactive oxygen species have been implicated in the pathogenesis of ischemic brain damage for many years. However, a more differentiated view of their role has emerged more recently with improved understanding of their sources, targets, and the particular pathophysiologic circumstances in which they may be most relevant.[185] It is increasingly clear that FRs populate the unstable terrain of the ischemic penumbra. FRs also participate in the particular patterns of injury observed in reperfused tissues.[186] A detailed discussion of FR chemistry is beyond the scope of this chapter, but in-depth reviews are available.[158,186]

As described previously, FRs are generated as byproducts of AA metabolism and polymorphonuclear leukocyte invasion and, as a result, may accumulate in tissues in which Ca^{2+} overload is established, lipolysis is advanced, and secondary vascular injury is under way. However, FRs may appear, at least theoretically, in earlier stages of tissue damage through a number of mechanisms. First, reactive oxygen species may accumulate in moderately ischemic tissue when the efficiency of aerobic glycolysis is compromised by the limited availability of molecular oxygen as a final acceptor of electrons within the mitochondria.[186] Second, FR formation may proceed from breakdown of metabolites of ATP via the xanthine oxidase pathway. This process is greatly facilitated by the Ca^{2+}-dependent activation of proteolytic enzymes, which in turn catalyze the conversion of xanthine dehydrogenase to xanthine oxidase. The break-

down of adenine nucleotides via xanthine oxidase yields superoxide and hydrogen peroxide as byproducts, and the quantity of these FRs are greatest in tissues with some capacity for ATP regeneration and turnover.[187]

Brain ischemia triggers the activation of various isoforms of NO synthase (NOS). These include the constitutively expressed neuronal (nNOS) and endothelial (eNOS) and the iNOS isoform. Excessive formation of NO may be cytotoxic by directly inhibiting enzymes that catalyze vital cellular functions involved in energy metabolism and DNA synthesis. The deleterious effects of NO are thought to be related to its well-known affinity for iron and thiol groups.[188,189] NO may also contribute to FR generation by forming peroxynitrite (ONOO-) ions, which are capable of generating the cytotoxic hydroxyl radical.[116] Development of mutant knockout mice with deletions of the gene encoding nNOS, eNOS, and iNOS, provided an opportunity to dissect the complex role of NO in cerebral ischemia. The data from these studies suggest that both nNOS- and iNOS-induced NO overproduction may be neurotoxic, whereas eNOS may protect brain tissue by improving blood flow and other hemodynamic factors.[115,116,190–192] NO may be a double-edged sword. Cytoprotective actions of NO have also been well documented. The salutary roles of NO could be related to its interaction with glutathione to form S-nitrosoglutathione, a highly potent antioxidant that may protect neurons against oxidative stress.[193] S-nitrosoglutathione is most likely generated in the endothelial and astroglial cells during oxidative stress and is transferred to neurons, where it neutralizes FRs via its c-guanosine monophosphate-independent nitrosylation actions.[194]

Until recently, FR injury was thought to involve vicious cycles of lipid catabolism and peroxidation occurring in neuronal membranes. Although membrane pathology is no doubt important, it is increasingly clear that FRs generated under ischemic conditions attack a wide variety of macromolecules, including enzymes and nucleic acids,[117,185] and are involved in the destruction of multiple cell types. FR formation may be a final common pathway of numerous immunocytologic processes that seem to mediate many aspects of ischemic microvascular damage. FRs may destroy the naturally occurring antioxidant activities present in neural tissues.[96,195,196] Significantly,

FR-mediated formation of DNA strand breaks may obligate ATP-consuming enzymatic repair activities, further depleting scarce energy reserves in partially ischemic tissues.[117,197]

An important insight linking the unique metabolic microenvironment of focal ischemia to FR injury is the observation that both the reduction of ferric to ferrous iron under acidic conditions and the release of iron from organic stores—delocalization—greatly enhance FR production.[185] Delocalized iron catalyzes the Haber-Weiss reaction, which in turn converts short-lived and weakly reactive superoxide anions and hydrogen peroxide to highly toxic hydroxyl radicals. The accumulation of lactate, hydrogen ions, and free iron under conditions of ischemia greatly facilitates FR injury and may promote the severe vasogenic edema that can attend reperfusion.[93,186] The best evidence to date of the relevance of FRs to focal ischemic injury rests with the demonstration that agents that neutralize[198] or prevent the formation[199] of FRs in vivo may substantially reduce the extent of infarction or postinfarct edema, at least when given before or shortly after an ischemic insult. Extensive studies in transgenic mice with overexpression or deletion of genes encoding FR scavenger enzymes also support the pivotal role of FRs in ischemic brain injury.[186]

Protein Metabolism and Gene Activation

The study of protein metabolism after pathologic stimuli, such as ischemia, is highly complex. However, several fundamental observations have been made. First, widespread depression of protein synthesis often precedes the failure of aerobic energy production resulting from focal reduction in CBF.[25,200] It is of considerable interest that amino acid incorporation can be completely arrested at degrees of CBF reduction well above the flow values required to maintain normal brain ATP concentrations and cell membrane polarity.[25] Faltering peptide chain initiation in mildly ischemic tissues may reflect subtle derangements in calcium-dependent regulatory enzymes as toxic substances (e.g., glutamate) or electrophysiologic disturbances (e.g., electrical spreading depression) that promote cellular calcium entry invade surrounding tissues from densely ischemic regions.[200] Despite the generalized reduction in protein synthesis, ischemia leads to the synthesis of potentially protective and damaging proteins via postischemic alteration of gene expression. It is remarkable that these unique families of "immediate-early genes" may be expressed in abundance, most notably by cells at the margins of dense ischemia or in functionally connected regions that do not themselves experience ischemia.[201] Mechanisms of ischemia-mediated gene activation are complex and involve several signaling processes and activation of transcription factors. Ca^{2+}, FRs, neurotrophins, platelet-activating factor (PAF), as well as neurotransmitters, are all capable of activating genes via the mitogen-activated protein kinase pathway or activation of transcription factors NF-κB and activator protein-1 (AP-1).[31,202] Genes expressed after ischemia have been conceived to be an adaptive response but can have a protective or a deleterious role. Their protective effects include promoting functional reorganization that enhances tolerance to mild ongoing ischemia, rebuilding damaged structures, or clearing away debris that may impair regrowth.[203] A specific example of a potentially adaptive response is the upregulation of expression of various neurotrophic factors.[204] Other genes, such as *c-fos*, *c-jun*, *junB*, *krox-20*, and *zif-268*, are expressed rapidly after ischemia.[201,202] Various heat shock proteins (hsp70, 72, 90) are increasingly expressed after ischemia. Overexpression of hsp70 reduces the extent of damage in hippocampal neurons after ischemia.[205] Anti-apoptotic genes, such as *bcl-2* and *bcl-xL*, have been shown to be expressed in the rat brain after global ischemia.[206] Pro-apoptotic genes of the *bcl*-family, including *bax* and *bcl-xS*, are also upregulated after cerebral ischemia.[207] The extent of neuronal apoptosis may be an interplay of anti-apoptotic and pro-apoptotic genes of the *bcl* family. Other genes that probably enhance damage and are increased after ischemia include COX-2, iNOS, nNOS, IL-1, and TNF-α. The roles of these genes and their products in ischemic brain injury are described in the sections Postischemic Inflammatory Reaction and Lipid Catabolism and the Arachidonic Acid Cascade.

Postischemic Inflammatory Reaction

Brain damage after cerebral ischemia-reperfusion may be accentuated by postischemic events, which constitute the secondary injury processes. Of the many pathophysiologic events that may contribute to secondary injury, cell-mediated processes in the postischemic inflammation have been extensively studied. Key features of inflammation have been characterized in the ischemic brain. These include accumulation of inflammatory mediators, including cytokines, prostaglandins, and leukotrienes; vascular injury entailing blood-brain barrier breakdown; edema formation; activation of microglia; and infiltration of inflammatory cells, including neutrophils and macrophage.[208]

Cerebral ischemia induces various pro-inflammatory genes by inducing the synthesis of transcription factors, such as NF-κB,[208] AP-1,[209,210] hypoxia inducible factor-1,[211] and interferon regulatory factor-1.[212] These transcription factors induce the production of mediators of inflammation, including IL-1β and TNF-α. IL-1β and TNF-α are expressed very early in cerebral ischemia and may contribute to initiating and perpetuating tissue inflammation. IL-1β messenger RNA levels are dramatically increased after ischemia,[177] starting at 3–6 hours, peaking at 12 hours, and declining at 5 days after ischemia.[213] It is likely that processing of IL-1β by IL-1β converting enzyme, one of the caspases involved in apoptosis, contributes to ischemic neuronal death. Transgenic mice that overexpress an IL-1β converting enzyme inhibitor, resulting in a deficiency in the production of mature IL-1β, had smaller infarctions and better neurologic outcomes after permanent middle cerebral artery occlusion.[214] Along with IL-1β, the level of IL-1 receptor antagonist—an inhibitor of IL-1 activity—also increases at approximately the same time. It is therefore the balance between the levels of IL-1β and IL-1 receptor antagonist expressed after ischemia that may be more critical for the degree of tissue injury. Increased TNF-α expression has been demonstrated after cerebral ischemia, starting at 1 hour, peaking at 12 hours, and declining at 5 days.[208] TNF-α acts as a local regulator of inflammatory reaction and stimulates the expression of adhesion molecules, chemokines, and pro-inflammatory transcription factor NF-κB. However, the roles of TNF-α in ischemic injury are complex, and evidence suggesting both deleterious as well as beneficial roles has been shown in different animal models.[208]

An important aspect of the postischemic inflammatory reaction, especially after reperfusion is leukocyte infiltration. The CD18 antigen on the surface of activated leukocytes binds to intercellular cell adhesion molecule-1 receptors on endothelial cells within the first few hours after ischemic injury. This results in leukocyte interaction with vascular endothelium, causing blood-brain barrier breakdown, plugging of capillaries, resulting in a "no-reflow" phenomenon, and release of deleterious factors, including proteases and oxygen FRs. These secondary effects of activated leukocytes can lead to additional injury beyond that caused by ischemia. Neutrophils are the primary effector leukocytes at the site of ischemia, entering 30 minutes after arterial occlusion and peaking at 24–48 hours, followed by other cells such as macrophages.[215] Thus, even if reperfusion occurs, the obstruction of the microvasculature and secondary tissue destruction may continue. Therefore, the postinflammatory reaction, especially neutrophil infiltration, may accentuate ischemic brain injury. Neuroprotective strategies directed at preventing neutrophil infiltration have been extensively reported. However, some animal studies from Washington University in St. Louis and elsewhere have suggested that neutrophils are not always detrimental in the settings of acute cerebral ischemia.[148,216] These findings cast doubt on the exclusively detrimental role of leukocytes in ischemic brain injury.

Some studies have implicated the activation of the complement system in the inflammatory mechanisms that lead to neuronal death after ischemia. Complement is a host defense mechanism, made up of plasma proteins that identify pathogens and injured cells, recruit inflammatory cells, and induce cell lysis. Huang and colleagues have shown that a hybrid molecule that simultaneously inhibits both complement activation and selectin-mediated endothelial-platelet-leukocyte interactions inhibited neutrophil and platelet accumulation, and reduced cerebral infarct volumes.[217]

Role of Apoptosis

Judging from the effects on protein synthesis, it would seem paradoxical that pharmacologic interference with protein synthesis has been advocated as a potential therapy for acute stroke. Administration of cycloheximide, a general protein synthesis inhibitor, during or shortly after a focal ischemic insult may reduce infarct volume or magnitude of neuronal depopulation with respect to controls.[218] It has been postulated that these findings support a role for specific products of postischemic gene expression in the pathogenesis of ischemic injury.[25,219] This scenario also points to the involvement of apoptosis in the cell death mechanisms after ischemia. Although ischemic neuronal death traditionally has been considered to be a necrotic process, it may involve both necrosis and apoptosis.[220,221] Animal models of ischemia have provided morphologic, biochemical, and pharmacologic evidence suggesting that apoptosis contributes to ischemic neuronal death.[104,220–226] Apoptosis after cerebral ischemia-reperfusion may be triggered by various factors, including growth factor deprivation, oxidative stress, impaired energy metabolism, kinase activation, and increased cytokine production. Mitochondria are considered to be the center of apoptosis[227] and are discussed in the following section. Studies in animal models suggest that inhibition of mitochondrial function and energy metabolism not only worsens excitotoxic injury but also triggers apoptotic neuronal cell death. Using animal models, the major steps involved in the apoptotic cascade, such as activation of caspases 8, 9, and 3, loss of mitochondrial barrier function, and release of cytochrome c, have been shown to contribute to cell death after ischemia.[228–230] Inhibitors of macromolecular synthesis and caspase activity have been noted to reduce infarct volume and improve neurologic outcome.[111,224–226] Further proof for an apoptotic process comes from studies showing that overexpression of *bcl-2*, an anti-apoptotic gene, in transgenic mice protects against neuronal death after cerebral ischemia.[231]

Hence, excitotoxicity and other molecular interactions resulting in disturbances of cellular calcium homeostasis after ischemia may trigger not only passive necrosis but also apoptosis. Apoptosis may contribute substantially to the overall magnitude of tissue attrition after ischemia. At the time of this writing, the specific mechanisms of apoptosis in the ischemic brain remain poorly defined, and a number of criticisms questioning its relevance to the pathophysiology of ischemia have been raised.[232,233] However, apoptosis after ischemia is an interesting concept, particularly as it relates to the phenomenon of delayed cell death: the curious dropping out of selectively vulnerable neurons subsequent to even brief ischemic insults (see Figure 2-6).

Role of Mitochondria

Mitochondria are assuming an increasingly important role in both apoptotic and necrotic cell death. The physiologic function of mitochondria is to generate ATP via oxidative phosphorylation. Mitochondria maintain a membrane potential by the movement of protons and products of mitochondrial respiration out of the mitochondrial matrix. A large amount of Ca^{2+} is stored in the mitochondria, as the negative membrane potential provides the driving force for the uptake of Ca^{2+} into the mitochondria and efflux occurs via a $2Na^+/Ca^{2+}$ exchanger. Various toxic cascades that are activated in ischemia converge on the mitochondria. Increase in intracellular Ca^{2+} level, production of FRs, and activation of upstream caspases and the Bcl-2 family genes all can induce disturbance in the mitochondrial homeostasis. The initial effect of ischemia is the inhibition of mitochondrial oxidative phosphorylation, and significant uncoupling results in lowered ATP levels, enhanced anaerobic metabolism, and production of lactate and H^+ from pyruvate. Mitochondria act as the major buffering system for the high intracellular Ca^{2+} levels in the initial stages of ischemia, but the loss of oxidative metabolism and the energy production disturbs the membrane potential required to drive Ca^{2+} uptake into the mitochondria. These changes also lead to increased mitochondrial FR production. Furthermore, the change in the membrane permeability transition and the opening of the membrane transition pore could result in the release of intramitochondrial molecules and ions that activate downstream cell death pathways. It is thought that probably two independent pathways are orchestrated in the mitochondria. One involves a change in the membrane permeability transition and the subsequent release of a 50 kDa protein apoptosis-inducing factor from the intermembrane space of mitochondria.[234] The other pathway involves the release of cytochrome c, an extrinsic protein found on the outer surface of the inner mitochondrial membrane, into the cytosol.[235,236] Some studies have revealed that this redistribution of cytochrome c from the intermembrane space could be a critical step in the apoptotic cell death pathway. A cytosolic protein fraction known as *apoptotic protease activating factor 1* has been obtained from the cytosol of apoptotic cells[234] and is also released from the intermembrane mitochondrial space. Apoptotic protease activating factor 1 in the presence of cytochrome c and dATP binds to the N-terminus of pro-caspase 9. The formation of this complex in vitro results in activation of caspase 9, which in turn activates caspase 3.[237] Caspase 3 is the common endpoint of all known apoptotic pathways, being responsible either wholly or partially for the proteolytic cleavage of many key proteins, which are cleaved in many different systems during apoptosis (see Figure 2-6).

The frontier defining the response of the neural genome to ischemia is just being opened. Absent so far from the bewildering array of neurogenetic data is an integrating theory that places the changes in gene expression into the context of the functional outcome of the whole organism after stroke. It is likely that the relative weight of destructive and restorative processes depends on the specific conditions producing or complicating the ischemic insult.[219] It is plausible that in defined circumstances, apoptosis may be a major component of the postischemic recovery response rather than its antithesis. Connections that retard or no longer subserve integrated function may be eliminated by way of apoptotic deletion of neurons in the way that the embryonic CNS systematically culls irrelevant or inefficient networks.

Consequences of Reperfusion

Outcome from focal ischemic injury can be determined not only by the depth and duration of the initial insult[238] but also by factors attending the restoration of blood flow. It has been estimated that spontaneous reperfusion occurs in at least one-third of thromboembolic strokes within 48 hours of the ictus, and may increase to half or more at 1 week.[239] Furthermore, advances in clinical pharmacology and interventional techniques have again raised the possibility of safe restoration of CBF in selected cases of acute stroke.[240] It is therefore relevant that in many animal models of both global and focal brain ischemia, return of inflow pressure can be associated with either frank failure of reperfusion ("no-reflow")[241,242] or a delayed period of hypoperfusion, the latter typically following a period of reactive hyperemia.[12,96,243] These patterns of no-reflow, reactive hyperemia, and delayed postischemic hypoperfusion (DPIH) are similar to phenomena observed in tissues outside the CNS. However, incomplete understanding of the mechanisms, timing, and magnitude of these CBF disturbances precludes any firm conclusions about their role in the development of primary focal ischemic brain injury.

No-Reflow and Delayed
Postischemic Hypoperfusion

Originally observed after global brain ischemia,[241] no-reflow has been reported in a number of focal ischemia models in small animals and primates.[244] No-reflow has been attributed to mechanical edema factors, intravascular activation of coagulation cascades, FR injury of endothelium, and interactions—adhesions—between endothelial cells and leukocytes. Brain endothelium may respond to a variety of inflammatory mediators produced during an ischemic episode (e.g., ILs, TNFs, platelet-activating factor) by changes in the expression of intercellular adhesion molecules that, in turn, modulate the infiltration and enzymatic activity of leukocytes in the microvasculature.[245] Leukocyte-mediated processes may compromise luminal patency and the functions of the blood-brain barrier. Novel therapeutic strategies, such as postischemic delivery of monoclonal antibodies against endothelial adhesion molecules, have been reported to reduce neurologic deficits after reversible spinal cord ischemia in a small-animal model.[246]

However, processes causing no-reflow seem to be most pronounced in tissues undergoing severe ischemia of long duration, possibly after the appearance of irreversible neuronal damage.[93] In general, there is limited evidence that no-reflow contributes significantly to primary focal ischemic brain injury.[12] An exception may be the circumstance of frank systemic hypotension complicating brain ischemia that may result in early and severe no-reflow.

The role of DPIH in focal ischemic injury is likewise ill-defined. The clinically relevant concern is that this phenomenon represents a treatable secondary increase in CVR-impairing residual blood flow, effectively extending the period of tissue ischemia and adversely affecting outcome. DPIH is undoubtedly multifactorial and, like no-reflow, has been reported to reflect phenomena as diverse as microcirculatory compression by swollen perivascular glial cells, formation of endothelial microvilli and "blebs," globally increased ICP from ischemic edema, disseminated intravascular coagulation, increased CVR from AA metabolites, and luminal obstruction by polymorphonuclear leukocytes.[96]

An alternative interpretation of depressed CBF after ischemia with reperfusion is appropriate coupling of flow to the decreased energy needs of irreversibly damaged or deafferented tissues. Distinguishing these equally plausible possibilities is a daunting task experimentally. To date, attempts at demonstrating a causal relationship between postischemic decreases in CBF and decreases in tissue metabolism that can be prevented by improvement in flow have generally produced negative results.[78] However, there are data suggesting that episodic mismatch between local metabolism and available flow may be the major determinant of the impact of DPIH in particular brain regions.[247] An aspect of the selective vulnerability of certain neuronal populations may lie in the development of episodic postischemic hypermetabolism.[248] This hypermetabolic response is likely multifactorial, but an intriguing candidate mechanism is the aforementioned wave of spreading depression that can expand from a region of severe focal ischemia, promote cellular Ca^{2+} loading, and potentially incite metabolic mismatch in hypoperfused adjacent brain regions.[49,52] Experimental therapeutic efforts designed to offset DPIH have produced results that are promising but controversial.[12,96] Convincing evidence of improved functional outcome from focal ischemia subsequent to "treated" DPIH remains unavailable.

Reperfusion Hyperemia

Ischemic tissues do not autoregulate blood flow normally and generate an array of substances capable of inducing vasodilatation (e.g., K^+, hydrogen ions, CO_2, adenosine, prostacyclin). Consequently, large increases in CBF, often several times normal levels and sustained over hours to days, frequently follow reperfusion.[96,249] Blood flow to reperfused brain often greatly exceeds the substrate demands of the tissue—so-called luxury perfusion.[14] This gross uncoupling of flow from metabolism limits the prognostic value of isolated CBF data obtained in the setting of acute stroke if partial or complete reperfusion has occurred (i.e., improved flow is not synonymous with improved tissue metabolism or function).[7,82] Reperfusion hyperemia itself can be viewed as a double-edged sword. Increased flow may bring substrate to marginal tissues and remove waste metabolites accumulated during ischemia. On the other hand, with reperfusion there is delivery of large quantities of oxygen to a biochemical environment primed to produce a "burst" of potentially damaging AA metabolites and FRs.[57,250] AA metabolites and FRs seem to have their major impact on the brain microvasculature. They can increase endothelial leukocyte adhesion and permeability, and promote vasogenic edema.[251] Restoration of vascular hydrostatic pressures to normal or supranormal levels may greatly facilitate brain edema as well.[252] Reperfusion injury may present a formidable challenge to acute stroke therapies that seek to restore CBF through thrombolysis, vascular reconstruction, or pharmacologic elevation of CPP. The clinical significance of the various reperfusion-related factors that modulate edema formation is potentially great: Vasogenic edema accounts for the majority of the deaths that occur shortly after acute ischemic stroke[253] (Figure 2-7).

Conclusion

Traditional concepts concerning blood flow and metabolism are an essential starting point for understanding the pathophysiology of ischemic injury. Stroke is foremost a disturbance of brain perfusion. Compensatory mechanisms involving changes in CVR and the extraction of circulating oxygen may maintain adequate rates of aerobic metabolism in the setting of decreased cerebral perfusion. Advances in the understanding of angio-

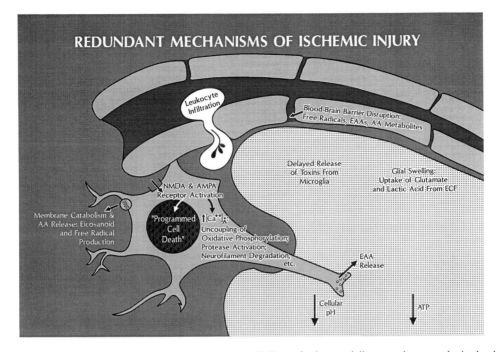

Figure 2-7. Redundant mechanisms of ischemic brain injury. Failure of substrate delivery to tissue results in the decline of aerobic metabolism and consequent decreases in tissue pH and adenosine triphosphate (ATP) levels. Excitatory amino acids (EAAs), such as glutamate, activate a number of specific neuronal (and possibly endothelial) receptors, such as those specifically targeted by N-methyl-D-aspartate (NMDA) and alpha-amino-3-hydroxy-5-methyl-4-isoxazole propionic acid (AMPA). Dissipation of normal transmembrane ionic gradients leads to the accumulation of calcium (Ca^{2+}) in cells with a number of pathologic consequences, including uncoupling of oxidative phosphorylation and unordered activation of numerous cellular enzyme systems. Ca^{2+}-activated phospholipase action results in the breakdown of cellular membranes with release of arachidonic acid (AA) metabolites and free radicals. Swelling of glia, leukocyte infiltration of the microvasculature, and breakdown of the blood-brain barrier may also contribute to the demise of neurons. Additionally, there may be specific derangements of genomic expression, leading to "programmed cell death." (ECF = extracellular fluid.)

genesis suggest that neovascularization may also be an important compensatory mechanism. Below critical levels of perfusion pressure, blood flow decreases, aerobic energy production fails, and a cascade of ionic and biochemical disturbances lead first to the loss of brain electrical activity and then cellular viability. Collateral blood flow variability largely accounts for the heterogeneous extent of infarction after otherwise similar disturbances of cerebral perfusion.

However, there is emerging awareness that classic hemodynamic and metabolic considerations are inadequate to fully explain many of the phenomena that occur during or after an ischemic insult. Traditionally, it has been assumed that the time-dependent deterioration of the ischemic penumbra reflects further decreases in CBF due to a variety of mechanical factors.

Experimental evidence suggests, however, that CBF can be stable for many hours in the steadily hypoperfused brain.[42,77,98] Furthermore, it has been difficult to rigorously define deterioration of the ischemic penumbra in terms of a predictable alteration of CBF, $CMRO_2$, or oxygen extraction in the clinical setting.[82] The critical determinant of deterioration of the penumbra, then, may not be the restriction of marginal blood flow but the proximity of vulnerable tissues to specific toxic threats. Densely ischemic tissue can be seen as a source of mediators of cellular injury that diffuse into the surrounding brain. For example, massive K^+ and glutamate release may trigger harmful waves of spreading depression that induce complex changes in Ca^{2+} homeostasis in surrounding tissues.[49,52] Additionally, regions of severe ischemia with damaged blood-brain barriers can serve as a source of edema fluid that, moving down hydrostatic gradients, exposes surrounding tissues to toxic materials from the plasma.[89] Recognizing the importance of factors independent of blood flow reduction to infarct evolution does not imply that the depth of ischemia in penumbral regions has no bearing on tissue outcome. The impact of excitotoxins and spreading depression in particular may be determined in large part by the tissue's capacity to mitigate disturbances of ion homeostasis, which directly reflects the efficiency of regional substrate delivery and energy-dependent regulatory mechanisms.[49] Therapies aimed at preventing deterioration of the ischemic penumbra, then, will probably need to encompass combined strategies that acutely improve CBF while reducing the toxicity of the microenvironment.

Currently, tissue plasminogen activator (t-PA) is the only U.S. Food and Drug Administration–approved therapeutic agent for the treatment of patients with acute ischemic stroke within a 3-hour window. t-PA, a thrombolytic agent, has been demonstrated to reduce ischemic brain injury in animal stroke models as early as 1985.[254] Based on the promising animal data, t-PA was tested in two phase III clinical trials sponsored by the National Institute of Neurological Disorders and Stroke and found to be efficacious in reducing functional impairment in selected populations of patients with ischemic stroke.[255,256] Intra-arterial thrombolysis with prourokinase has also been found to be of clinical benefit with a wider therapeutic window.[257] Ancrod, which lowers plasma fibrinogen levels and is presumed to improved perfusion, has also been shown to improve functional outcomes.[258] Reperfusion of the ischemic brain is a complex subject of increasing clinical importance. Future advances in clinical pharmacology and interventional techniques may permit the restoration of blood flow in acute stroke with a longer therapeutic window. A rigorous understanding of the various phenomena that may limit or follow from reperfusion is therefore essential. In conjunction with changes in the biochemical microenvironment, restoration of blood flow may promote edema and other forms of secondary tissue damage. The threat of reperfusion injury presents a formidable challenge to many acute stroke therapies.

References

1. Siesjo BK. Cerebral circulation and metabolism. J Neurosurg 1984;60:883–908.
2. Astrup J, Siesjo B, Symon L. Thresholds in cerebral ischemia: the ischemic penumbra. Stroke 1981;12:723–725.
3. Hossmann K-A, Kleihues R. Reversibility of ischemic brain damage. Arch Neurol 1973;29:375–382.
4. Hossmann K-A, Schmidt-Kastner R, Grosse Ophoff B. Recovery of integrative central nervous function after one hour global cerebrocirculatory arrest in normothermic cat. J Neurol Sci 1987;77:305–320.
5. Paulson OB, Strandgaard S, Edvinsson L. Cerebral autoregulation. Cerebrovasc Brain Metab Rev 1990;2:161–192.
6. Powers WJ, Raichle ME. Positron emission tomography and its application to the study of cerebrovascular disease in man. Stroke 1985;16:361–376.
7. Powers WJ. Cerebral hemodynamics in ischemic cerebrovascular disease. Ann Neurol 1991;29:231–240.
8. Grotta J, Ackerman R, Correia J, et al. Whole blood viscosity parameters and cerebral blood flow. Stroke 1982;13:296–301.
9. Wood JH, Kee DB. Hemorrheology of the cerebral circulation in stroke. Stroke 1985;16:765–772.
10. Powers WJ. Acute hypertension after stroke: the scientific basis for treatment decisions. Neurology 1993;43:461–467.
11. Brown MM, Wade JPH, Marshall J. Fundamental importance of arterial oxygen content in the regulation of cerebral blood flow in man. Brain 1985;108:81–93.
12. Hossmann K-A. Pathophysiology of Cerebral Infarction. In PJ Viken, GW Bruyn, HL Klawans (eds), Handbook of Clinical Neurology. New York: Elsevier, 1988;53:107–154.
13. Powers WJ, Tempel LW, Grubb RL Jr. Influence of cerebral hemodynamics on stroke risk: one year follow-up of 30 medically treated patients. Ann Neurol 1989;25:325–330.
14. Grubb RL Jr, Derdeyn CP, Fritsch SM, et al. Importance of hemodynamic factors in the prognosis of symptomatic carotid occlusion. JAMA 1998;280:1055–1060.
15. Olsen TS, Larsen B, Herning M, et al. Blood flow and vascular reactivity in collaterally perfused brain tissue: evidence of an ischemic penumbra in patients with acute stroke. Stroke 1983;14:332–341.
16. Wise R, Bernardi S, Frackowiak R, et al. Serial observations on the pathophysiology of acute stroke. Brain 1983;106:197–222.
17. Astrup J, Symon L, Branston NM, Lassen NA. Cortical evoked potential and extracellular K^+ and H^+ at critical levels of brain ischemia. Stroke 1977;8:51–57.
18. Harris R, Symon L. Extracellular pH, potassium, and calcium activities in progressive ischemia of rat cortex. J Cereb Blood Flow Metab 1984;4:178–186.
19. Plum F, Pulsinelli W. Cerebral Metabolism and Hypoxic-Ischemic Brain Injury. In A Asbury, G McKhann, A McDonald (eds), Diseases of the Nervous System. Philadelphia: Saunders, 1986;1086–1101.

20. Baron JC, Rougemont D, Soussaline F, et al. Local inter-relationships of cerebral oxygen consumption and glucose utilization in normal subjects and in ischemic stroke patients: a positron tomography study. J Cereb Blood Flow Metab 1984;4:140–149.

21. Naritomi H, Sasaki M, Kanashiro M, et al. Flow thresholds for cerebral energy disturbance and Na pump failure as studied by in vivo 31P and 23Na nuclear magnetic resonance spectroscopy. J Cereb Blood Flow Metab 1988;8:16–23.

22. Martin RL, Lloyd HG, Cowan AI. The early events of oxygen and glucose deprivation: setting the scene for neuronal death? Trends Neurosci 1994;17:251–257.

23. Tombaugh GC, Sapolsky RM. Evolving concepts about the role of acidosis in ischemic neuropathology. J Neurochem 1993;61:793–803.

24. Hansen AJ. Effect of anoxia on ion distribution in the brain. Physiol Rev 1985;65:101–148.

25. Jacewicz M, Kiessling M, Pulsinelli W. Selective gene expression in focal cerebral ischemia. J Cereb Blood Flow Metab 1986;6:263–272.

26. Duffy TE, Nelson SR, Lowry OH. Cerebral carbohydrate metabolism during acute hypoxia and recovery. J Neurochem 1972;19:959–977.

27. Mies G, Paschen W, Hossmann K-A, Klatzo I. Simultaneous measurement of regional blood flow and metabolism during maturation of hippocampal lesions following short-lasting cerebral ischemia in gerbils. J Cereb Blood Flow Metab 1983;3(Suppl 1):S329–S330.

28. Chopp M, Chen H, Ho KL. Transient hyperthermia protects against subsequent forebrain ischemic cell damage in the rat. Neurology 1989;39:1396–1398.

29. Glazier SS, O'Rourke DM, Graham DI, Welsh A. Induction of ischemic tolerance following brief focal ischemia in rat brain. J Cereb Blood Flow Metab 1994;14:545–553.

30. Matsushima K, Hogan MJ, Hakim AM. Cortical spreading depression protects against subsequent focal cerebral ischemia in rats. J Cereb Blood Flow Metab 1996;16:221–226.

31. Lipton P. Ischemic cell death in brain neurons. Physiol Rev 1999;79:1431–1568.

32. Semenza GL. Regulation of mammalian O_2 homeostasis by hypoxia-inducible factor 1. Ann Rev Cell Dev Biol 1999;15:551–578.

33. Iyer NV, Kotch LE, Agani F, et al. Cellular and developmental control of O_2 homeostasis by hypoxia-inducible factor 1 alpha. Genes Dev 1998;12:149–162.

34. Plate KH, Beck H, Danner S, et al. Cell type specific upregulation of vascular endothelial growth factor in an MCA-occlusion model of cerebral infarct. J Neuropathol Exp Neurol 1999;58:654–666.

35. Marti HJ, Bernaudin M, Bellail A, et al. Hypoxia-induced vascular endothelial growth factor expression precedes neovascularization after cerebral ischemia. Am J Pathol 2000;156:965–976.

36. Krupinski J, Issa R, Bujny T, et al. A putative role for platelet-derived growth factor in angiogenesis and neuroprotection after ischemic stroke in humans. Stroke 1997;28:564–573.

37. Speliotes EK, Caday CG, Do T, et al. Increased expression of basic fibroblast growth factor (bFGF) following focal cerebral infarction in the rat. Brain Res Mol Brain Res 1996;39:31–42.

38. Lin TN, Wang CK, Cheung WM, Hsu CY. Induction of angiopoietin and Tie receptor mRNA expression after cerebral ischemia-reperfusion. J Cereb Blood Flow Metab 2000;20:387–395.

39. Sharbrough FW, Messick JM, Sundt TM Jr. Correlation of continuous electroencephalograms with cerebral blood flow measurements during carotid endarterectomy. Stroke 1973;4:674–683.

40. Trojaborg W, Boysen G. Relation between EEG, regional cerebral blood flow and internal carotid artery pressure during carotid endarterectomy. Electroencephalogr Clin Neurophysiol 1973;34:61–69.

41. Heiss W-D, Hayakawa T, Waltz AG. Cortical neuronal fuction during ischemia: effects of occlusion of one middle cerebral artery on single-unit activity in cats. Arch Neurol 1976;33:813–820.

42. Jones TH, Morawetz RB, Crowell RM, et al. Thresholds of focal cerebral ischemia in awake monkeys. J Neurosurg 1981;54:773–782.

43. Gibson G, Pulsinelli W, Blass J, Duffy T. Brain dysfunction in mild to moderate hypoxia. Am J Med 1981;70:1247–1254.

44. Shimada N, Graf R, Rosner G, et al. Ischemic flow threshold for extracellular glutamate increase in cat cortex. J Cereb Blood Flow Metab 1989;9:603–606.

45. Bell BA, Symon L, Branston NM. CBF and time thresholds for the formation of ischemic cerebral edema, and effect of reperfusion in baboons. J Neurosurg 1985;62:31–41.

46. Staub F, Baethmann A, Peters J, Kempski O. Effects of lactic acidosis on volume and viability of glial cells. Acta Neurochir 1990;(Suppl 51):3–6.

47. Chan PH, Chu L. Mechanisms underlying glutamate-induced swelling of astrocytes. Acta Neurochir 1990;(Suppl 51):7–10.

48. Choi DW. Calcium-mediated neurotoxicity: relationship to specific channel types and role in ischemic damage. Trends Neurosci 1988;11:465–469.

49. Siesjo BK, Bengtsson F. Calcium fluxes, calcium antagonists, and calcium-related pathology in brain ischemia, hypoglycemia, and spreading depression: a unifying hypothesis. J Cereb Blood Flow Metab 1989;9:127–140.

50. Miller RJ. Multiple calcium channels and neuronal function. Science 1987;235:46–52.

51. Betz AL, Ianotti F, Hoff JT. Brain edema: a classification based on blood-brain barrier integrity. Cerebrovasc Brain Metab Rev 1989;1:133–154.

52. Back T, Kohno K, Hossmann K-A. Cortical negative DC deflections following middle cerebral artery occlusion and KCL-induced spreading depression: effect on blood flow, tissue oxygenation, and electroencephalogram. J Cereb Blood Flow Metab 1994;14:12–19.

53. Betz AL, Keep RF, Beer ME, Ren X. Blood-brain barrier permeability and brain concentration of sodium, potassium, and chloride during focal ischemia. J Cereb Blood Flow Metab 1994;14:29–37.

54. Madden KP. Effect of gamma-aminobutyric acid modulation on neuronal ischemia in rabbits. Stroke 1994;11:2271–2275.

55. Raichle ME. The pathophysiology of brain ischemia. Ann Neurol 1983;13:2–10.

56. Siesjo BK. Historical overview: calcium, ischemia, and death of brain cells. Ann N Y Acad Sci 1988;522:638–661.

57. Farber JL, Chien KR, Mittnacht S Jr. The pathogenesis of irreversible cell injury in ischemia. Am J Pathol 1981;102:271–281.

58. Carfoli E. Intracellular calcium homeostasis. Annu Rev Biochem 1987;56:395–433.

59. Van Nueten JM, Janssens WJ, Vanhoutte PM. Calcium Antagonism and Vascular Smooth Muscle. In PM Vanhoutte, R Paoletti, S Govoni (eds), Calcium Antagonists: Pharmacology and Clinical Research. New York: New York Academy of Sciences, 1988;234–247.

60. Mohamed A, Gatoh O, Graham D, et al. Effect of pretreatment with the calcium antagonist nimodipine on local blood flow and histopathology after middle cerebral artery occlusion. Ann Neurol 1985;18:705–711.

61. Meyer FB, Sundt TM Jr, Yanagihara T, et al. Ischemic Vasoconstriction and Parenchymal Brain pH. In PM Vanhoutte, R Paoletti, S Govoni (eds), Calcium Antagonists: Pharmacology and Clinical Research. New York: New York Academy of Sciences, 1988;502–515.

62. Deshpande JK, Wieloch T. Flunarizine, a calcium entry blocker, ameliorates ischemic brain damage in the rat. Anesthesiology 1986;64:215–224.

63. Gotoh O, Mohamed AA, McCulloch J, et al. Nimodipine and the hemodynamic and histopathological consequences of middle cerebral artery occlusion in the rat. J Cereb Blood Flow Metab 1986;6:321–331.

64. Petruk KC, West M, Mohr G, et al. Nimodipine treatment in poor grade aneurysm patients. J Neurosurg 1988;68:505–517.

65. The American Nimodipine Study Group. Clinical trial of nimodipine in acute ischemic stroke. Stroke 1992;23:3–8.

66. Ahmed N, Näsman P, Wahlgren NG. Effect of intravenous nimodipine on blood pressure and outcome after acute stroke. Stroke 2000;31:1250–1255.

67. Lennox WG, Gibbs FA, Gibbs EL. Relationship of unconsciousness to cerebral blood flow and to anoxemia. Arch Neurol Psych 1935;34:1001–1013.

68. Lowry OH, Passonneau JV, Hasselberger FX, Schulz DW. Effect of ischemia on known substrates and cofactors of the glycolytic pathway in brain. J Biol Chem 1964;239:18–30.

69. Kirino T. Delayed neuronal death in the gerbil hippocampus following ischemia. Brain Res 1982;239:57–69.

70. Brierly J. Cerebral Hypoxia. In W Blackwood, J Corsellis (eds), Greenfield's Neuropathology. London: Edward Arnold, 1976;43–85.

71. Coyle P. Diameter and length changes in cerebral collaterals after middle cerebral artery occlusion in the young rat. Anat Rec 1984;210:357–364.

72. Coyle P, Jokelainen PT. Differential outcome to middle cerebral artery occlusion in spontaneously hypertensive stroke-prone rats (SHRSP) and Wistar Kyoto (WKY) rats. Stroke 1983;14:605–611.

73. Leblanc R, Yamamoto YL, Tyler JL. Border zone ischemia. Ann Neurol 1987;22:707–713.

74. Carpenter DA, Grubb RL Jr, Powers WJ. Border zone hemodynamics in cerebrovascular disease. Neurology 1990;40:1587–1592.

75. Symon L, Pasztor E, Branston NM. The distribution and density of reduced cerebral blood flow following acute middle cerebral artery occlusion: an experimental study by the technique of hydrogen clearance in baboons. Stroke 1974;5:355–364.

76. Paulson OB. Regional cerebral blood flow in apoplexy due to occlusion of the middle cerebral artery. Neurology 1970;20:63–77.

77. Meyer FB, Anderson RE, Sundt TM Jr, Yaksh TL. Intracellular brain pH, indicator tissue perfusion, electroencephalography, and histology in severe and moderate focal cortical ischemia in the rabbit. J Cereb Blood Flow Metab 1986;6:71–78.

78. Welsh FA. Role of vascular factors in regional ischemic injury. Prog Brain Res 1993;63:19–27.

79. Zulch KJ. Cerebrovascular Pathology and Pathogenesis as a Basis of Neuroradiological Diagnosis. In L Diethelm, S Wende (eds), Handbuch der medizinischen Radiologie—Encyclopedia of Medical Radiology. Vol. XIV, part 1A. Berlin: Springer, 1981;1–192.

80. Kaplan B, Brint S, Tanabe J, et al. Temporal thresholds for neocortical infarction in rats subjected to reversible focal cerebral ischemia. Stroke 1991;22:1032–1039.

81. Hakim AM. The cerebral ischemic penumbra. Can J Neurol Sci 1987;14:557–559.

82. Powers WJ, Mintun MA. The Role of Positron Emission Tomography in Identification of the Ischemic Penumbra. In WJ Powers, ME Raichle (eds), Cerebrovascular Diseases. Fifteenth Princeton Research Conference. New York: Raven, 1987;273–281.

83. Plum F, Brown HW. The effect on respiration of central nervous system disease. Ann N Y Acad Sci 1963;109:915–931.

84. Ludwigs UG, Baehrendtsz S, Wanecek M, Matell G. Mechanical ventilation in medical and neurological diseases: 11 years of experience. J Intern Med 1991;229:117–124.

85. Hossmann K-A. Viability thresholds and the penumbra of focal ischemia. Ann Neurol 1994;36:557–565.

86. Fisher M, Garcia JH. Evolving stroke and the ischemic penumbra. Neurology 1996;47:884–888.

87. Ginsberg MD, Belayev L, Zhao W, et al. The acute ischemic penumbra: topography, life span, and therapeutic response. Acta Neurochir 1999;73(Suppl):45–50.

88. Ropper AH. Brain edema after stroke: clinical syndrome and intracranial pressure. Arch Neurol 1984;41:26–29.

89. Hatashita S, Hoff JT. Cortical tissue pressure gradients in early ischemic brain edema. J Cereb Blood Flow Metab 1986;6:1–7.

90. Marshall LF, Bruce DA, Graham DI, Langfitt TW. Alterations in behavior, brain electrical activity, cerebral blood flow, and intracranial pressure produced by triethyl tin sulfate induced cerebral edema. Stroke 1976;7:21–25.

91. Blasberg RG, Gazendam J, Patlak CS, Fenstermacher JD. Quantitative Autoradiographic Studies of Brain Edema

and a Comparison of Multi-Isotope Autoradiographic Techniques. In J Cervos-Navarro, R Ferszt (eds), Brain Oedema. New York: Raven, 1980;255–270.

92. Dirnagl U. Cerebral ischemia: the microcirculation as trigger and target. Prog Brain Res 1993;96:49–58.

93. Little JR, Kerr FWL, Sundt TM Jr. Microcirculatory obstruction in focal cerebral ischemia: relationships to neuronal alterations. Mayo Clin Proc 1975;50:264–270.

94. Barone FC, Feuerstein GZ. Inflammatory mediators and stroke: new opportunities for novel therapeutics. J Cereb Blood Flow Metab 1999;19:819–834.

95. Dietrich WD, Halley M, Valdes I, Busto R. Interrelationships between increased vascular permeability and acute neuronal damage following temperature-controlled brain ischemia in rats. Acta Neuropathol (Berl) 1991;81:615–625.

96. Ito U, Ohno K, Nakamura R, et al. Brain edema during ischemia and after restoration of blood flow. Stroke 1979;10:542–547.

97. Vise WM, Schuier FF, Hossmann K-A, et al. Cerebral microembolization. I. Pathophysiological studies. Arch Neurol 1977;34:660–665.

98. Hakim AM, Hogan MJ, Carpenter S. Time course of cerebral blood flow and histological outcome after focal cerebral ischemia in rats. Stroke 1992;23:1138–1144.

99. Choi DW. Cerebral hypoxia: some new approaches and unanswered questions. J Neurosci 1990;10:2493–2501.

100. Lemasters JJ, Diguiseppi J, Nieminen AL, Herman B. Blebbing, free Ca^{2+}, and mitochondrial membrane potential preceding cell death in hepatocytes. Nature 1987;325: 78–81.

101. Sato M, Paschen W, Pawlik G, Heiss W-D. Neurological deficit and cerebral ATP depletion after temporary focal ischemia in cats. J Cereb Blood Flow Metab 1984;4:173–177.

102. Yatsu FM, Lee L-W, Liao C-L. Energy metabolism during brain ischemia: stability during reversible and irreversible damage. Stroke 1975;6:678–683.

103. Pulsinelli WA. Selective neuronal vulnerability: morphological and molecular characteristics. Prog Brain Res 1985;63:29–37.

104. Du C, Hu R, Csernansky CA, et al. Very delayed infarction after mild focal cerebral ischemia: a role for apoptosis? J Cereb Blood Flow Metab 1996;16:195–201.

105. Hossmann K-A. Post-ischemic resuscitation of the brain: selective vulnerability versus global resistance. Prog Brain Res 1985;63:3–17.

106. McDonald JW, Johnston MV. Physiological and pathophysiological roles of excitatory amino acids during central nervous system development. Brain Res Brain Res Rev 1990;15:41–70.

107. Rothman SM. Synaptic activity mediates death of hypoxic neurons. Science 1983;220:536–537.

108. Choi DW. Glutamate neurotoxicity and diseases of the nervous system. Neuron 1988;1:623–634.

109. Choi DW. NMDA receptors and AMPA/kainate receptors mediate parallel injury in cerebral cortical cultures subjected to oxygen-glucose deprivation. Prog Brain Res 1993;96:137–143.

110. Choi DW. Ionic dependence of glutamate neurotoxicity in cortical cell culture. J Neurosci 1987;7:369–379.

111. Choi DW, Lobner D, Dugan LL. Glutamate Receptor-Mediated Neuronal Death in the Ischemic Brain. In CY Hsu (ed), Ischemic Stroke: From Basic Mechanisms to New Drug Development. Switzerland: Karger, 1998;2–13.

112. Rothman SM, Olney JW. Glutamate and the pathophysiology of hypoxic-ischemic brain damage. Ann Neurol 1986;19:105–111.

113. Olney JW. Neurotoxicity of Excitatory Amino Acids. In EG McGeer, JW Olney, PL McGeer (eds), Kainic Acid as a Tool in Neurobiology. New York: Raven, 1978;37–70.

114. Koh JY, Choi DW. Vulnerability of cultured cortical neurons to damage by excitotoxins: differential susceptibility of neurons containing NADPH–diaphorase. J Neurosci 1988;8:2153–2163.

115. Dawson VL, Dawson TM, London ED, et al. Nitric oxide mediates glutamate neurotoxicity in primary cortical cultures. Proc Natl Acad Sci U S A 1991;88:6368–6371.

116. Beckman JS, Beckman TW, Chen J, et al. Apparent hydroxyl radical production by peroxynitrite: implications for endothelial injury from nitric oxide and superoxide. Proc Natl Acad Sci U S A 1990;87:1620–1624.

117. Zhang J, Dawson VL, Dawson TM, Snyder SH. Nitric oxide activation of poly(ADP–ribose) synthetase in neurotoxicity. Science 1994;263:687–689.

118. Benveniste H, Drejer J, Schousboe A, Diemer NH. Evaluation of the extracellular concentrations of glutamate and aspartate in rat hippocampus during transient cerebral ischemia monitored by intracerebral microdialysis. J Neurochem 1984;43:1369–1374.

119. Swanson RA, Farrell K, Simon RP. Acidosis causes failure of astrocyte glutamate uptake during hypoxia. J Cereb Blood Flow Metab 1995;15:417–424.

120. Marrannes R, Willems R, De-Prins E, Wauquier A. Evidence for a role of the NMDA receptor in cortical spreading depression in the rat. Brain Res 1988;457:226–240.

121. McCulloch J, Ozyurt E, Park CK, et al. Glutamate receptor antagonists in experimental focal cerebral ischaemia. Acta Neurochir 1993;57(Suppl):73–79.

122. Simon RP, Swan JH, Griffiths T, Meldrum BS. Blockade of NMDA receptors may protect against ischemic damage in the brain. Science 1984;226:850–852.

123. Buchan A. Do NMDA antagonists protect against cerebral ischemia: are clinical trials warranted? Cerebrovasc Brain Metab Rev 1990;2:1–26.

124. Pulsinelli W, Sarokin A, Buchan A. Antagonism of the NMDA and non-NMDA receptors in global versus focal brain ischemia. Prog Brain Res 1993;96:125–135.

125. Park CK, Nehls DG, Graham DI, et al. The glutamate antagonist MK-801 reduces focal ischemic brain damage in the rat. Ann Neurol 1988;24:543–551.

126. Choi DW. Calcium-mediated neurotoxicity: relationship to specific channel types and role in ischemic damage. Trends Neurosci 1988;11:465–469.

127. Choi DW. Excitotoxicity in Cultured Cortical Neurons. In P Ascher, DW Choi, Y Christen (eds), Glutamate, Cell Death and Memory. Berlin: Springer, 1991.

128. Goldberg MP, Choi DW. Combined oxygen and glucose deprivation in cortical cell culture: calcium-dependent and calcium-independent mechanisms of neuronal injury. J Neurosci 1993;13:3510–3524.

129. Goldberg MP. Stroke trials database. Internet Stroke Center at Washington University (http://www.neuro.wustl.edu/stroke/stroke-trials.htm).

130. Olney JW. Neurotoxicity of NMDA receptor antagonists: an overview. Psychopharmacol Bull 1994;30:533–540.

131. Dyker AG, Lees KR. Safety and tolerability of GV150526 (a glycine site antagonist at the N-methyl-D-aspartate receptor) in patients with acute stroke. Stroke 1999;30:986–992.

132. Phase II studies of the glycine antagonist GV150526 in acute stroke: the North American experience. The North American Glycine Antagonist in Neuroprotection (GAIN) Investigators. Stroke 2000;31:358–365.

133. Xue D, Huang Z-G, Barnes K. Delayed treatment with AMPA, but not NMDA, antagonists reduces neocortical infarction. J Cereb Blood Flow Metab 1994;14:252–261.

134. Hollmann M, Hartley M, Heinemann S. Ca^{2+} permeability of KA-AMPA-gated glutamate receptor channels depends on subunit composition. Science 1991;252:851–853.

135. Schielke GP, Kupina NC, Boxer PA, et al. The neuroprotective effect of the novel AMPA receptor antagonist PD152247 (PNQX) in temporary focal ischemia in the rat. Stroke 1999;30:1472–1477.

136. Follis F, Scremin OU, Blisard KS, et al. Selective vulnerability of white matter during spinal cord ischemia. J Cereb Blood Flow Metab 1993;13:170–178.

137. Pantoni L, Garcia JH, Gutierrez JA. Cerebral white matter is highly vulnerable to ischemia. Stroke 1996;27:1641–1647.

138. David JC, Yamada KA, Bagwe MR, Goldberg MP. AMPA receptor activation is rapidly toxic to cortical astrocytes when desensitization is blocked. J Neurosci 1996;16:200–209.

139. McDonald JW, Althomsons SP, Hyrc KL, et al. Oligodendrocytes from forebrain are highly vulnerable to AMPA/kainate receptor-mediated excitotoxicity. Nat Med 1998;3:291–297.

140. Matute C, Sanchez-Gomez MV, Martinez-Millan L, Miledi R. Glutamate receptor-mediated toxicity in optic nerve oligodendrocytes. Proc Natl Acad Sci U S A 1998;94:8830–8835.

141. Kanellopoulos GK, Xu XM, Hsu CY, et al. White matter injury in spinal cord ischemia: protection by AMPA/kainate glutamate receptor antagonism. Stroke 2000;31:1945–1952.

142. Choi DW, Koh JY. Zinc and brain injury. Annu Rev Neurosci 1998;21:347–375.

143. Koh JY, Suh SW, Gwag BJ, et al. The role of zinc in selective neuronal death after transient global cerebral ischemia. Science 1996;272:1013–1016.

144. Muir KW. New experimental and clinical data on the efficacy of pharmacological magnesium infusions in cerebral infarcts. Magnes Res 1998;11:43–56.

145. Minamisawa H, Smith ML, Siesjo BK. The effect of mild hyperthermia and hypothermia on brain damage following 5, 10, and 15 minutes of forebrain ischemia. Ann Neurol 1990;28:26–33.

146. Dietrich WD, Busto R, Halley M, Valdes I. The importance of brain temperature in alterations of the blood-brain barrier following cerebral ischemia. J Neuropathol Exp Neurol 1990;49:486–497.

147. Busto R, Dietrich WD, Globus MY, et al. Small differences in intraischemic brain temperature critically determine the extent of ischemic neuronal injury. J Cereb Blood Flow Metab 1987;7:729–738.

148. Ahmed SH, He YY, Nassief A, et al. Effects of lipopolysaccharide priming on acute ischemic brain injury. Stroke 2000;31:193–199.

149. Ginsberg MD. Temperature Influences on Ischemic Brain Injury. In CY Hsu (ed), Ischemic Stroke: From Basic Mechanisms to New Drug Development. Switzerland: Karger, 1998;65–88.

150. Reith J, Jorgensen HS, Pedersen PM, et al. Body temperature in acute stroke: relation to stroke severity, infarct size, mortality, and outcome. Lancet 1996;347(8999):422–425.

151. Pulsinelli WA, Waldman S, Sigsbee B, et al. Experimental Hyperglycemia and Diabetes Mellitus Worsens Stroke Outcome. In E Betz (ed), Pathophysiology and Pharmacotherapy of Cerebral Vascular Disorders. Baden-Baden:Verlag Gerhard Witzstrock, 1980;196–199.

152. deCourten-Myers G, Myers R, Schoofield L. Hyperglycemia enlarges infarct size in cerebrovascular occlusion in cats. Stroke 1988;19:623–630.

153. Yip PK, He YY, Hsu CY, et al. Effect of plasma glucose on infarct size in focal cerebral ischemia-reperfusion. Neurology 1991;41:899–905.

154. Ginsberg MD. Mitochondrial metabolism following bilateral cerebral ischemia in the gerbil. Ann Neurol 1977;1:519–527.

155. Plum F. What causes infarction in ischemic brain? The Robert Wartenberg Lecture. Neurology 1983;33:222–233.

156. Siesjo BK, Katsura K, Mellergard P, et al. Acidosis-related brain damage. Prog Brain Res 1993;96:23–48.

157. Garcia JH, Liu K-F, Lian J, Xu J. Astrocytic and microvascular responses to the occlusion of a middle cerebral artery. J Neuropathol Exp Neurol 1993;52:288.

158. Rehncrona S, Hauge HN, Siesjo BK. Enhancement of iron-catalyzed free radical formation by acidosis in brain homogenates: difference in effect by lactic acid and CO_2. J Cereb Blood Flow Metab 1989;9:65–70.

159. Giffard RG, Monyer H, Christine CW, Choi DW. Acidosis reduces NMDA receptor activation, glutamate neurotoxicity, and oxygen-glucose deprivation neuronal injury in cortical cultures. Brain Res 1990;506:339–342.

160. Hara H, Onodera H, Yoshidomi M, et al. Staurosporine, a novel protein kinase C inhibitor, prevents postischemic neuronal damage in the gerbil and rat. J Cereb Blood Flow Metab 1990;10:646–653.

161. Madden KP, Clark WM, Kochhar A, Zivin JA. Effect of protein kinase C modulation on outcome of experimental CNS ischemia. Brain Res 1991;547:193–198.

162. Aronowski J, Grotta JC, Strong R, Waxham MN. Interplay between the gamma isoform of PKC and calcineurin in regulation of vulnerability to focal cerebral ischemia. J Cereb Blood Flow Metab 2000;20:343–349.

163. Wang KK. Calpain and caspase: can you tell the difference? Trends Neurosci 2000;23:20–26.

164. Aguilar HI, Botla R, Arora AS, et al. Induction of the mitochondrial permeability transition by protease activity in rats: a mechanism of hepatocyte necrosis. Gastroenterology 1996;110:558–566.

165. Lee KS, Frank S, Vanderklish P, et al. Inhibition of proteolysis protects hippocampal neurons from ischemia. Proc Natl Acad Sci U S A 1991;88:7233–7237.

166. Bartus RT, Baker KL, Heiser AD, et al. Postischemic administration of AK275, a calpain inhibitor, provides substantial protection against focal ischemic brain damage. J Cereb Blood Flow Metab 1994;14:537–544.

167. Markgraf CG, Velayo NL, Johnson MP, et al. Six-hour window of opportunity for calpain inhibition in focal cerebral ischemia in rats. Stroke 1998;29:152–158.

168. Horrocks L, Dorman R, Porcelati G. Fatty Acids and Phospholipids in Brain During Ischemia. In A Bes, P Braquet, R Paoletti, BK Siesjo (eds), Cerebral Ischemia. New York: Excerpta Medica, 1984;211–222.

169. Gardiner M, Nilsson B, Rehncrona S, Siesjo B. Free fatty acids in the rat brain in moderate and severe hypoxia. J Neurochem 1981;36:1500–1505.

170. Farber JL, Chi KR, Mittnacht S Jr. The pathogenesis of irreversible cell injury in ischemia. Am J Pathol 1981;102:271–281.

171. Chen ST, Hsu CY, Hogan EL, et al. Thromboxane, prostacyclin, and leukotrienes in cerebral ischemia. Neurology 1986;36:466–470.

172. Sairanen T, Ristimaki A, Karjalainen-Lindsberg ML, et al. Cyclooxygenase-2 is induced globally in infarcted human brain. Ann Neurol 1998;43:738–747.

173. Miettinen S, Fusco FR, Yrjanheikki J, et al. Spreading depression and focal brain ischemia induce cyclooxygenase-2 in cortical neurons through N-methyl-D-aspartic acid-receptors and phospholipase A_2. Proc Natl Acad Sci U S A 1997;94:6500–6505.

174. Nogawa S, Zhang F, Ross ME, Iadecola C. Cyclo-oxygenase-2 gene expression in neurons contributes to ischemic brain damage. J Neurosci 1997;17:2746–2755.

175. Crockard IIA, Bhakoo KK, Lascelles PT. Regional prostaglandin levels in cerebral ischaemia. J Neurochem 1982;38:1311–1314.

176. Hewett SJ, Uliasz TF, Vidwans AS, Hewett JA. Cyclooxygenase-2 contributes to N-methyl-D-aspartate-mediated neuronal cell death in primary cortical cell culture. J Pharmacol Exp Ther 2000;293:417–425.

177. Minami M, Kuraishi Y, Yabuuchi K, et al. Induction of interleukin-1 beta mRNA in rat brain after transient forebrain ischemia. J Neurochem 1992;58:390–392.

178. Lindgren JA, Hokfelt T, Dahlen SE, et al. Leukotrienes in the rat central nervous system. Proc Natl Acad Sci U S A 1984;81:6212–6216.

179. Moskowitz MA, Kiwak KJ, Hekimian K, Levine L. Synthesis of compounds with properties of leukotrienes C4 and D4 in gerbil brains after ischemia and reperfusion. Science 1984;224:886–889.

180. Valone F, Phillip R, Debs RJ. Enhanced human monocyte toxicity by platelet-activating factor. Immunology 1988; 166:715–718.

181. Hsu CY, Liu TH, Xu J, et al. Arachidonic acid and its metabolites in cerebral ischemia. Ann N Y Acad Sci 1989;559:282–295.

182. Hellenbeck JM, Furlow TW Jr. Prostaglandin I_2 and indomethacin prevent impairment of post-ischemic brain reperfusion in the dog. Stroke 1979;10:629–637.

183. Hsu CY, Faught RE, Furlan AJ, et al. Prostacyclin Study Group—Intravenous prostacyclin in acute non-hemorrhagic stroke: a placebo-controlled double blind study. Stroke 1987;18:353–358.

184. Martin JF, Hamdy N, Nicholl J, et al. Double-blind controlled trial of prostacyclin in cerebral infarction. Stroke 1985;16:386–390.

185. Chan PH. Role of oxidants in ischemic brain damage. Stroke 1996;27:1124–1129.

186. Traystman RJ, Kirsch JR, Koehler RC. Oxygen radical mechanisms of brain injury following ischemia and reperfusion. J Appl Physiol 1991;71:1185–1195.

187. Lindsay S, Liu T-H, Xu J, et al. Role of xanthine dehydrogenase and oxidase in focal cerebral ischemic injury to rat. Am J Physiol 1991;261:H2051–H2057.

188. Iadecola C. Bright and dark sides of nitric oxide in ischemic brain injury. Trends Neurosci 1997;20:132–139.

189. Dalkara T, Moskowitz MA. Nitric Oxide in Cerebrovascular Regulation and Ischemia. In CY Hsu (ed), Ischemic Stroke: From Basic Mechanisms to New Drug Development. Switzerland: Karger, 1998;28–45.

190. Huang Z, Huang PL, Panahian N, et al. Effects of cerebral ischemia in mice deficient in neuronal nitric oxide synthase. Science 1994;265:1883–1885.

191. Huang Z, Huang PL, Ma J, et al. Enlarged infarcts in endothelial nitric oxide synthase knockout mice are attenuated by nitro-L-arginine. J Cereb Blood Flow Metab 1996;16:981–987.

192. Iadecola C, Zhang F, Casey R, et al. Delayed reduction of ischemic brain injury and neurological deficits in mice lacking the inducible nitric oxide synthase gene. J Neurosci 1997;17:9157–9164.

193. Rauhala P, Lin AM, Chiueh CC. Neuroprotection by S-nitrosoglutathione of brain dopamine neurons from oxidative stress. FASEB J 1998;12:165–173.

194. Chiueh CC, Rauhala P. The redox pathway of S-nitrosoglutathione, glutathione and nitric oxide in cell to neuron communications. Free Radic Res 1999;31:641–650.

195. McCord JM. Oxygen-derived free radicals in postischemic tissue injury. N Engl J Med 1985;312:159–163.

196. Kontos HA, Wei EP, Povlishock JT, et al. Cerebral arteriolar damage by arachidonic acid and prostaglandin G_2. Science 1980;209:1242–1245.

197. Schraufstatter IU, Hyslop PA, Jackson J, Cochrane CC. Mechanisms of Oxidant Injury of Cells. In P Movat (ed), Leukocyte Emigration and Its Sequelae. Basel, Switzerland: Karger, 1987.

198. Liu T-H, Beckman JS, Freeman BA, et al. Polyethylene glycol-conjugated superoxide dismutase and catalase reduce ischemic brain injury. Am J Physiol 1989;256: H589–H593.

199. Itoh T, Kawakami M, Yamauchi Y. Effect of allopurinol on ischemia and reperfusion-induced cerebral injury in spontaneously hypertensive rats. Stroke 1986;17:1284–1287.

200. Hossmann K-A. Disturbances of cerebral protein synthesis and ischemic cell death. Prog Brain Res 1993;96:161–177.

201. An G, Lin T-N, Liu J-S, et al. Expression of c-fos and c-jun family genes after focal cerebral ischemia. Ann Neurol 1993;33:457–464.

202. Hsu CY, An G, Liu JS, et al. Expression of immediate early gene and growth factor mRNAs in a focal cerebral ischemia model in the rat. Stroke 1993;24(S):I78–I88.

203. Nowak TS. Protein synthesis and the heat shock/stress response after ischemia. Cerebrovasc Brain Metab Rev 1990;2:345–366.

204. Lindvall O, Ernfors P, Bengzon J, et al. Differential regulation of mRNAs for nerve growth factor, brain derived neurotrophic factor, and neurotrophin 3 in the adult rat brain following cerebral ischemia and hypoglycemic coma. Proc Natl Acad Sci U S A 1992;89:648–652.

205. Plumier JC, Krueger AM, Currie RW, et al. Transgenic mice expressing the human inducible Hsp70 have hippocampal neurons resistant to ischemic injury. Cell Stress Chaperones 1997;2:162–167.

206. Chen J, Graham SH, Nakayama M, et al. Apoptosis repressor genes Bcl-2 and Bcl-x-long are expressed in the rat brain following global ischemia. J Cereb Blood Flow Metab 1997;17:2–10.

207. Gillardon F, Lenz C, Waschke KF, et al. Altered expression of Bcl-2, Bcl-X, Bax, and c-Fos colocalizes with DNA fragmentation and ischemic cell damage following middle cerebral artery occlusion in rats. Brain Res Mol Brain Res 1996;40:254–260.

208. Schneider A, Martin-Villalba A, Weih F, et al. NF-kappaB is activated and promotes cell death in focal cerebral ischemia. Nat Med 1999;5:554–559.

209. Dai WJ, Funk A, Herdegen T, et al. Blockade of central angiotensin AT(1) receptors improves neurological outcome and reduces expression of AP-1 transcription factors after focal brain ischemia in rats. Stroke 1999;30:2391–2398.

210. Domanska-Janik K, Bong P, Bronisz-Kowalczyk A, et al. AP1 transcriptional factor activation and its relation to apoptosis of hippocampal CA1 pyramidal neurons after transient ischemia in gerbils. J Neurosci Res 1999;57:840–846.

211. Bergeron M, Yu AY, Solway KE, et al. Induction of hypoxia-inducible factor-1 (HIF-1) and its target genes following focal ischaemia in rat brain. Eur J Neurosci 1999;11:4159–4170.

212. Iadecola C, Salkowski CA, Zhang F, et al. The transcription factor interferon regulatory factor 1 is expressed after cerebral ischemia and contributes to ischemic brain injury. J Exp Med 1999;189:719–727.

213. Liu T, McDonnell PC, Young PR, et al. Interleukin-1 beta mRNA expression in ischemic rat cortex. Stroke 1993;24:1746–1750.

214. Friedlander RM, Gagliardini V, Hara H, et al. Expression of a dominant negative mutant of interleukin-1 beta converting enzyme in transgenic mice prevents neuronal cell death induced by trophic factor withdrawal and ischemic brain injury. J Exp Med 1997;185:933–940.

215. Kochanek P, Schoettle R, Uhl M, et al. Platelet-activating factor antagonists do not attenuate delayed posttraumatic cerebral edema in rats. J Neurotrauma 1991;8:19–25.

216. Hayward NJ, Elliott PJ, Sawyer SD, et al. Lack of evidence for neutrophil participation during infarct formation following focal cerebral ischemia in the rat. Exp Neurol 1996;139:188–202.

217. Huang J, Kim LJ, Mealey R, et al. Neuronal protection in stroke by an sLex-glycosylated complement inhibitory protein. Science 1999;285:595–599.

218. Linnik MD, Zobrist RH, Hatfield MD. Evidence supporting a role for programmed cell death in focal cerebral ischemia in rats. Stroke 1993;24:2002–2009.

219. Akins PT, Liu PK, Hsu CY. Immediate early gene expression in response to cerebral ischemia. Friend or foe? Stroke 1996;27:1682–1687.

220. Charriaut-Marlangue C, Margaill I, Represa A, et al. Apoptosis and necrosis after reversible focal ischemia: an in situ DNA fragmentation analysis. J Cereb Blood Flow Metab 1996;16:186–194.

221. MacManus JP, Linnik MD. Gene expression induced by cerebral ischemia: an apoptotic perspective. J Cereb Blood Flow Metab 1997;17:815–832.

222. Martin LJ, Al-Abdulla NA, Brambrink AM, et al. Neurodegeneration in excitotoxicity, global cerebral ischemia, and target deprivation: a perspective on the contributions of apoptosis and necrosis. Brain Res Bull 1998;46:281–309.

223. Linnik MD, Zobrist RH, Hatfield MD. Evidence supporting a role for programmed cell death in focal cerebral ischemia in rats. Stroke 1993;24:2002–2008.

224. Cheng Y, Deshmukh M, D'Costa A, et al. Caspase inhibitor affords neuroprotection with delayed administration in a rat model of neonatal hypoxic-ischemic brain injury. J Clin Invest 1998;101:1992–1999.

225. Endres M, Namura S, Shimizu-Sasamata M, et al. Attenuation of delayed neuronal death after mild focal ischemia in mice by inhibition of the caspase family. J Cereb Blood Flow Metab 1998;18:238–247.

226. Himi T, Ishizaki Y, Murota S. A caspase inhibitor blocks ischaemia-induced delayed neuronal death in the gerbil. Eur J Neurosci 1998;10:777–781.

227. Green DR, Reed JC. Mitochondria and apoptosis. Science 1998;281:1309–1312.

228. Krajewski S, Krajewska M, Ellerby LM, et al. Release of caspase-9 from mitochondria during neuronal apoptosis and cerebral ischemia. Proc Natl Acad Sci U S A 1999;96:5752–5757.

229. Ouyang YB, Tan Y, Comb M, et al. Survival- and death-promoting events after transient cerebral ischemia: phosphorylation of Akt, release of cytochrome C and Activation of caspase-like proteases. J Cereb Blood Flow Metab 1999;19:1126–1135.

230. Velier JJ, Ellison JA, Kikly KK, et al. Caspase-8 and caspase-3 are expressed by different populations of cortical neurons undergoing delayed cell death after focal stroke in the rat. J Neurosci 1999;19:5932–5941.

231. Martinou JC, Dubois-Dauphin M, Staple JK, et al. Overexpression of BCL-2 in transgenic mice protects neurons from naturally occurring cell death and experimental ischemia. Neuron 1994;13:1017–1030.

232. Deshpande J, Bergstedt K, Linden T, et al. Ultrastructural changes in the hippocampal CA1 region following transient cerebral ischemia: evidence against programmed cell death. Exp Brain Res 1992;88:91–105.

233. Colbourne F, Sutherland GR, Auer RN. Electron microscopic evidence against apoptosis as the mechanism of

neuronal death in global ischemia. J Neurosci 1999;19:4200–4210.

234. Susin SA, Zamzami N, Castedo M, et al. The central executioner of apoptosis: multiple connections between protease activation and mitochondria in Fas/APO-1/CD95- and ceramide-induced apoptosis. J Exp Med 1997;186:25–37.

235. Liu X, Kim CN, Yang J, et al. Induction of apoptotic program in cell-free extracts: requirement for dATP and cytochrome c. Cell 1996;86:147–157.

236. Kluck RM, Bossy-Wetzel E, Green DR, Newmeyer DD. The release of cytochrome c from mitochondria: a primary site for Bcl-2 regulation of apoptosis. Science 1997;275:1132–1136.

237. Susin SA, Lorenzo HK, Zamzami N, et al. Mitochondrial release of caspase-2 and -9 during the apoptotic process. J Exp Med 1999;189:381–394.

238. Heiss W-D, Rosner G. Functional recovery of cortical neurons as related to degree and duration of ischemia. Ann Neurol 1983;14:294–301.

239. del Zoppo GJ, Poeck K, Pessin MS, et al. Recombinant tissue plasminogen activator in acute thrombotic and embolic stroke. Ann Neurol 1992;32:78–86.

240. Brott T. Thrombolytic therapy for stroke. Cerebrovasc Brain Metab Rev 1991;3:91–113.

241. Ames A. Cerebral ischemia II: the no reflow phenomenon. Am J Pathol 1968;52:437–453.

242. Crowell RM, Olsson Y. Impaired microvascular filling after focal cerebral ischemia in the monkey. Neurology 1972;22:500–504.

243. Nagasawa H, Kogure K. Correlation between cerebral blood flow and histologic changes in a new rat model of cerebral artery occlusion. Stroke 1989;20:1037–1043.

244. Kagstrom E, Smith ML, Siesjo BK. Local cerebral blood flow in the recovery period following complete cerebral ischemia in the rat. J Cereb Blood Flow Metab 1983;3:170–182.

245. del Zoppo GJ. Microvascular changes during cerebral ischemia and reperfusion. Cerebrovasc Brain Metab Rev 1994;6:47–96.

246. Clark WM, Madden KP, Rothlein R, Zivin JA. Reduction of central nervous system ischemic injury by monoclonal antibody to intercellular adhesion molecule. J Neurosurg 1991;75:623–627.

247. Welsh FA, Durity F, Langfitt TW. The appearance of regional variations in metabolism at a critical level of cerebral oligemia. J Neurochem 1977;28:71–79.

248. Suzuki R, Yamaguchi T, Choh–Luh L, Klatzo I. The effects of 5-minute ischemia in Mongolian gerbils. II. Changes of spontaneous neuronal activity in cerebral cortex and CA1 sector of hippocampus. Acta Neuropathol (Berl) 1983;60:217–222.

249. Kuroiwa T, Ting P, Martinez H, Klatzo I. The biphasic opening of the blood brain barrier to proteins following temporary middle cerebral artery occlusion. Acta Neuropathol (Berl) 1985;68:122–129.

250. Ernster L. Biochemistry of reoxygenation injury. Crit Care Med 988;16:947–953.

251. Wei EP, Kontos HA, Dietrich WD, et al. Inhibition by free radical scavengers and by cyclooxygenase inhibitors of pial arteriolar abnormalities from concussive brain injury in cats. Circ Res 1981;48:95–103.

252. Kuroiwa T. Blood-brain barrier disruption and exacerbation of ischemic brain edema after restoration of blood flow in experimental focal cerebral ischemia. Acta Neuropathol (Berl) 1988;76:62–65.

253. Bounds JV, Wiebers DO, Whisnant JP, Okazaki H. Mechanism and timing of deaths from cerebral infarction. Stroke 1981;12:474–477.

254. Zivin JA, Fisher M, DeGirolami U, et al. Tissue plasminogen activator reduces neurological damage after cerebral embolism. Science 1985;230:1289–1292.

255. The National Institute of Neurological Disorders and Stroke rt-PA Stroke Study Group: tissue plasminogen activator for acute ischemic stroke. N Engl J Med 1995;333:1581–1587.

256. Kwiatkowski TG, Libman RB, Frankel M, et al. Effects of tissue plasminogen activator for acute ischemic stroke at one year. National Institute of Neurological Disorders and Stroke Recombinant Tissue Plasminogen Activator Stroke Study Group. N Engl J Med 1999;340:1781–1787.

257. Furlan A, Higashida R, Wechsler L, et al. Intra-arterial prourokinase for acute ischemic stroke. The PROACT II study: a randomized controlled trial. Prolyse in Acute Cerebral Thromboembolism. JAMA 1999;282:2003–2011.

258. Sherman DG, Atkinson RP, Chippendale T, et al. Intravenous ancrod for treatment of acute ischemic stroke: the STAT Study: a randomized controlled trial. JAMA 2000;283:2395–2403.

Chapter 3

New Magnetic Resonance Imaging Technologies for Stroke Diagnosis and Treatment Evaluation

Steven Warach and Alison E. Baird

The following is a typical scenario describing the initial management of patients presenting with acute stroke. The neurologist receives a call from the emergency room that a patient has arrived who had a sudden onset of aphasia and right hemiparesis 3 hours before. A computed tomography (CT) scan of the brain is performed; perhaps conventional T1- and T2-weighted magnetic resonance imaging (MRI) scans are performed if they are fortuitously available on short notice. The scans are normal. Because normal scans are consistent with the diagnosis of acute ischemic infarction at 3 hours, this clinical diagnosis is made. The patient is admitted to the hospital, the lesion is allowed to ripen for several days, the scan is repeated, and the diagnosis and localization are confirmed, corrected, or refined. The uncertainty inherent in the clinical diagnosis of stroke has long been accepted as the state of the clinical art. Similarly, in making a diagnosis of stroke based on neuroimaging, false-negative acute scans are accepted as part of the current standard of care.

However, this scenario has begun to change in many centers around the world. Since 1990, significant advances have occurred in stroke therapy and in brain imaging technologies. The 1990s, the "Decade of the Brain," saw the introduction of the first acute stroke treatment—recombinant tissue plasminogen activator—that must be administered

within 3 hours of onset.[1] Newer MRI techniques became available that can rapidly define areas of perfusion defects and localize regions of ischemic injury within minutes after onset of ischemia. These techniques include diffusion-weighted imaging (DWI), perfusion imaging, and fast types of MR angiography (MRA). Significant advances have occurred in CT and ultrasound methodologies that parallel many of the advances in MRI.[2]

The need for urgent and accurate brain imaging in acute stroke is being increasingly recognized. There is now a better understanding of the marked heterogeneity and dynamic nature of the ischemic process that exists in humans. Several ischemic patterns have been identified that could form the basis of therapeutic decision-making. These patterns were first recognized in positron emission tomography studies and subsequently with functional MRI.[2] It has recently been reported that the stroke treatment window for intra-arterial thrombolysis can be extended to six hours if patients are highly selected based on their pathophysiology.[3] Using imaging criteria might also help to solve the recent spate of negative stroke trials by allowing a smaller sample of highly selected patients to be studied.[4] The use of imaging patterns may help to reduce the excess risks associated with recombinant tissue plasminogen activator therapy in practice.[5] Brain imaging methods are also likely to have an important role in the development and testing of potential stroke therapies.[6] In this chapter, we provide an update on the new MRI methods and their potential applications in acute stroke therapy, starting with DWI, then proceeding to MR perfusion imaging and MRA.

Diffusion-Weighted Imaging

DWI allows the detection of ischemic stroke lesions as early as 39 minutes after the onset of symptoms.[7] This early detection of ischemic lesions, in combination with the quantitative information that is provided, makes DWI an appealing tool. DWI is quantitative both in that it measures a physiologic parameter—the apparent diffusion coefficient (ADC) of water in tissue—and in that it permits volumetric analysis of lesions that can be used to study ischemic pathophysiology in vivo.

The detection of ischemic stroke by DWI within minutes after vascular occlusion was first demonstrated in cats by Moseley and coworkers.[8,9] Diffusion is the random translational motion of molecules. Although the term is often used to describe microscopic movement of particles from a region of high concentration to a region of low concentration, such as a drop of ink in a bucket of water, MR diffusion imaging looks at self-diffusion of water, which is the mobility of water molecules among other water molecules. DWI is designed to detect the random molecular motion of water (Brownian motion) in tissue.[10] The diffusion-sensitive MRI pulse sequence involves the addition of a bipolar pair of diffusion-sensitizing magnetic field gradient pulses to a standard pulse sequence to cause a dephasing and then rephasing of the precessing protons in water molecules. This effectively marks the location of water molecules such that any net translational movement of water causes a net dephasing of spinning protons that move along the applied diffusion gradient. Because signal attenuation results from this dephasing, any net diffusion results in signal *loss* on diffusion-weighted images. The loss is greatest in tissue with the greatest fluid content, such as cerebrospinal fluid or watery cysts. On the other hand, tissues with decreased diffusion appear relatively bright because less signal is lost. In vivo diffusion of water in tissue can be quantified as the

physiologic variable—the ADC. The qualifier "apparent" is used as diffusion in tissue is not truly random but affected by biological barriers, such as cell membranes, which can cause restriction to diffusion.

The ADC is a function of two factors: the regional signal intensity (SI) in the images and a constant, called the *b value*, derived from the timings and strength of the diffusion-sensitizing gradients. The b value is indicative of the diffusion sensitivity of DWI. A minimum of two DWI acquisitions of different b values is required for ADC calculation. Calculation of ADC is based on the equation of Stejskal and Tanner,[11] as the negative slope of the linear regression line best fitting the points for b versus ln(SI). Thus, the greater the range and number of b values, the more accurate the ADC calculation. A synthetic image or map of ADC, which is a map of local water mobility, can be created by performing this calculation on a pixel-by-pixel basis. To control for individual differences in ADC due to uncontrolled variables that are known to affect ADC on a global basis, such as brain pulsations, temperature, or serum sodium concentration, a relative ADC value, such as the ratio of lesion ADC to control regions, is a useful measure for comparisons between individuals and within individuals at different times. One should note that DWIs and diffusion maps often have different visual appearance: Tissues that have high water mobility (e.g., cerebrospinal fluid and edema) have substantial signal attenuation in the diffusion-weighted image (and thus appear dark), but have a relatively high ADC value associated with its high mobility (and appear bright) in the diffusion map. Lesions that extend into white matter are best defined by controlling for anisotropy. *Anisotropy* in DWI refers to the dependence of diffusion measurements on the direction of the applied diffusion sensitizing gradient. For example, diffusion measured in a direction perpendicular to the long axis of axons is less (and appear more hyperintense) than that measured parallel, because in the former case more barriers to free diffusion are encountered.[12] The anisotropic effect can be minimized by looking at the so-called trace of the diffusion tensor, which is the average of the diffusion-weighted images with diffusion measured in each of the three orthogonal directions.[13–16] Diffusion trace imaging can be performed in a single acquisition,[16] and has now been incorporated into clinical DWI.

The earliest DWI studies were limited by long acquisition times and the restriction of imaging to a single brain slice. The echoplanar imaging technique allows ultrafast imaging of the whole brain and is now a standard part of the latest generation of MRI scanners.[17] DWI with echoplanar imaging and the higher magnetic field gradients that are associated with it (1) permit rapid whole-brain imaging in 2–3 seconds; (2) allow the use of multiple and higher diffusion sensitivities, which give more accurate calculations of ADC; (3) improve the sensitivity to detect diffusion abnormalities in acute stroke by allowing extremely high diffusion weighting; and (4) are free of degradation from motion artifact. New MR techniques that may be applied to the study of ischemic stroke include diffusion tensor imaging and DWI-fluid attenuated inversion recovery imaging. In diffusion tensor imaging,[18–20] the diffusion sensitizing gradients are applied in the six independent components of the diffusion tensor, not just in the x, y, and z directions as with trace imaging. This therefore allows determination of the directionality as well as the magnitude of water diffusion and could be used to quantify anisotropic effects within the gray and white matter[20] and to study remote effects of ischemic lesions such as wallerian degeneration of the motor tracts. DWI-fluid attenuated inversion recovery imaging may allow improved detection and quantification of ischemic lesions at the cortical edges and in the periventricular regions.[21–23] This is because the suppression of the cerebrospinal fluid signal reduces errors associated with partial volume effects in the ADC calculation in these regions.

Although the exact biophysical mechanism of the diffusion decrease in acute cerebral ischemia is not known with certainty—whether due to restriction of diffusion intracellularly or extracellularly, cellular swelling, contraction of the extracellular space, changes in membrane permeability, or, most likely, a combination of factors—many pathologic features associated with it have been identified. The hypothesis originally put forward by Moseley that the hyperacute decrease in ADC is associated with cytotoxic edema[8,9] has been supported by a number of lines of evidence, and it is generally accepted that the hyperacute diffusion changes occur along with a reduction in extracellular volume and an increase in

intracellular volume. Electrical impedance is increased in the acute stroke, consistent with decreased extracellular space.[24] Within minutes after the onset of ischemia in experimental models, there is a decrease of the energy-requiring Na^+-K^+-adenosine triphosphatase (ATPase) activity that maintains ionic gradients[25] and a corresponding drop in ADC of water measured with MR.[26] The hyperacute decrease in diffusion does not reflect change in water content of the lesion in the first few hours because there is no increase in SI on proton density–weighted imaging or T2-weighted imaging, and therefore, as there is concomitantly a change in the relative size of the intra- and extracellular compartments of water, there must be an associated change in the distribution of water from extracellular to intracellular. This decreased diffusion may also be reproduced by intraparenchymal infusions of ouabain, an inhibitor of Na^+-K^+-ATPase, and by infusions of glutamate or N-methyl-D-aspartate (NMDA) into the brain,[27] which activate NMDA receptors, mediators of ischemic neurotoxicity. There is a precise match between the ADC decrease at 7 hours in a model of a permanent middle cerebral artery occlusion and adenosine triphosphate depletion, histologic damage, and local tissue acidosis.[28] In animal models, sufficiently early reversal of ischemia causes reversal of the diffusion decrease that is not greater than a threshold value and prevents infarction.[29,30] Antagonists of NMDA receptors or calcium influx, mediators of ischemic neurotoxicity, and early reperfusion in animal models may cause reversal of some diffusion-weighted abnormalities.[31,32] Thus, the hyperacute decrease in ADC is considered a marker not only of cytotoxic edema but of failure of Na^+-K^+-ATPase activity in response to cerebral ischemia. ADC does not decrease until tissue perfusion falls below levels known to be critical for maintenance of Na^+-K^+-ATPase activity.[33] Transient decreases in ADC are seen during depolarizations associated with acute ischemic injury,[34] and these changes may also be a marker for spreading depression.[35] The significance of the decreased ADC as a marker of energy failure is that it may permit the definition of the ischemic penumbra: an area of reduced perfusion sufficient to cause potentially reversible clinical deficits but insufficient to cause either disrupted ionic homeostasis due to Na^+-K^+-ATPase failure[36,37] or ADC decrease.[33]

The earliest clinical reports of Warach et al.[17] using whole-brain echo planar MRI to identify and characterize diffusion abnormalities in acute cerebral ischemia have been replicated in many subsequent studies. Early ischemic lesions appear on DWI as hyperintense regions of decreased ADC in all patients who subsequently develop infarction before changes are evident on conventional MRI. Lesions as small as 4 mm in diameter can be identified. The mean ADC (± standard deviation) in the normal brain is typically approximately $9.15 (\pm 2.91) \times 10^{-4}$ mm^2 per second.[17,38] The mean ADC of ischemic regions is approximately 55–60% of control values and stays significantly reduced for 3–4 days after onset of ischemia.[17,39,40] The relative ADC increases progressively over time to become pseudonormalized at 5–10 days and elevated in the chronic state, making the distinction of acute lesions adjacent to chronic infarcts readily apparent. The rise in ADC toward control values most likely reflects a combination of various stages in the evolution of infarction, some that decrease and some that increase diffusion. As can be readily appreciated by the increased signal on T2-weighted imaging (indicative of increased water content) at these times, the brain is abnormal and an infarct is present and evolving. This observation points out that one cannot interpret the magnitude of diffusion change using only a diffusion-weighted image without knowledge of the T2-weighted image (b = 0) or calculation of the ADC. The presence of increased T2-weighted signal with normal ADC, subacutely, indicates that the tissue is not normal. Increased signal (hyperintensity) may be seen chronically in DWI in areas of increased diffusion if the T2-weighted image is sufficiently hyperintense, especially if the b value is intermediate.[17,39,40]

Sometimes normalization of the ADC may occur as early as 48 hours after stroke onset.[40–42] This is more likely to occur after early reperfusion. In some cases, this does appear to represent true DWI reversibility and tissue salvage after thrombolytic administration.[43,44] But in other cases, early normalization of the ADC may subsequently be followed by secondary decline in the ADC several days later, with the tissue progressing to infarction. The cause of the subsequent decline in the ADC is not yet determined but could represent secondary reperfusion injury or apoptosis. Other new pathophysiologic insights have been obtained from DWI. In DWI lesion evolution studies in humans, expansion of ischemic lesions occurs over 6–24 hours and beyond. There is often transient swelling between 3 to 7 days related to vasogenic edema.[45–48] Lesion expansion usually only occurs into a surrounding, larger area of hypoperfusion. DWI lesion evolution likely represents recruitment of penumbra into the core in most patients, but in some patients could also be due to processes such as delayed neuronal injury, apoptosis, reperfusion injury (as mentioned previously) or silent ischemia. To date, spreading depression in the evolution of human infarcts has not been found. Research has shown that the frequency of multiple silent ischemic lesions is much higher than previously realized. Multiple acute ischemic lesions occur in up to 17% of patients with acute stroke and may be due to simultaneous ischemia or to silent ischemia before and/or after the index clinical event. Patients with multiple acute lesions may be at greater risk for stroke recurrence.[42]

In clinical studies, DWI has proven highly sensitive and specific for the early detection of cerebral ischemia, including subcortical ischemia and lesions in the brain stem.[49,50] The earliest clinical reports did not find a high utility for DWI, but this might have related to the late time of imaging in many patients (mean time of 10.4 days post stroke onset).[39] With DWI performed within 24–48 hours of onset, a number of clinical applications have been identified. DWI lesion volumes correlate with acute clinical severity and outcome and may have prognostic value.[51–56] In one study, a simple three-tier algorithm for the early prediction of stroke recovery was developed that incorporated measurements of the National Institutes of Health Stroke Scale score, time in hours from onset, and DWI lesion volume. This allowed the recognition of patients likely to recover from their stroke as early as 3–6 hours after onset.[57] The pattern and distribution of lesions on DWI may provide clues to the ischemic stroke mechanism that can be valuable in immediately directing the clinical work-up and management of the patient.[42] Studies are in progress to determine if DWI can be used to identify patients at greatest risk for hemorrhagic transformation after thrombolytic therapy and for detection of hyperacute intracerebral hemorrhage.[42] DWI has been used to monitor thrombolytic therapy,[43,44] and DWI lesion evolution was used as an endpoint in a large study of citicoline therapy (see Stroke Treatment and Multimodality Magnetic Resonance Imaging for further discussion of this study).[6] The cost-effectiveness of DWI in acute stroke is an important issue that is yet to be determined, but studies are in progress.

Perfusion Imaging

Brain perfusion, defined in the broadest sense as some aspect of cerebral circulation, may be studied by various MR strategies. Two MR methods, one requiring the injection of contrast and the other not, have been used to study abnormal perfusion in human stroke. Dynamic contrast-enhancing blood volume imaging involves a bolus injection of gadolinium and T2*-weighted (susceptibility-weighted) gradient echo images rapidly acquired as a series. The intravascular passage of gadolinium in sufficiently high concentration distorts the local magnetic field due to magnetic susceptibility effects (shortening of the T2* relaxation time), causing dephasing of spins in brain tissue adjacent to the blood vessels and therefore signal loss. The amount of signal loss over time in a series of rapidly acquired images may be quantified and used to calculate the parameter $\int R2^*dt$, which has been shown to be proportional to cerebral blood volume (CBV) in healthy brain tissue.[58,59] The time it takes for the change in SI to reach a maximum is related to the mean transit time (MTT) of an idealized bolus of contrast. Because cerebral blood flow (CBF) in these intravascular models equals the ratio CBV/MTT, information about CBF can potentially be inferred with this technique.

The earliest MR perfusion studies reported qualitative maps of the relative MTT (rMTT), relative CBV (rCBV), and relative CBF (rCBF). The rMTT map or variants thereof have been the most reported because it affords the best contrast between a hypoperfused brain region and normal brain. Various algorithms for generating MTT maps are each theoretically justifiable; however, there is a paucity of data for comparing their respective ability for distinguishing the perfusion parameters. The clinical significance of these algorithms should be determined.[45,48,54] Nevertheless, in acute stroke patients these qualitative perfusion maps have permitted visualization of perfusion defects in acute infarcts,

correlation of perfusion defects distal to vascular occlusions, reperfusion of spontaneously recanalized vessels, and hyperperfusion of subacute infarcts.[42,45,60] The rCBV maps were also found to correlate with arterial patency on MRA.[42,60]

More recently, efforts have been under way to provide quantitative measurements of the CBF. This requires, amongst other factors, an accurate arterial input function so that the true MTT can be deconvolved from the observed transit time of the bolus. In most algorithms, the arterial input function is identified using the passage of the contrast agent into the middle cerebral artery. In volunteers, absolute quantification has been demonstrated; however, in patients with cerebrovascular disease, there may be substantial errors related to bolus delay and dispersion in large arteries, resulting in up to 30% underestimation of the CBF.[61–63] Methodologic improvement has been reported using modeling from residue data.[63] At present, derived perfusion parameters in cerebrovascular disease should be regarded as semiquantitative.

Arterial spin labeling methods use radio frequency inversion pulses to magnetically label spins in the arterial supply to brain regions, using arterial water as an endogenous diffusible tracer.[59] These methods have been applied both to produce perfusion images and to calculate quantitative rates of CBF, based on the assumptions of the diffusible tracer kinetic models. The method has the other advantages of being noninvasive, repeatable, and can now be performed on multiple brain slices.[64–68] Methods include flow-sensitive alternating inversion recovery, continuous arterial spin labeling,[65,68] and echoplanar imaging and signal targeting with alternating radio frequency (EPISTAR).[69] The result is a map of CBF at various phases, going from a proximal arterial phase at short delays to arteriolar, capillary, and parenchymal phases at longer delays. The tagged protons in the arterial water can diffuse out into the tissue once they have reached the capillaries. One therefore can visualize tissue perfusion. The method is useful not only in demonstrating relatively ischemic tissue[66–68] but also in functional activation studies, showing increases in cortical blood flow related to local increases in brain activity.[69] There has been a report of the use of separate coils for spin labeling and imaging, which allows selective labeling of blood in either carotid artery, by which an assessment can be made of each artery's perfusion territory.[70]

Magnetic Resonance Angiography

MRA uses the three-dimensional time-of-flight or phase contrast methods to provide imaging of the intracranial vasculature in the same imaging session as the DWI and MR perfusion acquisitions. MRA rivals conventional angiography for the detection of arterial stenoses and occlusions, although there is a tendency of MRA to overestimate the degree of stenosis.[71] This tendency may be reduced by performing the scans with shorter echo times, which decrease the opportunity of turbulent flow to cause dephasing of spins and artifactual signal loss. The most promising new approach for improved MRA is contrast-enhanced MRA, in which a rapid MR acquisition is timed to a bolus injection of contrast. Such an approach may permit routine acute imaging of the vasculature from the aortic arch through the branches of the circle of Willis within minutes.[72]

Stroke Treatment and Multimodality Magnetic Resonance Imaging

The *ischemic penumbra* was originally defined as an area of reduced perfusion that has become symptomatic, but in which energy-requiring processes to maintain ionic gradients are preserved.[36,37] The significance of the penumbra is that it is the area hypothesized to be at greatest risk for development of infarction and, therefore, a logical target for presumptive reperfusion and neuroprotective therapies. Because the diffusion decrease in acute ischemia is considered to reflect a failure of Na^+-K^+-ATPase activity and subsequent cellular swelling (see preceding discussion), the penumbra may be operationally defined by MR as an area of delayed or decreased perfusion that extends beyond the region of diffusion abnormality and is correlated with the severity of clinical deficit.[45,73]

From combined DWI and perfusion imaging, approximately 70% of patients have the pattern of the operationally defined ischemic penumbra during the first 24 hours of ischemic stroke. This has otherwise been called a *perfusion-diffusion mismatch*, in which the area of DWI abnormality is surrounded by a larger area of hypoperfusion. It has been proposed that this may form a template for guiding acute stroke therapy.[45,51,52,74] In other patients, the DWI lesion is larger than the perfusion lesion in approximately 10% (presumed partial or total reperfusion), and in another 10–15% of patients, the DWI and perfusion lesions are of equivalent size (operationally defined as a completed infarct).[45,51,52]

Studies to date provide support for the concept of the operationally defined ischemic penumbra. In infarcts that evolve over time, the lesions evolve into areas defined as the penumbra on earlier scans. Evolution of infarcts *without clinical worsening* has been observed in many cases days after onset, well beyond the therapeutic window generally accepted in clinical trial research.[45] Changes in mismatch size have been shown to correlate with changes in arterial patency as measured by MRA, providing support for a vascular basis for this signature pattern.[48] Clinical correlation studies have provided some supportive correlations of DWI and MR perfusion lesion volumes within the first 6 hours, although MR templates and signature patterns that could be used as surrogate markers for clinical trials are not yet standardized.[6,51–56] Several interesting studies have used the methodology to monitor thrombolytic therapy, demonstrating reversal of some DWI and perfusion lesions with successful thrombolysis.[43,44,75] In a large study of 100 patients randomized to receive the neuroprotective agent citicoline, there was a reduction in lesion growth from baseline to week 12 with citicoline, but not significantly so. Of import was the finding that there was a significant inverse relationship between MR lesion volume change over 12 weeks and clinical outcome for ischemic stroke, supporting the role of DWI as a surrogate marker of clinically meaningful lesion progression for stroke trials.[6]

Although functional MR provides the first practical and relatively widely available method for identifying potentially viable tissue in acute stroke, it should be noted that this pattern, as currently defined, is likely a marker for the ischemic penumbra. The rMTT map, as currently generated, overestimates the area of hypoperfusion, including tissue perfused above the infarct threshold. Also, the margins of the DWI lesion may be reversible. In a proportion of patients, evolution of infarcts may be due to other processes, such as apoptosis, spreading depression, delayed neuronal injury, reperfusion injury, and recurrent silent ischemia. Several authors have tried to identify the tissue at risk for infarct progression in more detail, coming up with a combination of rCBV, rCBF, and rMTT parameters[76-78]; it may be that a combination of time-based, quantitative perfusion and ADC thresholds will be required to accurately define the penumbra. In addition, the effects of spontaneous reperfusion should be realized when interpreting results: It may be that the penumbra can only be mapped accurately in patients without early reperfusion. The incorporation of MRA with perfusion and DWI lesions may also improve the accuracy of the ischemic patterns that have been proposed.[74,79] To advance this important application of functional multimodality MR for stroke therapy, we suggest that uniform methodologic approaches be defined, standardized imaging markers for surrogate endpoints be developed, and multicenter cooperative studies be undertaken.

Conclusion

The early promise of the new functional MRI methods is being realized. The technology has become widely available and is in use in many large hospital centers around the world. The goal of obtaining DWI, MR perfusion imaging, MRA, and structural imaging of the acute stroke patient within a 15-minute scanning session is routinely achieved in many centers. The results reported in early studies have been widely replicated, showing high sensitivity and specificity for the early detection of ischemia. General broad concepts have begun to emerge regarding the optimal use of these methods in practice and in clinical trials. However, there is still a need for a consensus on optimal methodology, improved and quantitative perfusion analyses, and multicenter cooperative studies. Furthermore, in this era of cost consciousness in medical practice, there is concern about the practicality of introducing new and expensive diagnostic tests, especially in light of advances in CT methodology. Cost-effectiveness analyses will be useful in showing the impact that MRI technology is actually having in practice. The methods have important potential applications in the setting of thrombolysis by allowing optimal patient selection on a pathophysiologic basis and helping minimize the risks of therapy. There is a compelling rationale for these methods to be used in drug development and for providing an objective, quantifiable method of assessing the neuroprotective effect of drugs. The integration of this type of imaging measurements in pharmacologic clinical trials has already been undertaken in one large study and is under way in several others.

Acknowledgments

The work from our institution referred to in this chapter was supported in part by grants from the National Institute of Neurological Diseases and Stroke (NS0163401) and the Doris Duke Charitable Foundation and was performed in collaboration with Dr. Robert Edelman.

References

1. The National Institute for Neurological Disorders and Stroke rt-PA Stroke Study Group Investigators. Tissue plasminogen activator for acute stroke. N Engl J Med 1995;333:1581–1587.
2. Baird AE, Warach S. Imaging developing brain infarction. Curr Opin Neurol 1999;12:65–71.
3. Furlan A, Higashida R, Wechsler L, et al. Intra-arterial prourokinase for acute ischemic stroke: the PROACT II Study: a randomized controlled trial. JAMA 1999;282:2003–2011.
4. Muir KW, Grosset DG. Neuroprotection for acute stroke: making clinical trials work. Stroke 1999;30:180–182.
5. Katzan IL, Furlan AJ, Lloyd LE, et al. Use of tissue-type plasminogen activator for acute ischemic stroke: the Cleveland area experience. JAMA 2000;283:1151–1158.
6. Warach S, Pettigrew LC, Dashe JF, et al. Effect of citicoline on ischemic lesions measured by diffusion-weighted MRI. Citicoline 101 Investigators. Ann Neurol 2000;48:713–722.
7. Yoneda Y, Tokui K, Hanihara T, et al. Diffusion-weighted magnetic resonance imaging: detection of ischemic injury 39 minutes after onset in a stroke patient. Ann Neurol 1999;45:794–797.
8. Moseley ME, Kucharczyk J, Mintorovitch J, et al. Diffusion-weighted MR imaging of acute stroke: correlation with T2-weighted and magnetic susceptibility-enhanced MR imaging in cats. AJNR Am J Neuroradiol 1990;11:423–429.
9. Moseley ME, Cohen Y, Mintorovitch J, et al. Early detection of regional cerebral ischemia in cats: comparison of diffusion- and T2-weighted MRI and spectroscopy. Magn Reson Med 1990;14:330–346.
10. Le Bihan D, Turner R, Douek P, Patronas N. Diffusion MR imaging: clinical applications. AJR Am J Roentgenol 1992;159:591–599.

11. Stejskal EO, Tanner JE. Spin diffusion measurements: spin echoes in the presence of a time-dependent field gradient. J Chem Phys 1965;42:288–292.

12. Merboldt KD, Hanicke W, Bruhn H, et al. Diffusion imaging of the human brain in vivo using high-speed STEAM MRI. Mag Reson Med 1992;23:179–192.

13. Warach S, Chien D, Li W, et al. Fast magnetic resonance diffusion-weighted imaging of acute human stroke. Neurology 1992;42:1717–1723.

14. Moseley ME, Cohen Y, Kucharczyk J, et al. Diffusion-weighted MR imaging of anisotropic water diffusion in cat central nervous system. Radiology 1990;176:439–445.

15. van Gelderen P, de Vleeschouwer MHM, DesPres D, et al. Water diffusion and acute stroke. Magn Reson Med 1994;31:154–163.

16. Mori S, van Zijl PCM. Single-scan magnetic resonance imaging of the trace of the diffusion tensor (abstract). Presented at Second Scientific Meeting of the Society of Magnetic Resonance. Berkeley, CA: Society of Magnetic Resonance, 1994;1:135.

17. Warach S, Gaa J, Siewert B, et al. Acute human stroke studied by whole brain echo planar diffusion weighted MRI. Ann Neurol 1995;37:231–241.

18. Shimony JS, McKinstry RC, Akbudak E, et al. Quantitative diffusion-tensor anisotropy brain imaging: normative human data and anatomic analysis. Radiology 1999;212:770–784.

19. Mukherjee P, Bahn MM, McKinstry RC, et al. Differences between gray matter and white matter in stroke: diffusion-tensor MR imaging in 12 patients. Radiology 2000;215:211–220.

20. Sorensen AG, Wu O, Copen WA, et al. Human acute cerebral ischemia: detection of changes in water diffusion anisotropy by using MR imaging. Radiology 1999;212:785–792.

21. Kwong KK, McKinstry RC, Chien D, et al. CSF-suppressed quantitative single-shot diffusion imaging. Magn Reson Med 1991;21:157–163.

22. Falconer JC, Narayana PA. Cerebrospinal fluid-suppressed high-resolution diffusion imaging of human brain. Magn Reson Med 1997;37:119–123.

23. Liu G, van Gelderen P, Duyn J, Moonen CT. Single-shot diffusion MRI of human brain on a conventional clinical instrument. Magn Reson Med 1996;35:671–677.

24. Hossmann K-A. Cortical steady potential, impedance and excitability changes during and after total ischemia of cat brain. Exp Neurol 1971;32:163–175.

25. Mintorovitch J, Yang GY, Shimizu H, et al. Diffusion-weighted magnetic resonance imaging in acute focal cerebral ischemia: comparison of signal intensity with changes in brain water content and Na+, K(+)-ATPase activity. J Cereb Blood Flow Metab 1994;14:332–336.

26. Davis D, Ulatowski J, Eleff S, et al. Rapid monitoring of changes in water diffusion coefficients during reversible ischemia in cat and rat brain. Magn Reson Med 1994;31:454–460.

27. Benveniste H, Hedlund LW, Johnson GA. Mechanism of detection of acute cerebral ischemia in rats by diffusion-weighted magnetic resonance microscopy. Stroke 1992;23:746–754.

28. Back T, Hoehn-Berlage M, Kohno K, Hossmann K-A. Diffusion nuclear magnetic resonance imaging in experimental stroke. Stroke 1994;25:494–500.

29. Mintorovitch J, Moseley ME, Chileuitt L, et al. Comparison of diffusion- and T2-weighted MRI for the early detection of cerebral ischemia and reperfusion in rats. Magn Reson Med 1991;18:39–50.

30. Hasegawa Y, Fisher M, Latour LL, et al. MRI diffusion mapping of reversible and irreversible ischemic injury in focal brain ischemia. Neurology 1994;44:1484–1490.

31. Minematsu K, Fisher M, Li L, et al. Effects of a novel NMDA antagonist on experimental stroke rapidly and quantitatively assessed by diffusion-weighted MRI. Neurology 1993;43:397–403.

32. Kucharczyk J, Mintorovitch J, Moseley ME, et al. Ischemic brain damage: reduction by sodium-calcium ion channel modulator RS-87476. Radiology 1991;179:221–227.

33. Busza AL, Allen KL, King MD, et al. Diffusion-weighted imaging studies of cerebral ischemia in gerbils. Potential relevance to energy failure. Stroke 1992;23:1602–1612.

34. Gyngell ML, Back T, Hoehn-Berlage M, et al. Transient cell depolarization after permanent middle cerebral artery occlusion: an observation between diffusion-weighted MRI and localized 1H-MRS. Magn Reson Med 1994;31:337–341.

35. Latour LL, Hasegawa Y, Formato JE, et al. Spreading waves of decreased diffusion coefficient after cortical stimulation in the rat brain. Magn Reson Med 1994;32:189–198.

36. Astrup J, Siesjo BK, Symon L. Thresholds in cerebral ischemia—the ischemic penumbra. Stroke 1981;12:723–725.

37. Hakim AM. The cerebral ischemic penumbra. Can J Neurol Sci 1987;14:557–559.

38. Ulug AM, Beauchamp N, Bryan RN, van Zijl PCM. Absolute quantitation of diffusion constants in human stroke. Stroke 1997;28:483–490.

39. Lutsep HL, Albers GW, de Crespigny A, et al. Clinical utility of diffusion-weighted magnetic resonance imaging in the assessment of ischemic stroke. Ann Neurol 1997;41:574–580.

40. Schlaug G, Siewert B, Benfield A, et al. Time course of the apparent diffusion coefficient (ADC) abnormality in human stroke. Neurology 1997;49:113–119.

41. Nagesh V, Welch KMA, Windham, JP, et al. Time course of ADCw changes in ischemic stroke: beyond the human eye! Stroke 1998;29:1778–1782.

42. Baird AE, Warach S. Magnetic resonance imaging of acute stroke. J Cereb Blood Flow Metab 1998;18:583–609.

43. Marks MP, Tong DC, Beaulieu C, et al. Evaluation of early reperfusion and IV tPA therapy using diffusion- and perfusion-weighted MRI. Neurology 1999;52:1792–1798.

44. Kidwell CS, Saver JS, Mattiello J, et al. Thrombolytic reversal of acute human cerebral ischemic injury shown by diffusion/perfusion magnetic resonance imaging. Ann Neurol 2000;47:462–469.

45. Baird AE, Benfield A, Schlaug G, et al. Enlargement of human cerebral ischemic lesion volumes measured by diffusion-weighted magnetic resonance imaging. Ann Neurol 1997;41:581–589.

46. Beaulieu C, de Crespigny A, Tong DC, et al. Longitudinal magnetic resonance imaging study of perfusion and diffusion in stroke: evolution of lesion volume and correlation with clinical outcome. Ann Neurol 1999;46:568–578.

47. Schwamm LH, Koroshetz WJ, Sorensen AG, et al. Time course of lesion development in patients with acute stroke. Serial diffusion- and hemodynamic-weighted magnetic resonance imaging. Stroke 1998;29:2268–2276.

48. Barber PA, Davis SM, Darby DG, et al. Absent middle cerebral artery flow predicts the presence and evolution of the ischemic penumbra. Neurology 1999;52:1125–1132.

49. Lovblad KO, Laubach HJ, Baird AE, et al. Clinical experience with DWI in acute ischemic stroke. AJNR Am J Neuroradiol 1998;19:1061–1066.

50. Singer MB, Chong J, Lu D, et al. Diffusion-weighted MRI in acute subcortical infarction. Stroke 1998;29:133–136.

51. Neumann-Haefelin T, Wittsack HJ, Fink GR, et al. Diffusion- and perfusion-weighted MRI: the DWI/PWI mismatch region in acute stroke. Stroke 1999;30:1591–1597.

52. Barber PA, Darby DG, Desmond PM, et al. Prediction of stroke outcome with echoplanar perfusion- and diffusion-weighted MRI. Neurology 1998;51:418–426.

53. Lovblad K, Baird AE, Schlaug G, et al. Ischemic lesion volumes in acute stroke by diffusion-weighted magnetic resonance imaging correlate with clinical outcome. Ann Neurol 1997;42:164–170.

54. van Everdingen KJ, van der Grond J, Kappelle LJ, et al. Diffusion-weighted magnetic resonance imaging in acute stroke. Stroke 1998;29:1783–1790.

55. Rordorf G, Koroshetz W, Copen W, et al. Regional ischemia and ischemic injury in patients with acute middle cerebral artery stroke as defined by early diffusion-weighted and perfusion-weighted MRI. Stroke 1998;29:939–943.

56. Tong DC, Yenari M, Albers GW, et al. Correlation of perfusion and diffusion weighted MRI with NIHSS score in acute (<6.5 h) ischemic stroke patients. Neurology 1998; 50:864–870.

57. Baird AE, Chaves C, Silver B, et al. Predictive value of diffusion-weighted imaging in acute stroke. Ann Neurol 1999;46:478–479.

58. Rosen BR, Belliveau JW, Chien D. Perfusion imaging by nuclear magnetic resonance. Magn Reson Q 1989;5:263–281.

59. Detre JA, Leigh JS, Williams DS, Koretsky AP. Perfusion imaging. Magn Reson Med 1992;23:37–45.

60. Warach S, Li W, Ronthal M, Edelman RR. Evaluation of acute cerebral ischemia using dynamic contrast-enhanced MR and MR angiography. Radiology 1992;182:41–47.

61. Ostergaard L, Weisskoff RM, Chesler DA, et al. High resolution measurement of cerebral blood flow using intravascular tracer bolus passages. Part I: mathematical approach and statistical analysis. Magn Reson Med 1996; 36:715–725.

62. Ostergaard L, Sorenson A, Kwong K, et al. High resolution measurement of cerebral blood flow using intravascular tracer bolus passages. Part II: Experimental comparison and preliminary results. Magn Reson Med 1996;36:726–736.

63. Ostergaard L, Chesler DA, Weisskoff RM, et al. Modeling cerebral blood flow and flow heterogeneity from magnetic

resonance residue data. J Cereb Blood Flow Metab 1999;19:690–699.

64. Wong EC, Buxton RB, Frank LR. Quantitative perfusion imaging using arterial spin labeling. Neuroimaging Clin N Am 1999;9:333–342.

65. Detre JA, Alsop DC. Perfusion magnetic resonance imaging with continuous arterial spin labeling: methods and clinical applications in the central nervous system. Eur J Radiol 1999;30:115–124.

66. Siewert B, Schlaug G, Edelman RR, Warach S. Comparison of EPISTAR and T2*-weighted gadolinium-enhanced perfusion in patients with acute cerebral ischemia. Neurology 1997;48:673–679.

67. Detre JA, Alsop DC, Vives LR, et al. Noninvasive MRI evaluation of cerebral blood flow in cerebrovascular disease. Neurology 1998;50:633–641.

68. Chalela JA, Alsop DC, Gonzalez-Atavales JB, et al. Magnetic resonance perfusion imaging in acute ischemic stroke using continuous arterial spin labeling. Stroke 2000;31:680–687.

69. Edelman RR, Siewert B, Darby DG, et al. Qualitative mapping of cerebral blood flow and functional localization with EPISTAR MRI. Radiology 1994;192:513–520.

70. Zaharchuk G, Ledden PJ, Kwong KK, et al. Multislice perfusion and perfusion territory imaging in humans with separate label and image coils. Magn Reson Med 1999;41:1093–1098.

71. Polak JF, Bajakian RL, Oleary DH, et al. Detection of internal carotid artery stenosis: comparison of MR angiography, color Doppler sonography, and arteriography. Radiology 1992;182:35–40.

72. Foo TK, Ho VB, Choyke PL. Contrast-enhanced carotid MR angiography. Imaging principles and physics. Neuroimaging Clin N Am 1999;9:263–284.

73. Schlaug G, Benfield A, Baird AE, et al. The ischemic penumbra operationally defined by perfusion and diffusion. Neurology 1999;53:1528–1537.

74. Albers GW. Expanding the time window for thrombolytic therapy in acute stroke. The potential role of acute MRI for patient selection. Stroke 1999;30:2230–2237.

75. Schellinger PD, Jansen O, Fiebach JB, et al. Monitoring intravenous recombinant tissue plasminogen activator thrombolysis for acute ischemic stroke with diffusion and perfusion MRI. Stroke 2000;31:1318–1328.

76. Sorensen AG, Copen WA, Ostergaard L, et al. Hyperacute stroke: simultaneous measurement of relative cerebral blood volume, relative cerebral blood flow, and mean tissue transit time. Radiology 1999;210:519–527.

77. Warach S, Wielopolski P, Edelman RR. Identification and characterization of the ischemic penumbra of acute human stroke using echo planar diffusion and perfusion imaging. Presented at the Twelfth Annual Scientific Meeting of the Society of Magnetic Resonance in Medicine, 1993;1(abstract):263.

78. Kidwell CS, Alger JR, Saver JS, et al. MR signatures of infarction vs. salvageable penumbra in acute human stroke: a preliminary model. Stroke 2000;31:285.

79. Koroshetz W, Gonzales G. Imaging stroke in progress: magnetic resonance advances but computed tomography is poised for counterattack. Ann Neurol 1999;46:556–558.

Chapter 4

Ultrasound Imaging in Ischemic Cerebrovascular Disease

Alejandro M. Forteza, Andrei V. Alexandrov, and Viken L. Babikian

Stroke is no longer considered an untreatable condition today because effective therapeutic strategies have been developed for most of the common causes of brain ischemia. These treatments are not without complications, however, and it is increasingly recognized that ischemic cerebrovascular disease is not a uniform condition, with each subtype requiring its own specific treatment. These considerations have led to an increased emphasis on accurate diagnosis based on an understanding of specific pathophysiology, and this, in turn, has stimulated research in technologies, such as computed tomography (CT), magnetic resonance imaging (MRI), ultrasonography, and contrast angiography, to image the brain and its arteries. This chapter focuses on the ultrasound-based evaluation of patients with ischemic cerebrovascular disease. A practical and therapy-oriented approach to the diagnostic process is presented.

Evaluation of Patients Who Present within Six Hours from Onset of Symptoms

The results of the study by the National Institute of Neurological Disorders and Stroke regarding the treatment of acute ischemic stroke with intravenous tissue plasminogen activator (t-PA) placed the disease in the list of emergencies amenable to effective therapy.[1] The American Heart Association and the American Academy of Neurology have issued guidelines for the implementation of the study's findings.[2,3] Their recommendations include a clinical examination based on the National Institutes of Health Stroke Scale (NIHSS), some blood tests, and a brain CT scan. The results of these tests determine whether a patient is a candidate for intravenous t-PA thrombolysis.

The preceding approach is relatively simple and pragmatic, and has the advantage of being applicable to a large number of patients. It should be remembered, however, that between 20% to 55% of patients do not have arterial occlusions when examined angiographically.[4–6] Thus, the "one treatment for all" approach may expose some individuals to the complications of thrombolysis without offering them a potential for any benefit, because they have no thrombi to be lysed. The "lumpers" approach has been criticized,[7,8] and a more thorough evaluation that includes imaging of the cerebral arteries and heart has been recommended.[7] The recommendation is even more relevant for patients who may be eligible for intra-arterial prourokinase or combined intravenous and intra-arterial thrombolytic therapy during the 6-hour window after the onset of symptoms.

Thus, imaging of the cerebral arteries is not routinely obtained before thrombolytic therapy. In the acute setting, ultrasound imaging can be clinically useful as a diagnostic aid and for monitoring the effects of specific interventions. It may also have a therapeutic potential. These applications are reviewed in the following paragraphs.

Extracranial Cerebral Arteries

The evaluation of the common carotid artery bifurcation with ultrasound in the acute setting is not well studied. An ultrasound-based approach has been proposed to evaluate the extracranial and intracranial circulation in acute ischemic stroke.[9] Imaging is indicated at centers with the capability to provide intra-arterial thrombolysis. The latter has been recommended for patients with carotid occlusion because it is difficult to establish patency with intravenous thrombolysis in the acute setting.[10–12] MR or CT angiography (MRA and CTA, respectively) are often obtained, but they have substantial limitations. When used in conjunction with transcranial ultrasonography, duplex imaging presents an alternative that needs further assessment.

Although controversial, urgent carotid artery endarterectomy is occasionally considered in selected patients with severe carotid stenosis, who have recurrent symptoms of cerebral ischemia despite medical treatment.[12–17] The approach seems reasonable given the poor outcome associated with unstable carotid syndromes.[10,11,15,17,18] Experience with early surgery remains limited. Duplex imaging is sufficient to establish a diagnosis in such cases.

Urgent ultrasound scanning of the common carotid artery bifurcation is not customarily performed in the acute stroke setting. Save for the exceptional circumstances presented in the preceding paragraphs, it is not recommended because it is unlikely to change the therapeutic approach.

Intracranial Arteries

Cerebral contrast angiography shows an arterial occlusion in 45–80% of patients with symptoms referable to the middle cerebral artery (MCA), if the study is performed within the initial 6 hours of symptoms.[4–6] Up to 70% of the occlusions are recanalized 1 week later.[4] Transcranial Doppler ultrasound (TCD) studies have confirmed these findings. TCD appropriately identifies a MCA or internal carotid artery (ICA) stenosis or occlusion in 70–88% of patients studied within 4–6 hours from the onset of symptoms,[19,20] with 86% recanalization 2 weeks later.[19] Absent MCA or supraclinoid ICA signals and severely "blunted" or asymmetric MCA signals strongly suggest arterial obstruction.[19,21] When compared to angiography, TCD's sensitivity in detecting ICA proximal or distal occlusions is 94% and 81%, respectively. TCD's sensitivity is 93% for MCA and 60% for basilar artery occlusions.[22–24] Specificity ranges from 96% to 98%.[22] In addition, when the TCD study is normal, there is a 94% chance that angiography will also fail to find an occlusion.[22] Contrast-enhanced transcranial color-coded duplex sonography (TCCD) may be even more sensitive than TCD in detecting ICA distribution occlusions.[25] These findings suggest that TCD can be used as an initial screening test when assessing patients presenting with acute stroke in the emergency room. TCD findings may help in the selection of candidates for intra-arterial or intravenous thrombolysis.

TCD findings during the first few hours after the onset of stroke symptoms may have prognostic value.[4,19,21,26,27] A normal or improving spectral pattern in consecutive studies is associated with a good prognosis, whereas an abnormal initial study is predictive of a poor outcome.[19,27]

TCD has been used to monitor spontaneous[28] and thrombolytic-induced[29–31] recanalization. The latter is diagnosed when low-resistance, stenotic, or normal flow patterns are found throughout the MCA with no other findings of persisting distal occlusion, such as a dampened distal signal. A low-resistance flow pattern correlates with angiographic patency, and persistence of absent, blunted, or dampened signals indicates unresolved occlusion. TCD is more than 90% accurate in discriminating between complete MCA recanalization and persisting occlusion.[32] Repeat testing several hours later, when the patient is no longer in the angiography suite and MRA and CTA are difficult to perform, can determine whether hyperemia has resolved, residual stenosis persists, or reocclusion has occurred. Recanalization can precede clinical recovery.[33] Based on the spectral pattern at the end of intravenous therapy,[32,34] TCD may also help in the decision regarding the need for further intra-arterial thrombolysis.

The following case report illustrates TCD's ability to monitor during thrombolysis. A 93-year-old man developed right hemiparesis and aphasia, and had an NIHSS score of 13 points at the time of presentation. Brain CT scan showed no early ischemic changes. Intravenous t-PA was started at 2 hours and 45 minutes from the onset of symptoms. TCD monitoring showed a reduced signal without an end-diastolic flow component, suggesting occlusion of the left MCA (Color Plate 1). Twenty-one minutes after the t-PA bolus was given, a partial improvement of the signal was noted with increased peak-systolic velocity, and microembolic signals were detected. This suggested the beginning of recanalization.[35] The neurologic deficit started improving, and the NIHSS score became 11. Eleven minutes later, the left MCA signal was restored, and the velocity and pulsatility values were equal to those from the nonaffected right MCA, indicating complete recanalization. By this time, the motor deficit had resolved, speech was improving rapidly, and the NIHSS score was 3. The neurologic deficit had completely resolved the next morning.

Compared to other neuroimaging technologies, TCD has substantial advantages for the purpose of assessing the effects of thrombolytic therapy. It offers continuous monitoring of the very variable that thrombolysis attempts to modify. Testing can be completed within minutes, at the bedside and in the emergency room, without causing delays in treatment. It also provides a means to monitor the efficacy of an essentially blind intravenous therapy. TCD's main limitations are its relatively low sensitivity in detecting occlusions in some arterial segments and an inability to assess the distal branches of basal cerebral arteries.

Ultrasound as a Therapeutic Adjuvant to Thrombolysis

Ultrasound is increasingly recognized as a therapeutic tool. High-intensity, low-frequency ultrasound is used routinely to disintegrate kidney and gallbladder stones.[36,37] An ultrasound scalpel has already been developed,[38] and therapeutic ultrasound is used to "clean" calcified mitral valves.[39] Although the concept of ultrasound-enhanced thrombolysis is not new,[40–42] its application to clinical vascular medicine is relatively recent. Since the mid-1980s, ultrasound has been used to lyse emboli.[43,44] Transcutaneous and catheter-delivered ultrasound is effective and can recanalize occluded coronaries and peripheral arteries.[45–47]

Low-frequency ultrasound administered through the temporal bone of human cadavers is able to enhance urokinase clot lysis.[48,49] Similar results have also been achieved in an in vitro model.[50] In a canine carotid occlusion model, Barnwell et al. showed that catheter-based ultrasound enhances the recanalization rate of urokinase.[51] Using standard TCD equipment, Alexandrov et al. reported on the arterial recanalization rate in acute ischemic stroke patients treated with intravenous t-PA. A higher number of patients than expected from historical controls achieved recanalization and clinical improvement.[52] These studies suggest that ultrasound-facilitated thrombolysis may have a role in the treatment of acute ischemic stroke. Further technologic advances are expected in this rapidly growing field.

Evaluation of Patients Who Present More Than Six Hours after Onset of Symptoms

The risk of "stroke in progression" or recurrent cerebral ischemic event is approximately 10–20% during the 3-week period after a brain infarct.[53,54] This risk is not uniform among the different subtypes of stroke.[55] Patients with large-vessel stenosis are at a higher risk for recurrence at 30 days than those with lacunes or infarcts of uncertain cause.[55] Also, lesions causing more than 50% stenosis of intracranial arteries are associated with a more than 10% yearly rate of recurrent ischemic events,[56,57] with most recurrences occurring soon after initial presentation. In symptomatic ICA extracranial severe disease, the risk is 44% at 2 years, and approximately one-half of recurrent infarcts occur during the first 2 months of follow-up.[58]

In addition to the early risk for recurrence, most stroke patients are at an increased, long-term risk for repeated cerebral infarction. Although the latter gradually decreases with the passage of time, it persists in certain conditions, such as nonvalvular atrial fibrillation,[59] and may actually increase as new arterial and cardiac lesions develop or old ones progress.

The evaluation of stroke patients who present more than 6 hours after the onset of stroke symptoms is focused on identifying arterial or cardiac lesions that increase the risk of early or late recurrence. Therapeutic options at this stage include antiplatelet agents, intravenous anticoagulation, and carotid endarterectomy or other revascularization procedures.

Extracranial Cerebral Arteries

ICA-origin stenoses constitute approximately 15–20% of all causes of brain infarction. Duplex imaging enables clinicians to portray the arterial wall and to assess corresponding intraluminal hemodynamic changes (Color Plate 2). Color-coded duplex imaging (CDI) is increasingly used because it improves the overall accuracy of duplex testing (see Color Plate 2). When compared to cerebral angiography, the sensitivity of CDI exceeds 95%, and its specificity ranges between 80% to 85%[60–62]; the overall accuracy is approximately 90%. Batteries of ultrasound criteria have been developed by several groups[63] to grade severity of ICA stenosis, but none is universally accepted. Most batteries combine several variables, including the peak-systolic and end-diastolic velocities, and ratios of velocities in the internal and common carotid arteries. A peak systolic velocity of 140 cm/sec or more, an end-diastolic velocity approaching (but not exceeding) 110 cm/sec, and an internal to common carotid artery velocity ratio exceeding 2 are often considered threshold criteria indicative of 50% stenosis or more (Color Plates 3 and 4).[64] Although the ability to detect complete occlusion is improved with CDI,[60] especially when an echocontrast agent is used,[65] cerebral angiography is still occasionally obtained to confirm the diagnosis. This is because the surgical option hinges on the demonstration of a patent artery, which ultrasound imaging can occasionally fail to detect. The ability of CDI to detect ICA dissection remains limited,[66] but CDI testing may be useful for the long-term monitoring of these patients. TCD can detect the intracranial hemodynamic effects of extracranial stenoses (Color Plate 5).

B-mode imaging has the unique capability of imaging the arterial wall (Figure 4-1) and the characteristics of atherosclerotic plaques. The finding of hypoechoic plaques is clinically relevant because they are associated with an increased risk of cerebral infarction, especially when the severity of stenosis exceeds 50%.[67,68] B-mode is also more sensitive than angiography in imaging plaque ulceration,[69] another feature associated with an increased risk of stroke.[70] Thus, although severity of stenosis remains the main criterion regarding the decision for carotid endarterectomy, the finding of hypoechoic plaque or ulceration on ultrasound imaging can help clinicians in further stratifying the risk for stroke and finalizing the decision for surgery.

The possibility of imaging the cerebral vasculature with MRA rather than ultrasound is an option available at most medical centers, and several studies have compared the accuracy of the two technologies to contrast angiography. At the time of this writing, available data do not permit a clear recommendation. Cost of testing, quality of equipment, experience of laboratory personnel, and the ability of a specific patient to cooperate are some of the factors that should affect the physician's decision regarding the diagnostic workup. Both technologies tend to overestimate the severity of stenosis,[71] and, as indicated in the preceding paragraphs, they can miss the presence of occlusion.[72] Most centers use a combination of duplex ultrasound and MRA to assess patients with carotid stenosis. It appears that the combination of the two tests, supplemented by cerebral angiography for disparate results, is associated with the lowest morbidity and mortality, and has a favorable cost-effectiveness ratio for the detection of lesions causing 70–99% stenosis.[73] The combination of MRA and ultrasound has increasingly replaced cerebral angiography in the preoperative evaluation of patients with symptomatic carotid stenosis. Ultrasound also offers a means for assessing the results of carotid endarterectomy and other interventional procedures (Color Plate 6).

Extracranial arterial lesions also include stenotic plaques of the vertebral artery origin, an arterial segment with substantial disease in approximately 20% of patients who present with ischemic symptoms of the posterior cerebral circulation.[74] Duplex imaging, TCD, and routine MRA do not

Figure 4-1. B-mode image of a common carotid artery (CCA) plaque. The noncalcified plaque (*arrow*) causes no significant luminal reduction. (RT = right.)

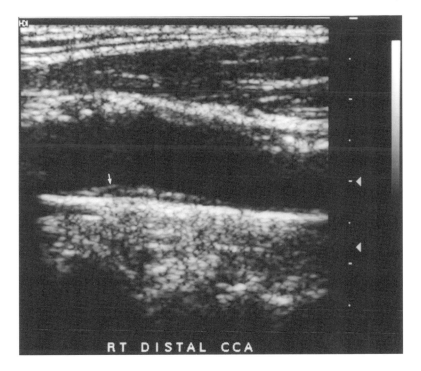

RT DISTAL CCA

assess the V1 portion of the vertebral artery. When clinically indicated, contrast MRA or cerebral angiography are obtained to further evaluate the original segments of the vertebral arteries.

Intracranial Arteries

Approximately 5–10% of brain infarcts are caused by stenotic lesions of intracranial arteries. Atherosclerotic plaques are frequently detected at the ICA siphon, MCA M1 segment, first half of the basilar artery, and V4 segment of the vertebral arteries.[56,57] Dissection[75] and arteritis can occur at these and other intracranial locations. TCD, MRA, CTA, and contrast angiography are technologies available to detect these lesions.

Transcranial ultrasound imaging includes the more traditional TCD method and, increasingly, TCCD. TCD criteria for intracranial stenoses have been published by several groups, but no battery is universally accepted. Lesions causing more than 50% luminal narrowing are associated with increased flow velocities at the site of stenosis, increased pulsatility indices proximal to the lesion, and arterial wall vibration (Color Plate 7). The

Stroke Outcome and Neuroimaging of Intracranial Atherosclerosis study, a research project funded by the National Institutes of Health, is testing the accuracy of TCD and MRA, as compared to cerebral angiography. Cutpoints for positive TCD studies include mean flow velocities of 100 cm/sec for the MCA, 90 cm/sec for the intracranial ICA, and 80 cm/sec for the V4 segment of the vertebral artery and the basilar artery. Published studies suggest that compared to cerebral angiography, TCD is more than 90% sensitive and 95% specific in detecting stenoses of the ICA siphon and MCA M1 segment.[76] Its sensitivity and specificity are lower when screening for lesions of the vertebrobasilar system (74% and 86%, respectively).[77] MRA may be more accurate when imaging lesions of the posterior cerebral circulation. Results are slightly better with TCCD testing (Color Plate 8). "Blind spots" include the distal third of the basilar artery.[78] The frequent tortuosity of the vertebral and basilar arteries is a common source of error. It should be noted that the accuracy of contrast angiography in detecting intracranial stenoses has been questioned, because angiography is often limited to a single lateral or anteroposterior view when imaging these arteries.

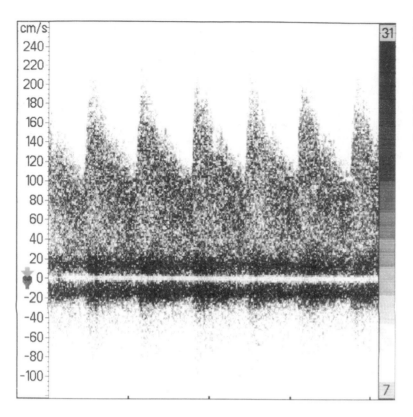

Figure 4-2. Sickle-cell disease in a patient with no history of stroke. The peak-systolic and end-diastolic velocities are 200 cm/sec and 110 cm/sec, respectively, at a depth of insonation corresponding to the distal internal carotid artery. They indicate the presence of an arteriopathy.

TCD testing has several limitations. In approximately 5–15% of patients, an adequate ultrasonic window is not present because of temporal bone hyperostosis, a limitation commonly encountered in elderly women. The Doppler signal can be substantially improved with the intravenous administration of ultrasonic contrast media, however.[79] Several contrast agents are either already available for clinical use or are undergoing phase III trials in western European countries. Although available in the United States for cardiac applications, no such agent has been approved by the U.S. Food and Drug Administration for use during the evaluation of neurologic disease. Limitations also include the lack of information regarding the angle of insonation during routine TCD testing. This angle can be measured with TCCD. In addition, several medications, the cardiac rhythm, and the hematocrit can affect TCD findings and should be taken into consideration when interpreting results.

Although not a common cause of stroke in adults, a cerebral arteriopathy occurs in sickle cell anemia and is associated with an increased risk for stroke in children. In the United States, the condition is predominantly seen in African Americans. TCD testing shows increased flow velocities in most intracranial arteries, particularly in the distal branches of the intracranial ICA. A time-averaged, maximum mean flow velocity exceeding 200 cm/sec in the MCA identifies asymptomatic children at an increased risk for stroke (Figure 4-2).[80] The risk is markedly reduced by periodic blood transfusions. A clinical alert from the National Heart, Lung and Blood Institute has recommended that patients with sickle-cell disease receive regular TCD testing to evaluate their stroke risk.[81]

Atherosclerotic stenoses of the intracranial arteries are dynamic lesions, and repeat angiographic or TCD studies show progression or regression over time.[82,83] Follow-up TCD studies are recommended for these patients. Further increases of flow velocities during follow-up or the development of arterial wall covibration indicate progression of disease. Criteria regarding progression of stenosis in intracranial arteries are not as well established as those for extracranial ICA disease.

Cerebrovascular Physiology

In the context of routine clinical care, the main purpose of cerebrovascular imaging is to detect stenotic or occlusive lesions. Ultrasound testing can also be used to detect cerebral microembolism and to assess vasomotor reactivity.

The ability to detect cerebral embolism in vivo is a unique capability of TCD testing. High-intensity, transient signals with specific characteristics correspond to particles composed of platelet-fibrinogen, cholesterol, and air in laboratory models and in clinical settings (Color Plate 9).[84] In patients with ICA or aortic arch stenosis, these particles are associated with symptoms of retinal or cerebral ischemia,[85] and their presence is a risk factor for future cerebral ischemic events.[86] Microembolic signals are also associated with plaque ulceration. They are helpful in identifying "active" athrosclerotic plaques, and can also be useful in other conditions, such as the fat embolism syndrome.[87] Monitoring during carotid endarterectomy can identify patients at an increased risk for infarction.[88,89]

Cerebrovascular reactivity refers to the response of the cerebral vasculature to vasoactive substances, such as acetazolamide and carbon dioxide. Cerebral blood flow (and velocity) changes in response to fluctuations in the level of carbon dioxide are mediated through dilatation or constriction of pial arteries, arterioles, and—to a lesser degree—large arteries at the base of the brain. The response is diminished in patients with hypertension, diabetes mellitus, and cerebral microangiopathy,[90] and is impaired distal to extracranial ICA occlusion or severe stenosis.[91,92] Long-term monitoring of patients with asymptomatic severe stenosis shows an association between impaired vasoreactivity and risk of ipsilateral ischemic events.[91] With the recently renewed interest in extracranial-intracranial bypass surgery, TCD testing may be potentially useful in selecting candidates for surgery.

Aortic Arch

The role of atherosclerotic plaques of the ascending aorta and aortic arch as a risk factor for recurrent cerebral ischemia is now well documented.[93,94] The prevalence of the condition was 25.6% in a study of patients referred for transesophageal echocardiography (TEE) after a stroke.[94] Plaques 4 mm or more in thickness and those with mobile thrombi or debris are associated with an increased risk of stroke (Figure 4-3),[95] and it is not unusual for patients to harbor tandem plaques at the aortic arch and the ICA origin. Because the incidence of recurrent brain ischemic events is in excess of 10% in symptomatic patients with thick aortic arch plaques, antiplatelet agents or anticoagulants are prescribed to prevent recurrence. Patients receiving anticoagulants may have a better outcome than those treated with antiplatelet agents.[94]

Although it tends to underestimate the severity of atherosclerosis,[96] TEE is the method of choice for noninvasive detection of plaques of the ascending segment and arch of the aorta. B-mode ultrasonography from the lateral supraclavicular fossa has been used at some centers,[97] but experience with the technique remains limited. TEE is associated with a small risk for complications, including cardiac arrhythmias and aspiration. The complication rate is higher in patients with swallowing difficulty and some esophageal or pulmonary disorders, conditions that are not uncommon in stroke patients.

Cardiac Chambers

The cardiac chambers are the source of cerebral emboli in approximately 15–20% of all ischemic strokes.[98–102] Thorough cardiac evaluations are especially indicated in patients younger than 45 years of age, in whom cardioembolism may be the cause of stroke in up to 36% of cases.[103,104] A cardiogenic mechanism may be suspected from the clinical presentation. A history of recent myocardial infarction, atrial fibrillation, and a deficit of sudden onset suggest cardiac embolism. The deficit tends to be maximal from the beginning, and at least some degree of cortical dysfunction is usually part of the symptom complex. In addition, CT and MRI show a wedge-shaped lesion that has a wider base toward the cortex and is prone to hemorrhagic transformation.

Cardiac testing usually starts after the first 24 hours, and in most cases includes an electrocardiogram and an ultrasound study. A limited review of

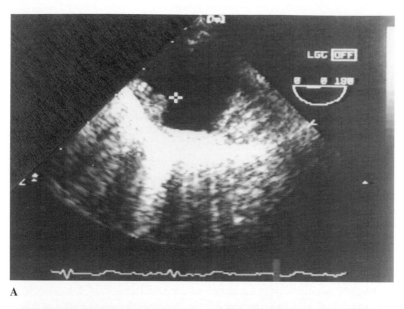

A

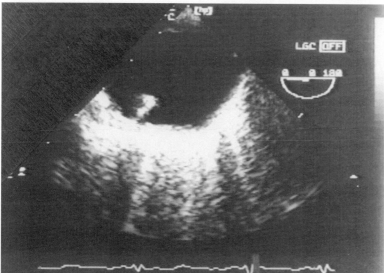

B

Figure 4-3. Aortic arch plaque. The transesophageal echocardiogram shows a 7-mm sessile plaque (*cursor*) in the proximal aortic arch of this patient with a history of transient monocular blindness (**A**). A mobile thrombus is detected in the ascending aorta of a patient with brain infarction (**B**).

the cardiac ultrasound evaluation is presented in the following paragraphs. More comprehensive reviews have been published elsewhere.[105–108]

Transthoracic echocardiography (TTE), a noninvasive and well-established technique that can be performed at the bedside, allows visualization of the cardiac chambers, and is the preferred method to estimate the left ventricular ejection fraction. It can also assess cardiac chamber configuration and dimensions, valvular abnormalities, left ventricular thrombi, and ventricular akinetic segments.[105,106] Acoustic attenuation caused by the lungs, subcutaneous tissues, and calcium are some of the limitations of TTE. TEE, a minimally invasive procedure requiring conscious sedation, is more accurate than TTE at identifying left atrial thrombi. It provides detailed views of the mitral valve structure and interatrial shunts and detects the presence of intra-atrial spontaneous echocontrast. The proximity of the esophagus to the left atrium is the main reason for this improved accuracy.[109–114] TEE is also an effective clinical method to evaluate the ascending aorta and aortic arch.

There is no consensus in the literature regarding the method of choice in the evaluation of patients with suspected cardioembolism. Most clinicians usually start with a TTE, and a TEE is obtained depending on TTE's results. This strategy is not necessarily correct, and it is the subject of much debate. TEE is unquestionably more accurate at detecting potential sources of embolism in patients with infarcts of unclear etiology.[113,115] Furthermore, the practice of initial TEE testing for all stroke patients, as opposed to only for those with a known cardiac disorder, may be more cost-effective than that of performing sequential TTE and TEE studies, based on clinical judgment.[116] The improved diagnostic capability does not consistently result in a change in therapy, however. It should also be remembered that negative echocardiographic studies do not rule out a cardioembolic etiology. Emboli may be too small and beyond the resolution of ultrasound, or they may no longer be in the cardiac chambers where they originated.[117] Table 4-1 presents the relative advantages of TTE and TEE as they relate to various cardiac lesions.

Paradoxical embolism through a patent foramen ovale is an increasingly recognized cause of stroke, and this is especially true in young adults in whom other causes of stroke cannot be found.[118,119] TEE, the gold standard, and TCD can both diagnose right to left cardiac shunts with high sensitivity and specificity.[120,121] A patent foramen ovale is usually diagnosed by TEE when microbubbles are seen crossing through the interatrial septum shortly after the injection of agitated saline in a peripheral vein (Color Plate 10). TCD testing involves insonation of one or both MCAs. The appearance of microembolic signals within 10 seconds from the injection of agitated saline in a peripheral vein is indicative of a right to left shunt (see Color Plate 10).

When compared to TEE, TCD has a sensitivity of 91–100% and a specificity that ranges between 65% to 93%. TCD has the advantage of being able to detect extracardiac shunts, such as pulmonary arteriovenous fistulas.[122] Because the latter cannot

Table 4-1. Relative Advantages of Transthoracic (TTE) and Transesophageal Echocardiography (TEE) as They Relate to Specific Cardiac Lesions

Cardiac Source	TTE	TEE
Valvular heart disease	++	+++
Endocarditis/vegetations	+	+++[134]
Mitral valve prolapse	++	++[135]
Valvular strands	±	+++[136,137]
Left atrial thrombi	+	+++[138]
Patent foramen ovale[a]	+	+++[139,140]
Atrial septal defects	+	+++[141]
Atrial septal aneurysm	+	+++[142]
Spontaneous echo contrast	+	+++[143]
Cardiac myxomas	+++	+++[144,b]
Left ventricular thrombi	+++[145]	++/+++[144,c]
Left ventricular hypokinesis/ LVEF	+++[105]	++
Apical aneurysm	+++	++
Cardioembolism of uncertain etiology	++	+++++[115,146]

LVEF = left ventricular ejection fraction; +, ++, +++, +++++, ± = compared sensitivity of method for specific conditions from less sensitive (+) to most sensitive (+++++).
[a]Need contrast.
[b]TTE and TEE can detect left-sided cardiac tumors at similar rates, but TEE is superior at detecting masses involving the right heart.[144]
[c]TEE is comparable but not superior to TTE in detecting left ventricular thrombi.[144]

be diagnosed with TEE, they can increase TCD's false positive rate and decrease its specificity when the two methods are compared. The administration of ultrasonic contrast agents and performance of the valsalva maneuver can improve the sensitivity of TCD.[120,123,124]

Evaluation of Patients with Vascular Risk Factors

The evaluation of patients with asymptomatic neck bruits is considered standard practice today, because bruits are associated with plaque formation at the common carotid artery bifurcation, and antithrombotic agents or carotid endarterectomy can be therapeutic options.[125] Duplex imaging is accurate, noninvasive, relatively inexpensive, and an appropriate means to assess the extracranial ICA in this setting. Duplex imaging is also useful to monitor patients with known disease. Disease progression is characterized by further increases of peak-systolic and end-diastolic velocities, and the development of turbulence. Asymptomatic patients with severe stenosis are considered candidates for endarterectomy.[125]

The timing of repeat testing must be individualized, however, because the rate of plaque progression is not well understood and varies among patients, and there are no published guidelines. The ultrasonic characteristics of a lesion, such as the presence of ulceration or hypoechoic plaque formation, can be helpful when making a decision. For patients with less than 50% stenosis, the authors obtain a first repeat study after 12–24 months, and for those with 50–75% disease, repeat testing is obtained within 12 months.

Whether patients with vascular risk factors should be screened for the presence of ICA stenosis remains a matter of debate. Screening large populations with ultrasound is not cost-effective, and patient selection is clearly indicated. Carotid stenosis of 60–99% is present in approximately 25% of patients with peripheral arterial disease,[126] and it is prevalent in elderly patients with coronary disease.[127,128] Screening is indicated at medical centers where carotid endarterectomy and coronary artery bypass graft surgery are regularly performed in the setting of one operation.

The extracranial carotid artery intima-media thickness, measured with high-resolution B-mode scanning, is a marker for diffuse atherosclerosis[129] and is an independent risk factor for myocardial infarction and stroke.[130–132] Because it can be measured noninvasively, the intima-media thickness can potentially be used as a surrogate endpoint to assess disease progression and to monitor the effects of therapy. The capability to measure the intima-media thickness is an exciting development, but its clinical value is still undetermined.[133]

Conclusion

This chapter summarizes the "state of the art" applications of ultrasound technology as they are relevant to the care of patients with ischemic cerebrovascular disease. The authors have taken a pragmatic approach, and they recognize that the chapter does not present a comprehensive review of the subject. Rather, it emphasizes the common uses and substantial diagnostic advantages and limitations of ultrasound technology, which should be taken into account by clinicians who rely on ultrasound testing.

To a large degree, advances in the medical sciences are driven by technological developments that enable clinicians to respond to previously unanswered questions. This is certainly true in stroke, in which contrast angiography, CT, MRI, ultrasound, and other technologies have framed the understanding of the disease process to such a profound degree that it is virtually impossible to take care of patients without some diagnostic testing. In spite of these advances, however, the understanding and available diagnostic capabilities remain limited. In an era of rapid change, ultrasound technology is expected to evolve and become increasingly responsive to the changing needs of patients.

References

1. The National Institute of Neurological Disorders and Stroke rt-PA Stroke Study Group. Tissue plasminogen activator for acute ischemic stroke. N Engl J Med 1995;333:1581–1587.
2. Adams HP Jr, Brott TG, Furlan AJ, et al. Guidelines for thrombolytic therapy for acute stroke: a supplement to the guidelines for the management of patients with acute ischemic stroke. A statement for healthcare professionals from a special writing group of the Stroke Council, American Heart Association. Stroke 1996;27:1711–1718.
3. Practice advisory: thrombolytic therapy for acute stroke—summary statement. Report of the Quality Standard Subcommittee of the American Academy of Neurology. Neurology 1996;47:835–839.
4. Fieschi C, Argentino C, Lenzi GL, et al. Clinical and instrumental evaluation of patients with ischemic stroke within the first six hours. J Neurol Sci 1989;91:311–321.
5. del Zoppo GJ, Higashida R, Furlan A, et al. PROACT Investigators: a phase II randomized trial of recombinant pro-urokinase by direct arterial delivery in acute middle cerebral artery stroke. Stroke 1998;29:4–11.
6. Horowitz SH, Zito JL, Donnarumma R, et al. Computed tomographic-angiographic findings within the first five hours of cerebral infarction. Stroke 1991;22:1245–1253.
7. Caplan LR. Stroke treatment: promising but still struggling. JAMA 1998;279:1304–1306.
8. Caplan LR, Mohr JP, Kistler JP, et al. Should thrombolytic therapy be first line treatment for acute ischemic stroke? Thrombolysis—not a panacea for ischemic stroke. N Engl J Med 1997;337:1309–1310.
9. Martin PJ, Pye IF, Abbott, RJ, Naylor AR. Color-coded ultrasound diagnosis of vascular occlusion in acute ischemic stroke. J Neuroimaging 1995;5:152–156.

10. Trouillas P, Nighoghossian N, Derex L, et al. Thrombolysis with intravenous rtPA in a series of 100 cases of acute carotid territory stroke: determination of etiological, topographic, and radiological outcome factors. Stroke 1998;29:2529–2540.

11. Endo S, Kuwayama N, Hirashima Y, et al. Results of urgent thrombolysis in patients with major stroke and atherothrombotic occlusion of the cervical internal carotid artery. AJNR Am J Neuroradiol 1998;19:1169–1175.

12. del Zoppo GJ, Poeck K, Pessin MS, et al. Recombinant tissue plasminogen activator in acute thrombotic and embolic stroke. Ann Neurol 1992;32:78–86.

13. Meyer FB, Sundt TM Jr, Piepgras DG, et al. Emergency carotid endarterectomy for patients with acute carotid occlusion and profound neurological deficits. Ann Surg 1986;203:82–89.

14. Mentzer RM Jr, Finkelmeier BA, Crosby IK, Wellons HA Jr. Emergency endarterectomy for fluctuating neurologic deficits. Surgery 1981;89:60–66.

15. Walters BB, Ojemann RG, Heros RC. Emergency carotid endarterectomy. J Neurosurg 1987;66:817–823.

16. Eckstein HH, Schumacher H, Klemm K, et al. Emergency carotid endarterectomy. Cerebrovasc Dis 1999;9:270–281.

17. Pikus HJ, Heros RC. Stroke: indications for emergent surgical interventions. Clin Neurosurg 1999;45:113–127.

18. Jansen O, von Kummer R, Forsting M, et al. Thrombolytic therapy in acute occlusions of the intracranial carotid artery bifurcation. AJNR Am J Neuroradiol 1995;16:1977–1986.

19. Alexandrov AV, Bladin CF, Norris JW. Intracranial blood flow velocities in acute ischemic stroke. Stroke 1994;25:1378–1383.

20. Camerlingo M, Casto L, Censori B, et al. Transcranial Doppler in acute ischemic stroke of the middle cerebral artery territories. Acta Neurol Scand 1993;88:108–111.

21. Halsey JH. Prognosis of acute hemiplegia estimated by transcranial Doppler ultrasonography. Stroke 1988;19:648–649.

22. Demchuk AM, Christou I, Wein TH, et al. Accuracy and criteria for localizing arterial occlusions with transcranial Doppler. J Neuroimaging 2000;10:1–12.

23. Brandt T, Knauth M, Wildermuth S, et al. CT angiography and Doppler sonography for emergency assessment in acute basilar ischemia. Stroke 1999;30:606–612.

24. Demchuk AM, Christou I, Wein TH, et al. Specific transcranial Doppler flow findings related to the presence and site of arterial occlusion. Stroke 2000;31:140–146.

25. Goertler M, Kross R, Baeumer M, et al. Diagnostic impact and prognostic relevance of early contrast-enhanced transcranial color-coded duplex sonography in acute stroke. Stroke 1998;29:955–962.

26. Kushner MJ, Zanette EM, Bastianello S, et al. Transcranial Doppler in acute hemispheric brain infarction. Neurology 1991;41:109–113.

27. Toni D, Fiorelli M, Zanette EM, et al. Early spontaneous improvement and deterioration of ischemic stroke patients. A serial study with transcranial Doppler ultrasonography. Stroke 1998;29:1144–1148.

28. Zanette EM, Roberti C, Mancini G, et al. Spontaneous middle cerebral artery reperfusion in ischemic stroke. A follow-up study with transcranial Doppler. Stroke 1995;26:430–433.

29. Kaps M, Link A. Transcranial sonographic monitoring during thrombolytic therapy. AJNR Am J Neuroradiol 1998;19:758–760.

30. Demchuk AM, Wein TH, Felberg RA, et al. Images in cardiovascular medicine. Evolution of rapid middle cerebral artery recanalization during intravenous thrombolysis for acute ischemic stroke. Circulation 1999;100:2282–2283.

31. Maurer M, Mullges W, Becker G. Diagnosis of middle cerebral artery occlusion and monitoring of systemic thrombolytic therapy with contrast enhanced transcranial duplex-sonography. J Neuroimaging 1999;9:99–101.

32. Burgin WS, Malkoff M, Felberg RA, et al. Transcranial doppler ultrasound criteria for recanalization after thrombolysis for middle cerebral artery stroke. Stroke 2000;31:1128–1132.

33. Demchuk AM, Felburg RA, Alexandrov AV. Clinical recovery from acute ischemic stroke after early reperfusion of the brain with intravenous thrombolysis. N Engl J Med 1999;340:894–895.

34. Lewandowski CA, Frankel M, Tomsick TA, et al. Combined intravenous and intra-arterial r-TPA versus intra-arterial therapy of acute ischemic stroke: Emergency Management of Stroke (EMS) Bridging Trial. Stroke 1999;30:2598–2605.

35. Alexandrov AV, Demchuk AM, Felberg RA, et al. Intracranial clot dissolution is associated with embolic signals on transcranial Doppler. J Neuroimaging 2000;10:27–32.

36. Puppo P. Percutaneous nephrolithotripsy. Curr Opin Urol 1999;9:325–328.

37. Howard DE, Fromm H. Nonsurgical management of gallstone disease. Gastroenterol Clin North Am 1999;28:133–144.

38. Trupka A, Hallfeldt K, Kalteis T, et al. Open and laparoscopic liver resection with a new ultrasound scalpel. Chirurg 1998;69:1352–1356.

39. Baumgartner FJ, Pandya A, Omari BO, et al. Ultrasonic debridement of mitral calcification. J Card Surg 1997;12:240–242.

40. Delaney LJ. Method for clot lysis. US Patent 3,352,303. July 28, 1965.

41. Kuris A. Ultrasonic method and apparatus for removing cholesterol and other deposits from blood vessels and the like. US Patent 3,565,062. June 3, 1968.

42. Sobbe A, Stumpff U, Trubestein G, et al. Die ultraschallauflosung von thromben. Klin Wochenschr 1974;52:1117–1121.

43. Siegel RJ, Fishbein MC, Forrester J, et al. Ultrasonic plaque ablation. A new method for recanalization of partially or totally occluded arteries. Circulation 1988;78:1443–1448.

44. Rosenschein U, Bernstein J, DiSegni E, et al. Experimental ultrasonic angioplasty: disruption of atherosclerotic plaques and thrombi in vitro and arterial recanalization in vivo. J Am Coll Cardiol 1990;15:711–717.

45. Rosenschein U, Rozenszajn A, Kraus L, et al. Ultrasonic angioplasty in totally occluded peripheral arteries. Initial clinical, histological, and angiographic results. Circulation 1991;83:1976–1986.

46. Siegel RJ, Gunn J, Ahsan A, et al. Use of therapeutic ultrasound in percutaneous coronary angioplasty. Experimental in vitro studies and initial clinical experience. Circulation 1994;89:1587–1592.

47. Luo H, Birnbaum Y, Fishbein MC, et al. Enhancement of thrombolysis in vivo without skin and soft tissue damage by transcutaneous ultrasound. Thromb Res 1998;89:171–177.

48. Akiyama M, Ishibashi T, Yamada T, Furuhata H. Low-frequency ultrasound penetrates the cranium and enhances thrombolysis in vitro. Neurosurgery 1998;43:828–832.

49. Harpaz D, Chen X, Francis CW, Meltzer RS. Ultrasound accelerates urokinase-induced thrombolysis and reperfusion. Am Heart J 1994;127:1211–1219.

50. Behrens S, Daffertshofer M, Spiegel D, Hennerici M. Low-frequency, low-intensity ultrasound accelerates thrombolysis through the skull. Ultrasound Med Biol 1999;25:269–273.

51. Barnwell SL, Eskridge JM, Pavenick D, et al. Ultrasound accelerated thrombolysis in a canine carotid model of ischemic stroke. Circulation 1999;l(abstract):100.

52. Alexandrov AV, Demchuk AM, Felberg RA, et al. High rate of complete recanalization and dramatic clinical recovery during tPA infusion when continuously monitored with 2-MHz transcranial Doppler monitoring. Stroke 2000;31:610–614.

53. Davalos A, Toni D, Iweins F, et al. Neurological deterioration in acute ischemic stroke: potential predictors and associated factors in the European cooperative acute stroke study (ECASS) I. Stroke 1999;30:2631–2636.

54. The International Stroke Trial (IST): a randomized trial of aspirin, subcutaneous heparin, both, or neither among 19,435 patients with acute ischemic stroke. International Stroke Trial Collaborative Group. Lancet 1997;349:1569–1581.

55. Petty GW, Brown RD, Whisnant JP, et al. Ischemic stroke subtypes. Stroke 2000;31:1062–1068.

56. Bogousslavsky J, Barnett HJM, Fox AJ, et al. Atherosclerotic disease of the middle cerebral artery. Stroke 1986;17:1112–1120.

57. Chimowitz MI, Kokkinos J, Strong J, et al. The Warfarin-Aspirin Symptomatic Intracranial Disease Study. Neurology 1995;45:1488–1493.

58. Streifler JY, Eliasziw M, Benavente OR, et al. The risk of stroke in patients with first ever retinal vs. hemispheric transient ischemic attacks and high-grade carotid stenosis. North American Symptomatic Carotid Endarterectomy Trial. Arch Neurol 1995;52:246–249.

59. Petersen P. Thromboembolic complications of atrial fibrillation. Stroke 1990;21:4–13.

60. Beebe HG, Salles-Cunha SX, Scissons RP, et al. Carotid arterial ultrasound scan imaging: a direct approach to stenosis measurement. J Vasc Surg 1999;29:838–844.

61. Horrow MM, Stassi J, Shurman A, et al. The limitations of carotid sonography: interpretive and technology related errors. AJR Am J Roentgenol 2000;174:189–194.

62. Neale ML, Chambers J, Kelly A, et al. Reappraisal of duplex criteria to assess significant carotid stenosis with special reference to reports from the North American Symptomatic Carotid Endarterectomy Trial and the European Carotid Surgery Trial. J Vasc Surg 1994;20:642–649.

63. Hood DB, Mattos MA, Mansour A, et al. Prospective evaluation of new duplex criteria to identify 70% internal carotid artery stenosis. J Vasc Surg 1996;23:254–262.

64. Babikian VL, Tegeler CH. Ultrasound Imaging of the Cerebral Vasculature. In WG Bradley, RB Daroff, GM Fenichel, CD Marsden (eds), Neurology in Clinical Practice (3rd ed). Boston: Butterworth–Heinemann, 2000;645–664.

65. Droste DW, Jurgens R, Nabavi DG, et al. Echocontrast-enhanced ultrasound of extracranial internal carotid artery high-grade stenosis and occlusion. Stroke 1999;30:2302–2306.

66. Sturzenegger M. Ultrasound findings in spontaneous carotid artery dissection. Arch Neurol 1991;48:1057–1063.

67. Polak JF, Shermanski L, O'Leary DH, et al. Hypoechoic plaque at US of the carotid artery: an independent risk factor for incident stroke in adults aged 65 years or older. Cardiovascular Health Study. Radiology 1998;208:649–654.

68. Geroulakos G, Domjan J, Nicolaides A, et al. Ultrasonic carotid artery plaque structure and the risk of cerebral infarction on computed tomography. J Vasc Surg 1994;20:263–266.

69. O'Donnell TF, Erdoes L, Mackey WC, et al. Correlation of B-mode ultrasound imaging and arteriography with pathologic findings at carotid endarterectomy. Arch Surg 1985;120:443–449.

70. Rothwell PM, Gibson R, Warlow CP. Interrelation between plaque surface morphology and degree of stenosis on carotid angiograms and the risk of ischemic stroke in patients with symptomatic carotid stenosis. On behalf of the European Carotid Surgery Trialists' Collaborative Group. Stroke 2000;31:615–621.

71. Levi C, Mitchell A, Fitt G, Donnan G. The accuracy of magnetic resonance angiography in the assessment of extracranial carotid artery occlusive disease. Cerebrovasc Dis 1996;6:231–236.

72. Furst G, Saleh A, Wenserski F, et al. Reliability and validity of noninvasive imaging of internal carotid artery pseudo-occlusion. Stroke 1999;30:1444–1449.

73. Kent KC, Kuntz KM, Patel MR, et al. Perioperative imaging strategies for carotid endarterectomy. An analysis of morbidity and cost-effectiveness in symptomatic patients. JAMA 1995;274:888–893.

74. Wityk RJ, Chang HM, Rosengart A, et al. Proximal extracranial vertebral artery disease in the New England Medical Center Posterior Circulation Registry. Arch Neurol 1998;55:470–478.

75. Le Tu PT, Zuber M, Meder JF, Mas JL. Dissection isolee de l'artere cerebrale posterieure. Rev Neurol 1996;152:542–547.

76. Ley-Pozo J, Ringelstein EB. Noninvasive detection of occlusive disease of the carotid siphon and middle cerebral artery. Ann Neurol 1990;28:640–647.

77. Tettenborn B, Estol C, DeWitt D, et al. Accuracy of transcranial Doppler in the vertebrobasilar circulation. J Neurol 1990;237(abstract):159.

78. Schulte-Altedorneburg G, Droste D, Popa V, et al. Visualization of the basilar artery by transcranial color-coded duplex sonography. Stroke 2000;31:1123–1127.

79. Gerriets T, Seidel G, Fiss I, et al. Contrast-enhanced transcranial color-coded duplex sonography. Neurology 1999;52:1133–1137.

80. Adams RJ, McKie VC, Hsu L, et al. Prevention of a first stroke by transfusions in children with sickle cell anemia

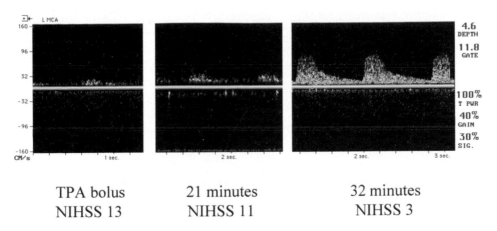

| TPA bolus | 21 minutes | 32 minutes |
| NIHSS 13 | NIHSS 11 | NIHSS 3 |

Plate 1. Middle cerebral artery recanalization during tissue plasminogen activator (t-PA) infusion. (LMCA = left middle cerebral artery; NIHSS = National Institutes of Health Stroke Scale.)

Plate 2. Duplex sonography of a normal distal common carotid artery (CCA). There is no evidence of plaque formation. The cursor is placed in the lumen of the artery, and the angle is corrected. The peak-systolic (PSV) and end-diastolic (EDV) flow velocities are 65 cm/sec and 20 cm/sec, respectively **(A)**. Color-coded sonography of the CCA bifurcation into internal (ICA) and external carotid arteries **(B)**.

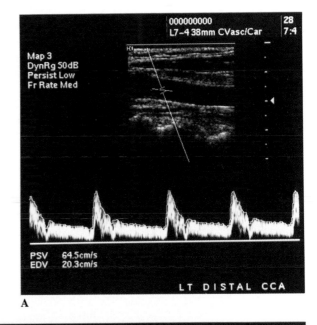

A

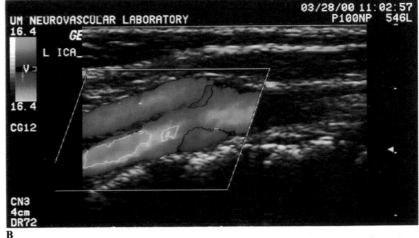

B

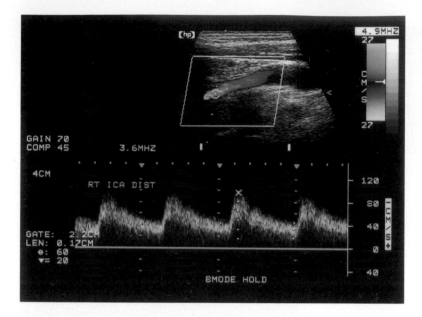

Plate 3. Color-coded duplex sonography of a normal internal carotid artery (ICA). The cursor identifies the region of the lumen being sampled. The peak-systolic and end-diastolic flow velocities are 98 cm/sec and 41 cm/sec, respectively. There is no ultrasonic evidence of flow turbulence. (Courtesy of Dr. James Menzoian, Boston Medical Center, Boston, MA.)

Plate 4. Color-coded duplex sonography of internal carotid artery (ICA) mild to moderate (**A**) and moderate (**B**) stenosis. The peak-systolic and end-diastolic velocities are respectively 175 cm/sec and 50 cm/sec (**A**), and 219 cm/sec and 39 cm/sec (**B**). (Courtesy of Dr. James Menzoian, Boston Medical Center, Boston, MA.)

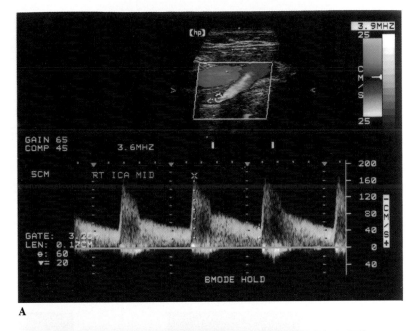

A

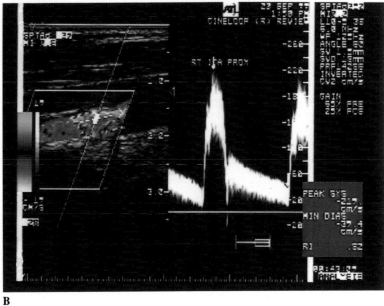

B

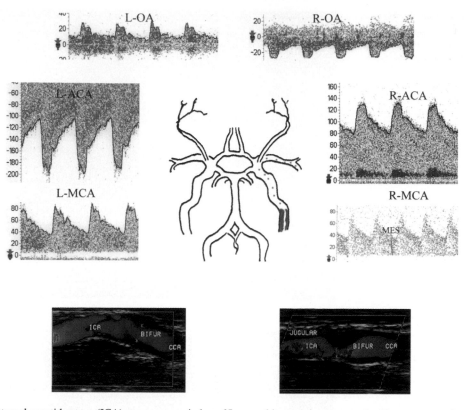

Plate 5. Internal carotid artery (ICA) severe stenosis in a 65-year-old man who presented with recurrent episodes of left hemiparesis and right monocular blindness. The color-coded duplex study shows right ICA severe stenosis (*right, lower corner*). The right ophthalmic (R-OA) and right anterior cerebral (R-ACA) arteries have retrograde flow. Flow velocities are increased in the left anterior cerebral artery (L-ACA), indicating collateral flow from the left to the right hemispheres through the anterior communicating artery. The right middle cerebral artery (R-MCA) spectra are dampened, and a micro-embolic signal (MES) (*in orange*) is seen. (L-OA = left ophthalmic artery; L-MCA = left middle cerebral artery; bifur = bifurcation; CCA = common carotid artery.)

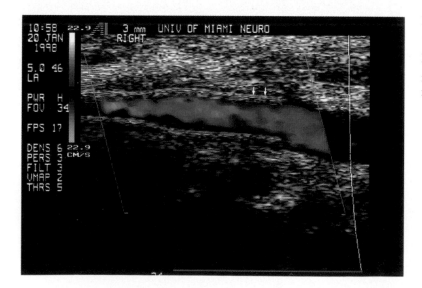

Plate 6. Internal carotid artery stent. The stent (*arrows*) is in good position, and the lumen of this previously severely stenotic internal carotid artery is now restored.

Plate 7. Transcranial Doppler ultrasound of middle cerebral artery stenosis. The peak systolic flow velocity is approximately 50 cm/sec at a depth of insonation of 56 mm (**A**). It increases to more than 300 cm/sec at 46 mm, indicating the presence of an area of focal stenosis (**B**).

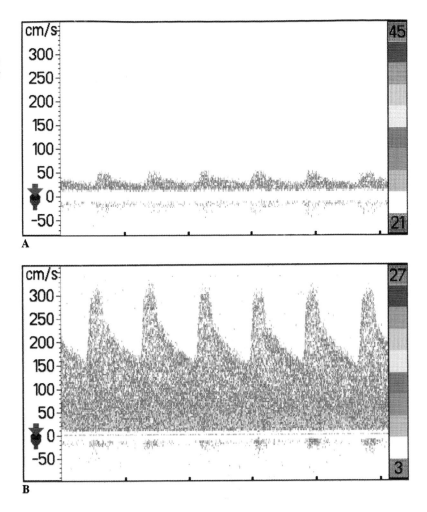

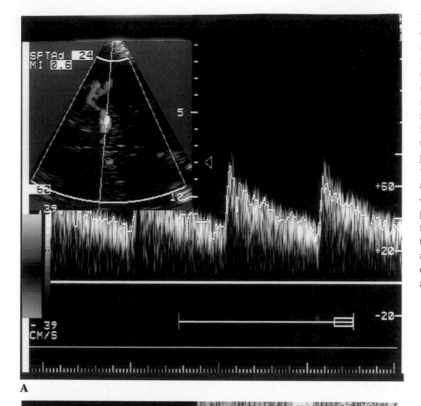

Plate 8. Transcranial color-coded duplex of the middle cerebral artery. Normal study (**A**) and middle cerebral artery stenosis (**B**). The color-coded image (*upper left corner*) shows the M1 segment of the artery and its two main branches (**A**). The cursor identifies the region of the lumen that is sampled. A normal Doppler study shows a peak-systolic velocity of less than 80 cm/sec and an end-diastolic velocity of 40 cm/sec (**A**). In another patient, the respective peak-systolic and end-diastolic velocities of approximately 450 cm/sec and 225 cm/sec confirm the presence of severe middle cerebral artery stenosis (**B**).

A

B

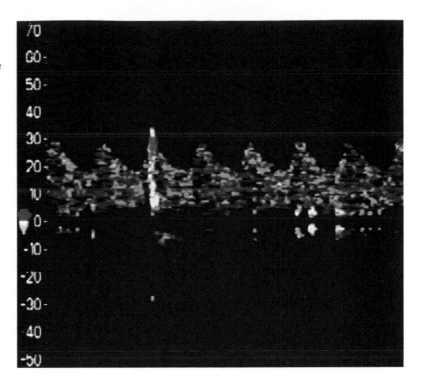

Plate 9. Microembolic signal. A microembolic signal (*in red and orange*) is detected with transcranial Doppler ultrasound during the third heartbeat.

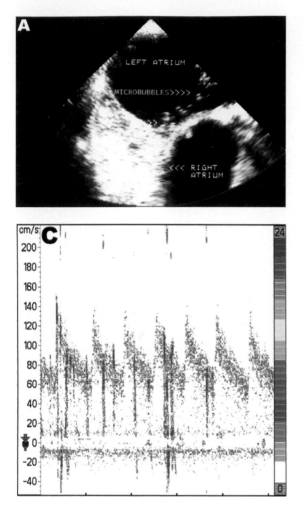

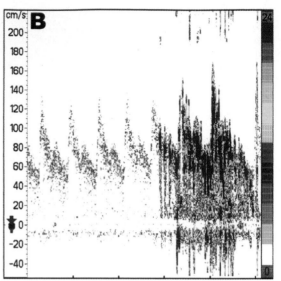

Plate 10. Patent foramen ovale in a 22-year-old woman who developed a cerebellar infarct after a long car trip. After the intravenous injection of agitated saline, the transesophageal echocardiogram shows the spontaneous passage of microbubbles (*arrows*) into the left atrium and confirms the presence of a patent foramen ovale (**A**). Seconds later, microembolic signals are detected in the right middle cerebral artery (**B** and **C**).

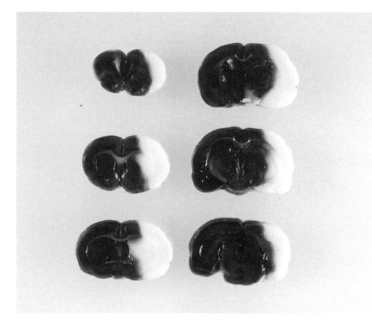

Plate 11. Triphenyltetrazolium chloride staining at 24 hours after permanent middle cerebral artery occlusion with the intraluminal suture occlusion method. Normal brain tissues stain red, whereas infarcted tissues do not stain (*white*), thus delineating good demarcation.

and abnormal results on transcranial Doppler ultrasonography. N Engl J Med 1998;339:5–11.

81. National Heart, Lung and Blood Institute. Clinical alert: periodic transfusions lower stroke risk in children with sickle cell anemia. September 18, 1997.

82. Akins PT, Pilgram TK, Cross DT, Moran CJ. Natural history of stenosis from intracranial atherosclerosis by serial angiography. Stroke 1998;29:433–438.

83. Schwarze JJ, Babikian VL, deWitt LD, et al. Longitudinal monitoring of intracranial stenoses with transcranial Doppler ultrasonography. J Neuroimaging 1994;4:182–187.

84. Babikian VL, Rosales R, Pochay V. Composition of particles associated with embolic signals on transcranial Doppler sonography. J Stroke Cerebrovasc Dis 1994;4:86–90.

85. Rundek T, DiTullio M, Sciacca R, et al. Association between large aortic arch atheromas and high-intensity transient signals in elderly stroke patients. Stroke 1999; 30:2683–2686.

86. Valton L, Larrue V, Pavy le Traon A, et al. Microembolic signals and risk of early recurrence in patients with stroke or transient ischemic attack. Stroke 1998;29:2125–2128.

87. Forteza A, Koch S, Romano JG, et al. Transcranial Doppler detection of fat emboli. Stroke 1999;30:2687–2691.

88. Spencer MP. Transcranial Doppler monitoring and causes of stroke from carotid endarterectomy. Stroke 1997;28: 685–691.

89. Ackerstaff RGA, Moons KGM, van de Vlasakker CJW, et al. Association of intraoperative transcranial Doppler monitoring variables with stroke from carotid endarterectomy. Stroke 2000;31:1817–1823.

90. Bakker SLM, de Leeuw FE, de Groot JC, et al. Cerebral vasomotor reactivity and cerebral white matter lesions in the elderly. Neurology 1999;52:578–583.

91. Silvestrini M, Vernieri F, Pasqualetti P, et al. Impaired cerebral vasoreactivity and risk of stroke in patients with asymptomatic carotid artery stenosis. JAMA 2000;283:2122–2127.

92. Kleiser B, Widder B. Course of carotid artery occlusions with impaired cerebrovascular reactivity. Stroke 1992;23: 171–174.

93. Atherosclerotic disease of the aortic arch as a risk factor for recurrent ischemic stroke. The French Study of Aortic Plaques in Stroke Group. N Engl J Med 1996;334:1216– 1221.

94. Ferrari E, Vidal R, Chevallier T, Baudouy M. Atherosclerosis of the thoracic aorta and aortic debris as a marker of poor prognosis: benefit of oral anticoagulants. J Am Coll Cardiol 1999;33:1317–1322.

95. Mitusch R, Doherty C, Wucherpfennig H, et al. Vascular events during follow-up in patients with aortic arch atherosclerosis. Stroke 1997;28:36–39.

96. Davila-Roman VG, Phillips KJ, Daily BB, et al. Intraoperative transesophageal echocardiography and epiaortic ultrasound for assessment of atherosclerosis of the thoracic aorta. J Am Coll Cardiol 1996;28:942–947.

97. Geraci A, Weinberger J. Natural history of aortic arch atherosclerotic plaque. Neurology 2000;54:749–751.

98. Bogousslavsky J, Van Melle G, Regli F. The Lausanne Stroke Registry: analysis of 1000 consecutive patients with first stroke. Stroke 1988;19:1083–1092.

99. Cardiogenic brain embolism. Cerebral Embolism Task Force. Arch Neurol 1986;43:71–84.

100. Cardiogenic brain embolism. The second report of the Cerebral Embolism Task Force. Arch Neurol 1989;46:727–743.

101. Foulkes MA, Wolf PA, Price TR, et al. The Stroke Data Bank: design, methods, and baseline characteristics. Stroke 1988;19:547–554.

102. Kittner SJ, Sharkness CM, Price TR, et al. Infarcts with a cardiac source of embolism in the NINCDS Stroke Data Bank: historical features. Neurology 1990;40:281–284.

103. Adams HP, Butler MJ, Biller J, Toffol GJ. Nonhemorrhagic cerebral infarction in young adults. Arch Neurol 1986;43:793–796.

104. Bevan H, Sharma K, Bradley W. Stroke in young adults. Stroke 1990;21:382–386.

105. Popp RL. Echocardiography I. N Engl J Med 1990;323: 101–109.

106. Popp RL. Echocardiography II. N Engl J Med 1990;323: 165–172.

107. Daniel WG, Mugge A. Transesophageal echocardiography. N Engl J Med 1995;332:1268–1279.

108. Cheitlin MD, Alpert JS, Armstrong WF, et al. ACC/AHA Guidelines for the Clinical Application of Echocardiography. A report of the American College of Cardiology/ American Heart Association Task Force on Practice Guidelines (Committee on Clinical Application of Echocardiography). Developed in collaboration with the American Society of Echocardiography. Circulation 1997;95:1686–1744.

109. Cujec B, Polasec P, Voll C, Shuaib A. Transesophageal echocardiography in the detection of potential cardiac sources of embolism in stroke patients. Stroke 1991;22:727–733.

110. Dressler FA, Labovitz AJ. Systemic arterial emboli and cardiac masses. Assessment with transesophageal echocardiography. Cardiol Clin 1993;11:447–460.

111. Lee RJ, Bartzokis T, Yeoh TK, et al. Enhanced detection of intracardiac sources of cerebral emboli by transesophageal echocardiography. Stroke1991;22:734–739.

112. Manning WJ, Weintraub RM, Waksmonski CA, et al. Accuracy of transesophageal echocardiography for identifying left atrial thrombi. Ann Intern Med 1995;123:817–822.

113. Pearson AC, Labovitz AJ, Tatieni S, Gomez CR. Superiority of transesophageal echocardiography in detecting cardiac source of embolism in patients with cerebral ischemia of uncertain etiology. J Am Coll Cardiol 1991;17:66–72.

114. Pop G, Sutherland GR, Koudstaal PJ, et al. Transesophageal echocardiography in the detection of intracardiac embolic sources in patients with transient ischemic attacks. Stroke 1990;21:560–565.

115. Rauh G, Fischereder M, Spengel FA. Transesophageal echocardiography in patients with focal cerebral ischemia of unknown cause. Stroke 1996;27:691–694.

116. McNamara RL, Lima JAC, Whelton PK, Powe NR. Echocardiographic identification of cardiovascular sources of emboli to guide clinical management of stroke: a cost-effectiveness analysis. Ann Intern Med 1997;127:775–787.

117. Caplan LR. Of birds and nests and brain emboli. Rev Neurol 1991;147:265–273.

118. Di Tullio M, Sacco RL, Gopal A, et al. Patent foramen ovale as a risk factor for cryptogenic stroke. Ann Intern Med 1992;17:461–465.

119. Webster MW, Chancellor AM, Smith HJ, et al. Patent foramen ovale in young stroke patients. Lancet 1988;2:11–12.

120. Droste DW, Kriete JU, Stypmann J, et al. Contrast transcranial Doppler ultrasound in the detection of right-to-left shunts: comparison of different procedures and different contrast agents. Stroke 1999;30:1827–1832.

121. Klotzsch C, Janssen G, Berlit P. Transesophageal echocardiography and contrast-TCD in the detection of a patent foramen ovale: experiences with 111 patients. Neurology 1994;44:1603–1606.

122. Kimura K, Minematsu K, Wada K, et al. Transcranial Doppler of a paradoxical brain embolism associated with a pulmonary arteriovenous fistula. AJNR Am J Neuroradiol 1999;20:1881–1884.

123. Albert A, Muller HR, Hetzel A. Optimized transcranial Doppler technique for the diagnosis of cardiac right-to-left shunts. J Neuroimaging 1997;7:159–163.

124. Zanette EM, Mancini G, De Castro S, et al. Patent foramen ovale and transcranial Doppler. Comparison of different procedures. Stroke 1996;27:2251–2255.

125. Carotid endarterectomy for patients with asymptomatic internal carotid artery stenosis. Asymptomatic Carotid Atherosclerosis Study Group. JAMA 1995;273:1421–1428.

126. Alexandrova NA, Gibson WC, Norris JW, Maggisano R. Carotid artery stenosis in peripheral vascular disease. J Vasc Surg 1996;23:645–649.

127. Eikelboom BE. Prevalence of Asymptomatic Carotid Artery Disease. In EF Bernstein, AD Callow, AN Nicolaides, EG Shifrin (eds), Cerebral Revascularization. London: Med-Orion, 1993;451–456.

128. Fowl RJ, Marsch JG, Love M, et al. Prevalence of hemodynamically significant stenosis of the carotid artery in an asymptomatic veteran population. Surg Gynecol Obstet 1991;172:13–16.

129. Adams MR, Celermajer DS. Detection of presymptomatic atherosclerosis: a current perspective. Clin Sci 1999;97:615–624.

130. Simons PC, Algra A, Bots ML, et al. Common carotid intima-media thickness and arterial stiffness: indicators of cardiovascular risk in high-risk patients. The SMART study (Second Manifestations of ARTerial disease). Circulation 1999;100:951–957.

131. O'Leary DH, Polak JF, Kronmal RA, et al. Carotid-artery intima and media thickness as a risk factor for myocardial infarction and stroke in older adults. Cardiovascular Health Study Collaborative Research Group. N Engl J Med 1999;340:14–22.

132. Chambless LE, Folsom AR, Clegg LX, et al. Carotid wall thickness is predictive of incident clinical stroke: the Atherosclerosis Risk in Communities (ARIC) study. Am J Epidemiol 2000;151:478–487.

133. Ubels FL, Terpstra WF, Smit AJ. Carotid intima-media thickness: influence of drug treatment and clinical implications. Neth J Med 1999;55:188–195.

134. Mugge A, Daniel WG, Frank G, Lichtlen PR. Echocardiography in infective endocarditis: reassessment of the prognostic implications of vegetations size determined by the transthoracic and transesophageal approach. J Am Coll Cardiol 1989;14:631–638.

135. Zenker G, Erbel R, Kramer G, et al. Transesophageal two-dimensional echocardiography in young patients with cerebral ischemic events. Stroke 1988;19:345–348.

136. Lee RJ, Bartzokis T, Yeoh TK, et al. Enhanced detection of intracardiac sources of cerebral emboli by transesophageal echocardiography. Stroke 1991;22:734–739.

137. Tice FD, Slivka AP, Walz ET, et al. Mitral valve strands in patients with focal cerebral ischemia. Stroke 1996;27:1183–1186.

138. Mugge A, Kuhn H, Daniel WG. The role of transesophageal echocardiography in the detection of left atrial thrombi. Echocardiography 1993;10:405–417.

139. Siostrzonek P, Zangeneh M, Gossinger H, et al. Comparison of transesophageal and transthoracic contrast echocardiography for detection of a patent foramen ovale. Am J Cardiol 1991;68:1247–1249.

140. Hausmann D, Mugge A, Becht I, Daniel WG. Diagnosis of patent foramen ovale by transesophageal echocardiography and association with cerebral and peripheral embolic events. Am J Cardiol 1992;70:668–672.

141. Kronzon I, Tunick PA, Freedberg RS, et al. Transesophageal echocardiography is superior to transthoracic echocardiography in the diagnosis of sinus venous atrial septal defect. J Am Coll Cardiol 1991;17:537–542.

142. Lucas C, Goullard L, Marchau M Jr, et al. Higher prevalence of atrial septal aneurysms in patients with ischemic stroke of unknown cause. Acta Neurol Scand 1994;89:210–213.

143. Black IW, Hopkins AP, Lee LCL, Walsh WF. Left atrial spontaneous echo contrast: a clinical and echocardiographic analysis. J Am Coll Cardiol 1991;18:398–404.

144. Mugge A, Daniel WG, Haverich A, Lichtlen PR. Diagnosis of noninfective cardiac mass lesions by two-dimensional echocardiography. Comparison of transthoracic and transesophageal approaches. Circulation 1991;83:70–78.

145. Stratton JR, Lighty GW Jr, Pearlman AS, Ritchie JL. Detection of left ventricular thrombus by two-dimensional echocardiography: sensitivity, specificity, and causes of uncertainty. Circulation 1982;66:155–166.

146. Pearson AC, Labovitz AJ, Tatineni S, Gomez CR. Superiority of transesophageal echocardiography in detecting cardiac source of embolism in patients with cerebral ischemia of uncertain etiology. J Am Coll Cardiol 1991;17:66–72.

Chapter 5
Animal Modeling for Developing Stroke Therapy

Fuhai Li and Marc Fisher

Animal modeling has played an important role in investigating the pathophysiology of ischemic stroke and developing preclinical stroke therapy. Combined with new magnetic resonance imaging (MRI) techniques, animal modeling provides opportunities to investigate early in vivo ischemic changes and monitor the temporal evolution of these changes. The introduction of transgenic and knockout mice into the stroke research arena has made it possible to study in vivo molecular changes after ischemia and to understand mechanisms of ischemic injury, leading to possible therapeutic strategies. Consequently, animal modeling is an indispensable step to develop effective pharmacologic compounds that recanalize the occluded artery (thrombolytic drugs), reduce ischemic damage (neuroprotective drugs), and restore neurologic function (restorative drugs).

General Criteria for Selecting Animal Models and Animals

Although the topographic location, extent, and pathogenesis of human ischemic stroke are quite variable, an ideal animal stroke model that is used to develop stroke therapy should be tightly controlled and satisfy these criteria[1,2]:

1. The ischemic process and pathophysiologic response should be relevant to human stroke.

2. The ischemic lesion size should be reproducible.
3. The technique used to perform the modeling should be relatively easy and minimally invasive.
4. Physiologic variables can be monitored and maintained within the normal range.
5. Brain samples are readily available for outcome measurements (e.g., histopathologic, biochemical, and molecular biological evaluation).
6. The cost and effort should be reasonable.

Generally, animal models of cerebral ischemia fall into two categories:

1. *Global cerebral ischemia*, with a widespread reduction or cessation in cerebral blood flow (CBF) that typically gives rise to selective neuronal death. This model is clinically relevant to human cardiac arrest.
2. *Focal cerebral ischemia*, with a local disturbance of CBF that may give rise to either selective neuronal death after brief period of transient focal ischemia (less than 30 minutes), or pannecrosis when focal ischemia is induced for more than 30 minutes.[3,4]

Focal ischemia is usually induced by occluding the middle cerebral artery (MCA) and is most frequently used to simulate human ischemic stroke, because human ischemic stroke is often caused by occlusion of the MCA or one of its branches.[5]

Focal cerebral ischemia models can be divided into transient ischemia and permanent ischemia, based on the duration of ischemia, whereas global ischemia is induced transiently. Focal ischemia is often used for developing neuroprotective agents, and permanent focal ischemia models should be studied first, followed by transient focal ischemia models in which 90 or 120 minutes of transient ischemia is usually used.[6] Less than 90 minutes of transient focal ischemia may not be appropriate for testing neuroprotective drugs because of large variability of infarct volumes.

The animals typically used in ischemia models include small animals, such as rats, mice, and gerbils, and higher animal species, such as cats, rabbits, dogs, pigs, and nonhuman primates. The rat is the most commonly used animal in stroke modeling because of its close resemblance to human cerebrovascular anatomy and physiology and its moderate size, which allows easy monitoring of physiologic parameters and collection of brain specimens.[7–9] For testing drug efficacy, the same strains of rats from the same vendor should be used throughout the experiment, because the histologic outcomes may be different between different strains and between the same strains but different vendors.[10,11] The mouse has been increasingly used because of the availability of transgenic technology. The introduction of transgenic mice has offered new insights into the molecular mechanisms involved in ischemic stroke. The gerbil may not be a good candidate for testing potential neuroprotective agents, because many neuroprotectants active in the gerbil fail to protect ischemic damage in other species.[6] Due to the relatively higher cost and greater difficulty in performing experiments, higher animal species are used in a more limited manner. However, it seems reasonable to consider testing neuroprotective agents in larger animal stroke models to determine if the compound is broadly effective before clinical trials begin.[6]

Precise control of physiologic variables, such as arterial blood pressure, blood gases (pH, P_{O_2}, and P_{CO_2}), serum glucose levels, body or brain temperature, or both, and hemoglobin, is essential to correctly interpret outcome, because fluctuations of these variables could introduce variability into the experimental data and confound the validity of the results.[1,2,12] Monitoring of these variables may be difficult in gerbils because of their small size. In addition, CBF should be measured by laser Doppler flowmetry or other techniques to ensure an appropriate induction of ischemia, thus avoiding modeling bias.

Global Cerebral Ischemia Models

Global cerebral ischemia can be induced by bilateral common carotid artery (CCA) occlusions, combined with hypotension induced by blood withdrawal or application of ganglion-blocking agents (two-vessel occlusion model),[12–14] or by bilateral CCA occlusion in combination with prior bilateral vertebral artery electrocoagulation (four-vessel occlusion model).[12,15–17] Other methods to produce global ischemia include occluding both CCAs in gerbils because of the incomplete circle of Willis,[18] ligating one carotid artery plus hypoxia (Levine model),[19] inducing cardiac arrest,[20,21] elevating cerebrospinal fluid pressure above blood pressure by infusing artificial cerebrospinal fluid into cistern magna,[22] or compressing both carotid arteries and veins by inflating a tourniquet.[12]

Global ischemia models are useful in investigating biochemical, metabolic, and physiologic responses after a transient decrease in CBF.[12] The primary histopathologic feature of transient global ischemia is delayed selective neuronal death.[23] Therefore, transient global ischemia is suitable for studying mechanisms associated with the process of selective neuronal vulnerability in the hippocampus after chronic survival. Global ischemia models were also previously used to test neuroprotective agents.[12] The results of therapeutic intervention tested by using global cerebral ischemia models are not applicable to human ischemic stroke, however, because the pathophysiologic and histopathologic features of human ischemic stroke are not reproduced by global ischemia models.

There are other disadvantages to using the global cerebral ischemia model.[12,14] First, the neuropathologic outcome is not easily standardized and not all occlusions induce ischemic neuronal injury, especially in the gerbil.[24,25] Second, postischemic seizures usually occur after longer durations of transient global ischemia, which may lead to neuronal damage and subsequently confound data analysis. Finally, global ischemia induced by cardiac arrest may be complicated by multiple organ insults, which subsequently can affect recirculation of the brain.

Focal Cerebral Ischemia Models

Focal cerebral ischemia can be induced by many approaches, including embolization of microspheres, photochemical thrombosis, endothelin-1 infusion, thromboembolus injection, direct surgical occlusion of the MCA, and intraluminal suture insertion. This review focuses on thromboembolic models, direct surgical MCA occlusion models, and the intraluminal suture MCA occlusion model because of their potential role and increasing popularity in developing thrombolytic drugs, restorative drugs, and neuroprotective drugs.

Embolus Model

Many materials, such as carbon, plastic microspheres, silicone cylinders, and air, can be used as emboli that induce ischemic damage after injection into the CCA or the internal carotid artery (ICA).[12,14,26–30] The magnitude and severity of ischemic damage induced by these models depend on the number and size of the emboli injected.[31] Diffuse distribution of infarction is the neuropathologic hallmark of these models and makes histologic evaluation difficult. The unpredictable location and extent of ischemic infarction in these models may preclude applying them for investigating mechanisms of ischemic injury and therapeutic interventions.

Photochemically Induced Thrombosis Model

The photochemically induced thrombosis model is induced by vascular injection of a photoactive dye, such as rose Bengal[32] or photofrin,[33–35] combined with irradiation with a light beam at a specific wavelength. Studies have shown that a reaction between the circulating dye and the light engenders free radicals, leading to platelet aggregation and thrombosis.[32] The location and extent of photochemically induced lesions can be controlled by selectively illuminating the brain tissue and by using different intensities of light and different doses of dye. A typical lesion in this model is a sharply circumscribed infarct that involves only the cortex. It is likely that there is only a small penumbra. In addition, breakdown of the blood-brain barrier and vasogenic edema occur early in this

model.[36–39] It is debatable whether the lesion induced by this model is secondary to an ischemic event.[34,35] Although this model was used to test neuroprotective agents,[40] its usefulness is limited, because the pathophysiologic processes it induces are less likely to be directly relevant to those in human ischemic stroke.[39]

Endothelin-Induced Middle Cerebral Artery Occlusion Model

Endothelin-1 is a 21–amino acid peptide that has a potent vasoconstrictor effect.[41] Application of endothelin-1 to the exposed MCA induces a significant decrease in CBF.[41] Furthermore, microinjection of endothelin-1 into areas near the MCA through a cannula also decreases CBF in the MCA territory. The distribution of ischemic infarct induced by this method is similar to that after permanent surgical ligation of the MCA.[42–44] CBF around the ischemic core significantly increases in this model. The advantage of this model is that ischemia can be induced in conscious rats, which excludes the confounding situation that anesthesia may cause. The ischemic damage is variable, due to different responses of vessels to endothelin-1,[41] however, and the duration of ischemia is not controllable because endothelin-1–mediated vasoconstriction may gradually disappear.[42] These limitations inhibit its use in drug development, although this model was used to test drug efficacy.[43,44]

Thromboembolic Model

Ischemia induced by thromboemboli is of great interest because of its resemblance to human ischemic stroke, approximately 80% of which are caused by thromboembolism,[45,46] and its role in seeking and evaluating thrombolytic therapy. One study demonstrated that thrombolytic therapy involving recombinant tissue plasminogen activator (rt-PA) administered within 3 hours after onset of ischemic stroke in humans improves neurologic outcomes.[47] Therefore, thromboembolic animal models are playing an increasingly important role in stroke therapy research.[48,49]

Thromboembolic ischemia can be produced by a photochemical approach, or by injection of autologous or heterologous thrombi. The photo-chemical method gives rise to an arterial lesion in the CCA that results in platelet-rich thrombus formation. This thrombus can dislodge, and thus embolize to distal vessels.[50–53] The photochemically induced thromboemboli are platelet-rich and, therefore, may not be amenable to thrombolytic therapy with rt-PA.

The most commonly used thromboembolic model is blood clot injection. This model was first described in the dog by Hill and colleagues[54] and subsequently was applied to the rat.[55,56] In the early iterations of this model, a suspension of microembolic clot was injected, causing diffuse and inhomogeneous infarction in the MCA territory because of peripheral branch microembolization. Scattered, multifocal lesions were also observed in the territories of the anterior cerebral artery and posterior cerebral artery, and even in the contralateral hemisphere.[55,56] In addition, early spontaneous recanalization frequently occurred, which made evaluation of thrombolytic therapy difficult. The early autolysis of blood clots may be due to a more fragile, red thrombus formed in vitro by whole blood. To overcome these problems, a more resistant, white thrombus was produced using a moving, high-pressure, closed-compartment system (PE-10 polyethylene tube with 0.28 mm in inner diameter).[57] Using white thrombi, Overgaard[57] demonstrated a substantial reduction of CBF in the affected region and no spontaneous recanalization at 2 hours after embolization—conditions necessary for studying thrombolytic treatment. Infarct size was variable, however, and ischemia caused by multiple small clots does not mimic typical clinical ischemic stroke. An ideal thromboembolic model should entail a blood clot that appropriately lodges in the proximal segment of the MCA, but the distal branches should remain open. Smaller clots embolize into the end-arterial trees, whereas larger clots may lodge in vessels too proximal from the origin of the MCA to occlude the MCA. Therefore, size (length and diameter), as well as the characteristics of blood clots (i.e., more rigid, fibrin-rich clot), is crucial in this model. Busch and colleagues[58] developed a rat clot model, in which 12 medium-sized (1.50×0.35 mm), fibrin-rich, autologous clots formed in a PE-50 catheter (0.58 mm in inner diameter) were injected to produce reliable occlusion of the proximal MCA. A consis-

tent reduction of CBF and histologic damage in the MCA territory were observed. Visual inspection demonstrated no early spontaneous clot lysis in the ipsilateral vessels at 3 hours after injection and no clots in the contralateral vessels. Thrombolytic therapy with rt-PA[58] or prourokinase[59] can recanalize the occluded MCA. By using a modified tube that was inserted into the ICA 2–3 mm proximal to the MCA origin, a single fibrin-rich clot (2.5×0.1 mm) can also be selectively introduced into the proximal part of the MCA[60] or a thrombosis can be induced at the origin of the MCA,[61] thus causing typical MCA occlusion. Using this single clot model, significant reduction of CBF in the MCA territory was demonstrated, and the blood clot in the MCA trunk was found at 24 hours after embolization.[61] This single clot was also applied to occlude the proximal MCA in mouse,[62] but one disadvantage was the relatively high incidence of subarachnoid and intraparenchymal hemorrhage.

In conclusion, these single clot or medium-sized clot models induce predictable and reproducible infarct in both extent and size in the MCA territory, similar to that caused by the intraluminal suture model.[58,60–62] Embolizing the proximal MCA trunk by a single, fibrin-rich clot bears similarity to human embolic stroke, because the majority of human ischemic strokes are caused by a single embolus in the MCA.[5] Therefore, the single clot model is promising for studying the pathogenesis of ischemic stroke and thrombolytic therapy.

Direct Surgical Middle Cerebral Artery Occlusion Model

Direct surgical MCA occlusion is invasive and requires a craniectomy. Ischemia can be induced by directly ligating, coagulating, clipping, or snaring the MCA trunk or its branches. The MCA occlusion in this model can be permanent or transient.[63–65] It has been performed in nonhuman primates,[66–68] dogs,[69] rabbits,[70] cats,[71–73] rats,[74–76] and mice.[77] Also, it can be performed under anesthesia or in awake animals.[14] The rat is the most common species to undergo surgical MCA occlusion.

Robinson and colleagues[74–76,78] first described direct ligation of the distal MCA at the rhinal fissure in the rat. The ischemic injury was demonstrated in the frontoparietal cortex, but the extent of lesion was quite variable. Through a subtemporal craniectomy, Albanese[79] and Tamura[80] performed surgical occlusion more proximally in the MCA trunk. Occluding the main trunk of the MCA proximal to the lenticulostriatal branches that supply the lateral caudoputamen results in an infarction involving both the cortex and caudoputamen. The infarction areas induced by proximal MCA occlusion appear to be larger and less variable compared with those induced by distal MCA occlusion.[80] This model is appropriate for investigating cerebrovascular function after focal ischemia.[81] Because focal occlusion of the MCA may not always produce infarction, even when the occlusion was performed at the proximal MCA trunk, Bederson[82] further refined this model and demonstrated that both the site and extent of MCA occlusion affect the neuropathologic outcome and are critical factors to produce reproducible infarction. Focal (1–2 mm) MCA occlusion results in wide variability of infarction, and the rate of infarction is low when focal MCA occlusion is performed at the origin of MCA. This may relate to the persistence of an abundant collateral circulation.[82] Furthermore, because MCA branching is variable,[83] such a focal occlusion at one point may not involve both the lenticulostriatal and cortical branches. In the young (36-day-old) rat, MCA occlusion beyond the point of origin of the striate branches does not cause neuronal injury, probably because of a better collateral blood supply in the young rat.[84]

Extensive (3 or 6 mm) MCA occlusion, however, induces uniform infarction in both size and location. This extensive occlusion involves the lenticulostriate and small cortical branches, and therefore produces reproducible infarction. Direct MCA occlusion can be combined with unilateral (two-vessel method) or bilateral CCA occlusion (three-vessel method). Studies have demonstrated that these combined two-vessel or three-vessel occlusions give rise to larger and more reproducible infarct.[85,86] Because the ischemic penumbra in this model may be small,[87] it may be less amenable to testing neuroprotective compounds. Due to higher long-term survival of rats, this model is feasible for investigations of stroke recovery drugs.[6]

There are some disadvantages to this direct surgical MCA occlusion model. First, performing this model is more difficult and requires more experience and skills, due to the variations of MCA anatomic pattern.[88] Second, direct exposure of brain to air after craniectomy may change intracranial pressure and blood-brain barrier permeability.[67,84] Third, a small amount of subarachnoid hemorrhage may occur around the MCA trunk.[80] Although this model has been extensively used, it has been largely replaced by the intraluminal suture MCA occlusion model.

Intraluminal Suture Middle Cerebral Artery Occlusion Model

In the suture model, the MCA is occluded by inserting a monofilament suture into the ICA to block blood flow to the MCA. The great advantage of this model is that it is relatively easy to perform and does not require a craniectomy. Physiologic complications of the procedure are minimal compared to the craniectomy models. Either permanent or transient MCA occlusion can be performed simply by maintaining or withdrawing the monofilament suture.

This model was originally described in rats by Koizumi and his colleagues in 1986[89] and modified by others thereafter. A 3-0 or 4-0 monofilament suture is usually used as an occluder either without coating,[90,91] or with coating by silicone[89,92] or poly-L-lysine.[93] The suture occluder can be inserted through the CCA, the external carotid artery, or the ICA. The length of suture inserted from the bifurcation of the CCA is approximately 17–22 mm,[94–96] depending on body weight, size of the suture tip, and location of the bifurcation.

The typical areas affected by this model include both the lateral caudoputamen and frontoparietal cortex. Generally, the infarct size induced by prolonged ischemia (>90 minutes) with the intraluminal suture method is relatively reproducible, making this suture model appropriate for testing neuroprotective agents. However, there are some factors that may affect infarct size. First, slight differences of the monofilament (i.e., diameter, tensile strength, and extensibility) may induce a significant difference in infarct volume.[97] Second, the ischemia induced by a silicone-coated suture is likely more profound and more reliable,[91,92] and, consequently, the infarct volume is more reproducible and larger than that achieved with an uncoated suture.[92,93] Third, a longer insertion distance of the monofilament suture gives rise to larger infarction, because the suture can also obstruct blood flow in some branches of the anterior cerebral artery.[95] Last, an inadvertent premature reperfusion is another factor that may cause variability of infarct volume.[98] It is important, therefore, that consistent and standardized surgical procedures and techniques be used to generate a reproducible lesion.

The suture MCA occlusion method can be also modified to induce ischemia in an MRI unit by remotely advancing the suture occluder, the so-called in-bore suture MCA occlusion model.[96,99–101] This enables researchers to monitor in vivo ischemic changes early after the onset of ischemia and to acquire both pre- and postischemic data for subsequent pixel-by-pixel comparison. This in-bore MCA occlusion method has been improved and has achieved high success rates.[96]

This suture method has been successfully applied to mice because transgenic or knockout mice provide a method for basic research into the molecular mechanisms contributing to ischemic cell damage and development of novel therapeutic interventions.[102–105] Usually, a 5-0 monofilament nylon suture or 8-0 suture coated with silicone is used to occlude blood flow to the MCA territory. The insertion depth from the bifurcation of CCA is 9–11 mm.[103,104] The lesion is reproducible and is similar to that in the rat.

There are some disadvantages and complications with the intraluminal suture MCA occlusion model. First, subarachnoid hemorrhage may occur because of inadvertent arterial rupture caused by the suture. This complication is likely to have a higher incidence with the uncoated suture than with silicone-coated suture.[91,98] Second, spontaneous hyperthermia occurs when the duration of ischemia is longer than 2 hours.[106–109] This may be associated with ischemic damage of the hypothalamus caused by suture insertion.[109] Finally, the inner surface of vessels may be mechanically injured by the suture, which may complicate reperfusion.[1]

Outcome Evaluation

Outcome measures are important for evaluating drug efficacy and should include both functional response and ischemic infarct volume.[6] The infarct volume can be evaluated by in vivo imaging techniques and by histologic techniques. If the outcome of drug testing is its effect on the volume of the lesion, then the animal must be sacrificed at an appropriate time point after the induction of ischemia. Many preclinical studies examined histopathologic outcomes only at 24 hours after the onset of ischemia. The acute evaluation of drug efficacy is essential, but outcome measures should be evaluated during both acute (1–3 days) and long-term phases (1–4 weeks). The evaluation of outcomes after a longer period is important, because it can determine that the initial effects observed during the acute phase persist, therefore disproving that the drugs only slow the maturation of histologic process.[110,111]

Functional Measures

Functional recovery is the main focus and interest for stroke patients and was thus used as a major endpoint in clinical trials.[47] Functional outcome is also usually evaluated in preclinical studies. It may have greater validity for efficient evaluation of functional recovery drugs (restorative drugs) that are desirable to improve functional outcome after experimental ischemic stroke, however, because drugs may merely stimulate the recovery of neuronal function without reducing infarct volume.[6] It is challenging to measure function and behavior in rats, although advanced techniques are available. Neurologic function can be evaluated by simply checking motor function.[82,94] More complicated methods to test sensorimotor function include paw-placing tasks, foot-fault tests, beam walking, beam-balance tests, cylinder tests, and reaching tests.[80,112–116] Cognitive status can also be tested by using the Morris water maze.[116]

In Vivo Evaluation by New Magnetic Resonance Imaging Techniques

A promising area for testing stroke therapies is the use of new MRI technologies to noninvasively measure ischemic changes over time. Diffusion-weighted imaging (DWI), superior to conventional MRI, is able to detect ischemic lesions within minutes after the onset of ischemia (Figure 5-1), and monitor the temporal evolution of ischemic lesions,[117,118] and it has been widely used in both experimental animal stroke models and stroke

Occ   1 hr   6 hr   12 hr

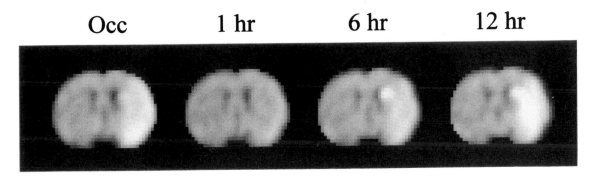

Figure 5-1. Serial diffusion-weighted images (DWI) after 30 minutes of transient middle cerebral artery occlusion. Ischemic DWI abnormalities are seen during occlusion (Occ), disappear 1 hour after reperfusion, and reappear gradually.

patients.[119–121] Because DWI allows measurement of a lesion in a real-time manner, it can be used to evaluate the efficacy of stroke therapy.[122–127] Thus, it is possible to know whether therapeutic approaches reverse ischemic changes or prevent growth of ischemic lesions.[124] Another advantage of in vivo monitoring of ischemic lesions is the ability to demonstrate a similar size of ischemic lesions in both the drug-treated and placebo-treated groups before the initiation of a pharmacologic treatment, thereby avoiding bias and variability of ischemic lesions.

Perfusion-weighted imaging (PWI) is another MRI technique that can monitor in vivo changes of CBF. PWI is able to demonstrate the benefit of thrombolytic therapy.[59,128,129] In addition to measuring therapeutic response in animals, DWI and PWI also can be used to measure response in humans.[120,121,130,131] Thus, the animal not only becomes a model for the ischemic event, but also a model for the monitoring method. This approach may strengthen the connection between animal testing and clinical conditions, and thereby promote effective development and evaluation of therapies. Furthermore, the combination of DWI with PWI can delineate differences, or abnormalities, on DWI and PWI (so-called DWI-PWI mismatch), and may thus identify subjects most likely to benefit from treatment.[120]

Our research group has developed a multispectral analysis (MSA) method, whereby each pixel is represented by a four-dimensional feature vector that is composed of the average apparent diffusion coefficient, CBF index, proton density, and T2 values. MSA has been shown to characterize the ischemic lesions over time and is able to differentiate between a region of more severe ischemia (*ischemic core*) and a region of less severe ischemia (*ischemic penumbra*).[132] The MSA technique, therefore, provides a multifaceted picture of how the ischemic tissue (core and penumbra) responds to pharmacologic therapy.[133]

It should be noted that in vivo evaluation of therapeutic efficacy by MRI techniques for longer periods may be necessary, because some studies showed that reversal of DWI abnormalities induced by reperfusion could be transient, and secondary DWI lesions develop later (see Figure 5-1).[134–136] Although the mechanisms responsible for these secondary DWI lesions are not understood, it is important to determine whether neuroprotection demonstrated by MRI is temporary or permanent. Furthermore, full recovery of DWI lesions may not necessarily indicate complete salvage of brain tissue from ischemic injury.[4,137]

Another novel imaging technique is functional MRI, which may have the potential to show efficacy of functionally restorative drugs. Functional MRI has been widely used to investigate brain function in humans, but has been restricted in animal research because of technical problems associated with animal movement or depression of functional activity in generally anesthetized animals. The introduction of head and body holders makes it possible to perform functional MRI in fully awake rats.[138] Studies have shown that some drugs can enhance neuronal sprouting in the uninjured area around the infarction site or in the contralateral hemisphere, thus stimulating the recovery of neuronal function.[139] Functional MRI may thus identify hyperactivation of some neurons and translocation of neuronal function induced by drugs promoting recovery.

In Vitro Histopathologic Evaluation

Histopathologic measures can be performed by 2,3,5-triphenyltetrazolium chloride (TTC) staining or by hematoxylin and eosin (H&E) staining. The lesion volume is usually used as a marker of the severity of ischemic damage. The lesion volume is calculated by multiplying the lesion area by the slice thickness, and it can be reported as direct (uncorrected) lesion volume or indirect (corrected) lesion volume. The direct lesion volume is obtained by summing the volumes of the lesion regions within the coronal sections, whereas the indirect lesion volume is obtained by subtracting the volume of the unaffected ipsilateral hemisphere from the volume of the contralateral hemisphere. The difference between these two methods is that corrected lesion volume is used to compensate for brain edema,[140,141] which is essential to exclude the possibility that pharmacologic intervention may reduce edema, but may not actually salvage ischemic brain tissue at risk of infarction. In addition to absolute lesion volumes, the percentage of the hemisphere involved with ischemia should also be provided, and it can be reported as a percentage of the ipsilateral or contralateral hemispheres. Finally, slice-by-slice lesion areas and cortical and subcortical lesion volumes should be reported. This provides insight into the anatomic distribution of ischemic damage and the location of reduction of the lesion by stroke therapy.

TTC staining (Color Plate 11) is easier, quicker, and less expensive for determining infarct volume as compared with H&E staining.[142,143] Usually, a 2% solution of TTC in normal saline is used to react with brain slices for 30 minutes at 37°C. Because the validity of TTC staining is based on mitochondrial enzyme damage,[144] caution must be used. TTC is reduced by mitochondrial enzymes to a red compound, and thus normal tissue stains red or dark red, whereas ischemic tissue with damaged mitochondrial enzymes does not stain (white) or faintly stains (pink), resulting in good contrast between normal and infarcted tissues. Studies have shown that TTC staining is useful between 6 to 72 hours after the onset of ischemia, and good correlation between TTC and H&E staining in delineating infarct volume exists.[141,142,145] When used earlier than 6 hours after ischemia onset, this technique may not accurately delineate the extent of irreversible ischemic

damage because destruction of mitochondrial enzyme requires time.[146,147] After 72 hours, the infarct volume determined by TTC staining may be underestimated, because gliosis, macrophage infiltration, and other proliferative inflammatory responses may obscure the periphery of ischemic damage.[144] In addition, delayed TTC staining within 8 hours after animals' deaths remains useful for determining infarct volume, because mitochondrial enzymes degrade slowly after death and can still reduce TTC in nonischemic tissues.[148]

H&E staining is a traditional technique for evaluating ischemic changes that may include both acute-type and delayed-type damage.[149,150] In the former, cellular swelling and neuropil spongiosis are prominent features, and the neurons exhibit a shrunken appearance during the first 6 hours after ischemia; in the latter, the neurons are irreversibly damaged and appear as red (eosinophilic) neurons or ghost neurons beginning 6–12 hours after ischemia.[149,150] Pannecrosis involving all cell types (neuronal, glial, and vascular cells) may not occur until 48–72 hours after ischemia.[149] Obviously, the temporal profile of ischemic cell damage depends on the severity and duration of the ischemic event. Short periods of transient ischemia may provide a profile of damage that is different from that caused by permanent ischemia, and the ischemic lesion increases in both intensity and extent with longer durations of ischemia. With the intraluminal suture MCA occlusion model, for example, it can evolve from selective neuronal damage (less than 30 minutes of ischemia) to focal infarction involving striatum (up to 60 minutes of ischemia) to widespread infarct encompassing both cortical and subcortical tissue (>90 minutes of ischemia).[3,151,152] These differences may have an impact on therapeutic intervention, and it is possible that a therapeutic intervention may be effective in reducing ischemic cell damage only for a particular duration of ischemic insult.

Some Concerns about Animal Models

Although animal modeling has provided much information about ischemic mechanisms and potential treatment of ischemic stroke, the relevance of animal stroke models to human stroke has been increasingly doubted, because many compounds showing neuroprotective effects in animal models have failed to show efficacy in stroke patients.[153] There are several concerns about animal modeling used to develop neuroprotective drugs.

Aged Animal

Most animal stroke models are performed in young adult animals, although some studies use aged rats.[154,155] In aged animals, the immune system, neurochemistry, vascular structure, and morphology may differ from those in young rats, and the neurochemical, morphologic, and behavioral changes resulting from ischemia may also be different.[156] Some evidence demonstrated that the infarct size is larger in older rats and that the lesion distribution is different between young and old rats,[157] although one study did not demonstrate bigger infarct size with aging.[10] In developing effective drugs, few experiments use aged animals to test the efficacy of compounds, which may in part explain failure in clinical trials in which elderly patients are the majority. It may be more important to determine whether a compound is still effective in aged animals, in addition to younger animals. However, it is not known what age in animals is comparable to the typical human stroke population.

Health Status

Animals used in most experimental stroke models are young and healthy, and are in contrast to most stroke patients who may also have diabetes mellitus, chronic hypertension, and hyperlipidemia.[153] These complicating factors may preclude response to therapy in humans. Therefore, experimental data from healthy animals may not be successfully extrapolated to sick and fragile patients. Although some attempts have been made to model "unhealthy status," such as using animals with atherosclerosis and hypertension, these circumstances are unlikely to be directly relevant to complicated human situations.

Animal Gender

One study demonstrated that infarct volume in stroke models is sex-related, and that female rats typically have smaller infarct size than male rats.[158] Because of difference in physiologic status, it is possible that response to treatment is different between the two genders. In preclinical assessments, male rats are predominantly used, and only a few studies have used female rats. It is important to know if the neuroprotective effect of compounds exists in both male and female animals.

Model-Related Neuroprotection

It is possible that neuroprotection may be model-related, because ischemic characteristics in different models may be different, and some models may not produce ischemic regions amenable to therapeutic regimens. This is confirmed by one study, in which neuroprotection was positive in one animal model but negative in the other model.[159] Therefore, choosing the proper model is important for developing drugs.

Strain- or Species-Related Neuroprotection

One reason for failure of data transition from the laboratory to bedside may be that neuroprotective effects are strain- or species-related. At least one study demonstrated that reduction in infarct size with calcium or N-methyl-D-aspartate antagonists depends on the rat strains used.[160] Although the reasons and mechanisms are not clear, it is essential that testing drug efficacy be performed in animal models with different strains and species. Even though drugs work in different animal strains and species, it is not easy to anticipate the effect that drugs may have on humans, due to their more complex pathophysiologic processes. However, such difficulties should not be a hurdle to prevent pursuit of effective treatment for human stroke, and intense efforts are being made continuously.

References

1. Macrae IM. New models of focal cerebral ischaemia. Br J Clin Pharmacol 1992;34:302–308.
2. Hsu CY. Criteria for valid preclinical trials using animal stroke models. Stroke 1993;24:633–636.
3. Memezawa H, Smith M-L, Siesjö BK. Penumbral tissues salvaged by reperfusion following middle cerebral artery occlusion in rats. Stroke 1992;23:552–559.

4. Li F, Han SS, Tatlisumak T, et al. Reversal of acute apparent diffusion coefficient abnormalities and delayed neuronal death following transient focal brain ischemia in rats. Ann Neurol 1999;46:333–342.

5. del Zoppo GJ, Poeck K, Pessin MS, et al. Recombinant tissue plasminogen activator in acute thrombotic and embolic stroke. Ann Neurol 1992;32:78–86.

6. Recommendations for standards regarding preclinical neuroprotective and restorative drug development. Stroke Therapy Academic Industry Roundtable (STAIR). Stroke 1999;30:2752–2758.

7. Coyle P. Arterial patterns of the rat rhinencephalon and related structures. Exp Neurol 1975;49:671–690.

8. Yamori Y, Horie R, Handa H, et al. Pathogenetic similarity of strokes in stroke-prone spontaneously hypertensive rats and humans. Stroke 1976;7:46–53.

9. Rieke GK, Bowers DE Jr, Penn P. Vascular supply pattern to rat caudoputamen and globus pallidus: scanning electronmicroscopic study of vascular endocast of stroke-prone vessels. Stroke 1981;12:840–860.

10. Duverger D, MacKenzie ET. The quantification of cerebral infarction following focal ischemia in the rat: influence of strain, arterial pressure, blood glucose concentration, and age. J Cereb Blood Flow Metab 1988; 8:449–461.

11. Oliff HS, Weber E, Eilon G, Marek P. The role of strain/vendor differences on the outcome of focal ischemia induced by intraluminal middle cerebral artery occlusion in the rat. Brain Res 1995;675:20–26.

12. Ginsberg MD, Busto R. Rodent models of cerebral ischemia. Stroke 1989;20:1627–1642.

13. Smith M-L, Bendek G, Dahlgren N, et al. Models for studying long-term recovery following forebrain ischemia in the rat. 2. A 2-vessel occlusion model. Acta Neurol Scand 1984;69:385–401.

14. Hossmann K-A. Animal models of cerebral ischemia. 1. Review of literature. Cerebrovasc Dis 1991;1(Suppl 1):2–15.

15. Pulsinelli WA, Brierley JB. A new model of bilateral hemispheric ischemia in the unanesthetized rat. Stroke 1979;10:267–272.

16. Pulsinelli WA, Buchan AM. The four-vessel occlusion rat model: method for complete occlusion of vertebral arteries and control of collateral circulation. Stroke 1988;19: 913–914.

17. Schmidt-Kastner R, Paschen W, Ophoff BG, Hossmann K-A. A modified four-vessel occlusion model for inducing incomplete forebrain ischemia in rats. Stroke 1989;20: 938–946.

18. Levine S, Sohn D. Cerebral ischemia in infant and adult gerbils. Relation to incomplete circle of Willis. Arch Pathol 1969;87:315–317.

19. Levine S. Anoxic-ischemic encephalopathy in rats. Am J Pathol 1960;36:1–17.

20. Hossmann V, Hossmann K-A. Return of neuronal functions after prolonged cardiac arrest. Brain Res 1973;60: 423–438.

21. Todd MM, Dunlop B, Shapiro HM, et al. Ventricular fibrillation in the cat: a model for global cerebral ischemia. Stroke 1981;12:808-815.

22. Kawakami S, Hossmann K-A. Electrophysiological recovery after compression ischemia of the rat brain. J Neurol 1977;217:31–42.

23. Pulsinelli WA, Brierley JB, Plum F. Temporal profile of neuronal damage in a rat model of transient forebrain ischemia. Ann Neurol 1982;11:491–498.

24. Levy DE, Brierly JB. Communications between vertebrobasilar and carotid arterial circulations in the gerbil. Exp Neurol 1974;45:503–508.

25. Mayevsky A, Breuer Z. Brain vasculature and mitochondrial responses to ischemia in gerbils. I. Basic anatomic patterns and biochemical correlates. Brain Res 1992;598: 242–250.

26. Siegel BA, Meidinger R, Elliott AJ, et al. Experimental cerebral microembolism. Multiple tracer assessment of brain edema. Arch Neurol 1972;26:73–77.

27. Kogure K, Busto R, Scheinberg P, Reinmuth OM. Energy metabolites and water content in rat brain during the early stage of development of cerebral infarction. Brain 1974; 97:103–114.

28. Kogure K, Busto R, Schwartzman RJ, Scheinberg P. The dissociation of cerebral blood flow, metabolism and function in the early stages of developing cerebral infarction. Ann Neurol 1980;8:278–290.

29. Garcia JH. Experimental ischemic stroke: a review. Stroke 1984;15:5–14.

30. Takeda T, Shima T, Okada Y, et al. Pathophysiological studies of cerebral ischemia produced by silicone cylinder embolization in rats. J Cereb Blood Flow Metab 1987;7(Suppl):S66.

31. Fukuchi K, Kusuoka H, Watanabe Y, Nishimura T. Correlation of sequential MR images of microsphere-induced cerebral ischemia with histologic changes in rats. Invest Radiol 1999;34:698–703.

32. Watson BD, Dietrich WD, Busto R, et al. Induction of reproducible brain infarction by photochemically initiated thrombosis. Ann Neurol 1985;17:497–504.

33. Chopp M, Glasberg MR, Riddle JM, et al. Photodynamic therapy of normal cerebral tissue in the cat: a noninvasive model for cerebrovascular thrombosis. Photochem Photobiol 1987;46:103–108.

34. Yoshida Y, Dereski MO, Garcia JH, et al. Neuronal injury after photoactivation photofrin II. Am J Pathol 1992;141: 989–997.

35. Yoshida Y, Dereski MO, Garcia JH, et al. Photoactivated photophrin II: astrocytic swelling precedes endothelial injury in rat brain. J Neuropathol Exper Neurol 1992;51:91–100.

36. Dietrich WD, Watson BD, Busto R, et al. Photochemically induced cerebral infarction. I. Early microvascular alterations. Acta Neuropathol (Berl) 1987;72:315–325.

37. Dietrich WD, Watson BD, Busto R, et al. Photochemically induced cerebral infarction. II. Edema and blood-brain barrier disruption. Acta Neuropathol (Berl) 1987;72:326–334.

38. van Bruggen N, Cullen BM, King MD, et al. T2- and diffusion-weighted magnetic resonance imaging of a focal ischemic lesion in rat brain. Stroke 1992;23:576–582.

39. Forsting M, Reith W, Dörfler A, et al. MRI monitoring of experimental cerebral ischaemia: comparison of two models. Neuroradiology 1994;36:264–268.

40. De Ryck M. Animal models of cerebral stroke: pharmacological protection of function. Eur Neurol 1990;3(Suppl): 21–27.

41. Robinson MJ, Macrae IM, Todd M, et al. Reduction of local cerebral blood flow to pathological levels by endothelin-1 applied to the middle cerebral artery in the rat. Neurosci Lett 1990;118:269–272.

42. Sharkey J, Ritchie IM, Kelly PA. Perivascular microapplication of endothelin-1: a new model of focal cerebral ischaemia in the rat. J Cereb Blood Flow Metab 1993;13: 865–871.

43. Sharkey J, Butcher SP, Kelly JS. Endothelin-1 induced middle cerebral artery occlusion: pathological consequences and neuroprotective effects of MK 801. J Auton Nerv Syst 1994;49:S177–S185.

44. Sharkey J, Butcher SP. Characterization of an experimental model of stroke produced by intracerebral microinjection of endothelin-1 adjacent to the rat middle cerebral artery. J Neurosci Methods 1995;60:125–131.

45. Sloan MA. Thrombolysis and stroke. Past and future. Arch Neurol 1987;44:748–768.

46. Albers GW. Antithrombotic agents in cerebral ischemia. Am J Cardiol 1995;75:348–388.

47. Tissue plasminogen activator for acute ischemic stroke. The National Institute of Neurological Disorders and Stroke rt-PA Stroke Study Group. N Engl J Med 1995; 333:1581–1587.

48. Overgaard K, Sereghy T, Boysen G, et al. Reduction of infarct volume by thrombolysis with rt-PA in an embolic rat stroke model. Scand J Clin Lab Invest 1993;53:383–393.

49. Overgaard K, Sereghy T, Pedersen H, Boysen G. Effect of delayed thrombolysis with rt-PA in a rat embolic stroke model. J Cereb Blood Flow Metab 1994;14:472–477.

50. Futrell N, Watson BD, Dietrich WD, et al. A new model of embolic stroke produced by photochemical injury to the carotid artery in the rat. Ann Neurol 1988;23:251.

51. Futrell N. An improved photochemical model of embolic cerebral infarction in rats. Stroke 1991;22:225–232.

52. Dietrich WD, Prado R, Waston BD, et al. Hemodynamic consequences of common carotid artery thrombosis and thrombogenically activated blood in the rats. J Cereb Blood Flow Metab 1991;11:957–965.

53. Dietrich WD, Prado R, Halley M, Watson BD. Microvascular and neuronal consequences of common carotid artery thrombosis and platelet embolization in rats. J Neuropathol Exp Neurol 1993;52:351–360.

54. Hill NC, Millikan CH, Wakim KG, et al. Studies in cerebrovascular disease. VII. Experimental production of cerebral infarction by intracarotid injection of homologous blood clot. Preliminary report. Mayo Clin Proc 1955;30:625–633.

55. Kudo M, Aoyama A, Ichimori S, Fukunaga N. An animal model of cerebral infarction. Stroke 1982;13:505–508.

56. Kaneko D, Nakamura N, Ogawa T. Cerebral infarction in rats using homologous blood emboli: development of a new experimental model. Stroke 1985;16:76–84.

57. Overgaard K, Sereghy T, Boysen G, et al. A rat model of reproducible cerebral infarction using thrombotic blood clot emboli. J Cereb Blood Flow Metab 1992;12:484–490.

58. Busch E, Krüger K, Hossmann K-A. Improved model of thromboembolic stroke and rt-PA induced reperfusion in the rat. Brain Res 1997;778:16–24.

59. Takano K, Carano RA, Tatlisumak T, et al. Efficacy of intra-arterial and intravenous prourokinase in an embolic stroke model evaluated by diffusion-perfusion magnetic resonance imaging. Neurology 1998;50:870–875.

60. Zhang RL, Chopp M, Zhang ZG, et al. A rat model of focal embolic cerebral ischemia. Brain Res 1997;766:83–92.

61. Zhang Z, Zhang RL, Jiang Q, et al. A new rat model of thrombotic focal cerebral ischemia. J Cereb Blood Flow Metab 1997;17:123–135.

62. Zhang Z, Chopp M, Zhang RL, Goussev A. A mouse model of embolic focal cerebral ischemia. J Cereb Blood Flow Metab 1997;17:1081–1088.

63. Shigeno T, Teasdale GM, McCulloch J, Graham DI. Recirculation model following MCA occlusion in rats. Cerebral blood flow, cerebrovascular permeability, and brain edema. J Neurosurg 1985;63:272–277.

64. Shigeno T, McCulloch J, Graham D, et al. Pure cortical ischemia versus striatal ischemia. Surg Neurol 1985;24: 47–51.

65. Takizawa S, Hakim AM. Animal models of cerebral ischemia. 2. Rat models. Cerebrovasc Dis 1990;1(Suppl 1):16–21.

66. Hudgins WR, Garcia JH. The effect of electrocautery, atmospheric exposure and surgical retraction on the permeability of the blood brain barrier. Stroke 1970;1:375–380.

67. Hudgins WR, Garcia JH. Transorbital approach to the middle cerebral artery of the squirrel monkey: a technique for experimental cerebral infarction applicable to ultrastructural studies. Stroke 1970;1:107–111.

68. Crowell RM, Marcoux FW, DeGirolami U. Variability and reversibility of focal cerebral ischemia in unanesthetized monkeys. Neurology 1981;31:1295–1302.

69. Suzuki J, Yoshimoto T, Tnanka S, Sakamoto T. Production of various models of cerebral infarction in the dog by means of occlusion of intracranial trunk arteries. Stroke 1980;11:337–341.

70. Slivka A, Pulsinelli W. Hemorrhagic complications of thrombolytic therapy in experimental stroke. Stroke 1987;18:1148.

71. Sundt TM, Waltz AG. Experimental cerebral infarction: retro-orbital, extradural approach for occluding the middle cerebral artery. Mayo Clin Proc 1966;41:159–168.

72. Hayakawa T, Waltz AG. Immediate effects of cerebral ischemia: evolution and resolution of neurological deficits after experimental occlusion of one middle cerebral artery in conscious cats. Stroke 1975;6:321.

73. Little JR. Implanted device for middle cerebral artery occlusion in conscious cats. Stroke 1977;8:258–260.

74. Robinson RG, Shoemaker WJ, Schlumpf M, et al. Effect of experimental cerebral infarction in rat brain on catecholamines and behaviour. Nature 1975;255:332–334.

75. Robinson RG. Differential behavior and biochemical effects of right and left hemispheric infarction in the rat. Science 1979;205:707–710.

76. Robinson RG, Coyle JT. The differential effect of right versus left hemispheric cerebral infarction on catecholamines and behavior in the rat. Brain Res 1980;188:63–78.

77. Backhauss C, Karkoutly C, Welsch M, Krieglstein J. A mouse model of focal cerebral ischemia for screening neuroprotective drug effects. J Pharmacol Toxicol Methods 1992;27:27–32.

78. Robinson RG, Bloom FE, Battenberg EL. A fluorescent histochemical study of changes in noradrenergic neurons following experimental cerebral infarction in the rat. Brain Res 1977;132:259–272.

79. Albanese V, Tommasino C, Spadaro A, Tommasello F. A transbasisphenoidal approach for selective occlusion of the middle cerebral artery in rats. Experientia 1980;36:1302–1304.

80. Tamura A, Graham DI, McCulloch J, Teasdale GM. Focal cerebral ischaemia in the rat. 1. Description of technique and early neuropathological consequences following middle cerebral artery occlusion. J Cereb Blood Flow Metab 1981;1:53–60.

81. Tamura A, Graham DI, McCulloch J, Teasdale GM. Focal cerebral ischaemia in the rat. 2: Regional cerebral blood flow determined by [^{14}C]iodoantipyrine autoradiography following middle cerebral artery occlusion. J Cereb Blood Flow Metab 1981;1:61–69.

82. Bederson JB, Pitts LH, Tsuji M, et al. Rat middle cerebral artery occlusion: evaluation of the model and development of a neurologic examination. Stroke 1986;17:472–476.

83. Fox G, Gallacher D, Shevde S, et al. Anatomic variation of the middle cerebral artery in the Sprague-Dawley rat. Stroke 1993;24:2087–2093.

84. Coyle P. Middle cerebral artery occlusion in the young rat. Stroke 1982;13:855–859.

85. Chen ST, Hsu CY, Hogan EL, et al. A model of focal ischemic stroke in the rat: reproducible extensive cortical infarction. Stroke 1986;17:738–743.

86. Brint S, Jacewicz M, Kiessling M, et al. Focal brain ischemia in the rat: methods for reproducible neocortical infarction using tandem occlusion of the distal middle cerebral and ipsilateral common carotid arteries. J Cereb Blood Flow Metab 1988;8:474–485.

87. Robinson RG, Shoemaker WJ, Schlumpf M, et al. In the rat: topography of hemodynamic and histopathological changes. Ann Neurol 1984;15:559–567.

88. Rubino G, Young W. Ischemic cortical lesions after permanent occlusion of individual middle cerebral artery branches in rats. Stroke 1988;19:870–877.

89. Koizumi J, Yoshida Y, Nakazawa T, et al. Experimental studies of ischemic brain edema: 1. A new experimental model of cerebral embolism in rats in which recirculation can be introduced in the ischemic area. Japan Stroke Journal 1986;8:1–8.

90. Longa EZ, Weinstein PR, Carlson S, Cummins R. Reversible middle cerebral artery occlusion without craniectomy in rats. Stroke 1989;20:84–91.

91. Laing RJ, Jakubowski J, Laing RW. Middle cerebral artery occlusion without craniectomy in rats. Which method works best? Stroke 1993;24:294–298.

92. Takano K, Tatlisumak T, Bergmann AG, et al. Reproducibility and reliability of middle cerebral artery occlusion using a silicon-coated suture (Koizumi) in rats. J Neurol Sci 1997;153:8–11.

93. Belayev L, Alonso OF, Busto R, et al. Middle cerebral artery occlusion in the rat by intraluminal suture. Neurological and pathological evaluation of an improved model. Stroke 1996;27:1616–1623.

94. Nagasawa H, Kogure K. Correlation between cerebral blood flow and histologic changes in a new rat model of middle cerebral artery occlusion. Stroke 1989;20:1037–1043.

95. Zarow GJ, Karibe H, States BA, et al. Endovascular suture occlusion of the middle cerebral artery in rats: effect of suture insertion distance on cerebral blood flow, infarct distribution and infarct volume. Neurol Res 1997;19:409–416.

96. Li F, Han S, Tatlisumak T, et al. A new method to improve in-bore middle cerebral artery occlusion in rats: demonstration with diffusion- and perfusion-weighted imaging. Stroke 1998;29:1715–1720.

97. Kuge Y, Minematsu K, Yamaguchi T, Miyake Y. Nylon monofilament for intraluminal cerebral artery occlusion in rats. Stroke 1995;26:1655–1658.

98. Schmid-Elsaesser R, Zausinger S, Hungerhuber E, et al. A critical reevaluation of the intraluminal thread model of focal cerebral ischemia: evidence of inadvertent premature reperfusion and subarachnoid hemorrhage in rats by laser-Doppler flowmetry. Stroke 1998;29:2162–2170.

99. Roussel SA, van Bruggen N, King MD, et al. Monitoring the initial expansion of focal ischemic changes by diffusion-weighted MRI using a remote controlled method of occlusion. NMR Biomed 1994;7:21–28.

100. Kohno K, Back T, Hoehn-Berlage M, Hossmann K-A. A modified rat model of middle cerebral artery thread occlusion under electrophysiological control for magnetic resonance investigations. Magn Reson Imaging 1995;13:65–71.

101. Röther J, de Crespigny AJ, D'Arceuil H, Mosley ME. MR detection of cortical spreading depression immediately after focal ischemia in the rat. J Cereb Blood Flow Metab 1996;16:214–220.

102. Kinouchi H, Epstein CJ, Mizui T, et al. Attenuation of focal cerebral ischemic injury in transgenic mice overexpressing CuZn superoxide dismutase. Proc Natl Acad Sci U S A 1991;88:11158–11162.

103. Yang G, Chan PH, Chen J, et al. Human copper-zinc superoxide dismutase transgenic mice are highly resistant to reperfusion injury after focal cerebral ischemia. Stroke 1994;25:165–170.

104. Hara H, Huang PL, Panahian N, et al. Reduced brain edema and infarction volume in mice lacking the neuronal isoform of nitric oxide synthase after transient MCA occlusion. J Cereb Blood Flow Metab 1996;16:605–611.

105. Hata R, Mies G, Wiessner C, et al. A reproducible model of middle cerebral artery occlusion in mice: hemodynamic, biochemical, and magnetic resonance imaging. J Cereb Blood Flow Metab 1998;18:367–375.

106. Warner DS, Mcfarlane C, Todd MM, et al. Sevoflurane and halothane reduce focal ischemic brain damage in the rat. Possible influence on thermoregulation. Anesthesiology 1993;79:877–880.

107. Kiyota Y, Pahlmark K, Memezawa H, et al. Free radicals and brain damage due to transient middle cerebral artery occlusion: the effect of dimethylthiourea. Exp Brain Res 1993;95:388–396.

108. Zhao Q, Memezawa H, Smith ML, Siesjo BK. Hyperthermia complicates middle cerebral artery occlusion induced by an intraluminal filament. Brain Res 1994;649:253–259.

109. Li F, Omae T, Fisher M. Spontaneous hyperthermia and its mechanism in the intraluminal suture middle cerebral artery occlusion model of rats. Stroke 1999;30:2464–2471.

110. Valtysson J, Hillered L, Andine P, et al. Neuropathological endpoints in experimental stroke pharmacotherapy: the importance of both early and late evaluation. Acta Neurochir 1994;129:58–63.

111. Coimbra C, Drake M, Boris-Moller F, Wieloch T. Long lasting neuroprotective effect of post-ischemic hypothermia and treatment with an anti-inflammatory/antipyretic drug. Evidence for chronic encephalopathic processes following ischemia. Stroke 1996;27:1578–1585.

112. Feeney DM, Gonzalez A, Law WA. Amphetamine, haloperidol, and experience interact to affect rate of recovery after motor cortex injury. Science 1982;217:855–857.

113. De Ryck M, Van Reempts J, Duytschaever H, et al. Neocortical localization of tactile/proprioceptive limb placing reactions in the rat. Brain Res 1992;573:44–60.

114. Markgraf CG, Green EG, Hurwitz BE, et al. Sensimotor and cognitive consequences of middle cerebral artery occlusion in rats. Brain Res 1992;575:238–246.

115. Jones TA, Schaller T. Use-dependent growth of pyramidal neurons after neocortical damage. J Neurosci 1994;14:2140–2152.

116. Kolb B, Cote S, Ribeiro-da-Silva A, Cuello AC. Nerve growth factor treatment prevents dendritic atrophy and promotes recovery of function after cortical injury. Neuroscience 1997;76:1139–1151.

117. Moseley ME, Cohen Y, Mintorovitch J, et al. Early detection of regional cerebral ischemia in cats: comparison of diffusion- and T2-weighted MRI and spectroscopy. Magn Reson Med 1990;14:330–346.

118. Minematsu K, Li L, Fisher M, et al. Diffusion-weighted magnetic resonance imaging: rapid and quantitative detection of focal brain ischemia. Neurology 1992;42:235–240.

119. Baird AE, Warach S. Magnetic resonance imaging of acute stroke. J Cereb Blood Flow Metab 1998;18:583–609.

120. Albers GW. Expanding the window for thrombolytic therapy in acute stroke. The potential role of acute MRI for patient selection. Stroke 1999;30:2230–2237.

121. Fisher M, Albers GW. Applications of diffusion-perfusion magnetic resonance imaging in acute ischemic stroke. Neurology 1999;52:1750–1756.

122. Minematsu K, Fisher M, Li L, Sotak CH. Diffusion and perfusion MRI studies to evaluate a noncompetitive N-methyl-D-aspartate antagonist and reperfusion in experimental stroke in rats. Stroke 1993;24:2074–2081.

123. Minematsu K, Fisher M, Li L, et al. Effects of a novel NMDA antagonist on experimental stroke rapidly and quantitatively assessed by diffusion-weighted MRI. Neurology 1993;42:397–403.

124. Lo EH, Matsumoto K, Pierce AR, et al. Pharmacologic reversal of acute changes in diffusion-weighted magnetic resonance imaging in focal cerebral ischemia. J Cereb Blood Flow Metab 1994;14:597–603.

125. Tatlisumak T, Takano K, Carano RA, Fisher M. Effect of basic fibroblast growth factor on experimental focal ischemia studied by diffusion-weighted and perfusion imaging. Stroke 1996;27:2292–2298.

126. Lo EH, Pierce AR, Mandeville JB, Rosen BR. Neuroprotection with NBQX in rat focal cerebral ischemia: effects on ADC probability distribution functions and diffusion-perfusion relationships. Stroke 1997;28:439–447.

127. Tatlisumak T, Carano RA, Takano K, et al. A novel endothelin antagonist, A-127722, attenuates ischemic lesion size in rats with temporary middle cerebral artery occlusion: a diffusion and perfusion MRI study. Stroke 1998;29:850–858.

128. Jiang Q, Zhang RL, Zhang ZG, et al. Diffusion-, T2-, and perfusion-weighted nuclear magnetic resonance imaging of middle cerebral artery embolic stroke and recombinant tissue plasminogen activator intervention in the rat. J Cereb Blood Flow Metab 1998;18:758–767.

129. Jiang Q, Zhang RL, Zhang ZG, et al. Magnetic resonance imaging indexes of therapeutic efficacy of recombinant tissue plasminogen activator treatment of rat at 1 and 4 hours after embolic stroke. J Cereb Blood Flow Metab 2000;20:21–27.

130. Warach S, Benfield A, Schlaug G, et al. Reduction of lesion volume in human stroke by citicoline detected by diffusion weighted magnetic resonance imaging: a pilot study. Ann Neurol 1996;40(abstract):527–528.

131. Marks MP, Tong DC, Beaulieu C, et al. Evaluation of early reperfusion and IV tPA therapy using diffusion- and perfusion-weighted MRI. Neurology 1999;52:1792–1798.

132. Carano RA, Li F, Irie K, et al. Multispectral analysis of the temporal evolution of cerebral ischemia in the rat brain. J Magn Reson Imaging 2000;12:842–858.

133. Li F, Carano RA, Irie K, et al. Neuroprotective effects of a novel broad spectrum channel blocker, LOE 908 MS, on transient focal ischemia: a multispectral study. J Magn Reson Imaging 1999;10:138–145.

134. Dijkhuizen RM, Knollema S, van der Worp H, et al. Dynamics of cerebral tissue injury and perfusion after temporary hypoxia-ischemia in the rat: evidence for region-specific sensitivity and delayed damage. Stroke 1998;29:695–704.

135. van Lookeren Campagne M, Thomas GR, Thibodeaux H, et al. Secondary reduction in the apparent diffusion coefficient of water, increase in cerebral blood volume, and delayed neuronal death after middle cerebral artery occlusion and early reperfusion in the rat. J Cereb Blood Flow Metab 1999;19:1354–1364.

136. Li F, Silva MD, Sotak CH, Fisher M. Temporal evolution of ischemic injury evaluated with diffusion-, perfusion-, and T2-weighted MRI. Neurology 2000;54:689–696.

137. Li F, Liu K-F, Silva MD, et al. Transient and permanent resolution of ischemic lesions on diffusion-weighted imaging after brief periods of focal brain ischemia in rat: correlation with histopathology. Stroke 2000;31:946–954.

138. Lahti KM, Ferris CF, Li F, et al. Imaging brain activity in conscious animals using functional MRI. J Neurosci Methods 1998;82:75–83.

139. Fisher M, Finklestein S. Pharmacological approaches to stroke recovery. Cerebrovasc Dis 1999;9(Suppl 5):29–32.

140. Swanson RA, Morton MT, Tsao-Wu G, et al. A semiautomated method for measuring brain infarct volume. J Cerebr Blood Flow Metab 1990;10:290–293.

141. Lin T-N, He YY, Wu G, et al. Effect of brain edema on infarct volume in a focal ischemia model in rats. Stroke 1993;24:117–121.

142. Bederson JB, Pitts LH, Germano SM, et al. Evaluation of 2,3,5-tryphenyltetrazolium chloride as a stain for detection and quantification of experimental cerebral infarction in rats. Stroke 1986;17:1304–1308.

143. Lundy EF, Solik BS, Frank RS, et al. Morphometric evaluation of brain infarcts in rats and gerbils. J Pharmacol Methods 1986;16:201–214.

144. Liszczak TM, Hedley-Whyte ET, Adams JF, et al. Limitations of tetrazolium salts in delineating infarcted brain. Acta Neuropathol (Berl) 1984;65:150–157.

145. Isayama K, Pitts LH, Nishimura MC. Evaluation of 2,3,5-triphenyltetrazolium chloride staining to delineate rat brain infarcts. Stroke 1991;22:1394–1398.

146. Park CK, Mendelow AD, Graham DI, et al. Correlation of triphenyltetrazolium chloride perfusion staining with conventional neurohistology in the detection of early brain ischaemia. Neuropathol Appl Neurobiol 1988;14:289–298.

147. Hatfield RH, Mendelow AD, Perry RH, et al. Triphenyltetrazolium chloride (TTC) as a marker for ischaemic changes in rat brain following permanent middle cerebral artery occlusion. Neuropathol Appl Neurobiol 1991;17:61–67.

148. Li F, Irie K, Anwer MS, Fisher M. Delayed triphenyltetrazolium chloride staining remains useful for evaluating cerebral infarct volume in a rat stroke model. J Cereb Blood Flow Metab 1997;17:1132–1135.

149. Garcia JH, Yoshida Y, Chen H, et al. Progression from ischemic injury to infarct following middle cerebral artery occlusion in the rat. Am J Pathol 1993;142:623–635.

150. Garcia JH, Liu K-F, Ho K-L. Neuronal necrosis after middle cerebral artery occlusion in Wistar rats progresses at different time intervals in the caudoputamen and the cortex. Stroke 1995;26:636–643.

151. Garcia JH, Wagner S, Liu K-F, Hu XJ. Neurological deficit and extent of neuronal necrosis attributable to middle cerebral artery occlusion in rats. Statistical validation. Stroke 1995;26:627–635.

152. Garcia JH, Liu K-F, Ye Z-R, Gutierrez JA. Incomplete infarct and delayed neuronal death after transient middle cerebral artery occlusion in rats. Stroke 1997;28:2303–2310.

153. Wiebers DO, Adams HP Jr, Whisnant JP. Animal models of stroke: are they relevant to human disease? Stroke 1990;21:1–3.

154. Wang LC, Futrell N, Wang DZ, et al. A reproducible model of middle cerebral infarcts, compatible with long-term survival, in aged rats. Stroke 1995;26:2087–2090.

155. Sutherland GR, Dix GA, Auer RN. Effect of age in rodent models of focal and forebrain ischemia. Stroke 1996;27:1663–1668.

156. Millikan C. Animal stroke models. Stroke 1992;23:795–797.

157. Davis M, Mendelow AD, Perry RH, et al. Experimental stroke and neuroprotection in the aging rat brain. Stroke 1995;26:1072–1078.

158. Alkayed NJ, Harukuni I, Kimes AL, et al. Gender-linked brain injury in experimental stroke. Stroke 1998;29:159–166.

159. Takamatsu H, Kondo K, Ikeda Y, Umemura K. Neuroprotective effects depend on the model of focal ischemia following middle cerebral artery occlusion. Eur J Pharmacol 1998;362:137–142.

160. Sauter A, Rudin M. Strain-dependent drug effects in rat middle cerebral artery occlusion model of stroke. J Pharmacol Exp Ther 1995;274:1008–1013.

Chapter 6
Clinical Trial Design for Cerebrovascular Disorders

Lawrence M. Brass

The focus of this book is what is known about the treatment of cerebrovascular diseases. This chapter deals with how that knowledge is gained. Information on stroke therapies is growing rapidly,[1] as is knowledge about gathering this data. Most clinicians are aware of how rapidly knowledge of new stroke therapies is advancing; however, few are aware of the rapid evolution of clinical trial design and methodology that has taken place at the same time.

The effort in selecting the appropriate investigative tool to answer a specific clinical question should be as rigorous as designing an experiment to measure an ion flux across a neuronal membrane.[2] Without the proper setup, design, and execution, bad data are equally likely to result. Unlike bench research, in which clear standards and rigorous controls have emerged for most methods, the same caliber of standards has not been widely applied to clinical methods in neurology. This is changing, however.

The evaluation of the efficacy and safety of a (potential) new agent for stroke therapy requires well designed clinical trials. The design, execution, and analysis of clinical trials are the focus of this chapter. It is important that clinicians who make use of new agents have a better understanding of the design, performance, and interpretation of clinical trials. This chapter overviews some of the basic principles of clinical studies and expands on a previous review.[3]

Clinical Research

Clinical research has been divided into three broad areas: (1) epidemiologic research, (2) outcomes and health services research, and (3) patient-oriented research. *Clinical epidemiology* has been referred to as the basic science for clinical medicine.[4] Epidemiologic principles and methods are applied to problems encountered in the practice of medicine. Most often, clinicians think of randomized clinical trials when clinical studies are mentioned. This is only one small part of clinical research (Table 6-1).[5]

Although clinical studies have been described as far back as the Old Testament, rigorous methods for evaluating clinical phenomena and measuring therapeutic benefit have only recently been applied in medicine. Many widely held clinical beliefs related to clinical management have not been rigorously tested.[6] For example, it is widely believed that magnetic resonance imaging (MRI) is well established as superior to computed tomography (CT) scanning for the management of patients with ischemic stroke. A review of clinical studies of MRI shows that the evidence for the superiority of MRI is weak.[7] Although there is promise, especially with newer MR techniques, there are little data to support the superiority of MRI over CT. There are even less data to show a beneficial effect on patient outcome.

Table 6-1. Key Questions in the Practice of Medicine

Topic	Typical Clinical Question
Normality	Is the person sick or well?
	What abnormalities are associated with the disease?
Diagnosis	How accurate is a diagnosis or specific test?
Frequency	How often does a disease occur?
Risk	What factors are associated with the likelihood of disease?
Prognosis	What happens to the patient?
Treatment	Does a treatment alter the course of the disease?
Prevention	Is detection of those at risk and treatment possible?
Cause	What conditions result in disease?
	What mechanisms are involved?

Source: Modified from RH Fletcher, SW Fletcher, EH Wagner. Clinical Epidemiology: The Essentials (2nd ed). Baltimore: Williams & Wilkins, 1988.

Outcomes and health services research deals with the clinical course after a completed stroke and the associated use of health services.[8,9] Given the large portion of stroke patients with long-term disability and the complex nature of recovery, the need for clinical research to go beyond traditional endpoints or recurrent stroke or death seems obvious.

Patient-oriented research is defined as research conducted with human subjects (or on material of human origin, such as tissues, specimens, and cognitive phenomena), in which an investigator (or colleague) directly interacts with human subjects. This patient-oriented research includes four broad areas: (1) mechanisms of human disease, (2) therapeutic interventions, (3) development of new technologies, and (4) clinical management. This chapter focuses on clinical trials.

Introduction to Clinical Trials

Neuroscientists who develop new drugs using animal models may be unfamiliar with the best methods of testing these new therapies in humans. Medications with dramatic benefits in vitro or in animal models may fail to demonstrate significant clinical efficacy when applied to patients, or may be associated with significant adverse events.[10] A bet-

ter understanding of the clinical aspects of new drug development can enhance chances for discovery of new and better treatments for neurologic disorders.[2]

Understanding clinical research methods is important for clinical practice. It allows a physician to better interpret how and when new research findings should be applied in his or her practice. It is also important that clinicians have a basic understanding of how to assess the quality of a clinical trial. The assessment and application of results from randomized clinical trials is unfamiliar to most clinicians. Checklists for assessing the quality of clinical trials exist but are often too technical in detail to be useful for the practicing physician.[11,12] This chapter attempts to fill these gaps by introducing some of the basic concepts associated with the design and application of clinical trials. Several excellent, comprehensive reviews of clinical trial design exist,[13–17] and a useful approach to the assessment of clinical trials has been provided by Ellenberg.[18] This list is shown in Table 6-2.

What Is a Clinical Trial?

A clinical trial is an experiment with a specified number of patients designed to determine the effects of an intervention in those patients. However, the results of the trial have potential implications for larger populations of patients. Most of the techniques, experiments, and results described in the neuroscience of brain ischemia deal with explication investigations. Explication investigations try to identify phenomena and explain or understand the underlying mechanisms of stroke. Clinical trials fall into a different category of scientific investigation referred to as *interventional studies*. Interventional studies try to change a phenomenon, such as the amount of neuronal injury associated with a stroke or the risk of a recurrent stroke.[19,20]

History of Clinical Trials

The idea of clinical trials is not new.[15] An early description of a clinical trial that is surprisingly sophisticated by modern standards dates back to the Book of Daniel 1:1–21. Nebuchadnezzar, king of Babylon, had conquered Judah. He selected captured Israeli youths to learn the ways of the

Table 6-2. Considerations in the Design or Review of a Clinical Trial

Key Element	Issues Related to Key Element	Specific Items to Evaluate
Question	Therapy being tested	Method, route, and timing of administration; substances used for placebo; use of concurrent therapies
	Dose duration	Maximum tolerated dose, fixed dose per kg, extent of surgery
	Patient characteristics	Age, stage of disease, comorbidity
	Criteria for success	Cure, stop progression, reduce frequency, period of evaluation
Outcome	Primary outcome	Measurement recording procedures
	Secondary outcomes and definitions	Same as above
	Complications	Expected/unexpected toxicity in treatment arm
	Censoring	Competing risks with primary outcome death; cases lost
Study design	Randomization	Simple, stratified, blocked
	Blinding	None, single, double, triple
	Control	Historical, concurrent
	Type of design	Factorial, crossover, two-arm comparison
Cohort	Target population	Source of patients, description of patient pool (referrals)
	Screening process	Criteria used; procedures implementation
	Eligibility	Reasons for inclusion and exclusion
	Cascade	Accounting for patient numbers and characteristics as far back in the screen as possible
	Final number of patients randomized	Given by treatment arm
Study protocol	Follow-up schedule	Duration, periodicity, comparison of workups, bias control, observers/evaluations
	Procedures for call back	Reminder cards, phone calls
	Number of missed visits	Comparison of baseline characteristics of patients who missed visits, number of missed visits by treatment arm, efforts to improve compliance with follow-up and protocol
Quality control	Randomization	Comparison of treatment arms for baseline control variables
	Evaluation of endpoints	Repeat evaluations, review of responses for time bias
	Data entry	Cross-validation, range checks, double key entry
	Blindness	Comparison of treatment arms for blindness and break of blind
Analysis	Statistical methods	Actual methods with references to standard texts; power of statistical tests used; report the "p" values and confidence intervals; degree of statistical expertise used in design and analysis of clinical trial

Source: JH Ellenberg. Clinical trials. Neurol Clin 1990;8:15–30.

Chaldeans. A portion of the king's food and wine was provided to the youths. Daniel, a Judean youth, rejected the king's largesse and preferred to eat a simple mixture of leguminous crops, including peas, beans, and lentils, called *pulse*. To support the efficacy and safety of his choice, Daniel proposed to the steward, "Try thy servants . . . (for) ten days; and let them give us pulse to eat, and water to drink. Then let our countenances be looked on before thee, and the countenances of the youths that eat the king's food." The steward agreed to try this. After 10 days, those eating pulse "appeared fairer, and they were fatter of flesh, than all of the youths that did eat of the king's food." Daniel's "clinical trial" was successful in demonstrating that the diet of pulse was better than the king's menu. The stewards took away the king's food and wine and gave Daniel and the other Judean youths pulse to eat.

After this, the king invited Daniel to join his council, where he remained throughout the remainder of Nebuchadnezzar's reign. In this way, Daniel also shared an experience common to many modern trialists: After the completion of a successful clinical trial, he was called on to serve for extended terms on a sponsor's council and study sections.

Daniel included in his proposal one of the most important features of modern clinical trials—a control group. Although controls were included in this very early clinical trial, the selection of treatments throughout most of medical history was usually based on uncontrolled and anecdotal clinical observations. The idea of comparing groups treated with one drug against others who did not have this treatment was rarely implemented. Observers relied on pathophysiologic rationales provided by experts in justifying a new treatment, *not* on documented evidence of greater efficacy compared with other treatments. For example, the idea that certain diseases are blood-borne was reasonable but not necessarily correct. Physicians were taught the reasonable theory that diseases were in the blood, and, therefore, bleeding was a rational way of letting these substances escape the body. However, this theory was incorrect.

The appeal of reasoned theory still persists. If a treatment ought to work by virtue of its pathophysiologic mechanism, it may seem intuitively that a formal clinical trial is unnecessary. An example might be use of steroids for ischemic stroke; there is no evidence of efficacy, but it seems intuitively reasonable. Not only does this approach often result in the use of inappropriate therapies, but it also hampers implementation of well-designed clinical trials that could provide unequivocal answers to key questions about the benefit of a new treatment. Clinical investigators are repeatedly frustrated by clinicians who "know" that an untested therapy "works" and, therefore, will not withhold it from their patients. This intuitive "reasonable" approach posed a problem during the recruitment of patients for many trials, including those of extracranial-intracranial (EC-IC) bypass surgery, carotid endarterectomy, anticoagulation, and hormone replacement therapy. A strong pathophysiologic rationale and good preliminary data does not ensure a positive clinical trial. This has been well documented in some studies of acute ischemic stroke.[21–24]

During the first part of this century, investigators began applying blinding, controls, and randomization in clinical trials when evaluating a new treatment. After World War II, there was great interest in the methods of clinical testing and the accurate determination of clinical efficacy of new agents because an expanding pharmaceutical industry was interested in how best to determine whether to invest in, develop, and market a new drug.[25]

During the 1950s, the public became aware of the need for improved testing of new medical treatments. This awareness was largely the result of the birth defects associated with the use of thalidomide. A direct consequence of this in the United States was the passage of the Food and Drug Administration (FDA) Act in 1962, which required that the efficacy and safety of new drugs be demonstrated before they were approved for marketing. Efficacy of new therapeutic agents is best demonstrated by a randomized clinical trial.

The documentation and regulations involved in developing a new medication are complex.[26] In the United States, the testing of a new agent begins with submission of an Investigational New Drug Application to the FDA. Clinical testing usually involves three phases, although there may be overlap depending on the design of the clinical trial.[27] Phase I studies are initial tests of a new agent in humans, usually normals (i.e., without the target disease). Goals include the measurement of pharmacokinetics and determination of tolerated doses, ranges, and regimens. Phase II studies are relatively smaller studies of patients with the target disease. The goal is to examine the safety of a medication and begin to measure effectiveness. Controls are not always used in phase II studies. Phase III studies are controlled studies designed to compare the new therapy to no treatment or to a current standard treatment. Both efficacy and safety are assessed in a phase III trial. Most of the clinical trials referred to in this chapter are phase III trials.

Two additional phases of testing are commonly discussed. A phase IIIb study is done after the sponsoring company has completed a phase III study and submitted a New Drug Application to the FDA, but before receiving approval for marketing. These studies are usually done to expand the approved indications or investigate other measures of efficacy (e.g., functional outcome or quality of life). Finally, phase IV studies may be performed.

These are studies of a therapy after approval for marketing by the FDA. These studies may provide additional information on efficacy, safety, dosing regimens, or drug interactions.

Key Elements of Clinical Trials

An understanding of the key elements of a randomized clinical trial is important not only for designing one but also for assessing and applying the results. The reader not only has to assess the scientific merit of a trial but also must be aware of how to interpret the results. Clinicians also must decide whether the results apply to any particular clinical situation of their patients.

The Question

The clinical question addressed by a given clinical trial is critical. This question influences nearly all aspects of the trial (e.g., the number of patients required as well as the tests that should be used to determine statistical significance).

Process Affected

First, the process to be affected by a potential therapy should be considered. Therapies directed at a common vascular risk factor, such as hypertension, could be applied to most types of cerebrovascular disease. In contrast, a trial of an *N*-methyl-D-aspartate blocker might be limited to stroke patients with gray matter ischemia, where glutamate is released.[23]

Even if the therapy is directed at an appropriate target, other factors must be considered. For example, what is the contribution of the targeted process to the overall outcome among stroke patients, and hence, the potential impact of a therapy directed at this process. This principle is illustrated by the use of anticoagulation in the setting of acute ischemic stroke. Neurologic deterioration may occur in up to one-fourth of patients with acute ischemic stroke. This was often attributed to recurrent stroke and thromboembolism. It is logical to think that intravenous anticoagulation might reduce the risk of this common problem. Other data, including those from clinical trials, suggest that recurrent or progressing stroke occurs in only a small percentage of patients.

If a large portion of patients should be treated (and exposed to an increased risk of bleeding) to ensure that those who would have a recurrent or progressing stroke are treated (assuming intravenous heparin was effective), then the net result might still be negative (or harmful).[28] For example, if 100 patients are treated with a 4% risk of intracranial bleeding, and heparin reduces the risk of recurrent stroke—which occurs in 4% of cases—by 50%, for each 100 patients treated, treatment causes four intracranial hemorrhages to prevent two recurrent strokes. In this example, although heparin is effective in reducing recurrent stroke because there is a risk associated with its use, the low frequency of recurrent stroke results in no net benefit (and, in fact, harm). With these same numbers, if recurrent stroke occurred in 20% of cases, there would be a strong net benefit. It is important to avoid looking at the results of a trial in isolation.

It is also important to define clearly the purpose of a trial. The European Carotid Surgery Trial (ECST)[29] and North American Symptomatic Carotid Endarterectomy Trial[30] both reported a dramatic reduction in the rate of recurrent stroke and death in patients with 70% or greater carotid stenosis treated with carotid endarterectomy after a transient ischemic attack (TIA) or nondisabling stroke. Surgeons selected to participate in those trials had to have a low rate of complications, centers had to have low angiographic morbidity, and patients with low surgical risk were selected. How these results can be generalized to the community at large may require further study because these studies were not designed to decide if endarterectomy should be done everywhere; rather, they were designed to see if the procedure should be done anywhere.[31,32]

Dosing

Some agents have shown profound protective effects only if already present at the time of injury or immediately thereafter.[33] Thus, the protection occurs in limited situations, such as when the agent can be given before a planned operation such as coronary artery bypass grafting. The timing of administration of a therapeutic agent is critically important.[34] Seat belts, no matter how effective if applied before a car collision, have no protective effect when they are put on after the impact. For example, the level of hydroxyl radical formation is highest during the first few hours after cerebral ischemia and falls dramatically after 60 minutes.[35] Lipid peroxidation occurs later, particularly after 60 minutes following onset of ischemia. Therapeutic agents are being developed that could be given at each of these metabolic steps and potentially ameliorate adverse effects of the ischemia. Even if inhibition of hydroxyl radical formation showed dramatic results when given early after the onset of ischemia in animal models, however, an antiperoxidation agent (with a less potent effect in animal studies) could have far greater clinical benefit because it can be given later, when most patients are enrolled in clinical trials, and still be effective.

The time interval between onset of the stroke and beginning therapy influences therapeutic efficacy.[10,33] Neuroprotective agents, like nimodipine, have been given in clinical trials up to 48 hours after onset without a clear benefit. In the few patients who were enrolled within a few hours after the ictus and received a dose of 120 mg per day, however, there was a slight improvement in neurologic recovery.[36] The analysis of the efficacy in early treated patients was not planned when the study was designed. Post hoc analyses have much less weight than the planned analyses. Thus, many years passed and much money was spent on this nimodipine trial, but no definitive proof of efficacy was found. As a result, and because of the additional expense associated with further testing, a decision was made not to test further, and a potentially useful therapy may never be approved for marketing. On the other hand, patients with stroke may have been spared from using an unproven, expensive treatment and from its possible side effects.

When a therapy is given after an ictus, the rate of complications can be affected. For example, thrombolytic agents for stroke appear to be associated with a significantly higher rate of intracranial hemorrhage when given more than 3–6 hours after the onset of recognized stroke.[37,38]

Lack of attention to the details of the dosing could lead to unnecessary toxicity (dose too high) or a lack of efficacy (too little medication or medication given too late). This may have been the case with nimodipine. It may have also accounted for the higher rate of hemorrhage seen in the European thrombolytic trials.[39,40] Given the costs and time associated with the development of new therapies, attention to the timing of treatment and to the dose given is essential to minimize the chance that an effective medication will be missed. As in all experimental work, however, there is no substitute for experience, and one of the important outcomes of a clinical trial is learning how to do another trial better.

Patient Characteristics

It is important that the patients included in a trial are appropriate for the proposed therapy. As an example, before 1991, the Joint Study of Extracranial Arterial Occlusion[41] was the only randomized trial of carotid endarterectomy to enroll a large number of patients. The design of this trial reflected the evolving science of clinical trials. In this trial, only 316 patients were randomized. This sample size was inadequate because of the many patients who were lost to follow-up. Moreover, the primary analysis did not include stroke occurring in the hospital, and less than one-half of the patients who were included had stroke symptoms referable to the more stenotic carotid circulation.

Usually, characteristics of the patients included are determined by the pathophysiology of stroke and the proposed mechanism of action of the therapeutic agent, but this is not always necessary. Unexpected benefits of the drug might be discovered if broader selection criteria for eligibility of patients were used. For example, there are many mechanisms for recurrent stroke (e.g., lacunar disease, embolism, distal field ischemia),[42] and aspirin reduces the overall risk of recurrent stroke by approximately 20%. Those patients who have a recurrent stroke while taking aspirin are often referred to as *aspirin failures*. It may not be aspirin's failure but failure to identify those patients who are most likely to benefit. In contrast, patients with atrial fibrillation (AF) have a relatively uniform pathophysiology for recurrence (i.e., cardioembolic stroke). Anticoagulation with warfarin, which may be effective in preventing thrombus formation or extension, reduces the risk of stroke by 60–80%.

All known factors that could affect the action of a therapy or influence the pathophysiology and prognosis of the disease should be considered in selecting the characteristics of patients included in a clinical trial. Among the most common factors considered are age, stage of the disease, and comorbid conditions.

Criteria for Success

With the great interest in neuroprotective agents, there is a tendency to forget that there are many ways to treat a stroke. Effects in one area or concomitant therapies could complicate the design of a trial. Even for acute strokes, there are many types of treatments and therapies that could potentially improve outcome.[9,13,43] The following are specific therapies:

- Increase cellular resistance to ischemia
- Minimize neurotoxic effects of dying neurons
- Reduce edema or inflammation
- Improve blood flow to ischemia penumbra via collaterals or reperfusion
- Enhance neuronal repair
- Prevent early deterioration from thrombus extension
- Prevent early recurrence (e.g., recurrent cerebral embolus)

The following are nonspecific treatments:

- Improve wakefulness (may reduce aspiration pneumonia)
- Prevent secondary complications (e.g., venous thrombosis)
- Prevent depression after stroke (occurs in approximately 40%)
- Manage sequelae of stroke (e.g., physical/occupational therapy)

Outcome

A second group of key elements in the design and interpretation of clinical trials pertains to the selection of appropriate outcomes.[44] Data on many clinical variables may be collected during the clinical trial; however, it is important to identify clearly what outcomes will be used to measure efficacy and to do so before starting the trial. Identifying the primary outcomes guides the trial design and influences the duration of the trial, frequency of assessment, details of follow-up examinations, and required sample size.[45] It also allows interpretation of the results reported.

If too many outcomes are examined, some are likely to show a positive effect of a treatment solely by chance (type I error). The outcomes selected should be clinically important and not trivial. Minor changes in an outcome or how it is measured can result in a trial going from being "statistically significant" to not meeting the threshold of $P < .05$ commonly used in clinical trials. For example, in the European Cooperative Acute Stroke Study II trial, the prespecified endpoint of a score on the Rankin Scale of 0 or 1 was not reduced in the group treated with tissue plasminogen activator (t-PA)[39]; however, in a post hoc analysis, a Rankin Scale score of 0, 1, or 2 (a measure used in other studies) achieved statistical significance.[46] The results of a single trial should not be given too much weight when minor differences in an endpoint can make the difference between success and failure. The interpretation of such results must be done in the context of the larger amount of data available on the therapy.

Outcomes and Definitions

The outcome variable(s) selected should be easily, reliably, and objectively measured on all subjects. A continuous and easily quantifiable variable, such as blood pressure, is relatively easy to measure and makes a good outcome variable. The endpoint should also be responsive to useful clinical improvement.[45] For stroke, however, selection of an appropriate outcome is more difficult because stroke type, severity, location, and rate of recovery are highly variable among individuals.

The selection of appropriate outcomes or endpoints for stroke may not be immediately obvious. Death may occur after the earlier stroke and remove individuals who might otherwise—had they lived—developed a second stroke. Thus, a therapy could reduce the risk of a recurrent stroke simply by increasing mortality. "Dead patients cannot have strokes."[47] Elevated serum cholesterol in a high-fat diet could conceivably reduce the rate of stroke during follow-up simply by increasing death from coronary artery disease. Because many deaths after a stroke are related to cardiac disease, and therapies for stroke may influence the heart, the combined endpoint of stroke or death (i.e., stroke-free survival) may be more appropriate for trials than test drugs that purportedly prevent cerebrovascular disease. However, controversy exists on which endpoint(s) are the most appropriate for a clinical trial designed to detect a beneficial effect of a new medication or determine the likelihood of benefit when applied in clinical practice.[48]

Similarly, all types of strokes, including cerebral hemorrhage, should be reported in the analysis. This is especially important for therapies that might decrease the risk of ischemic stroke by increasing the risk for intracranial hemorrhage (e.g., anticoagulants). For example, investigators from the Stroke Prevention in Atrial Fibrillation (SPAF) II study looked at differences in stroke rates for those randomized to either aspirin or warfarin.[49] In all categories, patients treated with warfarin had lower rates of ischemic stroke. For this perspective, warfarin does reduce the risk of ischemic stroke more than aspirin in patients with AF. Clinically, it is important to account for the risks. A decrease in the rate of ischemic stroke is undesirable if it is offset by an increase in intracerebral hemorrhage. This was the case in older patients who were at higher risk for bleeding, and in those without vascular risk factors who were at lower risk for ischemic stroke but still subjected to the risk of hemorrhage while being treated with warfarin.

The importance of using stroke-free survival, as opposed to frequency of recurrent stroke alone, is illustrated in one of the ticlopidine studies. The Ticlopidine-Aspirin Stroke Study compared ticlopidine and aspirin for the secondary prevention of stroke after a TIA or minor stroke.[50] The investigators reported a 21% relative risk reduction in recurrent stroke frequency with ticlopidine compared to aspirin. In contrast, when stroke or death was the endpoint, there was only a 12% reduction, and the 95% confidence interval included zero (i.e., the relative risk reduction was not statistically significant).

At an additional level of refinement and clinical relevance, outcomes can be viewed as hierarchical. This means that some of the endpoints are less desirable. For example, if a therapy did not change the rate of the combined endpoints of nonfatal myocardial infarction (MI) or death, but did significantly increase the portion of those with nonfatal MI, it would probably be a desirable therapy. Similarly, if a therapy decreased the severity of the stroke, this would also likely be viewed as beneficial. This emphasis on a functional outcome is especially important when there are multiple endpoints that could occur in survivors. For example, if the rate of brain hemorrhages increased in the SPAF II trial, but those with brain hemorrhages tended to have minor strokes, warfarin might still be a desirable treatment. The SPAF II investigators did include among their endpoints disabling and nondisabling stroke. Although these endpoints are not as helpful in understanding *how* warfarin changes the rate of stroke (as looking at hemorrhage versus ischemic stroke may be), however, they are helpful for deciding *whether* warfarin therapy should be used.[49]

Beyond death and disease, there are four additional categories of outcome that should be considered[5]: (1) disability, the functional status of the patient; (2) discomfort, undesirable symptoms experienced by the patient or his or her family; (3) dissatisfaction, unpleasant emotional and mental states such as sadness or anger; (4) dollars, the cost to the patient, family, or society for an intervention or management strategy. Many of these are included under the rubric of "patient-oriented" outcomes.[51]

Since 1990, there has been growing interest in developing valid and reliable tools to measure patient-oriented outcomes in clinical studies. These measures assess the overall impact of a treatment or a disease on the physical, emotional, and social aspects of a patient's life.[52] They supplement the tools available to investigators but do not replace other stroke measures. Although generic tools, such as the Short-Form-36 General Health Survey, are commonly used, stroke-specific measures are more sensitive to meaningful changes in poststroke function.[52] Although patient-oriented and quality of life outcomes are rarely reported in randomized controlled trials, they are likely to play a greater role in future studies as reporting standards emerge. They may be of special importance for therapies such as neuroprotectants, in which the major impact will not be on mortality or disease progression, but severity of deficit.[53]

Reliability of Outcome Measures

Non-neurologists may assume that making a diagnosis of stroke or TIA is easy and reliable. It is also widely believed that a "standard neurologic examination" is, in fact, well standardized. Neither is the case. The difficulties in diagnosing stroke clinically or even with special neuroimaging aids introduces difficulties in planning a clinical trial. Also, standardizing the neurologic examination to measure clinical deficits from stroke is far from easy. The reliability of outcomes or endpoints can be

Table 6-3. Reproducibility of Components of the Neurologic Examination (Mathews Scale)

Examination Item	Kappa Score
Orientation	0.189
Speech, aphasia	0.758
Homonymous hemianopsia	0.159
Facial weakness	0.126
Right arm strength	0.909
Right leg strength	0.637
Left arm strength	0.455
Left leg strength	0.399
Sensory	0.265

Table 6-4. Reproducibility of Common Diagnosis in Cerebrovascular Disease

Diagnostic Item	Kappa Score
TIA	0.65
Location of TIA	0.36
Previous TIA	0.19
Previous stroke	0.40
Normal CT with stroke	0.68
Small deep infarct on CT	0.76
ICH on CT	1.00

TIA = transient ischemia attack; CT = computed tomography; ICH = intracerebral hemorrhage.
Source: Data from D Shinar, CR Gross, JP Mohr, et al. Interobserver variability in the assessment of neurological history and examination in the Stroke Data Bank. Arch Neurol 1985;42: 557–565.

improved by using unequivocal events for which there is little or no variability (e.g., death). This type of endpoint is appropriate for some trials of secondary prevention but is of little value for a therapy designed to improve functional outcome. For some clinical trials designed to measure functional improvement, investigators trying to improve outcome measures have used only those patients whose deficits persisted for longer than 7 days.[29] This was done to eliminate those patients who are most likely to improve spontaneously without treatment. For standardized assessment of functional improvement, a functional assessment scale is needed.[54]

There are many ways to test the use of a clinical assessment scale. These include determining the ability of the scale to grade severity, detect change, predict outcome, and guide therapeutic decisions. The scale must also show consistent and reproducible results (i.e., it must be reliable).[55] One measure of reproducibility is the kappa score, which is a measure of agreement among observers beyond what is due to chance. For example, if two neurologists examine the same patient, how likely are they to report the same degree of arm weakness? A kappa score of 1.00 is perfect agreement, 0.00–0.20 is slight, 0.21–0.40 is fair, 0.41–0.60 is moderate, 0.61–0.80 is substantial, and 0.81–0.99 is near perfect. Reliability measures of one scale used in stroke trials, the Mathews Scale,[56] are shown in Table 6-3.

There is significant variability in the interobserver reliability of the usual bedside neurologic examination. As mentioned, even making a diagnosis of cerebrovascular disease is subject to some interobserver variability. Locating the area of ischemic stroke damage is even more problematic,

especially for transient ischemia. An accurate determination of the site of the brain ischemia with TIAs is necessary for determining whether carotid endarterectomy is indicated, but, as seen in Table 6-4, the interobserver reliability is not good (kappa = 0.36). The difficulty in localizing the ischemic area has important implications for a clinical trial because the patients studied tend to be more heterogeneous. The heterogeneity makes the application of trial results more difficult in practice. The kappa scores for some other common stroke conditions are shown in Table 6-4.[57]

This issue has impacted the results of clinical trials. For example, in the Veterans Affairs Cooperative Studies Program High-Density Lipoprotein Cholesterol Intervention Trial, a trial comparing gemfibrozil with placebo among men with coronary artery disease and low levels of high-density lipoprotein cholesterol,[58] there was a significant reduction in stroke endpoints reported by the investigators. However, it did not remain statistically significant after the stroke endpoints were adjudicated by vascular neurologists.

Not only are there potential problems in determining stroke endpoints for clinical trials, but issues may also exist for determining adverse events. In a review of studies assessing the risk for carotid endarterectomy, studies in which neurologists reviewed a case were several times more likely to report major adverse events (i.e., stroke or death) than those studies in which cases were reviewed by surgeons.[59]

Censoring

Censoring refers to the loss of patients from follow-up. This attrition of patients is often ignored when designing and interpreting a clinical trial's results. An example of how the results of a trial are influenced by patients lost to follow-up is seen in data reported by Temkin[60] on phenytoin for the prevention of post-traumatic seizures. In that study, the investigators concluded that phenytoin exerted a beneficial effect by reducing seizures, but only during the first week after the head trauma responsible for the seizure. There was no significant difference in seizure frequency between treated and control groups after the first week following head trauma.

To conclude that phenytoin is ineffective in reducing seizures 1 week after head trauma requires an understanding of the effect of censoring. In longitudinal studies of traumatic brain injury, there are potential problems with outcome measures and the ability of investigators to detect them. Patients with severe head injury often die early. This censors the cohort by restricting it to survivors of head trauma. Depending on when the traumatized patients die, the surviving group of patients may be less severely affected and, thus, less likely to have a seizure. In addition, there is a high frequency of associated alcohol and drug abuse in most cohorts of traumatic brain-injured patients, which can also affect risk of seizures. Trauma may tend to occur more frequently in lower socioeconomic groups. Alcohol and drug abuse are factors that increase the dropout rate in a trial. Dropouts may be the patients with the worst prognosis. However, dropouts could also be the group most likely to benefit from long-term treatment with anticonvulsants.

In Temkin's clinical trial, there was a 25% dropout rate. It is certainly possible that among dropouts from this group, phenytoin may have had a beneficial effect. Just as it is important to know who enrolls in a trial, it is also important to know who drops out. If there is a significant loss to follow-up, a comparison of baseline features between those completing the protocol and those lost to follow-up may provide useful clues for interpreting the effect of the trial on outcome measures and endpoints.

Intermediate (Surrogate) Outcomes

For diseases in which the study outcomes occur infrequently, large numbers of patients and longer follow-up are usually required to ensure that a trial has adequate power to test a new therapy. Similarly, when functional outcomes such as severity of neurologic deficits are used, the less precise the measure, the larger the number of patients needed. In animal studies of neuroprotective agents, few animals are needed to demonstrate an effect because the animals are usually sacrificed. Volume of infarction can be easily quantified and is highly reproducible. Intermediate outcomes are commonly used in studies of vascular disease for factors that are well established, as risk factors or mechanisms of disease.

New imaging techniques, including MRI, are opening up new views of the brain.[61] For example, signal abnormalities present on brain MRI at the time of development of optic neuritis are associated with a risk of developing multiple sclerosis. Therapy with an intravenous methylprednisolone regimen reduces the rate of new demyelinating events.[62] If the development of lesions is reliably associated with the development or progression of multiple sclerosis, then a change in the appearance of sequential MRI studies may be able to demonstrate a beneficial effect of a proposed therapy.[63]

Similarly, measures of the volume of infarction can be made with increasing precision on brain imaging studies. This is certainly an appealing measure for clinical trials, but important questions remain. For example, if there is a 5% reduction in stroke volume but no change in neurologic outcome, how much effort, expense, or risk should be undertaken when introducing a therapy into clinical management? There may also be effective measures for assessing brain damage, such as *N*-acetyl aspartate or brain lactate.[64] Preliminary investigations in animal models suggest that diffusion-weighted imaging is a potential intermediate endpoint for acute stroke therapies,[65] but caution is needed.[66]

An intermediate outcome can be very sensitive to the biological effects of a therapy, but is a poor index of a clinical effect.[45] For example, arrhythmia is associated with death after acute MI. Antiarrhythmic medications can reduce the rate of cardiac arrhythmias (ventricular ectopy) after MI;

however, use of antiarrhythmic medications dramatically increases mortality.[67] It does not follow that just because an intermediate outcome is correlated with a clinical outcome in observational studies, it will respond in the same way to a new treatment.

The decision of which endpoint to use still should be based on how good a therapy needs to be to influence clinical practice.[68] This is true whether the effect is measured by a stroke outcome measure or an intermediate outcome.[69] A quote attributed to Gertrude Stein summarizes much of the design and interpretation of clinical trials[15]: "For a difference to be a difference, it has to make a difference."

Study Design

Many complex issues are involved in designing clinical trials. Although the importance of study design in such trials is generally appreciated by practitioners, some concepts may be misunderstood.

Control Group

A clinical trial needs an untreated group or a group on standard therapy to which the new therapy can be compared. The group not on new therapy is called the *control group*. One major goal in setting up a trial is to ensure that the control and treated groups are as similar as possible. This is done so that at the termination of the trial any differences between the two groups can be attributed to the actions of the new therapy and not to differences in the two groups. The control group can be given standard therapy (e.g., aspirin for secondary prevention of stroke). If there is no standard therapy, then a placebo (inactive substance made to resemble the new therapy) is often used.

In diseases in which the natural history is well established and stable, historical controls may be used in some instances. When historical controls are used, however, bias may be introduced. Sacks et al.[70] compared 50 randomized clinical trials involving randomized assignment and treated control groups with 56 trials using historical controls for six different therapies and procedures. For each intervention, the results "were more dependent on the method of selection of the control group than on the therapy under study . . . historical controls were much more likely than randomized clinical trials to find a difference, despite similar outcomes in the treated patients in the two types of study."

Historical controls are almost never appropriate for therapeutic trials in stroke for several reasons. First, the frequency of stroke has declined since the 1980s, and the mortality from cerebrovascular disease has been falling since the earliest part of the nineteenth century. Second, new therapies have been introduced into practice that may have altered the outcome rate from stroke over time (e.g., aspirin, ticlopidine, anticoagulation therapy for stroke, or improved intensive care management). Finally, evolving diagnostic criteria and imaging technology for stroke as well as refinements in identifying stroke subtype have changed the apparent pattern of stroke types since the 1950s.

The effect of inappropriate controls is illustrated in a study of gastric cooling for duodenal ulcer disease. Wagensteen[71] recognized that gastric cooling decreased acid secretion. The first few patients treated in this way described sharp reductions in their symptoms and had radiologic evidence of healing. Wagensteen described this as dramatically different from his previous experience, in effect relying on historical controls and stating, "Since 1961, no patients with duodenal ulcer referred for elective operation have been operated on in the senior author's surgical service. This circumstance in itself bespeaks the confidence in the method by patients as well as surgeons."[71]

As a result of this report, more than 2,500 gastric freezing machines were purchased before a randomized clinical trial could be completed. The subsequent clinical trial used concomitant controls and documented subsequent surgery for ulcer disease, gastrointestinal bleeding, or hospitalization for pain. In the sham frozen (control) group, 44% had one of these undesirable endpoints compared with 51% of patients undergoing actual gastric freezing.[72] Thus, the gastric freezing was clearly not beneficial and may have been worse than nonfreezing. This report illustrates not only the importance of appropriate controls and follow-up, but also the advantage of planning for the possibility that gastric freezing was, in fact, worse than a sham procedure.

Randomization

Randomization is a process applied in clinical trials to help ensure that the clinical characteristics of the group receiving the test agent and the control group are similar.[73,74] Randomized controlled trials are the most vigorous way to determine a cause-effect relationship between a therapy and an outcome.[75] Through randomization, the factors that might affect outcome, whether known or unknown, tend to become distributed equally between the groups being compared so that (ideally) only the treatment differs consistently. Randomization was first proposed in 1923 for use in agricultural research and applied to medical trials in 1926 with sancrysin for the treatment of tuberculosis.[15]

After World War II, there was a great interest in the process of randomization and the accurate determination of clinical efficacy for new therapeutic agents. This interest was prompted, in large part, by the rapidly growing pharmaceutical industry. Drug manufacturers were interested in how best to decide whether to invest in, develop, and market a new drug. Many new therapeutic agents were available only in limited supply. To minimize cost of development, risk stratification was applied in studies. For example, in 1946 streptomycin was scarce. A trial in the United Kingdom was designed to treat patients with tuberculosis using streptomycin, but the trial was restricted to only the most severely ill cases. In effect, a group of patients was selected among whom an effective therapy would show the most dramatic results (i.e., survival). If a clear beneficial effect was achieved, the number of cases needed would be relatively few, but a small beneficial effect could easily be missed in a small study. Randomization would balance extraneous variables that might dilute the ability to recognize a beneficial effect.

Randomization is a process, not a result.[76] By chance, a perfectly appropriate randomization scheme could, theoretically, still be associated with an imbalance between groups for an important risk factor, although in large series, the likelihood of such an occurrence becomes negligible. Nonetheless, it is always useful to test the effectiveness of randomization in a separate analysis. The larger the study, the more likely it is that the randomization process effectively balances comparison groups. In small studies or when individual sites each com-

pare only a small number of patients, however, balance could be disturbed.

There are research questions that, when applied to humans, cannot be tested with a randomized, controlled trial.[77] For example, smoking may be associated with a small protective effect against Parkinson's disease. Few people would volunteer to participate in a randomized trial, and the ethical concerns could make such a trial unfeasible. This limitation is more often encountered in studies of vascular risk factors or hazardous agents. For studies of stroke risk factors, the case control method, with careful attention to choosing cases and controls, can help define the etiology or suggest new therapeutic approaches to vascular disease.[78]

Stratification. When there are strong prognostic risk factors, a stratified randomization scheme may be appropriate. In that scheme, prognostic factors are measured at the time of randomization and a patient is assigned to a risk stratum. For example, in patients with carotid disease in which severity of stenosis is important in determining outcome (i.e., the likelihood of recurrent stroke), one could stratify the selection of patients by severity of carotid stenosis to ensure balance in the comparison. Patients are then randomized to a treatment within a risk stratum (degree of carotid stenosis).

Blocked Randomization. Another method to ensure a more equal distribution between the group receiving the active agent and controls is blocked randomization.[79] With blocking, there are a specified number of patients with certain characteristics within a group (block) of patients. Within each block, there is an equal number of patients treated with each agent. For example, if a block size of four is selected, then there are six possible assignments for this group of patients: AAPP, APAP, PPAA, APPA, PAAP, and PAPA (A = active agent, P = placebo). These possible assignments within each sequential block of six patients are determined randomly.

Blinding

Bias introduces a systematic error into a trial and can occur at any point in a trial, from its initial design through the final data interpretation. There are guidelines for reducing bias in clinical trials.[80,81] Two of these used as illustrations include randomization and the design of the blinding process. Bias can be introduced at the start of a trial by an uneven distribution of patients within the treatment groups. For example, if there were a greater number of severely ill patients in the control group and they therefore improved less, a "better response" could be seen with the new agent even if it were not more effective for all patients. Randomization schemes are used to minimize such sources of bias.

Another type of bias results from knowing which therapy a patient is receiving. Nonblinding can influence the sensitivity of detecting the effect of an outcome variable.[82] For example, if a physician knows that a patient is on warfarin, he or she might inquire more diligently whether the patient has bleeding while shaving. By blinding the patients and the physicians to the therapy received, these effects should be minimized. The impact of blinding was illustrated in a clinical trial involving treatments for multiple sclerosis compared to a placebo. The unblinded but not the blinded neurologists' scores demonstrated an apparent benefit for one of the treatments.[83] A similar result was seen for stroke endpoints in the Veterans Affairs Cooperative Studies Program High-Density Lipoprotein Cholesterol Intervention Trial.

There are different degrees of blinding. In single-blind studies, the patient is unaware of the treatment (i.e., active agent versus placebo). In double-blind studies, the patient and the treating physician are both unaware of the treatment. In triple-blind studies, those analyzing the data are also blinded. They evaluate treatment A and treatment B looking for evidence that one is superior to the other. At the end of the analysis, the blind may be broken.

Blinding is especially important in studies in which the endpoints are subjective, but problems with bias can arise even in studies with "hard" endpoints. For example, deciding whether a patient had a TIA or a minor stroke is often difficult. Blinding would help prevent the bias that could assign TIA disproportionately to the new treatment group and thus give an unfair advantage to this treatment over placebo or standard therapy in measuring efficacy. Blinding should therefore be an integral part of all therapeutic trials in stroke. Even if the treating physician is different from the trial's principal investigator, blinding should be maintained for both when possible. An unblinded treating physician could unintentionally favor one of the groups with extra or different care (e.g., by performing additional diagnostic testing, eliciting more detailed interval histories that detected extra endpoints, or providing additional therapies that influence outcome or side effects). Despite the importance of blinding in a clinical trial, patient safety remains the foremost consideration, and mechanisms should always be in place to "break" the blind if necessary to protect the patient.

In some studies, blinding is not practical (e.g., carotid surgery). In such studies, objective endpoints are especially important.[84] Also, for studies with an objective endpoint, such as death, blinding is less important. Practical, ethical, or fiscal concerns may outweigh the scientific desirability of a double-blind design.[85,86] The investigators chose an open-label (unblinded) strategy for the Global Utilization of Streptokinase and Tissue Plasminogen Activator for Occluded Coronary Arteries trial, which showed a decreased 30-day mortality for inpatients presenting with acute MI treated with accelerated-dose t-PA compared with streptokinase.[87] Also, as described in Intent-to-Treat Analysis, local law prohibited the use of placebo for a nutritional study of vitamin A therapy.

Types of Design

There are many ways to design a clinical trial. The design chosen depends heavily on the natural history of the disease. One widely used design is the parallel trial, in which a group of patients is selected for a new therapy while another group concomitantly serves as a control. Both groups are chosen by some randomized method and treated during the same time interval. Patients should remain in the category to which they were assigned throughout the trial. A disadvantage of the parallel design is that the control group is denied the new medication. For promising new therapies in stroke, especially because no other approved therapy exists, patients and their families are often reluctant to agree to the possibility of being randomized to a placebo group. This issue exists for other diseases as well and has, for example, been raised forcibly by autoimmune deficiency syndrome advocacy groups because any possibly effective treatment is deemed better than no treatment and inevitable, early death.

Crossover trials are another common study design.[88] Patients are assigned to a new treatment group or to a placebo group, but sometime during the trial the groups switch. Those originally taking placebo begin taking the new agent, whereas those taking the new agent receive placebo. Crossover trials have the advantage that all patients in the trial receive the new therapy at some point. Also, fewer patients are usually needed to detect a therapeutic effect. Despite these advantages, crossover trials are usually not suitable for stroke trials because the risk of reaching an endpoint, such as recurrent stroke or improvement, changes over time, and therefore, some patients are being treated when their risk profile for a recurrent stroke or further improvement has changed. Parallel studies are more appropriate for stroke studies. Yet another disadvantage of the crossover trial is that the effect of the treatment may persist for an indefinite period beyond when it is stopped and could influence results even when patients are receiving only placebo. Crossover trials are more suited to chronic diseases in which the risk of change in status is less variable over time (e.g., epilepsy or migraine).

Other trial designs may be used in special settings. Withdrawal studies can be used for chronic disease therapies (e.g., withdrawal of aspirin a decade after a stroke). A factorial design is used when testing more than two therapies (e.g., the Canadian Cooperative Trial[89] that compared aspirin with sulfinpyrazone and each individually to placebo). Group allocation trials consist of those in which an individual study site treats all patients with a given therapy, with the results compared with centers using a different treatment. Group allocation has the advantage of treating all patients at one site with the same agent. Subjects may feel more comfortable with this approach, but patient differences across sites in socioeconomic, nutritional, or ethnic characteristics could invalidate comparisons or bias results for the trial as a whole.

Study Population

In performing a clinical trial, it is not enough to propose that a new therapy will be effective for "stroke" in general. One must also specify the types of stroke patients in the population. For example, patients experiencing hemorrhagic and ischemic strokes are likely to benefit from different therapies. Not only is the type of stroke important to consider but also the severity of the deficit. For example, in the Sygen Acute Stroke Study, there was no statistically significant overall effect of ganglioside GM-1 in improving functional outcome after an ischemic stroke.[90] In this trial, patients with minor deficits were enrolled, many of whom returned to normal, even in the control group. If too many patients in the control group make full recoveries (as measured on the stroke rating scales) in a study, then there is no difference to detect between the active therapy and placebo. By restricting their analysis to those patients with greater deficits (i.e., who could benefit from the proposed therapy) a greater therapeutic effect was seen. A statistically significant beneficial effect for the cohort was only seen in post hoc analyses using motor improvement as the outcome measure.

A study population is really a subset of the general population with stroke, and the cohort studied is defined by the competing goals of inclusion and exclusion criteria. It is important that clinicians interpreting and applying the results of a clinical trial know how representative subjects in the trial are of the general population with the disease. A thorough description of the cohort of patients actually included in the trial is therefore important.

Because of the need to meet both inclusion and exclusion criteria for enrollment, only a fraction of patients (usually less than 10%) with a stroke qualify for enrollment in any given therapeutic trial. In addition, not all patients who qualify agree to participate, so that those who refuse or are disqualified should be described. As an illustration, it is useful to consider the ECST,[29] in which a subtle selection bias may have occurred. Patients were enrolled in this trial only if their referring physician was "reasonably uncertain" whether to recommend carotid endarterectomy. If the physician was confident that the patient should, or should not, have an endarterectomy, the patient was excluded from the trial. It is possible that the general medical status (e.g., presence of coronary disease) influenced clinicians to refer only less representative patients for surgical intervention. For a trial with results favoring intervention like ECST, the group not having intervention may have been sicker and thus surgery could have been given a spurious advantage in the analysis. Alternatively, it is possible that the physicians were able to identify a group who would not benefit from surgery, but this could not be proven if such patients were excluded from analysis. By not characterizing those excluded from the trial (and ideally, their outcome), the ability to generalize the results of the ECST trial is limited.

From a practical point of view, it is also important for physicians at participating study centers to recognize that if they believe that they "know" that a given therapy works in certain patients, systematically excluding such patients from participation in a clinical trial could result in treating only patients who respond less favorably. This could have the effect of eliminating a treatment that is, in fact, effective for some individuals. An example is EC-IC bypass, which was once a common procedure for treating some stroke patients. A randomized clinical trial of EC-IC bypass failed to show any efficacy.[91] Surgeons at some participating institutions criticized the results, stating that appropriate patients had been operated on in the participating institutions but were excluded from the trial.[91,92] The argument of those who favored EC-IC bypass was not accepted,[93] and this surgical procedure is now seldom performed. Citing study results, many insurers no longer reimburse for the cost of this procedure. Yet, the procedure may still be appropriate for some patients.

Study Protocol

In organizing a formal clinical trial, availability of a reasonable therapy is only the first step. The day to-day operations of a trial are critical to its success. The procedures for formal data collection are described in the study protocol. Some key elements of such a protocol are listed in Table 6-2. The importance of the study protocol is illustrated by examples from other studies, including follow-up in a trial of phenytoin for post-traumatic seizures[60] and compliance in the Coronary Drug Research Group.[94]

Quality Control

Although the scientific validity of randomized controlled trials has received great attention, the management of such trials has received little attention.[95] A clinical trial can be only as good as the data it collects. Such data are collected from several sources, are varied in type, and are derived from different centers. Detailed discussion of quality control of clinical trial data are not presented in this chapter, but, at every stage, methods are needed to help ensure the data are accurate. Methods include monitoring by outside reviewers who visit each center to check the completed protocols against the clinical records, duplicate entry of data into computerized files, and consistency checking of the data to detect out-of-range values and biologically impossible combinations (e.g., the left carotid territory stroke cannot produce left body weakness).

Analysis

A detailed discussion of the methods of analysis of clinical trials is also beyond the scope of this chapter but, in brief, there are at least four topics that commonly arise in analyzing clinical trials: (1) whether to use one- or two-tailed testing for significance of results, (2) the hazards of post hoc analysis, (3) intent-to-treat versus efficacy analysis, and (4) factors contributing to power and sample size requirements.

One- and Two-Tailed Tests

A one-tailed test is usually applied to answer the question of whether a given therapy is superior to another agent or to a placebo. The advantage of a one-tailed test is that fewer patients are required to achieve statistical significance. A disadvantage is that the trial is not designed to detect whether the new therapy is worse than the control. The clinical situation often determines whether a one- or two-tailed test is the appropriate statistical comparison. For example, if a pharmaceutical company were developing a new antiplatelet agent that was more expensive or possibly more dangerous than aspirin, it would be primarily interested in developing and marketing the agent only if the new medication were substantially more effective than aspirin. Unquestionably, the control or existing therapy (i.e., aspirin in this example) would continue to be recommended if the new therapy were more costly or more dangerous.

The two-tailed test requires more patients but has the advantage of being able to determine an effect for better or worse, if it exists. A two-tailed statistical test is appropriate for studies in which two therapies are roughly equivalent in cost and risk in that it allows the investigator to determine which therapy is superior and not just whether the test agent is superior.

Hazards of Post Hoc Analysis

Once a clinical trial is completed and the data set is available to an investigator, he or she may be tempted to perform additional analyses not planned before the trial began. These are termed *post hoc analyses*. There are often hidden biases in such analyses. For example, an investigator might be tempted to look at the results only in those patients who complied with the therapy as prescribed (analysis as treated).

Although this seems sensible, there may be biasing factors associated with the tendency to comply with a treatment schedule, such as younger age, better health habits, and more education. Such a bias could favor compliant over noncompliant patients, independent of drug effect. For example, the Coronary Drug Research Group reported that men with MI were started on a therapy and followed subsequently until they had another MI or died. Men who took 80% or more of the prescribed medication had a mortality rate of 16%. This group was compared to those who took less than 80% of the prescribed medication, in whom the mortality rate was 26%. This difference was statistically significant. All of the patients who were more compliant were taking placebo.[94]

This "analysis as treated" usually selects out certain subgroups and affects the randomization process. Because reasons for noncompliance may influence outcome, as shown in the preceding example, the more acceptable method, an intent-to-treat analysis, is to analyze by the group to which patients were originally (randomly) assigned, regardless of compliance with the regimen.[96]

Subgroup analyses within a trial must be viewed with great caution.[97] Even within a well-designed and well-executed trial, such analyses are prone to random error. If enough variables are examined, some will cross the threshold for statistical significance. For example, in the Second International Study of Infarct Survival trial, the response to thrombolytic therapy varied by astrological sign.[98] The danger in this result being incorporated into the clinical practice is small because it is not believable by most educated individuals. Statisti-

cally, the result is no less valid than the finding that ticlopidine may be more effective in women, as noted in the Ticlopidine-Aspirin Stroke Study.[99] Even when "fishing expeditions" result in biological variables associated with increased efficacy, most readers do not recognize the large number of variables usually required to achieve the few positive associations.[99] Reports of subgroup analyses tend to emphasize variables that are associated with a greater therapeutic effect and not lesser effects. For example, ticlopidine has been reported to be more effective in blacks,[100] women,[99] and diabetics,[101] and patients with posterior circulation strokes,[99] patent carotids,[99] or minor strokes.[102] Yet, among the conclusions of such reports, it is seldom mentioned that a therapy would be less helpful among white men with a TIA who have significant carotid disease. Subsequent studies based on selected subgroups, analyses, or endpoints, however appealing, must be viewed with great caution.[103] The credibility of their conclusions is built on the stability of their assumptions.[104]

Subgroup analyses can be helpful but should always be viewed with caution. Belief in the results of subgroup analyses should be strictly limited to those that are biologically plausible, defined in advance, and reproducible.[104] An example of a relevant, predefined, and biologically plausible subgroup analysis is the evaluation of the degree of carotid stenosis in the trials of endarterectomy for symptomatic carotid stenosis.[30]

Intent-to-Treat Analysis

As mentioned, analysis of a therapy can be based on the group to which patients were randomized (intent to treat) or the group on the therapy as taken (analysis as treated). The difference between these two strategies is well illustrated in the Canadian-American Ticlopidine Study.[105] The investigators reported an efficacy analysis based on analysis as treated. In this analysis, there was a relative reduction of 30% for recurrent stroke, MI, or vascular death after a stroke. This was a placebo-controlled trial. The casual reader might think that the 30% risk reduction was even greater than the 20% usually reported with aspirin treatment. He or she might conclude that patients treated with ticlopidine did approximately 50% better ([30%–20%]/20%). An intent-to-treat analysis, however, showed that 12% of patients had to discontinue ticlopidine due to side effects, whereas only 3% discontinued aspirin. In an intent-to-treat analysis, the risk reduction of stroke recurrence for ticlopidine was 23%, a number similar to the risk reduction usually reported for aspirin. It is important for the reader to be aware that the most dramatic results reported in a trial may not be the most meaningful. Intent-to-treat analyses often reflect the real problems physicians may encounter when giving the drug and thus give a more accurate, if not the most favorable, results of treatment.

The importance of the intent-to-treat analysis is widely accepted in theory but not always implemented in practice.[106] There are rare exceptions in which intent-to-treat analysis is not imperative. In discussing the results of a randomized trial of vitamin A supplementation in Indonesian children, Sommer and Zeger described uncommon circumstances in the control group and among noncompliant patients.[107] In their trial, local Indonesian law prohibited the use of a placebo, control patients were not treated, and there was "100% compliance." In the treatment arm (vitamin A tablets), noncompliers (approximately 20%) were sicker and more likely to die. The authors argued that if a placebo had been used, a similar noncompliance problem would have occurred in the placebo group. Using simple proportions, they estimated the portion and outcome of noncompliance among the controls. This group was subtracted, and an efficacy analysis was performed. The authors pointed out the importance of this analysis in discussing the effects of introducing vitamin A into a staple food everyone would eat (i.e., 100% compliance). This circumstance is not likely to arise in trials of stroke therapies, and the standard remains intent to treat.

Sample Size

When determining the number of patients that should be included in a trial (sample size calculation), the investigators should answer a series of questions. The first is, "What is the frequency of endpoints that can be expected to occur in the control group?" The smaller this rate, the greater the number of patients needed to detect a significant difference between the test agent and the control. The next task is to select the magnitude of the effect of the test agent the investigator would consider clinically meaningful. For example, a postulate might be that warfarin reduces the risk of recurrent stroke or death in patients with a first stroke by 25% compared with aspirin (325 mg/day) when prothrombin time is maintained between 1.3 and 1.5 times the control level. The third task is to specify the levels for type I and type II errors. These "errors" reflect the random fluctuation that will be seen in results if the same experiment is repeated several times. It can never be determined with certainty that even a beneficial agent will always show a positive effect or that an ineffective agent will show no "beneficial" effect. In setting up a clinical trial of a new therapy, the investigators should decide how willing they are to miss potentially significant results. Conventionally, a value of 5% is set, but a more stringent criterion (e.g., only once in 100 trials) or a less stringent criterion (once in 10 trials) can be set. Formal testing for significance in a clinical trial is stated as a null hypothesis (i.e., it is hypothesized that there is no statistically significant difference between the test therapy and a control agent). If the results of the trial allow one to reject the null hypothesis that the test therapy and the control therapy are equivalent, then investigators can conclude that one therapy is different than another within certain confidence limits.

A type I (also called *alpha*) error occurs when the results of the trial suggest there is a difference when the true result is no difference. This could lead to accepting the new agent as more effective, when it is, in fact, not. If the probability of this occurring was set at 0.05, then the chance is that such an error will occur only five times in 100 comparisons. A type II (beta) error occurs when the null hypothesis is accepted (i.e., that there is no difference) when it is wrong. This means that an effective therapy is rejected as ineffective. Conventionally, the probability of making a type II error is usually set at less than 0.20. The power of the trial (1-beta) is then said to be 80%.

These elements form the basis of a sample size calculation. In general, the sample size is directly proportional to the outcome rate in the placebo group and inversely proportional to the size of the type I and II errors. Thus, these elements set the sensitivity of the trial. A sample size calculation is given in Table 6-5 for an agent that reduces the risk of stroke or death by 30% in a group of patients

Table 6-5. Sample Size Estimates for a Randomized, Double-Blind, Controlled Trial in Stroke

Length of Patient Accrual Phase (yrs)	Total Trial Duration (yrs)					
	3	4	5	6	7	8
1	1,285*	935	741	618	533	470
2	1,594	1,082	827	674	572	499
3	2,119	1,291	938	743	619	534
4	—	1,609	1,089	831	676	574
5	—	—	1,304	945	747	622

*Number of patients.

with a 5-year event rate of 20% in the control group. The calculation is for a one-tailed test (alpha = 0.05 and beta = 0.10). Table 6-5 also gives the number of patients required in each group (placebo or control) to meet the preceding conditions.[108] Most physicians and many investigators are surprised to learn of the large number of patients required to test a promising new therapy.

Depending on the outcome measure, the number of patients required may be even greater than shown in Table 6-5. For example, with an outcome such as death, there is little variation in the determination of the endpoint. With other endpoints, such as TIA, less precisely defined criteria of occurrence are available. This difficulty works to increase the sample size required to show a statistically significant difference in the results.

Design Problems Related to Cerebrovascular Disease

In addition to the guidelines for clinical trials discussed that apply to all randomized clinical trials, there are some problems unique to neurologic studies[109] and especially to cerebrovascular disease.

Lack of Adequate Animal Models

Animal models for brain ischemia are limited,[110] especially for lacunar disease and infarction in the distal bed of a vessel. The small vessels at the base of the brain where occlusion is associated with lacunar disease have a different configuration in animals compared to humans. Although it has been possible to produce small deep infarction in subhuman animal models, the relevance of such lesions to lacunar infarction in humans is still unknown. Similarly, the low-flow states presumably associated with distal ischemic infarct have not been adequately reproduced in animal models because collateral flow in animals is usually much greater than in humans.

Hemodynamic Classification

Neurodiagnostic procedures have tended to focus on anatomic, not physiologic or hemodynamic, changes. Although several classifications of stroke subtypes have been proposed, none have been correlated with hemodynamic changes. Although sophisticated techniques, such as positron emission tomography and single-photon emission CT, are available and provide hemodynamic information, relatively few studies have used such techniques to look at stroke classification or outcome. The necessary equipment is expensive, not universally available, and technically difficult to use.

Etiologic Classification

Strokes and TIAs are clinical phenomena that can be caused by many different processes. For example, a stroke related to low flow from a narrowed carotid artery could be due to atherosclerotic narrowing, mural thrombus, hemorrhage into a plaque, dissection, or a combination of these factors. The outcome and best therapies for these various causes of stroke are likely to be different. Currently, the technology or knowledge to classify these etiologic mechanisms consistently in clinical trials is not widely available.

Magnitude of Effect

The effects for many therapeutic agents are not likely to be as dramatic for stroke as those seen for serious infectious diseases or nutritional deficiencies. This increases the number of patients required for studies of stroke therapies. It also increases the complexity and cost of a clinical trial for stroke.

Clinimetrics

Clinimetrics involves indices, rating scales, and other measures used to describe or assess symptoms, physical signs, and other distinctly clinical phenomena.[55] Clinical trials are particularly suited for diseases, treatments, and patients in which the observed results do not take long to occur, the measures are easily and reliably quantified, and large sample sizes are not required to achieve statistical significance. Fasting blood sugar would be an example of an easily determined value in a clinical trial using such a measure; few patients are needed to show an effect of insulin on hyperglycemia. However, such measures are not very well developed for stroke. Many rating scales for stroke have been proposed, but all have limitations and few have been adequately tested for validity and reliability.[55,111–113] Better measures are needed for assessing neurologic and functional deficits. Also, adequate severity ratings and precise criteria for the diagnosis of TIA and stroke are needed.[55]

Lack of Prognostic Information

Prognostic information and risk stratification can help select the groups most likely to benefit from a given therapy. This becomes especially important for therapies that are costly or dangerous. Few studies of stroke have adequately addressed prognosis.[114] However, some studies suggest that effective risk stratification can be achieved.[115]

Lack of Pathophysiologic Knowledge

Advances in the understanding of the cellular and molecular mechanisms of injury associated with cerebral ischemia have been dramatic.[116,117] This new understanding has provided the basis for some of the most promising therapies for acute ischemic stroke. Nevertheless, key questions remain. Among the most pressing is how long after the onset of a stroke a given therapy can be applied. Another area of active debate concerns the effectiveness of thrombolytic therapy.

In trials of acute myocardial ischemia, 4–6 hours is usually recognized as the upper limit for thrombolysis to be effective.[118] It seems likely that a similar limit exists for brain ischemia; however, differences between the cerebral and myocardial circulation exist and the "window of opportunity" may extend beyond this time for some patients.[119] The maximum time to treat for a stroke clinical trial depends on the proposed mechanism of the therapy. Trials of revascularization or for blocking the effects of excitatory neurotransmitters seem likely to have an effect only during the first minutes or hours after the onset of ischemia. For agents intended to inhibit the migration of leukocytes into an infarction (which may extend the area of injury), treatment for stroke for up to the first 48 hours may be appropriate.[117]

Are Clinical Trials Ethical?

By the time a new therapy reaches the point of testing in a randomized clinical trial, physicians may already have strong feelings about previously reported evidence for clinical efficacy, based on their clinical experience with therapy or preclinical testing in vitro or in animal models. The literature on therapy contains many examples of widely used therapies that, when subjected to a randomized clinical trial, were shown not to be efficacious. Sometimes those treated with untested drugs actually did worse in a clinical trial than those who were not treated. This was the case with IC-EC bypass surgery, a procedure widely used before the results of a randomized clinical trial were published that failed to show the procedure was effective.[91]

It has been argued that to participate in a clinical trial, researchers should modify their ethical commitments to the individual patient because the results of clinical trials are not available to physicians on an ongoing basis during the testing of a new therapy.[120] It takes time to collect data in a clinical trial, and the hazards of bias introduced by an early look at interim results is discussed previously. Many years may pass before the effectiveness and safety of a new therapy can be identified. Without randomized clinical trials, however, the process of finding truly better and safer drugs is likely to be even more difficult. Alternatives to a full-scale clinical trial can be considered, especially with a rapidly fatal disorder like autoimmune deficiency syndrome, but these new techniques should be subjected to rigorous testing before they are widely applied without a randomized clinical trial to avoid harm.

Several features should be part of ethically sound trials.[121–123] The first is informed consent. Patients should be aware that they are participating in a randomized trial and feel comfortable with the potential risks and benefits. Second, a state of clinical equipoise should exist,[124] meaning that a group of competent, informed physicians would be content to have a patient take either therapy or placebo as a treatment as neither has been demonstrated to be superior. Third, the study should be well designed and well executed. It should include a data monitoring committee to stop the trial if new evidence arises that provides clear evidence for a benefit (or hazard) of the test therapy.[125–127] Fourth, the trial's procedures, consent forms, and ongoing safety and efficacy results should be monitored by a group with diverse expertise, both clinical and ethical (an internal review board), as well as scientific experts with biostatistical and clinical training (an external monitoring committee).[128] Given all of these needs, it is clear that the clinical trial is costly, not only in time but also in money.

Are Clinical Trials Cost Effective?

Whether clinical trials are cost effective depends on the target population, severity of the disease, and the effects of the therapy. Given that cerebrovascular disease costs the U.S. economy approximately $25 billion per year, a study that significantly benefits even a portion of these patients is likely to pay for itself in a short period.

As an example, the SPAF study demonstrated that warfarin reduced the incidence of stroke for patients with AF by as much as 80%.[129] If the results of this trial were applied to the more than 1 million people in the United States with AF, 100–150 strokes per day could be prevented. The poten-

tial savings are estimated at more than $200 million per year.[130] This study cost approximately $4.6 million, meaning that it could pay for itself in less than a week with savings from the strokes prevented.

In the United States, less than 1% of national health expenditures is spent on randomized clinical trials. Rigorous fiscal analyses confirm the conclusion of the preceding example.[131] These cost analyses can help to target health spending more appropriately and should help refine health priorities.

Problems with Randomized Clinical Trials

It is worth mentioning some general limitations of randomized clinical trials.[15,132–134] The main clinical problem is that they are designed to answer questions of therapeutic efficacy rather than questions regarding clinical practice. In almost all forms of medical therapy, there is controversy about the best management strategy. Common topics include the best dosage, timing of administration, risks and benefits, costs, and use of expensive diagnostic or imaging technology. Although clinical trials can answer some questions about clinical management (e.g., which drug is most effective), a clinical trial is not a panacea for all management problems. Clinical trials are an extremely powerful tool, but they can address only a limited range of clinical questions. For example, some trials have demonstrated the efficacy of carotid endarterectomy,[29,30] but many important problems in clinical management of severe carotid disease still remain. These include how to treat patients with carotid stenosis with progressive stroke (stroke in evolution), progressive retinal ischemia, stroke associated with acute carotid occlusion, global ischemia with multiple large-vessel narrowing, tandem lesions, and asymptomatic lesions. Moreover, the risks and costs of carotid surgery are far from trivial.

A fundamental scientific problem with clinical trials is that they tend to ignore challenges of taxonomy and patient variability. Patients in a randomized clinical trial are grouped to average out clinical differences, and the patients are usually assumed to have the identical disease. Important clinical differences are often ignored in the "melting pot." If included patients are identified who may have especially high or low risk for an important outcome, the results of a randomized clinical trial may not apply as well to them. Moreover, death from unrelated causes can affect the magnitude of the endpoint and other interventions, especially when there is considerable variation in how a disease is treated. Death can also modify effects attributable to the therapy being tested. In addition, compliance with the intended drug regimen is often variable. An intent-to-treat analysis is important to eliminate bias (as illustrated previously), but it minimizes the clinical sense of the results because patients for whom treatment was intended, but to whom treatment was never given, are analyzed as if they were treated. For example, patients who have a recurrent stroke while awaiting an endarterectomy have not had the opportunity to benefit from the surgical procedure. Why should they be classified as a surgical failure of endarterectomy simply because they were randomized to have the operation? This is a criticism of the intent-to-treat analysis. Many argue that if it were known which procedure was efficacious and risk of early recurrence of stroke were high, clinical practice could be modified to perform endarterectomies. In a clinical study, in which up to a few weeks may pass before a patient is recruited, enrolled, randomized, and operated on, the effect of these early recurrences tends to minimize the apparent therapeutic effect of endarterectomy.

Randomized clinical trials are also not feasible for the direct comparison of all possible therapeutic agents and their combinations. Clinical trials are also cumbersome and expensive for examining long-term effects of treatment because such studies usually require follow-up of large numbers of patients for many years. Not only does the expense become limiting, but also the refined analytic techniques that can separate therapeutic effects due to the primary agents from those due to other interventions that may be introduced during prolonged follow-up are not well developed. How to apply the results of clinical trials to optimize clinical management cannot easily be derived from randomized clinical trials. Perhaps new science must be developed to study clinical care.[19,55]

Interpreting Trials

Even when the trial results are available, the meaning of the results may not be clear. Even if an inter-

vention works well in the setting of a clinical trial, it many not work well when applied in the community.[135] Effectiveness of stroke therapy in the community depends on diagnostic accuracy, provider compliance with treatment protocols, patient adherence to medications, and coverage of health services. For example, carotid endarterectomy was demonstrated to be highly effective in clinical trials. This result was dependent on low surgical morbidity and mortality; however, this may not be the case in all communities.[136] Similar concern has been raised about the use of acute thrombolytic therapy in the community, in which protocol deviations are common, and the rate of hemorrhage is much higher than reported in the clinical trials.[137]

Often it is difficult to put the results of a trial into clinical perspective. A clinician must decide if a treatment is worth the time, expense, danger, and discomfort for a given effect in his or her practice. There is wide variation among clinicians in interpreting results, even for well-designed studies. One reason for this is that randomized clinical trials do not address all aspects of patient management.[138] Another reason is the lack of readily apparent meaning for measures such as percent reduction or relative risks for the average clinician.

This trend has changed more recently, and new measures are being devised and reported with therapeutic trials. One of the most popular is the number of patients needed to treat with a specific regimen to prevent one adverse clinical event.[139] The number needed to treat is equal to the inverse of the difference between two treatment groups. For example, in the Global Utilization of Streptokinase and Tissue Plasminogen Activator for Occluded Coronary Arteries trial the 1-month mortality after MI was 6.3% on t-PA and 7.3% on streptokinase. This is a 1% absolute difference and a 14% relative reduction. The number needed to treat (to save one additional life) is [1/(0.073–0.063)] = 100. It is easier for most people to think in these terms. If 100 patients are treated with t-PA instead of streptokinase, one less person would die within 1 month of the MI. This also makes it easier to calculate the cost differences. For example, if the cost of t-PA were $2,400 and streptokinase $400, an additional $240,000 for medications would need to be spent to save one additional life.[140] These calculations, although often useful conceptually, must be viewed with caution because the costs associated with one therapy may extend far beyond just those of the medication. In addition, as discussed earlier, the patients who are included in clinical trials and their causes of stroke (or other clinical outcome) may be different than in general practice. Other concerns about determining whether the results of a trial will help a clinician care for his or her patients are discussed by Guyatt and associates.[141]

Finally, it is worth noting that a clinical trial may demonstrate that a therapy of procedure currently used in clinical practice is ineffective or unnecessary.[142] This occurred with the EC-IC bypass surgery,[93] for example, and may also be occurring with the use of intravenous anticoagulation for acute ischemic stroke.[28]

Alternatives to Clinical Trials

Randomized clinical trials have been viewed as the gold standard for testing new therapies, but because of the limitations of their application to many practical areas of clinical management, scientifically sound new methods should be developed and applied in situations inappropriate or impossible to evaluate with clinical trials.[15] In fact, techniques are being developed to minimize the possible biases of nonrandomized treatment assignment by defining prognostically similar groups. Improved observational cohort methods using many of the principles of a randomized clinical trial may achieve results similar to those of randomized clinical trials.[78,143,144] Although controversy exists,[145] many more developments are expected in this dynamic and rapidly expanding research area as a new century for clinical research unfolds.[146]

Conclusions

Randomized clinical trials are a powerful tool for clinical investigation of the effects of new treatments. Like other scientific techniques, they have clear uses and limitations. As was found in basic research, the technique of patch clamping is a powerful tool for examining the behavior of ion channels in 10-mm round isopotential cells, but the technique is less practical for those studying those same receptors on the dendrites of a highly branched neuron. Similarly, randomized clinical trials are useful for testing whether a new therapy is superior to a control therapy, but the method has little value in understanding the natural history of a disease and may not give the optimal answers about how to treat patients. For example, decreasing mortality from stroke may actually increase morbidity and the cost to society. Also, quality of life for those saved from stroke recurrence must be considered when applying information about preserving brain tissue injured by stroke.

Randomized clinical trials are likely to emerge as one of the main scientific advances in clinical neuroscience during the twentieth century. As advances in basic neuroscience are applied in clinical studies, there will be many opportunities for interaction between basic and clinical research in the nervous system. Effective therapies for some of the most serious and heretofore incurable human diseases can be anticipated. The testing of new candidate therapies surely depends, in part, on the proper application of the principles of randomized clinical trials. The better the medical community understands the principles of these trials, the easier it is to move from bench research to clinical trials and ultimately to new and more effective therapies for stroke.

References

1. Brott T, Bogousslavsky J. Treatment of acute ischemic stroke. N Engl J Med 2000;343:710–722.
2. Stroke Therapy Academic Industry Roundtable (STAIR). Recommendations for standards regarding preclinical neuroprotective and restorative drug development. Stroke 1999;30:2752–2758.
3. Brass LM, Alter M. Clinical Trial Design for Cerebrovascular Disorders. In Fisher M (ed), Stroke Therapy. Boston: Butterworth–Heinemann, 1995;135–170.
4. Sackett DL, Haynes RB, Guyatt GH, Tugwell P. Clinical Epidemiology: A Basic Science for Clinical Medicine (2nd ed). Boston: Little, Brown, 1991.
5. Fletcher RH, Fletcher SW, Wagner EH. Clinical Epidemiology (2nd ed). Baltimore: Williams & Wilkins, 1988.
6. Jaeschke R, Guyatt G, Sackett DL. Users' guides to the medical literature: III. How to use an article about a diagnostic test. A. Are the results of the study valid? Evidence-Based Medicine Working Group. JAMA 1994;271: 389–391.
7. Magnetic resonance imaging of the brain and spine: a revised statement. American College of Physicians. Ann Intern Med 1994;120:872–874.
8. Symposium recommendations for methodology in stroke outcome research. Task Force on Stroke Impairment

TFoSD, and Task Force on Stroke Handicap. Stroke 1990;21(Suppl II):68–73.

9. Quality Enhancement Research Initiative (QUERI) for Stroke Toolbox. QUERI Stroke Executive Committee. In EZ Oddone, L Kaplan, (eds),1999.

10. Fisher M, Bogousslavsky J. Further evolution toward effective therapy for acute ischemic stroke. JAMA 1998; 279:1298–1303.

11. Gardner MJ, Machin D, Campbell MJ. Use of check lists in assessing the statistical content of medical studies. BMJ 1986;292:810–812.

12. Weintraub M. How to critically assess clinical drug trials. Drug Therapy 1982;12:131–148.

13. Capildeo R, Orgogozo JM. Methodology of Clinical Trials in Neurology: Vascular and Degenerative Brain Disease. London: Macmillan, 1988.

14. Pocock SJ. Clinical Trials: A Practical Approach. New York: John Wiley & Sons, 1983.

15. Feinstein AR. Clinical Epidemiology: The Architecture of Clinical Research. Philadelphia: Saunders, 1985.

16. Friedman LM, Furberg CD, DeMets DL. Fundamentals of Clinical Trials. Littleton, MA: PSG Publishing Co., Inc., 1985.

17. Spilker B. Guide to Clinical Trials. New York: Raven Press, Ltd., 1991.

18. Ellenberg JH. Clinical trials. Neurol Clin 1990;8:15–30.

19. Feinstein AR. Basic Clinimetric Science in the 21st Century. In MA Hardy, RKH Kinne (eds), Biology and Medicine into the 21st Century. New York: Karger, 1991;178–195.

20. Marshall FJ, Kieburtz K, McDermott M, et al. Clinical research in neurology. From observation to experimentation. Neurol Clin 1996;14:451–466.

21. Tirilazad mesylate in acute ischemic stroke: a systematic review. Tirilazad International Steering Committee. Stroke 2000;31:2257–2265.

22. Clark WM, Williams BJ, Selzer KA, et al. A randomized efficacy trial of citicoline in patients with acute ischemic stroke. Stroke 1999;30:2592–2597.

23. Muir KW, Grosset DG. Neuroprotection for acute stroke: making clinical trials work. Stroke 1999;30:180–182.

24. Low molecular weight heparinoid, ORG 10172 (danaparoid), and outcome after acute ischemic stroke: a randomized controlled trial. The Publications Committee for the Trial of ORG 10172 in Acute Stroke Treatment (TOAST) Investigators. JAMA 1998;279:1265–1272.

25. Doll R. Controlled trials: the 1948 watershed. BMJ 1998;317:1217–1220.

26. Zivin J. Understanding clinical trials. Sci Am 2000;282: 69–75.

27. U.S. Food and Drug Administration. Clinical investigations: proposed establishment of regulations on obligations of sponsors and monitors. Fed Reg 1977:35210–35236.

28. Swanson RA. Intravenous heparin for acute stroke. Neurology 1999;52:1746–1750.

29. MRC European Carotid Surgery Trial: interim results for symptomatic patients with severe (70–99%) or with mild (0–29%) carotid stenosis. European Carotid Surgery Trialists' Collaborative Group. Lancet 1991;337:1235–1243.

30. Beneficial effect of carotid endarterectomy in symptomatic patients with high-grade carotid stenosis. North American Symptomatic Carotid Endarterectomy Trial Collaborators. N Engl J Med 1991;325:445–454.

31. Rothwell PM. Interpretation of variations in outcome in audit of clinical interventions. Lancet 2000;355:4–5.

32. Barnett HJM, Broderick JP. Carotid endarterectomy: another wake-up call. Neurology 2000;55:746–747.

33. Zivin JA. Factors determining the therapeutic window for stroke. Neurology 1998;50:599–603.

34. Heiss WD, Thiel A, Grond M, Graf R. Which targets are relevant for therapy of acute ischemic stroke? Stroke 1999;30:1486–1489.

35. Hall ED, Braughler JM. Free radicals in CNS injury. Research Publications—Association for Research in Nervous and Mental Disease. 1993;71:81–105.

36. Clinical trial of nimodipine in acute ischemic stroke. American Nimodipine Study Group. Stroke 1992;23:3–8.

37. del Zoppo GJ, Poeck K, Pessin MS, et al. Recombinant tissue plasminogen activator in acute thrombotic and embolic stroke. Ann Neurol 1992;32:78–86.

38. Clark WM, Wissman S, Albers GW, et al. Recombinant tissue-type plasminogen activator (Alteplase) for ischemic stroke 3 to 5 hours after symptom onset. The ATLANTIS Study: a randomized controlled trial. Alteplase Thrombolysis for Acute Noninterventional Therapy in Ischemic Stroke. JAMA 1999;282:2019–2026.

39. Hacke W, Kaste M, Fieschi C, et al. Randomised double-blind placebo-controlled trial of thrombolytic therapy with intravenous alteplase in acute ischaemic stroke (ECASS II). Second European-Australasian Acute Stroke Study Investigators. Lancet 1998;352:1245–1251.

40. Hacke W, Kaste M, Fieschi C, et al. Intravenous thrombolysis with recombinant tissue plasminogen activator for acute hemispheric stroke: The European Cooperative Acute Stroke Study (ECASS). JAMA 1995;274: 1017–1025.

41. Fields WS, Maslenikov V, Meyer JS, et al. Joint study of extracranial arterial occlusion. V. Progress report of prognosis following surgery for or nonsurgical treatment for transient cerebral ischemic attacks and cervical carotid artery lesions. JAMA 1970;211:1993–2003.

42. Hier DB, Foulkes MA, Swiontoniowski M, et al. Stroke recurrence within 2 years after ischemic infarction. Stroke 1991;22:155–161.

43. Kurtzke JF. On the role of clinicians in the use of drug trial data. Neuroepidemiology 1982;1:124–136.

44. Roland M, Torgerson D. Understanding controlled trials: what outcomes should be measured? BMJ 1998;317:1075.

45. Rothwell PM. Responsiveness of outcome measures in randomized clinical trials in neurology. J Neurol Neurosurg Psychiatry 2000;68:274–275.

46. Wardlaw JM, Sandercock PA, Warlow CP, Lindley RI. Trials of thrombolysis in acute ischemic stroke: does the choice of primary outcome measure really matter? Stroke 2000;31:1133–1135.

47. Sackett DL. The Canadian trial of aspirin and sulphinpyrazone in threatened stroke (letter). N Engl J Med 1978; 301:955.

48. Albers GW. Choice of endpoints in antiplatelet trials: which outcomes are most relevant to stroke patients? Neurology 2000;54:1022–1028.

49. Warfarin versus aspirin for prevention of thromboembolism in atrial fibrillation: Stroke Prevention in Atrial Fibrillation II Study. Stroke Prevention in Atrial Fibrillation Investigators. Lancet 1994;343:687–691.

50. Hass WK, Easton JD, Adams HPJ, et al. A randomized trial comparing ticlopidine hydrochloride with aspirin for the prevention of stroke in high-risk patients. N Engl J Med 1990;321:501–507.

51. Vickrey BG. Getting oriented to patient-oriented outcomes. Neurology 1999;53:662–663.

52. Williams LS, Weinberger M, Harris LE, Biller J. Measuring quality of life in a way that is meaningful to stroke patients. Neurology 1999;53:1839–1843.

53. Sanders C, Egger M, Donovan J, et al. Reporting on quality of life in randomised controlled trials. BMJ 1998;317:1191–1194.

54. Duncan PW, Jorgensen HS, Wade DT. Outcome measures in acute stroke trials: a systematic review and some recommendations to improve practice. Stroke 2000;31:1429–1438.

55. Feinstein AR. Clinimetrics. New Haven, CT: Yale University Press, 1987.

56. Gelmers HJ, Gorter K, de Weerdt CJ, Wiezer HJA. Assessment of interobserver variability in a Dutch multicenter study on acute ischemic stroke. Stroke 1988;19:709–711.

57. Shinar D, Gross CR, Mohr JP, et al. Interobserver variability in the assessment of neurological history and examination in the Stroke Data Bank. Arch Neurol 1985;42:557–565.

58. Rubins HB, Robins SJ, Collins D, et al. Gemfibrozil for the secondary prevention of coronary heart disease in men with low levels of high-density lipoprotein cholesterol. Veterans Affairs High-Density Lipoprotein Cholesterol Intervention Trial Study Group. N Engl J Med 1999;341:410–418.

59. Rothwell PM, Slattery J, Warlow CP. A systematic comparison of the risks of stroke and death due to carotid endarterectomy for symptomatic and asymptomatic stenosis. Stroke 1996;27:266–269.

60. Temkin NR, Dikmen SS, Wilensky AJ, et al. A randomized, double-blind study of phenytoin for the prevention of post-traumatic seizures. N Engl J Med 1990;323:497–502.

61. Prichard JW, Brass LM. New anatomical and functional imaging methods. Ann Neurol 1992;32:395–400.

62. Beck RW, Cleary PA, Trobe JD, et al. The effect of corticosteroids for acute optic neuritis on the subsequent development of multiple sclerosis. The Optic Neuritis Study Group. N Engl J Med 1993;329:1764–1769.

63. McDonald WI, Thompson AJ. Are magnetic resonance findings predictive of clinical outcome in therapeutic trials in multiple sclerosis? The dilemma of interferon-β. Ann Neurol 1994;36:14–18.

64. Graham GD, Blamire AM, Rothman DL, et al. Early temporal variation of cerebral metabolites after human stroke: a proton magnetic resonance spectroscopy study. Stroke 1993;24:1891–1896.

65. Minematsu K, Fisher M, Li L, et al. Effects of a novel NMDA antagonist on experimental stroke rapidly and quantitatively assessed by diffusion-weighted MRI. Neurology 1993;43:397–403.

66. Powers WJ, Zivin J. Magnetic resonance imaging in acute stroke: not ready for prime time. Neurology 1998;50:842–843.

67. Preliminary report: effect of encainide and flecainide on mortality in a randomized trial of arrhythmia suppression after myocardial infarction. The Cardiac Arrhythmia Suppression Trial (CAST) Investigators. N Engl J Med 1989;321:406–412.

68. Raju TNK, Langenberg P, Sen A, Aldana O. How much "better" is good enough? The magnitude of treatment effect in clinical trials. Am J Dis Child 1992;146:407–411.

69. Johnston KC. What are surrogate outcome measures and why do they fail in clinical research? Neuroepidemiology 1999;18:167–173.

70. Sacks H, Chalmers TC, Smith HJ. Randomized versus historical controls for clinical trials. Am J Med 1982;72:233–240.

71. Wagensteen OH, Peter ET, Nicoloff DM. Achieving "physiological gastrectomy" by gastric freezing: a preliminary report of an experimental and clinical study. JAMA 1962;180:439.

72. Ruffin JM, Grizzle JE, Hightower NC, et al. A cooperative double-blind evaluation of gastric "freezing" in the treatment of duodenal ulcer. N Engl J Med 1969;281:16.

73. Altman DG. Treatment allocation in controlled trials: why randomise? BMJ 1999;318:1209.

74. Roberts C, Torgerson D. Randomisation methods in controlled trials. BMJ 1998;317:1301.

75. Sibbald B, Roland M. Understanding controlled trials. Why are randomised controlled trials important? BMJ 1998;316:201.

76. Chalmers TC, Celano P, Sacks HS, Smith H. Bias in treatment assignment in controlled clinical trials. N Engl J Med 1983;309:1358–1361.

77. Feinstein AR, Horwitz RI. Choosing cases and controls: the clinical epidemiology of "clinical investigation." J Clin Invest 1988;81:1–5.

78. Horwitz RI, Viscoli CM, Clemens JD, Sadock RT. Developing improved observational methods for evaluating therapeutic effectiveness. Ann Intern Med 1990;89:630–638.

79. Altman DG, Bland JM. How to randomise. BMJ 1999;319:703–704.

80. Sackett DL. Bias in analytic research. J Chronic Dis 1979;32:51–63.

81. Imperiale TF, Horwitz RI. Scientific standards and the design of case-control research. Biomed Pharmacother 1989;43:187–189.

82. Day SJ, Altman DG. Blinding in clinical trials and other studies. BMJ 2000;321:504.

83. Ebers JH, Vandervolt MK, Farguhar RE, et al. The impact of blinding on the results of a randomized, placebo-controlled multiple sclerosis clinical trial. Neurology 1994;44:16–20.

84. Study design for randomized prospective trial of carotid endarterectomy for asymptomatic atherosclerosis. Asymptomatic Carotid Atherosclerosis Study Group. Stroke 1989;20:844–849.

85. Lee KL, Califf RM, Simes J, et al. Holding GUSTO up to the light. Global Utilization of Streptokinase and Tissue

Plasminogen Activator for Occluded Coronary Arteries. Ann Intern Med 1994;120:876–881.

86. Ridker PM, O'Donnell CJ, Marder VJ, Hennekens CH. A response to "Holding GUSTO up to the light." Ann Intern Med 1994;120:882–885.

87. An international randomized trial comparing four thrombolytic strategies for acute myocardial infarction. The GUSTO investigators. N Engl J Med 1993;329:673–682.

88. Sibbald B, Roberts C. Understanding controlled trials. Crossover trials. BMJ 1998;316:1719–1720.

89. A randomized trial of aspirin and sulfinpyrazone in threatened stroke. The Canadian Cooperative Study Group. N Engl J Med 1978;299:53–59.

90. Ganglioside GM1 in acute ischemic stroke. The SASS trial. Stroke 1994;25:1141–1148.

91. Failure of extracranial-intracranial arterial bypass to reduce the risk of ischemic stroke. Results of an international randomized trial. Extracranial-Intracranial Bypass Study Group. N Engl J Med 1985;313:1191–1200.

92. Goldring S, Zervas H, Langfitt T. The extracranial-intracranial bypass study. A report of the committee appointed by the American Association of Neurological Surgeons to examine the study. N Engl J Med 1987;316:817–820.

93. Barnett HJ, Sackett D, Taylor DW, et al. Are the results of the extracranial-intracranial bypass trial generalizable? N Engl J Med 1987;316:820–824.

94. Influence of adherence to treatment and response of cholesterol on mortality in the coronary drug project. Coronary Drug Project Research Group. N Engl J Med 1980;303:1038–1041.

95. Farrell B. Efficient management of randomised controlled trials: nature or nurture. BMJ 1998;317:1236–1239.

96. Armitage P. Controversies and achievements in clinical trials. Control Clin Trials 1984;5:67–72.

97. Yusuf S, Wittes J, Probstfield J, Tyroler HA. Analysis and interpretation of treatment effects in subgroups of patients in randomized clinical trials. JAMA 1991;266:93–98.

98. Randomised trial of intravenous streptokinase, oral aspirin, both, or neither among 17,187 cases of suspected acute myocardial infarction: ISIS-2. ISIS-2 (Second International Study of Infarct Survival) Collaborative Group. Lancet 1988;2:349–360.

99. Grotta JC, Norris JW, Kamm B. Prevention of stroke with ticlopidine: who benefits most? TASS Baseline and Angiographic Data Subgroup. Neurology 1992;42:111–115.

100. Weisberg LA. The efficacy and safety of ticlopidine and aspirin in non-whites: analysis of a patient subgroup from the Ticlopidine Aspirin Stroke Study. Neurology 1993;43:27–31.

101. Grotta J. Is aspirin effective in preventing strokes in diabetic patients? Stroke 1993;24:760.

102. Harbison JW. Ticlopidine versus aspirin for the prevention of recurrent stroke. Analysis of patients with minor stroke from the Ticlopidine Aspirin Stroke Study. Stroke 1992;23:1723–1727.

103. Oster G, Huse DM, Lacey MJ, Epstein AM. Cost-effectiveness of ticlopidine in preventing stroke in high-risk patients. Stroke 1994;25:1149–1156.

104. van Gijn J, Algra A. Ticlopidine, trials, and torture. Stroke 1994;25:1097–1098.

105. Gent M, Blakely JA, Easton JD, et al. The Canadian American Ticlopidine Study (CATS) in thromboembolic stroke. Lancet 1989;1:1215–1220.

106. Newell DJ. Intention-to-treat analysis: implications for quantitative and qualitative research. Int J Epidemiol 1982;21:837–841.

107. Sommer A, Zeger SL. On estimating efficacy from clinical trials. Stat Med 1991;10:45–52.

108. Taylor DW, Sackett DL, Haynes RB. Sample size for randomized trials in stroke prevention. How many patients do we need? Stroke 1984;15:968–970.

109. McKhann GM. The trials of clinical trials. Arch Neurol 1989;46:611–614.

110. Wiebers DO, Adams HPJ, Whisnant JP. Animal models of stroke: are they relevant to human disease? Stroke 1989;21:1–3.

111. Brass LM, Kernan WN. Canadian Neurological Scale. Neurology 1989;39:1556–1558.

112. Goldstein LB, Bertels C, Davis JN. Interrater reliability of the NIH stroke scale. Arch Neurol 1989;46:660–662.

113. Adams RJ, Meador KJ, Sethi KD, Grotta JC. Graded neurological scale for use in acute hemispheric stroke treatment protocols. Stroke 1987;18:665–669.

114. Kernan WN, Feinstein AR, Brass LM. A methodological appraisal of research on prognosis after transient ischemic attacks. Stroke 1991;22:1108–1116.

115. Kernan WN, Horwitz RI, Brass LM, et al. A prognostic system for patients with TIA or minor stroke. Ann Intern Med 1991;114:552–557.

116. Pulsinelli W. Pathophysiology of acute ischaemic stroke. Lancet 1992;339:533–536.

117. Fisher M, Bogousslavsky J. Evolving toward effective therapy for acute ischemic stroke. JAMA 1993;270:360–364.

118. ISIS-3: a randomized comparison of streptokinase vs tissue plasminogen activator vs anistreplase and of aspirin plus heparin vs aspirin alone among 41,299 cases of suspected acute myocardial infarction. ISIS-3 (Third International Study of Infarct Survival) Collaborative Group. Lancet 1992;339:753–770.

119. Albers GW. Expanding the window for thrombolytic therapy in acute stroke. The potential role of acute MRI for patient selection. Stroke 1999;30:2230–2237.

120. Hellman S, Hellman DS. Of mice but not men. Problems with the randomized clinical trial. N Engl J Med 1991;324:1585–1589.

121. Passamani E. Clinical trials—are they ethical? N Engl J Med 1991;324:1589–1592.

122. Edwards SJL, Lilford RJ, Hewison J. The ethics of randomised controlled trials from the perspectives of patients, the public, and healthcare professionals. BMJ 1998;317:1209–1212.

123. Ethical issues in clinical research in neurology: advancing knowledge and protecting human research subjects. The Ethics and Humanities Subcommittee of the American Academy of Neurology. Neurology 1998;50:592–595.

124. Freedman B. Equipoise and the ethics of clinical research. N Engl J Med 1987;317:141–145.

125. Barnett HJM, Sackett DL. Monitoring clinical trials. Neurology 1993;43:2437–2438.

126. Abrams KR. Monitoring randomised controlled trials. BMJ 1998;316:1183–1184.

127. Hampton JR. Clinical trial safety committees: the devil's spoon. BMJ 2000;320:244–245.

128. Alves WA, Macciocchi SN. Ethical considerations in clinical neuroscience. Current concepts in neuroscience trials. Stroke 1996;27:1903–1909.

129. Preliminary report of the Stroke Prevention in Atrial Fibrillation Study. Stroke Prevention in Atrial Fibrillation Investigators. N Engl J Med 1990;322:863–868.

130. Hooper C. Stroke study calls attention to atrial fibrillation. J NIH Res 1990;2:41–42.

131. Detsky AS. Are clinical trials a cost-effective investment? JAMA 1989;262:1795–1800.

132. Feinstein AR. An additional basic science for clinical medicine: II. The limitations of randomized trials. Ann Intern Med 1983;99:544–550.

133. Yusuf S. Randomised controlled trials in cardiovascular medicine: past achievements, future challenges. BMJ 1999;319:564–568.

134. Beto R, Baigent C. Trials: the next 50 years. BMJ 1999; 317:1170–1171.

135. Haynes B. Can it work? Does it work? Is it worth it? BMJ 1999;319:652–653.

136. Goldstein LB, Moore WS, Robertson JT, Chaturvedi S. Complication rates for carotid endarterectomy. A call to action. Stroke 1997;28:890–891.

137. Katzan IL, Furlan AJ, Lloyd LE, et al. Use of tissue-type plasminogen activator for acute ischemic stroke: the Cleveland area experience. JAMA 2000;283:1151–1158.

138. Laupacis A, Sackett DL, Roberts RS. Therapeutic priorities of Canadian internists. CMAJ 1990;142:329–333.

139. Laupacis A, Sackett DL, Roberts RS. An assessment of clinically useful measures of the consequences of treatment. N Engl J Med 1988;318:1728–1733.

140. Farkouh ME, Lang JD, Sackett DL. Thrombolytic agents: the science of the art of choosing the better treatment. Ann Intern Med 1994;120:886–888.

141. Guyatt GH, Sackett DL, Cook DJ. Users' guides to the medical literature. II. How to use an article about therapy or prevention. B. What were the results and will they help me in caring for my patients? Evidence-Based Medicine Working Group. JAMA 1994;271:59–63.

142. Ilstrup DM. Randomized clinical trials: potential cost savings due to the identification of ineffective medical therapies. Mayo Clin Proc 1995;70:707–710.

143. Concato J, Shah N, Horwitz RI. Randomized, controlled trials, observational studies, and the hierarchy of clinical designs. N Engl J Med 2000;342:1887–1892.

144. Barton S. Which clinical studies provide the best evidence? BMJ 2000;321:255–256.

145. Pocock SJ, Elbourne DR. Randomized trials or observational tribulations? N Engl J Med 2000;342:1907–1909.

146. Benson K, Hartz AJ. A comparison of observational studies and randomized, controlled trials. N Engl J Med 2000;342:1878–1886.

Chapter 7
Endpoints and Statistical Concerns for Acute Stroke Therapy Trials

Stephen M. Davis

Acute stroke therapy has been transformed by a general acceptance of the principles of evidence-based medicine and the rapid translation of high-quality evidence into clinical practice.[1] This process has been facilitated by the development and dissemination of clinical practice guidelines.[2,3] The fundamental rationale of evidence-based medicine is that there is a hierarchy of the strength and quality of evidence that should be used by clinicians in treatment decisions, with the strongest evidence (Level 1) generated from well designed and executed randomized, controlled clinical trials. The lowest level of evidence (level 4 or 5, depending on the scale used) is based on case series and anecdote. Based on the level of evidence, guidelines are used to generate strength of recommendations, usually graded A–C.[2] In acute stroke therapy, grade A recommendations include the admission of acute stroke patients to a geographical stroke unit, routine acute aspirin therapy for ischemic stroke, and the use of tissue plasminogen activator (t-PA) within 3 hours of onset of ischemic stroke in selected patients.[2,3]

Conversely, negative trial results can also have a significant effect on clinical practice. Anticoagulation of acute stroke is a good example. Although heparin is still the most widely used—yet unproven—acute stroke therapy, some trials have shown that any benefits from subcutaneous, unfractionated heparin, or intravenous low molecular-weight heparin and heparinoids, appear to be outweighed by the risk of major hemorrhage.[4–7] As a result, some reviews have emphasized the lack of evidence for anticoagulation in acute stroke,[8] and many clinicians have re-evaluated their longstanding protocols for anticoagulation in stroke. Similarly, a series of well conducted and adequately powered trials of neuroprotective strategies have been negative, leading to questions about the failure of promising compounds in animal studies to translate to positive results in phase III clinical trials.[9–11]

Despite their impact on practice, these and other influential stroke trials have used disparate designs, which illustrate many of the issues and controversies surrounding trial methodology at the present time. For example, the National Institute of Neurological Disorders and Stroke (NINDS) trial of t-PA was a rigorously conducted trial performed in a relatively small number of expert stroke centers in the United States, involving a sample size of more than 600 patients.[12] With some exceptions, a trial size of between 600 (e.g., NINDS trial)[12] and 1,800 patients (e.g., Glycine Antagonist [gavestinel] in Neuroprotection trial)[10] has been the norm in most acute stroke trials of intravenous thrombolysis, antithrombotic, and neuroprotective therapies.[6,9,10,12,13] Conversely, the International Stroke Trial (IST) represented the first acute stroke megatrial, involving 20,000 patients in a factorial design.[4] It was, therefore, analogous to the large myocardial infarction (MI) trials of thrombolytic and antithrombotic therapies, which changed clinical practice.[14] The IST was performed in both expert and nonexpert centers in 36 countries, and the large patient numbers allowed more robust statistical analysis of a number of prespecified secondary outcomes, as well as post hoc subgroup analyses. Even with this large number, the evidence favoring acute aspirin therapy was only marginal, although it was made more robust by the aspirin benefits shown by the Chinese Acute Stroke Trial (CAST), another mega-trial involving a similar number of patients.[15,16] The evidence in favor of acute stroke units was generated by another different approach, namely the meta-analysis of many individual trials, a substantial number of which showed no statistically significant benefit of stroke units.[17,18]

In addition to the debate about trial size, there has also been disagreement as to the most appropriate endpoints for use in acute stroke trials. In trials of acute MI, mortality is the accepted primary endpoint. In stroke trials, it is generally agreed that reduction in disability is the most important endpoint. Stroke trials have generally not been powered to evaluate reduction in mortality, although a therapy that significantly increases mortality, despite attenuation of disability, is unlikely to be licensed. Disability can be measured in terms of neurologic impairment, dependency in activities of daily living, and global handicap.[19] Most stroke trials have used activity scales measuring dependency, usually the well validated Barthel Index (BI) or the Rankin Scale.[20–22] Given that prespecified endpoints and statistical methods are an accepted part of good trial design, choice of the primary endpoint is crucial. Minor variation in the choice of endpoint can have a critical effect on the analysis of a trial result, as is seen later in the section Measuring Stroke Trial Outcomes and Endpoints. Other issues in stroke trial design include consent procedures and randomization strategies.

Stroke investigators are also questioning the overall development strategy for new compounds. The 1990s witnessed the negative results of a series of trials of neuroprotective strategies, despite positive results in validated animal models.[11] This challenged investigators to question the traditional sequence of phase I and II trials that precede definitive phase III trials.[23]

It is widely held that *proof of concept* trials using surrogate measures, such as infarct volume

on magnetic resonance imaging, might have an important role in indicating a substantial probability of success as a prelude to the larger scale of phase III trials. Finally, there is controversy and debate concerning the organization of large, expensive trials and the relationships between investigators and the pharmaceutical industry.

What Is Generally Agreed on and What Are the Issues in Stroke Trials?

Stroke investigators agree that clinical trials should address important questions (usually whether a novel agent is effective and safe, compared with placebo or best available therapy in most cases); be ethically conducted with appropriate consent procedures; be adequately powered; be performed in experienced centers that are carefully monitored for protocol adherence; and have a randomized, controlled design and validated endpoints.[24] Some of the current issues in trial methodology include the choice of randomization protocols, consent procedures and the role of surrogate consent, trial size and conduct, choice of endpoints, the use of meta-analyses and systematic overviews, the difficulties in translation from animal to human trials and the use of surrogate endpoints, and the alliances between academic investigators and pharmaceutical companies (Table 7-1).

Randomization Procedures

Randomization is an essential feature of trial design, intended to protect against systematic bias in treatment allocation. Two main concepts have been used in stroke trial randomization. The traditional approach emphasizes sequential randomization of all eligible, consenting patients. Because there must be clinical equipoise in any ethical study, explained as a genuine uncertainty that a novel strategy is or is not safe and efficacious, the patient and clinician must accept the random allocation of therapy. The treatment is usually administered in a double-blind design, although procedural and operative interventions are often open and single-blind. In single-blind design, assessment of the primary endpoint is usually performed by an observer who should be unaware of the patient's treatment allocation and clinical course.

The other strategy, mainly advocated in British-based trials such as the IST[4] and European Carotid Endarterectomy study,[25] involves the *uncertainty principle*. This technique is useful in testing treatments that are available but unproven, such as heparin or aspirin, or procedural interventions, such as carotid endarterectomy or arterial stenting. The methodology is based on the assumption that any trial involves a small sample of eligible patients at any time, in part because of the random nature of patients being admitted to an institution involved in the trial, as well as variation in patient and physician consent. The underlying principle is that the patients not enrolled in a trial are unimportant, provided that those actually enrolled are typical of the target population, so that the results can be reasonably generalized. In this randomization strategy, patients whom the clinician believes are likely to benefit from the strategy are excluded and treated openly, whereas those thought unlikely to benefit are also excluded, so that they are not treated. When there is clinical uncertainty about treatment benefit versus risk, the patient is randomized. Because there is such a range of opinion concerning controversial and unproven treatment decisions, the area of uncertainty varies enormously between clinicians, so that the patients actually randomized tend to be representative of the target trial population.

Whatever the randomization technique, any trial involves only a small proportion of eligible patients. There are still those who dispute, for example, the results of the Extracranial-Intracranial Bypass Study Group trial, claiming that patients likely to benefit from the surgical intervention tended not to be enrolled by participating clinicians.[26] This proposition is generally irrelevant if the trial involved a population typical of the target population for the intervention, as in the case of the Extracranial-Intracranial Bypass Study Group trial. Similarly, it is notable that the two different approaches to randomization used in the North American Symptomatic Carotid Endarterectomy Trial and European Carotid Surgery Trial produced remarkably consistent results.[25,27]

Consent Procedures and Surrogate Consent

Simplified, ethically sound consent procedures are most important for trial enrollment and conduct.

Table 7-1. Issues in Trial Methodology

Topic	Controversy
Randomization procedures	Sequential randomization versus randomization based on uncertainty
Consent procedure	Should surrogate consent be permitted?
Trial size and conduct	Mega-trials versus small, focused trials
Choice of endpoints	Simple versus more complex outcome scales
	Emphasis on reduction of poor outcome versus achievement of good outcome
Meta-analyses and systematic overviews	Power of meta-analysis versus application to individual patients
	Limitations of meta-analysis versus definitive trials
Investigator/pharmaceutical company alliances	Academic and scientific safeguards in partnerships between academic investigators and the pharmaceutical industry

The two key issues of relevance to stroke trials are (1) the complexity of the consent procedure, and (2) whether surrogate consent is permitted in patients with aphasia or impaired conscious state. For example, the huge disparity between accrual for the Second International Study of Infarct Survival acute MI trial in the United Kingdom and United States was thought to have reflected the more complex consent protocol required in the United States.[14] The British approach is typically a less formal one than in the United States, allowing far greater discretion by the individual doctor, with the view that excessively detailed consent can be inhumane and can impair trial recruitment. Furthermore, by delaying the discovery of effective treatments, complex consent protocols might potentially cause many deaths.[28]

Although virtually all countries require some form of informed consent, most institutional ethics committees allow surrogate consent by spouse or next of kin if the patient cannot provide consent because of dysphasia or depressed conscious state. For example, post-treatment consent is sometimes permitted in France if the patient is unable to consent and the family is not immediately available. In some Asian countries, such as Singapore, discussion and consent by the family is paramount.

In contrast, in some countries, only the patient can consent to involvement. Hence, patients with dysphasia or altered conscious state are excluded from acute trials. In the United States, there are differences in legislation between states and policies by individual institutional review boards, but evolving legal policies might well prohibit surrogate consent. Various patient advocacy and guardianship acts, which prohibit surrogate consent, are already in place in some Australian states. One American study indicated that such policies could reduce acute trial accruals by one-third and particularly affect entry of patients with more severe or language-impairing strokes.[29]

Trial Size: Mega-Trials versus Small, Focused Trials

Two of the pivotal stroke trials evaluating thrombolytic and antithrombotic therapies, the NINDS t-PA trial and the IST, have had a major impact on clinical practice, despite their radically different size and design. The IST was the first acute stroke mega-trial.[4] Proponents of mega-trial design emphasize the greatly increased statistical power generated by large study numbers, and the greater generalizability of the trial results to other stroke populations. Smaller, yet biologically important differences can be detected. For example, the IST and CAST mega-trials indicated that acute aspirin therapy was an effective therapy, and were able to detect only a 1% treatment effect.[4,15,16] These large trials showed that there would be 10 fewer deceased or dependent patients for every 1,000 patients treated with aspirin, the number needed to treat (NNT) therefore being 100.[4,15] The usual trial size of between 600 and 1,200 patients would not show this treatment benefit, and a potentially valuable therapy could have been discarded. The smaller, focused trials have been designed to show a 10–20% difference in outcomes between the investigational therapy and placebo, an NNT of only five to 10. It has been suggested that such designs might miss smaller but biologically important benefits, in which the NNT is significantly larger. Another advantage of mega-trials is that they usually have a simpler trial design, because prognostic variables tend to be better balanced at baseline.

Stroke trials are expensive. Large trials have been used to evaluate secondary prevention strategies. For example, the CAPRIE trial involved nearly 20,000 patients to demonstrate a small benefit of clopidogrel over aspirin.[30] Mega-trials in acute stroke have thus far generally been investigator-driven, rather than organized by pharmaceutical companies. Critics of this approach point out that such design necessitates the involvement of large numbers of less experienced acute stroke centers, and hence inherently less rigorous monitoring of trial quality and compliance. Auditing and data validation are logistically more difficult. Advocates of the mega-trial approach illustrate the advances in therapy of acute MI, based on trial sizes of 20,000–50,000 patients, concluding that new investigational therapies in stroke should be tested on large numbers of patients.[14,31]

Proponents of small, focused trials point out that stroke is a far more heterogeneous disease than MI. There may be important differences between therapeutic responses in those with small versus large vessel disease, cardioembolic versus atherothrombotic pathologies, anterior versus posterior circulation ischemia, or infarction versus hemorrhage. As a result, there is an argument that any putative stroke therapy should be targeted to a specific pathology. For example, some would advocate that thrombolytic therapy should be used chiefly in those with demonstrated vessel occlusion, avoiding the risks of the treatment in those patients with patent vessels.[32] There has been speculation that the time threshold for basilar thrombolysis may be different than that for thrombolysis in the middle cerebral artery. Examples of small, focused trials aimed at specific stroke subtypes include the Prolyse in Acute Cerebral Thromboembolism II trial in the United States,[33] which found that intra-arterial thrombolysis was an effective strategy for middle cerebral artery occlusion, and the ongoing Australian Urokinase Stroke Trial, which is investigating intra-arterial thrombolysis for basilar thrombosis.[34]

Advocates of smaller stroke trials point out that mega-trials tend to lump together patients with diverse pathologies and time intervals from stroke onset. In addition, stroke trials use disability as the primary endpoint, whereas mortality is usually a secondary endpoint. Hence, stroke trial size is lower than the acute MI trials that use mortality as the primary endpoint. Mega-trials may pose greater risks to patients than small, focused trials, and it has been suggested that these should be performed when safety parameters are better established.

Table 7-2. Controversies in Size of Acute Stroke Trials

	Mega-Trials	**Small, Focused Trials**
Advantages	Large statistical power	Recognize heterogeneity of stroke subtypes
	Able to detect small, biologically important differences	May be more rigorously conducted
	More likely to change clinical practice	May be safer for accrued patients
Disadvantages	May be less rigorous monitoring	May not detect small but significant treatment effect
	Safety issues for therapies with small risk/ benefit ratio (e.g., t-PA)	May be less generalized to stroke populations
	Lumps together stroke subtypes	May be less likely to change clinical practice

t-PA = tissue plasminogen activator.

There is likely to be a place for both types of trial design in the evaluation of acute stroke therapies, depending on the hypothesis and specific agent to be studied. For example, the IST and CAST both required large patient numbers to show a modest but biologically important benefit from aspirin; an inexpensive, widely available, and relatively safe treatment.[4,15] In contrast, evaluation of thrombolytic therapy in trials has occurred in closely vetted patients in expert stroke centers with strict protocol adherence.

The controversial role of t-PA in acute stroke encapsulates the argument concerning the level of evidence necessary to establish or reject a new therapy. Based on the NINDS trial, t-PA was licensed in the United States and more recently in Canada.[12] No other t-PA trial has been unequivocally positive, although subset benefits were evident in both European Cooperative Acute Stroke Study (ECASS) 1[35] and ECASS 2.[36] Indeed, ECASS 1 was positive in the target population (those who were eligible and received the protocol, rather than intention to treat), and was positive if the NINDS dichotomized outcome endpoint was used.[37] Similarly, ECASS 2 showed a strong trend in favor of therapy, and would have been positive if a slightly different definition of good outcome was used with the dichotomized Rankin Scale in the prespecified analysis.[36] Meta-analysis shows significant benefits of t-PA within 6 hours.[38] At the time of this writing, however, the drug is not licensed for ischemic stroke in most countries outside of North America.

It has been proposed that this uncertainty can only be resolved if t-PA is evaluated in a mega-trial design. Proponents of mega-trial evaluation of thrombolysis point out that any licensed acute stroke therapy would, in fact, be conducted in less experienced centers and raise doubts about the generalizability of the t-PA trial results, given that the trial was performed in experienced academic centers. Conversely, many would argue that there is an adequate level of proof of benefit within 3 hours, provided that the therapy is only administered within experienced stroke units, employing the safeguards used in the NINDS trial. Indeed, post-marketing experience with t-PA indicates the hazards of the therapy when these guidelines are breached. In one open study in which there were protocol violations in 50% of patients, the symptomatic intracerebral hemorrhage rate reached 16%, compared with 6.4% in NINDS.[39] In contrast, the hemorrhage rate in experienced centers was found to be only 3.3% in the Standard Treatment with Alteplase to Reverse Stroke study, which evaluated t-PA experience with strict protocol adherence.[40] Given that the balance between risk and benefit is so highly poised, there is strong argument that any further thrombolytic trials should only be conducted in highly experienced centers, with rigorous monitoring of protocol compliance. The risk of testing of thrombolysis in a mega-trial design is the real potential for discarding an important therapy, which—unlike aspirin—should only be administered in expert centers (Table 7-2).

Measuring Stroke Trial Outcomes and Endpoints

Broadly, stroke outcomes can be categorized into neurologic impairment (signs elicited by examination due to the disease), disability (the functional effects of the impairment), and handicap (the social consequences of the disability).[18,41] They can be more simply classified as impairment measures and activity measures.[42] Neurologic impairment scales, such as the National Institutes of Health Stroke Scale (NIHSS), the Canadian Stroke Scale, or the Scandinavian Stroke Scale, measure neurologic signs elicited by examination. They are routinely used to determine and often stratify neurologic severity at entry and ensure balance at baseline between treatment and control groups. They also have validated prognostic value.[43,44] The NIHSS is a widely used and well validated scale, measuring speech and language, cognition, visual field deficits, motor and sensory impairments, and ataxia.[43,45] Standardized videotapes are used for training and certification of examiners. Non-neurologic physicians and nurse study coordinators can be reliably trained to use the scale in clinical trials.[46]

Change in the NIHSS was used as one endpoint in the NINDS trial, but most stroke trials have used activity measures to measure functional outcome after stroke. The most commonly used are the BI and the Modified Rankin Scale (MRS). The BI was first published in 1965[20] and later modified to measure dependency in 10 activities of daily living.[21] Most clinicians use the 0–100 scaled BI, where 0 equals total dependency and 100 represents complete independence. The majority of stroke trials have used a dichotomized endpoint (good vs. bad outcome), although a wide variation of cutoff scores have been chosen to indicate the criterion for favorable outcome.[22] For example, many trials have used a BI >60 to represent reasonable functional independence.[9] A BI >60 is equivalent to a patient who may have significant disability, but is functionally independent. More recently, trials have used the concept that a stroke therapy should, if successful, produce minimal disability. Hence, the NINDS trial used a BI >95 to represent excellent outcome.[12] Another approach, used in the Glycine Antagonist (gavestinel) in Neuroprotection trials, is to use a trichotomized outcome of the BI.[10] This approach used 0–55 to represent poor outcome, 60–90 as a reasonable outcome or moderate recovery, and >95 as excellent outcome. The advantage of trichotomy is that a shift from one group to another may be detected. In theory, a therapy might move patients from poor to moderate outcome without a significantly greater number of excellent outcomes.[10] Other studies have used up

to six subdivisions of the BI.[47] It has been pointed out that many of the cutoff scores have never been validated.[22] Sulter et al. argued that given the disparity between definitions of good outcome, there could be greater consistency if reduction in poor outcome was chosen as the primary endpoint, defined as death, institutionalization, MRS >3, or BI <60.[22] In support of this argument, it has been pointed out that an arbitrary choice of good outcome as the endpoint naturally excludes patients with premorbid disability from participating in acute stroke trials.[48]

It has been argued that simplicity of design is important in stroke trials,[49] but this is not a universal opinion.[50] For example, the IST investigators chose a simple but clinically meaningful outcome scale that could be conducted by telephone.[51] This scale simply grades the patient as 1 (alive, fully recovered), 2 (alive, residual symptoms but independent), 3 (alive, dependent), or 4 (deceased). The MRS also measures independence on a simple 0–6 scale, where 0 = no symptoms, 5 = severe disability, and 6 = deceased. Dichotomized outcome based on the MRS has been widely used, whereby either 0–1 or 0–2 are considered to represent good outcome, with the remainder regarded as poor outcome. An alternative view is that predominantly motor scales may be relatively insensitive outcome measures, given that motor function only represents a small part of the cerebral hemisphere. It has been argued that scales that incorporate higher level functions, such as language, skilled motor acts, and sensory discrimination, might provide a more relevant measure of the effects of some acute therapies.[50]

Choice of the definition of favorable outcome is crucial, as exemplified by the ECASS 2 trial. This trial found no statistical benefit for t-PA using the prespecified 0–1 MRS definition of favorable outcome. In post hoc analysis, however, shifting the endpoint to a MRS of 0–2 for good outcome produced a statistically significant result.[22,36,52,53]

A further innovation in trial design was the development of a global test as a test of the primary hypothesis of the NINDS trial. This global test was a composite endpoint, using a consistent and persuasive difference in the proportion of patients achieving a favorable outcome on the BI, MRS, Glasgow Outcome Scale, and the NIHSS.[12,54] The NINDS data and safety monitoring committee chose this composite approach, considering that a positive result would be more robust than the use of a single endpoint.[54]

Clearly, greater rigor in acute stroke trial design, performance, and choice of primary endpoints is desirable (Table 7-3). A review of 174 acute stroke trials performed over 40 years concluded that many used outcome measures that were inadequate in terms of content, blinding, reliability, validation, and statistical analysis.[55] For example, some trials did not report mortality; some trials employed unique and unvalidated scales; parametric statistics were often used for skewed data distributions; blinding was often suboptimal; and primary and secondary endpoints were frequently not clearly stated.[55] Another review concluded that dichotomization of outcome should be avoided and that nonparametric statistics should be used to analyze the whole range of outcome data to assess shifts in disability.[42]

Meta-Analysis and Systematic Reviews

Meta-analyses of published trials and systematic reviews, which include unpublished results as well, have had a substantial impact on clinical practice. Systematic reviews are needed to allow the clinician and those devising clinical guidelines to draw conclusions about therapy. Furthermore, the results of such reviews can change clinical practice, and they require frequent updating.[56] Meta-analyses increase power and precision and can produce a definitive answer, even when the results of individual trials are inconclusive. They can reduce the bias of individual trials and allow testing of questions that cannot be reliably addressed in individual trials.[57] The proof of the substantial benefit of stroke units shown in the 1993 meta-analysis by Langhorne, in which many of the rather small individual trials had been underpowered, is a striking example.[17] The introduction of stroke units, shown to reduce mortality by at least 20%, is the single most important change in acute stroke management and a key plank of published expert guidelines around the world.

Another important and often cited example of the importance of frequent, systematic overviews of all the available data[58] was the delay in the recommendations for the introduction of thrombolytic therapy for MI years after it was evident that the therapy was effective, based on cumulative meta-analysis.[31] Systematic reviews in stroke, which

Table 7-3. Endpoints and Statistical Concerns in Stroke Trials

Issue	Example
Primary endpoint	One endpoint or a composite endpoint
	Disability score or simple outcome scale
Primary trial analysis	Dichotomy, trichotomy, or analysis of the full range of outcomes
	Proportion achieving good outcome versus proportion achieving poor outcome
Statistical analysis	Parametric versus nonparametric statistics in analysis of often skewed outcome data

include all retrievable data (published and unpublished), are performed and regularly updated by the Cochrane Stroke Collaborators.[58]

There are also limitations of meta-analysis. These include the potential for excessive heterogeneity between trial results due to major differences in trial design and conduct, variations in trial quality, and publication and reporting bias.[57] Even with the powerful data generated by meta-analysis, care has to be taken in applying the conclusions to individual patients, as treatment effect is dependent on baseline risk, which varies considerably within trials.[59] Few meta-analyses evaluate the quality of individual trials, despite the potential for low-quality trials influencing the estimate of treatment effect.[60] Large randomized trials may not agree with previous meta-analyses. Despite these reservations, most investigators would consider that the strengths of meta-analyses outweigh their weaknesses, provided that their limitations are also considered.[61]

Translation of Animal Models to Clinical Trials: Lessons from Failed Trials and Use of Surrogate Endpoints

In the treatment of acute ischemic stroke, the two major strategies that have been used to limit the degree of the ischemic insult and infarct size are reperfusion (particularly thrombolysis) and neuroprotection. Both of these strategies rely on the presence of functionally impaired but potentially viable and salvageable tissue in the ischemic penumbra. The successful clinical trials in thrombolysis[12] represented the first success in translating animal model studies[62] into positive human trials.

Table 7-4. Lessons from Failed
Neuroprotective Trials

Issue	Example
Validity of animal models	Poor translation of animal models to human stroke trials
Time windows	Time windows of 6–12 hours are probably too long
Drug dosage and bioavailability	Poor penetration of drugs into the ischemic penumbra
Neuroprotection as a single strategy	Neuroprotection without reperfusion may convey little therapeutic benefit
Traditional drug development strategy	"Proof of concept" surrogate endpoint trials (e.g., DWI) would increase probability of success in phase III trials

DWI = diffusion-weighted imaging.

The second strategy, neuroprotection, is based on attenuation of the pathobiochemical sequelae of ischemia. In animal studies, chiefly using rats, reduction of infarct size by up to 50% has been demonstrated with the use of strategies that attenuate the excitotoxic cascade, impair free radical toxicity, reduce harmful inflammatory reactions, or attenuate cell death by apoptosis. The positive results in animal models using neuroprotection, however, unlike the thrombolytic studies, have not been translated into positive phase III human trials.[9–11]

Explanations for the difficulty in translating animal stroke models to human brain ischemia include critique of the actual models (chiefly rats), and the poor penetration of neuroprotective drugs into the hypoperfused penumbral region. Some trials may have been underpowered. In many, the time window was probably too long. It has been suggested that, compared with the amount of tissue destroyed directly by hypoperfusion, the secondary and delayed biochemical cascade may be responsible for relatively little additional brain damage.[63] Other strategies suggested include reperfusion therapy preceding neuroprotection and sequences of neuroprotective agents, such as initial modification of excitotoxicity (e.g., N-methyl-D-aspartate antagonists), followed by treatments to reduce the delayed sequelae of stroke, such as inflammation and apoptosis (Table 7-4).[63]

Because of the failures of these trials, many investigators have questioned the traditional sequence of the evaluation of novel compounds, whereby effective agents that limit infarct size in animal models move through a rapid process of safety, feasibility, and dose-ranging studies in limited numbers of subjects, followed typically by two pivotal phase III trials. It is appealing to first determine whether the animal evidence of infarct volume limitation can be confirmed in human studies as a prelude to definitive clinical trials. Hence, an attractive strategy is to use diffusion-weighted imaging (DWI) and perfusion-weighted imaging (PWI) as surrogate markers of outcome.[64,65] In general, the acute DWI lesion represents the irreversibly damaged ischemic core, whereas the difference between the hypoperfusion boundary measured by PWI and the DWI core is postulated to represent tissue at risk in the putative ischemic penumbra.[64–66] The penumbra is present in the great majority of patients in the first few hours after stroke,[67] and the frequency of the penumbra subsequently progressively declines. In patients with acute stroke, there is typically substantial growth of the DWI ischemic core between acute and outcome studies.[64,68,69] This is chiefly confined to those patients with the penumbral pattern, in which the PWI lesion is larger than the DWI ischemic core.

Attenuation of the increase in the volume of the ischemic core is a surrogate endpoint that can be used in proof of concept stroke trials as the intermediate step bridging the animal evidence of infarct limitation and definitive large clinical trials. Such trials can be performed with approximately 100–200 patients randomized between a placebo and putative interventional strategy.[69] A positive proof of concept result should provide a better indication of the likely efficacy of a new treatment in definitive phase III trials. In addition to cost savings, large numbers of patients would not be treated with an experimental compound with a low probability of success.

Investigator-Pharmaceutical Issues in Trial Conduct

In essence, stroke trial organization and management ranges from investigator-driven studies, often poorly funded from national grant agencies, to pharmaceutical industry-sponsored "in-house" studies. The great majority of trials involve some form of partnership between academic investigators and the pharmaceutical industry. Most stroke trials of novel compounds necessitate industry involvement, in large part because of the huge costs in conducting large clinical trials. Many investigators have expressed concerns about such relationships, citing problems associated with in-house management and statistical control of trial databases, and particularly publication bias, when there is less urgency to report negative trial results.[70] Although trial size is prespecified, based on predicted treatment effects and power calculations, there is a tendency for pharmaceutical trials to have built-in interim analyses for testing of futility. This can lead to commercial considerations influencing trial completion, with the potential for discarding a potentially useful therapy (type 2 error). The credibility of trial results is often directly related to these organizational and procedural issues.

Most stroke investigators would consider that safeguards for partnerships with industry for the evaluation of novel compounds should include an independent, expert steering committee with only minority company representation, an independent and experienced data and safety monitoring committee without company representation, and, ideally, independent access and statistical evaluation of the trial database in the testing of the hypotheses. The steering committee should be involved with development of the trial protocol. A priority in selection of investigators should be their involvement in nonpharmaceutically sponsored research. The data and safety monitoring committee should have predetermined stopping rules and then recommend continuation, cessation, or interim analysis of the results to the steering committee. Because of publication bias toward positive trial results, there should be a publication policy before analysis of the trial results and agreement that publication of negative results should proceed. Because the licensing of a new compound, as well as the scientific acceptance of a positive trial, are so dependent on scientific credibility, these types of trial guidelines are likely to become more common.

Conclusion

The design of stroke trials has been a controversial issue in recent years, particularly with a recent series of negative results using compounds that appeared theoretically attractive and promising in animal models. Probably the most contentious issues have included trial size, endpoints, and overall design. There are currently vigorous proponents of mega-trials and smaller, focused trials. Even the definitions of these terms are unresolved and both types of trials are likely to be conducted in the next few years. Most acute stroke trials now use a fairly simple design. The global outcome test, used in the NINDS trial,[12] is particularly attractive, rather than reliance on a single endpoint.

It is interesting that the only positive acute stroke trials (NINDS[12] and the aspirin trials IST[4] and CAST[15]) have been investigator driven. This has generated considerable discussion about the relationships between academic investigators and the pharmaceutical industry. The credibility of trial results is dependent on the perception of an independent academic steering committee and rigorous trial conduct, including an agreement to publish negative as well as positive results in a timely manner. There is also a widely held view that there are frequently inadequate animal and phase II data before pivotal phase III trials have been commenced. Surrogate endpoints, particularly using new MRI techniques such as DWI, are now starting to be used in "proof-of-concept" studies. These trials test whether infarct attenuation can be confirmed with a putative stroke compound, in relatively small studies, as a prelude to definitive clinical trials. In summary, the lessons learned from both the positive trial results, together with many disappointments, should increase the chances of successfully designed stroke trials with positive outcomes in the future.

References

1. Ellrodt G, Cook DJ, Lee J, et al. Evidence-based disease management. JAMA 1997;278:1687–1692.
2. Adams HP Jr, Brott TG, Crowell RM, et al. Guidelines for the management of patients with acute ischemic stroke. A statement for healthcare professionals from a special writing group of the Stroke Council, American Heart Association. Stroke 1994;25:1901–1914.
3. Adams HP, Brott TC, Furlan AJ. Guidelines for thrombolytic therapy for acute stroke. A statement for healthcare professionals from a special writing group of the Stroke Council, American Heart Association. Stroke 1996;27:1711–1718.

4. The International Stroke Trial (IST): a randomized trial of aspirin, subcutaneous heparin, both, or neither among 19,435 patients with acute ischaemic stroke. International Stroke Trial Collaborative Group. Lancet 1997;349:1569–1581.

5. Swanson RA. Intravenous heparin for acute stroke: what can we learn from the megatrials? Neurology 1999;52:1746–1750.

6. Low molecular weight heparinoid, Org 10172 (danaparoid), and outcome after acute ischemic stroke: a randomized controlled trial. The Publications' Committee for the Trial of Org 10172 in Acute Stroke Treatment (TOAST) Investigators. JAMA 1998;279:1265–1272.

7. Gubitz G, Counsell C, Sandercock P, et al. Anticoagulants in acute ischaemic stroke (Cochrane Review). In: The Cochrane Library, Issue 3, 1999. Oxford: Update Software.

8. Bath PMW, Lees KR. ABC of arterial and venous disease. Acute stroke. BMJ 2000;320:920–923.

9. Davis SM, Lees KR, Albers GW, et al. Selfotel in acute ischemic stroke: possible neurotoxic effects of an NMDA antagonist. Stroke 2000;31:347–354.

10. Lees KR, Asplund K, Carolei A, et al. Glycine antagonist (gavestinel) in neuroprotection (GAIN International) in patients with acute stroke: a randomized controlled trial. GAIN International Investigators. Lancet 2000;355:1949–1954.

11. Gorelick PB. Neuroprotection in acute ischaemic stroke: a tale of for whom the bell tolls? Lancet 2000;355;1925–1926.

12. Tissue plasminogen activator for acute ischemic stroke. The National Institute of Neurological Disorders and Stroke rt-PA Stroke Study Group. N Engl J Med 1995;333:1581–1587.

13. Donnan GA, Davis SM, Chambers BR, et al. Streptokinase for acute ischemic stroke with relationship to time of administration: Australian Streptokinase (ASK) Trial Study Group. JAMA 1996;276:961–966.

14. Randomized trial of intravenous streptokinase, oral aspirin, both or neither among 17,187 cases of suspected acute myocardial infarction: ISIS-2. ISIS-2 (Second International Study of Infarct Survival) Collaborative Group. Lancet 1988;2:349–360.

15. CAST: randomized placebo-controlled trial of early aspirin use in 20,000 patients with acute ischaemic stroke. CAST (Chinese Acute Stroke Trial) Collaborative Group. Lancet 1997;349:1641–1649.

16. Chen ZM, Sandercock P, Pan HC, et al. Indications for early aspirin use in acute ischemic stroke: a combined analysis of 40,000 randomized patients from the Chinese Acute Stroke Trial and the International Stroke Trial. On behalf of the CAST and IST collaborative groups. Stroke 2000;31:1240–1249.

17. Langhorne P, Williams BO, Gilchrist W, Howie K. Do stroke units save lives? Lancet 1993;342:395–398.

18. Collaborative systematic review of the randomized trials of organized inpatient (stroke unit) care after stroke. Stroke Unit Trialists' Collaboration. BMJ 1997;314:1151–1159.

19. International Classification of Impairments, Disabilities, and Handicaps. Geneva, Switzerland: World Health Organization, 1980.

20. Mahoney FI, Barthel DW. Functional evaluation: the Barthel Index. Md Med J 1965;14:61–65.

21. Collins C, Wade DT, Davies S, et al. The Barthel ADL Index: a reliability study. Int Disabil Stud 1988;10:61–63.

22. Sulter G, Steen C, De Keyser J. Use of the Barthel Index and modified Rankin Scale in acute stroke trials. Stroke 1999;30:1538–1541.

23. Zivin JA. Understanding clinical trials. Sci Am 2000;282:69–75.

24. Brass LM, Alter M. Clinical Trial Design for Cerebrovascular Disorders. In M Fisher (ed), Stroke Therapy. Butterworth–Heinemann, 1995:135–170.

25. Randomized trial of endarterectomy for recently symptomatic carotid stenosis: final results of the MRC European Carotid Surgery Trial. Lancet 1998;351:1379–1387.

26. Failure of extracranial-intracranial arterial bypass to reduce the risk of ischemic stroke. Results of an international randomized trial. Extracranial-Intracranial Bypass Study Group. N Engl J Med 1985;313:1191–2000.

27. Beneficial effect of carotid endarterectomy in symptomatic patients with high-grade carotid stenosis. North American Symptomatic Carotid Endarterectomy Trial Collaborators. N Engl J Med 1991;325:445–453.

28. Collins R, Doll R, Peto R. Ethics of Clinical Trials. In CJ Williams (ed), Introducing New Treatments for Cancer: Practical, Ethical, and Legal Problems. Chichester: Wiley, 1992;49–65.

29. Saver JL, Starkman S, Fox S, et al. The impact upon clinical stroke trials of restricting informed consent. Stroke 1995;26(abstract):157.

30. A randomized, blinded, trial of clopidogrel versus aspirin in patients at risk of ischaemic events (CAPRIE). CAPRIE Steering Committee. Lancet 1996;348:1329–1339.

31. Antman EM, Lau J, Kupelnick B, et al. A comparison of results of meta-analyses of randomized control trials and recommendations of clinical experts. Treatments for myocardial infarction. JAMA 1992;268:240–248.

32. Caplan LR, Mohr JP, Kistler JP, Koroshetz W. Should thrombolytic therapy be the first-line treatment for acute ischemic stroke? Thrombolysis—not a panacea for ischemic stroke. N Engl J Med 1997;337:1309–1310.

33. Furlan AJ, Higashida R, Wechsler L, et al. Intra-arterial prourokinase for acute ischemic stroke. The PROACT II study: a randomized controlled trial. Prolyse in Acute Cerebral Thromboembolism. JAMA 1999;282:2003–2011.

34. Mitchell PJ, Gerraty RG, Donnan GA, et al. Thrombolysis in the vertebrobasilar circulation. The Australian Urokinase Stroke Trial (AUST) Pilot Study. Cerebrovasc Dis 1997;7:94–99.

35. Hacke W, Kaste M, Fieschi C, et al. Intravenous thrombolysis with recombinant tissue plasminogen activator for acute hemispheric stroke. The European Cooperative Acute Stroke Study (ECASS). JAMA 1995;274:1017–1025.

36. Hacke W, Kaste M, Fieschi C, et al. Randomized double-blind placebo-controlled trial of thrombolytic therapy with intravenous alteplase in acute ischaemic stroke (ECASS II). Second European-Australasian Acute Stroke Study Investigators. Lancet 1998;352:1245–1251.

37. Hacke W, Bluhmki E, Steiner T, et al. Dichotomized efficacy end points and global end-point analysis applied to the ECASS intention-to-treat data set: post hoc analysis of ECASS 1. Stroke 1998;29:2073–2075.

38. Hacke W, Ringleb P, Stingele R. Thrombolysis in acute cerebrovascular disease: indications and limitations. Thromb Haemost 1999;82:983–986.
39. Katzan IL, Furlan AJ, Lloyd LE, et al. Use of tissue-type plasminogen activator for acute ischemic stroke: the Cleveland area experience. JAMA 2000;283:1151–1158.
40. Albers GW, Bates VE, Clark WM, et al. Intravenous tissue-type plasminogen activator for treatment of acute stroke: the Standard Treatment with Alteplase to Reverse Stroke (STARS) study. JAMA 2000;283:1145–1150.
41. Wade DT. Measurement in Neurological Rehabilitation. New York: Oxford Medical Publications, 1992.
42. Duncan PW, Jorgensen HS, Wade DT. Outcome measures in acute stroke trials: a systematic review and some recommendations to improve practice. Stroke 2000;31:1429–1438.
43. Brott T, Adams HP Jr, Olinger CP, et al. Measurements of acute cerebral infarction: a clinical examination scale. Stroke 1989;20:864–870.
44. Chua MG, Davis SM, Infeld B, et al. Prediction of functional outcome and tissue loss in acute cortical infarction. Arch Neurol 1995;52:496–500.
45. Goldstein LB, Bertels C, Davis JN. Interrater reliability of the NIH stroke scale. Arch Neurol 1989;46:660–662.
46. Goldstein LB, Samsa GP. Reliability of the National Institutes of Health Stroke Scale. Extension of non-neurologists in the context of a clinical trial. Stroke 1997;28:307–310.
47. De Deyn PP, Reuck JD, Deberdt W, et al. Treatment of acute ischemic stroke with piracetam. Members of the Piracetam in Acute Stroke Study (PASS) Group. Stroke 1997;28:2347–2352.
48. Gray CS, Scott JF, O'Connell JE. Measuring outcome in acute stroke trials (letter). Stroke 2000;31:232.
49. Adams IIP Jr. Trials of trials in acute ischemic stroke. The Humana Lecture. Stroke 1993;24:1410–1415.
50. Mohr JP. Are more complex study designs needed for future acute stroke trials? Cerebrovasc Dis 1998;8(Suppl 1):17–22.
51. Van Gijn J, Warlow C. Down with stroke scales! Cerebrovasc Dis 1992;2:244–246.
52. Mohr JP. Thrombolytic therapy for ischemic stroke: from clinical trials to clinical practice. JAMA 2000;283: 1189–1191.
53. Wardlaw JM, Sandercock PA, Warlow CP, Lindley RI. Trials of thrombolysis in acute ischemic stroke: does the choice of primary outcome measure really matter? Stroke 2000;31:1133–1135.
54. Tilley BC, Marler J, Geller NL, et al. Use of a global test for multiple outcomes in stroke trials with application to the National Institute of Neurological Disorders and Stroke t-PA Stroke Trial. Stroke 1996;27:2136–2142.
55. Roberts L, Counsell C. Assessment of clinical outcomes in acute stroke trials. Stroke 1998;29:986–991.
56. Wardlaw JM, Warlow CP, Counsell C. Systematic review of evidence on thrombolytic therapy for acute ischaemic stroke. Lancet 1997;350:607–614.
57. Buyse M, Piedbois P, Piedbois Y, Carlson RW. Meta-analysis: methods, strengths, and weaknesses. Oncology (Huntingt) 2000;14:437–447.
58. Counsell C, Warlow C, Sandercock P, et al. Meeting the need for systematic reviews in stroke care. The Cochrane Collaboration Stroke Review Group. Stroke 1995;26:498–502.
59. Rothwell PM. Can overall results of clinical trials be applied to all patients? Lancet 1995;345:1616–1619.
60. Moher D, Pham B, Jones A, et al. Does quality of reports of randomized trials affect estimates of intervention efficacy reported in meta-analysis? Lancet 1998;352:609–613.
61. Lau J, Ioannidis JP, Schmid CH. Summing up evidence: one answer is not always enough. Lancet 1998;351:123–127.
62. Zivin JA, Fisher M, DeGirolami U, et al. Tissue plasminogen activator reduces neurological damage after cerebral embolism. Science 1985;230:1289–1292.
63. Heiss WD, Thiel A, Grond R. Which targets are relevant for therapy of acute ischemic stroke? Stroke 1999;30: 1486–1489.
64. Barber PA, Darby DG, Yang Q, et al. Prediction of stroke outcome with echoplanar perfusion- and diffusion-weighted MRI. Neurology 1998;51:418–426.
65. Fisher M, Albers GW. Applications of diffusion-perfusion magnetic resonance imaging in acute ischemic stroke. Neurology 1999;52:1750–1756.
66. Davis SM, Tress B, Barber PA, et al. Echoplanar magnetic resonance imaging in acute stroke. J Clin Neurosci 2000;7:3–8.
67. Darby DG, Barber PA, Gerraty RP, et al. Pathophysiological topography of acute ischemia by combined diffusion-weighted and perfusion MRI. Stroke 1999;30:2043–2052.
68. Barber PA, Davis SM, Darby DG, et al. Absent middle cerebral artery flow predicts the presence and evolution of the ischemic penumbra. Neurology 1999;52:1125–1132.
69. Warach S, Pettigrew LC, Dashe JF, et al. The effect of citicoline on lesion volume in acute stroke: a multicenter double blind placebo controlled trial. Stroke 1999; 30(abstract):243.
70. Dorman PJ, Counsell C, Sandercock P. Reports of randomized trials in acute stroke, 1955–1995: what proportions were commercially sponsored. Stroke 1999;30:1995–1998.

Chapter 8
Atherosclerosis

Fenwick T. Nichols III

Atherosclerosis is a major contributor to the pathogenesis of heart attack, cerebral infarction, and peripheral vascular disease. It is currently estimated to contribute to 600,000 deaths per year in the United States. Although it has been the subject of great interest, it is not a disease unique to modern time. It has been identified in Egyptian mummies more than 2,000 years old. In 1904, Shattock described plaque-like lesions in the arteries of the mummy of Menephthah, purportedly the pharaoh of the Exodus.[1]

Atherosclerosis begins early in life. Fatty streaks are found in the majority of children,[2] and plaque has been found in asymptomatic young soldiers.[3–5] Its presence is usually not recognized until relatively late in its development, when there may be an acute thrombotic event, typically an ischemic event affecting the heart, brain, or legs. As in all of medicine, the best therapy is prevention, rather than intervening after injury has occurred. To prevent the development of this disease, a better understanding of the primary events in the atherosclerotic process is needed. This chapter offers an overview of the current understanding of atherosclerosis by presenting a review of its anatomy, pathology, initiating events, progression, and potential interventions.

This chapter focuses primarily on the cellular aspects of atherosclerosis and potential evaluation and management of early atherosclerosis. It does not address the various therapeutic interventions for acute ischemic episodes with antiplatelet, antithrombotic, anticoagulant, and fibrinolytic agents. Nor does it address the use of antiplatelet agents for either primary or secondary prevention of the ischemic events associated with atherosclerosis. These discussions are beyond the scope of this chapter.

"Standard" atherosclerosis development follows a relatively reproducible pattern. In early lesions, an excess of lipid is found in the arterial intima. This is associated with an influx of monocytes and T cells (e.g., involvement of the immune system with an inflammatory response). Monocytes are converted into macrophages and ingest lipids, becoming foam cells. Some smooth muscle cells undergo a transition from a contractile state to a secretory state, with the production of matrix proteins that are deposited in the plaque. Foam cell necrosis occurs with the formation of a lipid pool with an overlying fibrous cap. At this point, thrombotic complications may begin to play a major role in the occurrence of clinical events. In advanced plaques, there may be central necrosis and associated changes, such as fibrosis, intraplaque hemorrhage, ulceration, and mineralization.

Atherosclerosis growth results from a complex interaction between injurious and reparative agents and events. The severity of the atherosclerosis and the actual local morphology and histology of the plaque are determined by these interactions. A large number of seemingly disparate processes may be associated with the development of atherosclerosis. It is apparent that if one process (e.g., severe hypercholesterolemia, severe hypertension) is the predominant or "driving" force, it will be the major contributor to the development of atherosclerosis. However, it is also apparent that in many cases no single identifiable agent is primarily responsible for plaque development, and that atherosclerosis has developed in response to the cumulative effects of multiple processes. For example, cholesterol in combination with hypertension results in more atherosclerosis than either alone; the addition of cigarette smoking further increases the risk of atherosclerosis. A wide variety of processes can result in the development of atherosclerosis, including mechanical (hemodynamic), metabolic, and immunologic injuries. The responses of the hemostatic system, cytokine-induced alterations in cell growth and differentiation, and the production of extracellular matrix proteins also play a role in the development of atherosclerosis. This suggests that the different manifestations of arterial injury may simply represent parts of a spectrum of pathologic change, with the difference in lesion size and clinical manifestations being more quantitative than qualitative.

The histologic variation of atherosclerotic plaques may range from lesions that are almost purely fibrous to lesions with atheromatous gruel in the center to lesions that are heavily calcified.[6] In addition, there may be intraplaque hemorrhage, ulceration, or superficial thrombosis. These differences in plaque morphology may occur within an individual patient, suggesting that hemodynamic factors or local structural variations may account for some of the variability. Plaque morphology and extent may also vary among populations, with some having more fibrous lesions and others having more typical atheronecrotic lesions. On a population level, some of this variation may be due to genetic differences in responses to similar stimuli or to different triggering events. For example, U.S. data suggest that diets high in animal fat are more atherogenic, yet the Masai warriors in Africa, whose caloric intake is 60% animal fat, have low serum lipids and a low incidence of atherosclerosis.[7] This would argue against diet alone as a necessary substrate for the development of atherosclerosis.

Similarly, animal experiments have demonstrated that there are differences between species in response to the same stimuli.[8] When fed the same high-cholesterol diet, rhesus monkeys develop a readily reversible atherosclerosis, whereas cynomolgus monkeys develop what is essentially an atheroarteritis, with inflammation of all three layers of the arterial wall and circulating immune complexes that affect endothelial function. In addition, different types of plaque may develop when similar degrees of hypercholesterolemia are induced in the same animal model using different dietary cholesterol sources, such as peanuts, corn or coconut oils, or butter.[9]

The discovery of the large number of cytokines, growth factors, and prothrombotic, antithrombotic, and vasoactive agents in cell culture that are potentially involved in the atherosclerotic process is extremely exciting, because these observations potentially offer insight into cellular mechanisms of atherosclerosis. However, the relative importance of each or all of these factors in the human arterial milieu is unknown. It should also be recognized that the development of plaque and the associated ischemic symptomatology may be two separate but related processes (e.g., ischemia may more often be the result of thrombosis, vasospasm, or both, than of progressive plaque development), and that processes that induce atherosclerosis may or may not be involved in the production of ischemic symptoms. Many animal models of atherosclerosis do not develop ischemic phenomena.[10]

The understanding of the initiation, development, and associated symptoms of atherosclerosis is reminiscent of the blind men's understanding of the size and shape of the elephant: The observations of the clinical, pathologic, and biochemical aspects of atherosclerosis are all valid, but they do not necessarily relate to each other in a pattern that we recognize. The relative importance of individual observations and the inter-relationships among them remain less than perfectly understood.

We have identified a number of risk factors for the development of clinically recognized atherosclerosis. The best accepted of these are age, elevated low-density lipoprotein (LDL) cholesterol, low high-density lipoprotein (HDL) cholesterol, hypertension, and smoking. In detailed reviews of cases of atherosclerosis that identified the recognized "risk factors," it appears that the reason for its development remains unexplained in a significant (more than 50%) percentage of cases.[11,12] Elevated lipids clearly increase the risk of atherosclerosis but do not guarantee its development.[13] This indicates that the understanding of many aspects of atherosclerosis is limited and that further research is needed to clarify these problems. (A number of possible explanations for these observations have been proposed, based on the understanding of atherosclerosis induction. It is possible that some cases with normal cholesterol levels have low HDL or other lipid abnormalities that may trigger plaque formation.)[14,15]

Anatomy

Three articles summarizing the understanding of the anatomy and basics of early and late atherosclerosis have been published by the American Heart Association (AHA) and should be consulted for more details.[16–18]

Atherosclerotic plaque formation has a predilection for particular sites in the arterial bed. Although in an individual, the severity of atherosclerosis in one vascular bed may not predict the severity in others,[19] there is a pattern to the sites of atherosclerosis development. In general, fatty streaks first affect the aorta and the carotid arteries, initially appearing in infancy and childhood, with virtually 100% of the population having fatty streaks by age 10 years. Although plaques do develop at the sites of fatty streaks, not all fatty streaks progress to plaques. Fatty streaks and plaques usually develop in and around flow dividers, suggesting involvement of hemodynamic factors. Fatty streaks that do progress may begin to do so during puberty. Fatty streaks in the coronary arteries develop slightly later, during adolescence, with almost 100% of the population having them by age 20 years. In high-risk populations, these may progress to typical fibrous plaques by the age of 20–30 years. The vertebral and intracranial arteries begin to develop fatty streaks at approximately the same time as the coronary arteries, but advanced lesions do not appear until much later.[20] The renal, mesenteric, and pulmonary arteries are the least likely to develop atherosclerosis.[19,21–25]

Structural Pathology

Stary has reported on the detailed pathology of coronary arteries in 691 patients younger than 40 years old coming to autopsy.[26] These data are the first to clearly demonstrate the lesion that is intermediate between the fatty streak and the more typical plaque. Stary described the development of atherosclerosis as proceeding through five stages:

1. *Type I lesion.* This was found in infants and consisted of a small number of macrophages, with some containing lipid droplet inclusions (foam cells). These were found almost exclusively in eccentric thickenings at bifurcations. Eccentric thickenings occur on the arterial wall opposite the flow divider; they have also been referred to as *intimal cushions* and *adaptive thickening.*[16] Foam cells occurred in up to 45% of infants in the first 8 months but decreased in frequency to 17% by 5 years of age. Around puberty, these lesions again increased in frequency. Lipid-laden smooth muscle cells were not a part of this lesion.

2. *Type II lesions (fatty streak).* These lesions, which occurred in eccentric thickenings, were composed of multiple layers of macrophages and smooth muscle cells overloaded with lipid droplets. There were two types of fatty streaks: a superficial macroscopically visible one and a submerged, macroscopically invisible one in the depths of the eccentric thickening. These were found in 43% of patients between the ages of 10–14 years. In the early stages, the lipid was located primarily in the macrophages; as the lesions became larger, the number of smooth muscle cells containing lipid began to outnumber the macrophages. Not all fatty streaks progressed to the next type. Type I and type II peaked at approximately age 14, at which time they were present in almost 70% of the population, then gradually decreased, with some lesions being replaced by more advanced ones.

3. *Type III (preatheroma, intermediate lesion, transitional lesion).* Not all fatty streaks progress to atheroma. Numerous studies have documented that some populations have a high incidence of fatty streaks and a low incidence of atherosclerosis. This has caused concern that the fatty streak might not be the true precursor to typical atherosclerosis.[27] Stary described the lesion that links fatty streaks to typical atherosclerosis. In young people, only fatty streaks in eccentric thickenings evolved into this intermediate lesion. The intimal lesions developed many separate "pool-like aggregates" of extracellular lipid particles deep to the foam cell layer, with disruption of the musculoelastic intima. There was an associated change from a contractile toward a synthetic state in the smooth muscle cells at this level. Starting after puberty, there was a progressive increase in their frequency, being present in 66% of cases by age 39 years. Fibroatheroma began to appear in the third decade of life.

4. *Type IV (atheroma).* By this stage, a macroscopically visible lipid core had developed. It appeared to be a coalescence of the extracellular lipid first noted in the type III lesions. Lipid cores were only found in the eccentric thickenings and did not contain any macrophages. Macrophage

foam cells, including dead and decomposing ones, were found on the luminal side of the lipid core. It was suggested the lipid core was derived from macrophage foam cell death with release of lipids. There was approximately a 10-year lag between the development of type III and type IV lesions. A compensatory dilation of the arterial wall at this level occurred so that there was no reduction in luminal area. This has been found by a number of other investigators.[28,29]

5. *Type V (fibroatheroma)*. This lesion was distinguished by the development of a fibrous cap immediately overlying the lipid core. The cap, which extended a variable distance beyond the surface of the lipid core, was composed of smooth muscle cells in a collagen matrix. The formation and thickening of the cap was accelerated when platelets and fibrin originally deposited on the intima were incorporated into the intima. This is the plaque that provides the base for the complications of atherosclerosis.[30,31]

In a subsequent publication, Stary described additional plaque types.[32] Type VI, the complicated fibroatheroma, has intraplaque hemorrhage, surface thrombus formation, or both. Type VII is the calcific lesion, in which calcium replaces the necrotic cell remnants and the extracellular lipid; although calcium is present to some extent in most advanced plaques, in type VII, calcium is the dominant plaque component. Type VIII, the densely fibrotic lesion, has minimal lipid. Stary noted that type VIII is most typically seen in the lower extremities.

The AHA Committee on Vascular Lesions uses a modification of this classification. Types I, II, III, and IV are the same in both classifications,[33] but the classification of the more advanced lesions is somewhat different. The classification is as follows:

I. Early lesions:
   A. *Type I*: Initial lesion, also referred to as *fatty streak* or *early lesion*; consists of isolated macrophage foam cells
   B. *Type IIa and IIb (progression-prone and progression-resistant type II)*: Also referred to as *fatty streak* or *early lesions*; primarily intracellular lipid accumulation
   C. *Type III*: Intermediate lesion or preatheroma; type II lesions plus extracellular lipid accumulations

The AHA article classified the more advanced lesions slightly differently than Stary did in his research, as follows:

I. Advanced lesions (lesions that disrupt intimal structure):
   A. *Type IV (atheroma)*: Type II changes plus a central core of lipid; also referred to as *atheromatous plaque*, *fibrolipid plaque*, or *fibrous plaque*
   B. *Type V*:
      1. *Va (fibroatheroma)*: Type IV changes plus prominent new fibrous connective tissue; may be multilayered with several lipid cores separated by thick layers of fibrous connective tissue stacked irregularly
      2. *Vb*: Characterized by heavy mineralization (calcification) (type VII in Stary's classification)
      3. *Vc (fibrotic lesions)*: Normal intima is replaced and thickened with fibrous connective tissue, with minimal lipid accumulation (type VIII in Stary's classification)
   C. *Type VI (complicated lesions)*: Type IV or V lesions with superimposed changes
      1. *VIa*: Disruption of the surface (fissures, ulcerations)
      2. *VIb*: Hemorrhage or hematoma
      3. *VIc*: Thrombosis

The lesion-prone sites, particularly the eccentric thickenings, appear to differ structurally and functionally from nonlesion-prone sites. These differences may contribute to the localization of plaque in these areas. These sites have increased endothelial permeability to blood macromolecules, such as albumin,[34,35] fibrinogen,[36] and LDL cholesterol,[37] and are the same sites at which animals fed high-cholesterol diets demonstrate increased intimal cholesterol.[38] The increased cholesterol in the arterial wall may be the result of increased serum levels or "trapping" of cholesterol in the wall by modification (oxidation) once it has entered the intima. Other differences in the lesion-prone areas include (1) the glycocalyx endothelial coating is thinner (13 nm) than normal (44 nm) in these areas,[39] (2) endothelial cell turnover is greater,[40] (3) the endothelial cells display a different morphology, being larger and more rounded than cells from non-lesion areas,[41] (4) there is lesion-site–

specific chemotactic recruitment of monocytes even before there is microscopic evidence of plaque formation,[42] and (5) the subendothelial space is consistently larger in the lesion-prone areas.[43]

Gerrity has suggested that in these areas of different macromolecule uptake, an injury to the endothelium may not be needed to produce local lipid accumulations and that the local lipid accumulations may simply represent the superimposition of altered blood composition on areas of normally different structural and functional characteristics.[44] The resulting local accumulation of lipids may then trigger the event leading to lesion formation.

Cellular Aspects of Atherosclerosis

Endothelium

For plaque to develop, the endothelium must be involved. For many years, the endothelium was thought of as an inert cell layer that lined the vascular system and transported various substances into or out of the bloodstream. The endothelium is now recognized to be extremely active in regulating a number of different systems[45] and in maintaining a delicate balance between the competing processes of vasodilation and constriction, platelet adhesion and removal, coagulation and fibrinolysis, and the immune-mediated adhesion of white cells. Imbalances between these competing processes may result in a number of different tissue stimuli or injuries that contribute to the development of atherosclerosis.

The endothelium has a complex array of functions. The endothelium of muscular and elastic arteries is a smooth monolayer, with the long axis of the cells oriented in the direction of flow, except for bifurcations in regions of oscillating shear stress. The endothelium produces a variety of substances that are potentially competitive in function, and it must maintain a balance between them for proper functioning.[46] It manufactures vasoconstrictors (endothelin and superoxide anions and thromboxane)[47,48] as well as vasodilators (endothelial-derived relaxation factor [EDRF] and prostacyclin [PGI_2]). When there is an imbalance, as in coronary atherosclerosis, there may be impaired endothelial relaxation, and there may be paradoxic arterial constriction with administration of acetylcholine, a vasodilator.

The endothelium is normally nonthrombogenic, balancing the competing processes of coagulation and fibrinolysis: It synthesizes and releases von Willebrand's factor and factor V; it produces heparin sulfate and dermatan sulfate, both anticoagulants; it interacts with coagulation factors, thrombomodulin, thrombin, and plasminogen activator inhibitors, all of which facilitate coagulation; and it interacts with protein C, protein S, heparin, antithrombin III, plasminogen, and plasminogen activators, all of which interfere with the coagulation process. These compounds are involved in a complex series of interactions and feedback loops to prevent the development of ongoing coagulation or fibrinolytic activity.[49]

The endothelium also synthesizes and secretes two compounds that have both vasodilator activity and platelet inhibition activity: PGI_2 and EDRF. In addition, it metabolizes the platelet-aggregating agents adenosine diphosphate, serotonin, prostaglandin F_1, and angiotensin. All of these actions interrupt platelet activation and adherence.[50,51]

The endothelium interacts with the immune system, with both pro- and anti-inflammatory products. Intercellular adhesion molecule (ICAM) and vascular cell adhesion molecule (VCAM) may be produced in response to activation by cytokines, such as interleukin-1 (IL-1), tumor necrosis factor (TNF), or oxidized LDL. These adhesion molecules mediate endothelial cell adhesion to monocytes and T lymphocytes.[52] As noted, the earliest abnormality in plaque-prone lesions is monocyte adherence to the endothelium.[53]

The endothelium also produces growth stimulators (basic fibroblast growth factor [FGF]) and tissue growth factor beta-1,[54] which may contribute to plaque growth by stimulating cell replication.

In addition, the endothelium is involved in transport of substances from the plasma and is permeable to all plasma proteins via transcytosis and passage through intercellular junctions.

It has also become clear that endothelium from different organs and from different sized vessels within organs behaves differently. This may account for some organ-specific differences in the development of atherosclerosis and its complications.[55,56]

Smooth Muscle Cells

Smooth muscle cells primarily exist as contractile cells in the tunica media. Under certain situations, such as hypercholesterolemia or balloon injury, smooth muscle cells migrate into the intima and become secretory cells, which then manufacture matrix proteins (connective tissue matrix proteins: elastic fiber proteins, collagen, proteoglycans) that are necessary for plaque development. A variety of stimuli have been demonstrated in in vitro and in vivo animal models to trigger this conversion; the relative importance of each of these stimuli (growth hormones, cytokines, etc.) remains to be defined. A smooth muscle cell variant is the basement membrane–rich intimal smooth muscle cell, which is usually located in the region between the lipid core and the arterial lumen. The basement membrane may be up to 10 times thicker than the cell body, which may be thinner than usual. It has been proposed that these cells represent an attempt to restore normal tissue architecture, provide anchor points for cells, and possibly guide repair processes.[57] Smooth muscle cells may also become macrophages and contribute to the formation of fatty streaks.[58] It has been noted that these smooth muscle cells are usually monoclonal in origin, raising the suggestion that the plaque is a tumor-like growth.[59]

Fibrinogen

There is a significant accumulation of fibrinogen, which contributes to the volume of most advanced lesions. Some of the fibrinogen probably arises from the infiltration of plasma; however, some probably arises from incorporation of thrombi.[60]

Cytokines and Growth Factors

Cytokines are cell-secreted peptides that affect cell activation or protein synthesis in both paracrine and autocrine fashions. A number of cytokines and growth factors have been identified in vitro that potentially play a role in atherosclerosis development; however, the relative contribution of any or all of these in in vivo human atherosclerosis has not been fully investigated. Cytokines may participate in the initiation of endothelial injury through IL-1 or TNF-α, which trigger the production of cell surface adhesion molecules (ICAM and VCAM). Cytokines also may promote monocyte adhesion and activation (monocyte chemotactic

protein-1 [MCP-1]), and may be involved in LDL oxidation through a variety of pathways.[61]

Among the vascular cells involved in atherosclerosis (the endothelium, smooth muscle cells, and monocytes), there is potential for the elaboration of many cytokines and growth factors that may stimulate transformation and proliferation of cells and stimulate smooth muscle migration and matrix deposition. These include IL-1 α, IL-1 β, IL-6, IL-8, MCP-1, monocyte colony stimulating factor (M-CSF), granulocyte-macrophage colony stimulating factor, platelet-derived growth factor (PDGF), TNF-α, interferon-γ, transforming growth factor β (TGF-β), acidic FGF, basic FGF, and epidermal growth factor.[62,63] Of the different growth factors, PDGF has probably received the most attention. Although originally identified as a product of platelets, PDGF has been found to be produced by other cells, including monocytes and smooth muscle cells. It stimulates smooth muscle migration from the media into the intima and activates DNA synthesis.[64]

It is possible that future antiatherogenic therapies will be directed at specific cytokines or growth factors.

Immune System

The immune system is involved from the earliest stages of the development of atherosclerosis. Although most of the data center on the role of the monocyte, there are data to support the involvement of other parts of the immune system, including T lymphocytes and circulating autoimmune complexes. Ross has summarized the data on inflammatory aspects of atherosclerosis.[65] He proposes that injurious processes cause endothelial changes. These changes affect the endothelium's adhesiveness for platelets and white blood cells, and may cause the endothelium to manifest procoagulant properties rather than anticoagulant properties. These changes may also result in the endothelium releasing cytokines, growth factors, and vasoactive substances. Ross proposes that the inflammatory system attempts to neutralize the triggering process, providing the stimulus for smooth muscle cell migration and proliferation and later stimulating migration of lymphocytes and macrophages into the lesion.[65] Infectious agents have also been demonstrated to be associated with the development of atherosclerosis, perhaps by triggering the initiating injury and immune response.

Monocytes

In atherosclerosis-prone regions, the earliest change noted is monocyte recruitment, in which monocytes adhere to the endothelium in an essentially inflammatory process. Various endothelial adhesion factors, such as ICAM-1, VCAM-1, and others, are involved in this process.[66–69] Both CD4 (T helper cells) and CD8 (T killer cells) are found in atherosclerotic lesions.

After attachment, monocytes penetrate the endothelium. MCP-1, which is produced by both endothelium and smooth muscle cells, is involved in monocyte migration from the lumen to the subendothelial region.[70–73]

Many mediators may be involved in the differentiation of monocytes into macrophages. One of these factors is M-CSF, which binds to the M-CSF receptor on monocytes and induces changes leading to macrophage differentiation and activation.[74] Macrophages may also be derived from smooth muscle cells.[75]

Monocyte-derived macrophages can generate cytokines (TNF-α, IL-1, and TGF-β), growth factors (PDGF, insulin-like growth factor I), free radicals, proteases, and lipases. These free radicals may then oxidize LDL. When this occurs, the oxidized LDL is no longer recognized by the normal macrophage receptor, but is recognized by the macrophage scavenger receptor. The scavenger receptor differs from the normal LDL receptor in that it does not down-regulate in response to cellular cholesterol accumulation. This may result in a progressive accumulation of LDL, with eventual development of foam cells. These cells may continue to accumulate oxidized LDL to the point of cell death and rupture, with release of the LDL into the extracellular space and the formation of an extracellular lipid core (e.g., there is progression from the foam cell to the more advanced atherosclerotic lesion). During this phase, there is smooth muscle cell proliferation, with the manufacture of matrix proteins and a resultant increase in lesion size.[76] Oxidized LDL causes an increase in MCP-1

production. MCP-1 is cytotoxic, has chemotactic properties, inhibits monocyte migration, inactivates EDRF, and is antigenic, possibly contributing to the development of autoimmune inflammation.

Other Immune Interactions

Although T cells are routinely found in small numbers in both early fatty lesions and advanced plaques, their presence is of uncertain significance. T cells may be attracted to the plaque by a variety of factors, including modified lipoproteins, partially denatured or degraded cellular or matrix constituents released into the necrotic core, intracellular components released on cell death, or viral proteins. Experimentally, T cells have been shown to modulate the atherosclerotic response and may down-regulate the scavenger receptor, preventing the development of foam cells.[77–82]

In addition, some evidence indicates that infectious agents can potentially contribute to the initiation or development of atherosclerosis. Histologic studies have identified cytomegalovirus and herpes virus particles in some plaques; epidemiologic studies using antibody data and, occasionally, histologic data have raised the possibility that infections with cytomegalovirus, herpes, *Chlamydia pneumoniae*, and *Helicobacter pylori*[83] increase the risk of developing atherosclerosis. These observations, in conjunction with the recognized immune-mediated aspects of atherosclerosis, suggest that viral or antigenic injury may trigger or promote the development of atherosclerosis.[84–90] Circulating immune complexes play a role in atherosclerosis in some animal models, but their role in human atherosclerosis is unknown.[91]

The endothelial adhesion factors ICAM-1 and VCAM-1, which are important in monocyte adhesion to endothelial cells, are members of the immunoglobulin gene super-family of adhesion receptors. Both molecules have immunoglobulin-like domains.

Hemodynamics

Intimal proliferation typically is first seen in the regions of bifurcations, with an eccentric thickening of the side opposite the bifurcation. This has been noted in a number of different vascular systems, including the coronary and the cerebral vessels.[92,93] The intimal proliferation is unequal in asymmetric bifurcations. Stehbens attributes this to "hemodynamic stress."[94]

Ku and Giddens[95] developed a flow model of the carotid bifurcation, demonstrating that atherosclerosis occurs in regions of low or oscillating shear stress, areas that correspond to the eccentric thickenings described by Stehbens in the intracranial arteries and to those described by Stary for the coronary arteries.[30,96] Ku and Giddens proposed that the oscillating shear stress causes the eccentric thickening. In addition, in the region of oscillating shear stress, clearance of blood and its components is delayed, allowing prolonged contact of potentially toxic substances with the intima in this region. This could potentiate intimal injury.

As plaque develops, there is an increase in the shear stress at the level of the stenosis. Arterial remodeling with compensatory dilation may occur in these regions to reduce the shear stress to normal levels. The artery may dilate to a point at which the patent lumen remains unchanged from its original size, but there is a 40% stenosis of the actual (enlarged) lumen. After plaque has developed, hemodynamic changes at the level of the stenosis may play a role in plaque destabilization, progression, and rupture.[96]

Lipids

Even at "normal" levels, LDL appears to enter the arterial wall. Once within the wall, it may undergo oxidation, by either the adjacent endothelial or smooth muscle cells or by macrophages-monocytes, thus becoming trapped in the wall.[97] Higher circulating levels of LDL appear to increase the amount transported into the arterial wall.[98,99] The oxidized LDL may injure the endothelium, triggering MCP-1 production as well as causing monocyte-binding molecules to develop on the luminal surface. In its nonoxidized state, LDL may be transported out of the arterial wall by HDL via the reverse cholesterol transport system. This may be the basis for HDL's apparent antiatherogenic activity.[100] Antibodies to oxidized LDL are found in atherosclerotic plaques in rabbits and humans, sug-

gesting another level of immune system participation in plaque development.[101]

Although most oxidized LDL has been identified in the arterial wall,[102–104] circulating oxidized LDL has been described by some investigators.[105,106] In one publication, the presence of circulating antibodies to oxidized LDL was identified as increasing the risk for atherosclerosis progression.[107]

Another lipoprotein that has attracted attention is lipoprotein (a) (Lp[a]). Lp(a) consists of one molecule of apolipoprotein B-100 and two molecules of apolipoprotein (a). It shares a strong homology with plasminogen and can competitively inhibit plasminogen binding to endothelium, thereby interfering with surface-associated plasmin generation.[108] This suggests that it promotes a hypercoagulable state, which could precipitate thrombosis, resulting in acute ischemia or eventual incorporation of the thrombus into the plaque, with progressive plaque enlargement.[109,110]

Platelets

The actual contribution of platelets, fibrin, and fibrinogen to the development of the early plaque has remained controversial,[111] but it is clear that the coagulation system may play a significant role in the later stages of atherosclerosis.

Platelets are active participants in atherosclerosis.[112] There are data suggesting that platelets may initiate atherosclerosis, but this appears to be unusual.[113] Experimentally, it has been demonstrated that platelets may provide the cholesterol necessary for foam cell formation.[114–117] It appears that platelets may actively contribute to plaque growth by several mechanisms. One involves the release of cytokines and growth factors such as PDGF, TGF-β, and acidic and basic FGF, all of which are involved in plaque growth. Another mechanism involves platelet adhesion to the plaque, with subsequent incorporation into the plaque.[118–121] This may occur with or without fibrin. Bini has demonstrated the presence of fibrin and fibrin-related products in intima, neointima, and deeper medial layer, particularly around areas of plaque incorporation, which is consistent with incorporation of thrombus into the plaque.[60] Additionally, when there is plaque denudation or rupture, platelets actively participate in the production of ischemic symptoms by involvement in thrombus formation.

Hypercholesterolemia has been shown to influence platelet activity and is associated with increased platelet adhesion and aggregation, increased serotonin levels,[122,123] increased levels of circulating thromboxane A_2,[124] and decreased sensitivity to the platelet-inhibiting property of PGI_2.[125] In patients whose hyperlipidemia is controlled by either diet or medication, the platelet activity may return to normal.[126,127]

Another observation potentially related to platelet function is that occlusive events, such as myocardial infarction (MI) and ischemic stroke, occur more frequently in the early morning, at a time of increased sympathoadrenal activity.[128] Badimon demonstrated that the baseline catecholamine levels significantly correlated with the extent of platelet deposition; this effect was only apparent at high shear rates, such as those expected to be found at the site of a stenosis.[129]

As discussed under Clinical Events, Falk has demonstrated that the plaque in coronary arteries of patients dying of MI had thrombi in layers of different ages, suggesting that repeated episodes of mural thrombosis with organization contributed to plaque growth.[120]

Clinical Aspects of Atherosclerosis

Risk Factors

Atherosclerosis can be thought of as scar formation in response to injury to the endothelium or smooth muscles of the arterial wall. Unlike most situations in which there is a single injury with healing, atherosclerosis may occur in an environment of ongoing insult or injury, resulting in progressive development of plaque. Each factor may contribute, with a cumulative effect that may be greater than that from a single factor taken in isolation (e.g., hypertensive patients who smoke have higher plaque scores than those who do not).[130,131]

Numerous processes have been proposed as risk factors for the development of atherosclerosis.[132] Although some of these factors appear to directly affect the atherosclerotic process, others have a less clearly defined relationship to symptomatic atherosclerosis. A number of studies have demonstrated that patients with symptomatic atherosclerosis have an increased frequency of risk factors, such as elevated LDL, depressed HDL, hypertension, and cigarette smoking. However, a risk factor's presence is a poor predictor of the presence of atherosclerosis. It is this phenomenon that causes them to be labeled *risk factors* rather than causative agents.[133] The following discussion reviews some of the better-recognized risk factors for atherosclerosis.

One study conducted in New Orleans provided an interesting pathologic observation. There was a documented decrease in the frequency of atherosclerotic lesions over time, raising the optimistic possibility that interventions in patients with risk factors may be decreasing the frequency of atherosclerosis.[134]

Age

That the risk of having atherosclerosis increases with increasing age may represent the cumulative effect of a number of processes over time.[135]

Genetics

It is well documented that patients with strong family histories of premature atherosclerosis have an increased risk for the development of symptomatic atherosclerosis. There may be a variety of causes (such as different lipid abnormalities, endothelial dysfunction, and abnormal cytokines) for this, including a large number of potential genetic and environmental contributions.

Hypertension

Hypertension increases the risk of atherosclerosis development, presumably by altering the hemodynamics of the arterial system. Hypertension is more closely associated with fibrous plaques than with fatty streaks and has been shown to be associated with increased atherosclerosis in both animals and humans.[136] When hypertension occurs with hypercholesterolemia, the effect on atherosclerosis development is additive.[130,131,137–142] Hypertension also appears to be an accelerant for the development of atherosclerosis[141,142] and the major factor in the development of intracranial atherosclerosis.[131]

Lipids

As discussed in the previous Lipids section, elevated LDL and depressed HDL are risk factors for the development of clinically symptomatic atherosclerosis.[143] It has been shown that for comparable levels of LDL, the risk of atherosclerosis varies in different populations. This indicates the importance of other factors in the development of symptomatic atherosclerosis.

Elevated triglyceride levels are usually seen in association with elevated LDL and low HDL levels. Single triglyceride measurements have shown poor correlation with the development of atherosclerosis. However, postprandial triglyceride levels appear to be predictive of the development of coronary artery disease (CAD).[144–146]

Smoking

Cigarette smoking has been associated with an increased risk of symptomatic atherosclerosis. Smoking clearly increases the incidence and severity of coronary heart disease.[147] Several possible mechanisms may be involved. Nicotine may inhibit prostacyclin (PGI_2) release and promote platelet adhesion.[148] Smokers have lower HDL levels and elevated fibrinogen levels and can have platelet function abnormalities, all of which may predispose to a hypercoagulable state.[149] Smokers also have an increased number of white cells. Elevated numbers of white cells have been found in some studies to be a risk factor for CAD.[150] Cigarette smokers also appear to more frequently have raised lesions of the basilar artery.[151] Smoking has also been found to be an independent risk factor for increased thickness of atherosclerosis in the carotid bifurcation.[152]

Hyperglycemia

Hyperglycemia can result in glycosylation of LDL, rendering it more atherogenic via the macrophage scavenger pathway.[153] Glycosylation may predispose LDL to oxidation. Glycosylation and oxidation can also affect collagen, resulting in increased cross-linking, with increased stiffness of the arterial wall.[154] In addition, patients with elevated glucose levels have altered lipid levels that may predispose them to accelerated atherosclerosis.

Homocysteine

Increased homocysteine levels have been associated with symptomatic atherosclerosis. Homocysteine increases the risk of thrombosis. Thrombosis, with subsequent incorporation into the plaque, can result

in progressive plaque growth. Hyperhomocystinemia could also contribute to the symptomatology by increasing the risk of acute thrombotic episodes.[155–158] This topic has been reviewed by Welch.[159]

Two other observations have been made that focus more attention on the inflammatory aspects of symptomatic atherosclerosis. Ridker reported that the level of high-sensitivity C-reactive protein (CRP) correlated with the risk of vascular events. In a large study of postmenopausal women, high-sensitivity CRP was as predictive of risk of cardiovascular events as the HDL/total cholesterol ratio.[160] In a prior publication, Ridker reported a similar correlation between CRP and stroke and MI in men.[161] In the same study, Ridker demonstrated that the use of aspirin was associated with a significant reduction in the risk of MI and a decrease in CRP, and suggested that some of aspirin's benefit in risk reduction was related to its anti-inflammatory actions.

Circulating levels of ICAM-1 and E-selectin were found to be higher in patients with coronary heart disease (204 patents) and carotid artery disease (272 patients) than in age-matched normal controls (316 patients). Compared to patients in the lowest quartile, those in the highest quartile of ICAM-1 levels had a 5.5-fold increased risk of developing clinical coronary heart disease, and a 2.33-fold increased risk of carotid artery atherosclerosis. There was no significant difference in the levels of VCAM between any of the groups. The authors suggested that the plasma levels of these adhesion molecules could serve as molecular markers for atherosclerosis.[162]

Clinical Events

Although atherosclerosis appears to be ubiquitous, the frequency of development of clinically obvious ischemic events varies widely.[163] The actual composition of plaques also varies widely, and data suggest that different plaque composition or morphology is associated with different risks for ischemic events. As acute ischemic syndromes have been studied primarily in the coronary arteries, the following discussion of acute events is based primarily on the coronary artery literature. In general, plaques that produce the greatest degree of stenosis are more fibrotic and have a lower lipid content than those associated with acute thrombosis. Plaques associated with rupture, thrombosis, and acute ischemia tend to be less stenotic and have an eccentrically placed lipid core with a thin fibrous cap. Although the reason for rupture remains conjectural, there are several possibilities. Some authors have noted increased numbers of macrophages and T lymphocytes in the caps that rupture, suggesting a proteolytic injury to the cap.[164,165] Others have suggested a hemodynamic injury to the endothelium, with loss of structural integrity resulting in plaque rupture. Or, if the cap is at the maximum stenosis, the shear stress on the cap, which lacks underlying collagen support, may be sufficient to cause rupture.[166–168] Rupture of plaque with thrombosis has been documented to occur in the carotid artery.[169–172]

Most clinical events are associated with either thrombosis over the plaque or with a sudden increase in the plaque size. Thrombosis may occur over a plaque that appears to be structurally intact or over the point of rupture of a fibrous cap. Mural thrombosis can then undergo a fibrous transformation caused by ingrowth and organization of smooth muscle cells, thereby expanding the connective tissue mass.[173] Hemorrhage into a plaque may result in an acute increase in the severity of stenosis or in local thrombosis with occlusion of the vessel.[174] Intraplaque hemorrhage may be the result of blood tracking from the lumen into the plaque or may arise from rupture of vaso vasorum vessels supplying the plaque. Although there are a large number of publications on intraplaque hemorrhage, disagreement remains concerning not only the significance of the hemorrhage in symptom production but also the actual source of the hemorrhage. Detailed studies in both the carotid and the coronary arteries suggest that most of the intraplaque hemorrhage is from the lumenal surface.[174,175] Hemorrhage may also occur from rupture of neovascular vessels that grow into the plaque; some of these are from the lumenal surface, although the majority appear to derive from the vaso vasorum. The relative contribution of hemorrhage from these vessels is unknown.[176,177]

Plaques may develop fissures, triggering local thrombosis. In a review of coronary arteries of patients dying from MIs, many plaques appeared to have previously healed fissures with different states of thrombus formation, suggesting that most fissures reseal with incorporation of thrombus without manifestation of clinical symptoms.[178–181]

Treatment

As noted, the best treatment is prevention. Once ischemic symptoms have developed, a different approach may be required. One potentially realistic therapeutic goal is to induce plaque stabilization, regression, or both. This could be accomplished by modification of the risk factors, by treating hypertension and diabetes mellitus, smoking cessation, and decreasing LDL levels. Increases in HDL to improve removal of lipid from the arterial wall might also be effective. The removal of lipid from plaque potentially may have beneficial effects by also decreasing the risk of rupture and acute thrombosis.[182]

Therapy for symptomatic acute rupture with thrombosis has used a variety of antiplatelet agents, anticoagulants, and fibrinolytic agents. This chapter does not discuss these interventions.

Clinical Measurement of Atherosclerosis

Review of the data cited in the preceding sections suggests a variety of potential interventions to prevent atherosclerosis development and its ischemic complications. There are several different ways to approach evaluation of atherosclerosis therapy. One is an epidemiologic method that follows clinical events. Although this type of study specifically addresses the clinical concerns about the disease process (the actual events secondary to the disease process), it has the disadvantage of requiring the entry of large numbers of patients at risk for atherosclerosis and then following them for extended periods to detect a small number of clinical events. For many reasons, these trials are technically difficult to run, time consuming, and expensive. The Multiple Risk Factor Intervention Trial, which followed 366,000 men for a period of 12 years, is an example of a study of this type.[183] An alternative approach is to identify and follow a surrogate endpoint that parallels the severity of the disease. It has been hoped that atherosclerosis could be measured and quantified and that changes in plaque in response to interventions could be followed. The actual pattern (rate, location, etc.) of plaque growth is not known. Whether it is slow and continuous or episodic with rapid progression and even occasional regression has not been defined.[184]

Although it is generally assumed that there is a linear relationship between the amount of plaque and the development of symptomatology, this may not be the case. As described, highly stenotic plaques tend to be more fibrotic, whereas those associated with acute occlusion tend to be slightly smaller with a more rupture-prone, eccentrically located lipid core.

One goal has been to develop a technique that would permit repeated measurements of plaque and its change over time, allowing assessment of its natural history and its response to intervention. Two major techniques have been used in clinical trials: angiography and ultrasound. Several reviews of each technique's problems have been published.[185–187] As these publications point out, the measurement of atherosclerosis is fraught with potential problems.

Angiography

A number of investigators have used coronary angiography to identify the presence and extent of atherosclerosis and then to follow the change in stenosis over time. The Program on the Surgical Control of the Hyperlipidemias study[188] has demonstrated a parallel between angiographic measurements of atherosclerosis and the clinical event rate, and validates the use of angiography as a surrogate endpoint. Angiography is an invasive technique with potential for significant complications and is generally not used to assess asymptomatic patients. Because of its potential risks, frequent or repeated evaluations are difficult to justify. Therefore, most studies either use only a single measurement to assess the presence and severity of disease or perform measurements at the beginning and termination of the study, so that the actual rate and manner of progression cannot be assessed. Another problem with angiographic assessment of atherosclerosis lies in the fact that atherosclerosis is a disease of the arterial wall, and angiography only measures the arterial lumen, providing at best only second-order information about the arterial wall. Arterial lumenal reduction could be from local atherosclerosis, from clot superimposed on atherosclerosis, or from vasospasm. Apparent regression, or lack of progression, of atherosclerosis can occur

as a result of compensatory arterial enlargement in response to the development of local atherosclerosis.[28,29,189] There are also problems of accurately measuring the degree of arterial stenosis as imaged by coronary angiography.[190] Intermediate degrees of stenosis may be either over- or underestimated, depending on the angle of the x-ray beam in relationship to both the artery and the plaque.

Ultrasound

Another approach has been to use ultrasound, a noninvasive technique, as a surrogate endpoint to follow atherosclerosis. The carotid artery wall can be easily imaged, and measurements of the adventitia, media, and intima can be obtained using high-resolution ultrasound.[191] B-mode ultrasound is safe and painless, and repeat examinations can be performed frequently. B-mode ultrasound directly measures the arterial wall, the site of atherosclerosis, rather than the lumen, which is only secondarily involved. Although the coronary arteries cannot be well visualized by noninvasive ultrasound, the carotid arteries are readily accessible for ultrasound examination and have been evaluated in a number of studies. There is a strong association between the presence and severity of carotid atherosclerosis and the presence and severity of coronary atherosclerosis, indicating the former is a marker for large-vessel atherosclerosis.[192] Patients with carotid atherosclerosis have an increased risk for stroke, transient ischemic attack, angina, and MI. Its presence as detected by carotid ultrasound has been demonstrated to be an independent risk factor for the presence of coronary atherosclerosis.[193] In addition, the risk factors for carotid atherosclerosis are the same as those for coronary artery atherosclerosis: increasing age, male sex, white race, tobacco use, hypertension, left ventricular hypertrophy on electrocardiogram, diabetes, and elevated LDL and low HDL cholesterol. All these observations suggest that the ultrasonic measurement of carotid atherosclerosis is a potentially viable technique for assessment of systemic atherosclerosis and a means to follow changes in plaque over time.

B-mode ultrasound can be used to measure the carotid artery's intimal medial thickness (IMT) at the sites most predisposed to atherosclerosis development: the distal common carotid artery (CCA), the bifurcation of the CCA, and the proximal portion of the internal carotid artery. The Multicenter Isradipine Diuretic Atherosclerosis Study (MIDAS), using high-resolution B-mode measurement of small plaques, demonstrated that it was possible to reproducibly measure plaque with a mean absolute difference of +0.3 mm on repeat measurements.[194]

A number of studies have been published that have measured IMT in the cervical CCA and demonstrated a relationship between increasing IMT and risk of atherosclerosis.[195–198]

Potential problems also exist with ultrasound. It provides only a two-dimensional representation of a complex three-dimensional structure, and consequently may over- or underestimate plaque size or volume, particularly in large, complex plaques, which may have irregular contours. In addition, B-mode resolution is best when the ultrasound beam is perpendicular to the plaque; resolution decreases when the angle of insonation is less than 90 degrees. This means that measurement is best in the distal CCA and may be less precise in the bifurcation where the vessel is angled obliquely to the skin surface. Several studies have attempted to address the problem of measurement variability in individual plaque thickness by employing a scoring system using summation of plaque thickness measurements made at several locations, assuming that the variation around the mean would result in a reproducible, average score.[199] This also allows development of the concept of *plaque extent* or *burden* in the area studied. An additional problem is that thicker plaques tend to be mineralized, resulting in complete reflection of the ultrasound beam at that point (called *shadowing*), so that no information can be gathered from tissue at depths greater that the site of mineralization.

In other studies that evaluated plaques regardless of size and B-mode characteristics, there was a much larger variation in measurement reproducibility. In the Atherosclerosis Risk in Communities Study (ARIC), there was a 0.29–0.74-mm range of average absolute differences between replicate scans on the far wall of the CCA.[200,201] In the Multicenter Validation Study, the mean absolute single maximum thickness, as measured both by the same reader or by different readers, varied between 0.81 and 1.30 mm.[202] These studies included patients with large plaques. The scans of these plaques were subject to the previously mentioned problems of variable surface contour and shadowing.

There is interest in identifying plaque characteristics that may predict progression. It appears that the more homogeneous plaques are fibrotic and less likely to progress during the time of observation, and that the more heterogeneous plaques are more likely to progress during observation.[203] Criteria for classification into plaque subtypes are not exact, making it difficult to compare studies.

It may be that ultrasound is best for identifying and following interventions in early plaque, before the development of complex lesions. From a therapeutic perspective, it may be easier to stabilize or even regress smaller plaques, so that their identification and measurement may prove to be useful in future studies.

Other Imaging Techniques

Several different measurements should be tracked by imaging techniques of atherosclerosis. One is a global assessment of plaque volume to determine the response of atherosclerosis to therapy. The other is a measure of the severity of local stenosis, because this may be a better measure for potential local tissue ischemic events in an individual patient. To follow plaque progression, a potentially better technique would be a three-dimensional imaging one (ultrasound, computed tomography, or magnetic resonance imaging) that essentially provided a topographic map of the atherosclerosis and allowed tracking of the total volume of plaque. The thickness of the plaque at a given site (i.e., the severity of stenosis produced by the plaque) could also be measured and tracked.

A number of other techniques are being evaluated for measurement of atherosclerosis. These include intravascular ultrasound, magnetic resonance imaging, and spiral computed tomography; however, none of these have been used in large prospective studies of the measurement of atherosclerosis.[204–209]

Clinical Trials in Atherosclerosis

Lipid Lowering

Because cholesterol plays such an important role in the development, progression, and complications of plaque, a number of cholesterol-lowering trials have been designed and carried out. Many (but not all) have demonstrated that reduction in total cholesterol may decrease the clinical event rate. Studies using angiographic estimates of changes in plaque size have failed to consistently demonstrate a significant change in the degree of stenosis but have clearly demonstrated a decrease in clinical event rates.[210–212]

This decrease in events may be seen within a few weeks after lowering cholesterol, suggesting that there has been an alteration in the coagulation system (or some other process).[213] It also suggests that it is not plaque regression or lack of progression that results in the decreased frequency of clinical events, but perhaps some other phenomenon, such as decreased plaque rupture, decreased vasospasm, improved microvascular function, improved collateral flow, or decreased thrombosis at the level of the plaque.

It has been hoped that vigorous lipid-lowering therapy would result in plaque regression. Although lipid regression has been demonstrated to cause regression in some animal models, most of these improvements have occurred in animals that have developed atherosclerosis while on a high-cholesterol diet. These lesions are generally extremely lipid-laden, and a decrease in the atheroma size can be accomplished by reducing the amount of plaque cholesterol.[214–218] In most of these models, during the high-cholesterol diet phase there is a marked accumulation of arterial collagen, elastin, and cholesterol. With regression, the lipid content as well as the elastin in the atheroma decrease dramatically, but the collagen content is only minimally decreased. Based on comparisons with expected degrees of atherosclerosis in matched animals, the plaques appear to regress from their maximal extent. This differs from the human lesion, which tends to become more complex before becoming symptomatic. In complex lesions there may be cholesterol pools in conjunction with fibrosis, intraplaque hemorrhage, and mineralization (calcification). Although it is still possible to decrease the intraplaque cholesterol content, it is unlikely that these other changes can be reversed. For this reason, plaque stabilization may be a more realistic goal for symptomatic lesions.

A number of studies have used angiographic assessment of coronary artery lesions in lipid-lowering trials.[219–227] Although the angiographic changes are relatively small, each study demonstrated a clinical benefit with a decreased number of ischemic events in the group receiving lipid-lowering therapy. Reduction of lipid levels by diet[223] and lifestyle changes have also been shown to have benefit. Numerous lipid-lowering therapies have been evaluated in clinical trials and documented to have at least some clinical efficacy in the studied populations. Drugs used include niacin,[220,228] cholestyramine,[229] gemfibrozil,[230] colestipol,[222] hepatic 3-methylglutaryl coenzyme A reductase inhibitors,[213,231–233] and probucol (which is also an antioxidant).

Another approach has been to raise HDL as well as lowering LDL. HDL is thought to promote reverse cholesterol transport, potentially removing it from the arterial wall. In studies of rabbits fed high cholesterol and then given homologous HDL, fatty streaks and localized lipid deposits were decreased.[234] It is thought that converting HDL-3 to HDL-2[235] improves reverse transport.[236] Gemfibrozil and nicotinic acid may raise HDL, especially in hypertriglyceridemic patients.

Several studies evaluating the efficacy of statins in patients with CAD have found not only a reduction of myocardial ischemic events, but also a reduction of stroke risk.[237–241] The absolute numbers of stroke in each series have been small, but the series have all reported approximately a 30% reduction in stroke. This reduction has only been noted in studies of secondary MI prevention and not in primary MI prevention studies. There are a number of possible explanations for this observation of decreased stroke risk in these populations, including the fact that fewer MIs result in fewer cardioembolic strokes. A number of interesting observations have been made that suggest statins may have other potentially beneficial actions. Statins have also been reported to improve endothelial vasomotor function, increase endothelial fibrinolytic activity, block platelet activation,[242] inhibit the expression of macrophage tissue factor, reduce matrix metalloproteinase secretion, lower CRP levels,[243] and decrease smooth muscle migration and proliferation.[244] Statins also may have a neuroprotective effect.[245]

Antioxidants

Because oxidation of LDL appears to be an important step in the transition from fatty streak to atherosclerotic plaque (because of foam cell necrosis or rupture due to uptake of oxidized LDL), there has been great interest in the possible beneficial effects of antioxidants. Probucol, a lipid-lowering agent, has also been shown to have an antioxidant effect and may function as a free-radical scavenger. Probucol, which is lipophilic, is transported in LDL, HDL, and very-low-density lipoprotein particles. Vitamin E and probucol are incorporated into the lipoprotein particles and can potentially protect them from oxidative modification.[246] Probucol has been shown to retard lesion development in the Watanabe rabbit model of familial homozygous hypercholesterolemia,[247,248] as well as reduce intimal proliferation in response to balloon catheter–induced injury in swine.[249] This appeared to be independent of any lipid-lowering effect, as there was minimal change in the cholesterol level.[250] The Probucol Quantitative Regression Swedish Trial (PQRST) compared angiographic changes in the estimated atheroma volume based on change in lumen volume of the femoral artery in hypercholesterolemic patients. All patients were treated with cholestyramine and diet and then randomized to probucol or placebo. There was no statistical difference in change in lumen volume between the two treatment groups. The probucol group had a 17% reduction of total cholesterol, 12% reduction of LDL, 24% reduction of HDL, and a 34% reduction in HDL2b.[251–253]

Vitamin E and beta carotene are antioxidants that are normally present in circulation. Animals fed a high-cholesterol diet and supplemented with vitamin E have been shown to develop less atherosclerosis than those fed a similar diet without vitamin E.[254] Studies of vitamin E in human atherosclerosis have had mixed results. Stocker discusses that, depending on the fate of the α-tocopherol radical, vitamin E can have antioxidant, neutral, or pro-oxidant activity.[255,256]

Antiproliferative Agents

A variety of drugs may inhibit the arterial proliferative response to different forms of injury. All of these have been found to decrease atherosclerosis in experimental models, but their potential usefulness in human atherosclerosis intervention has not yet been clearly demonstrated. These include heparin (which may interfere with platelet adhesion and may also decrease smooth muscle proliferation),[257] cyclosporin A (which may block smooth muscle replication in plaque),[258] calcium antagonists (which may decrease matrix protein production, decrease platelet adhesion, and interfere with calcium uptake by plaque),[259–261] and angiotensin-converting enzyme inhibitors (which may inhibit smooth muscle proliferation and matrix protein synthesis).[262]

Two studies used angiographic progression data in patients treated with calcium channel blockers and demonstrated that, although there was no difference between groups treated with calcium channel blockers and other agents in plaque progression for the larger plaques, it appeared that fewer small plaques developed or progressed in the calcium channel blocker group,[263,264] again raising the hope that early intervention might be more effective in preventing the development of atherosclerosis.

Omega-3 Fatty Acids

Another novel approach to atherosclerosis intervention was prompted by the recognition of the low mortality rate from CAD in Greenland Eskimos. This population eats primarily a fish diet that is high in omega-3 fatty acids (n-3 class of polyunsaturated fatty acids).[265] These fatty acids have been demonstrated to have a number of interesting effects. They have inhibitory effects on white blood cells, particularly monocytes,[266] and on platelets. In animal models, they have been shown to reduce the development of atherosclerosis.[267,268] They also appear to decrease the frequency of thrombotic events associated with atherosclerosis. There are at least two different mechanisms for their beneficial effects: They interfere with coagulation by affecting platelet function, and they may also decrease the intimal proliferative response to injury. In experimental models in nonhuman primates, n-3 fatty acids are rapidly incorporated into blood and vascular tissue, are found to decrease the thrombotic response of flowing blood to thrombogenic surfaces, and can eliminate both the thrombotic and proliferative responses of mechanically damaged arteries without causing a significant platelet hemostatic dysfunction.[269,270] They also decrease the platelet membrane concentration of arachidonic acid, thus preventing thromboxane A_2

synthesis, and may compete with arachidonic acid for cyclooxygenase, leading to the formation of three biologically inactive compounds (inactive prostanoids). In a swine atherosclerosis model, with hypercholesterolemia induced before balloon abrasion of a coronary artery, the animals on a high-cholesterol diet all developed moderate to severe lesions, whereas those receiving cod-liver oil had minimal disease; levels of abnormal lipids were similar, but platelet arachidonic acid levels were much lower and eicosapentanoic levels were higher in treated pigs.[267] One study evaluated the effect of omega-3 fatty acids on patients with angiographically documented CAD. Patients were followed for 2 years and then had repeat quantitative angiography. There was no statistically significant difference between the angiographic change in coronary atherosclerosis, and there was a trend toward fish oil recipients having fewer clinical cardiovascular events.[271]

Conclusion

The development of the understanding of atherosclerosis at a cellular level should allow investigators to target specific processes for intervention. It is possible that antibodies to specific cytokines or growth factors may be used to prevent the development of the initial lesions, or simply blocking the effects of the growth factors may prevent the development of plaque. Anti-inflammatory agents directed at the monocyte-endothelial interaction could potentially be used to prevent one of the initial steps in atherosclerosis. Antibodies to the scavenger receptor, or "turning off" the scavenger receptor, could prevent the progression to typical plaque. Antioxidant therapies to prevent the oxidation of LDL may prove useful in preventing the secondary problems of atherosclerosis. Development of agents to improve LDL transport out of the plaque may allow plaque stabilization. Identification of the atherogenic components of lipids may allow targeting of them, as, for example, via reduction of LDL or interference with LP(a).

As these therapies are developed, they may be tested using techniques that can measure atherosclerosis presence and extent safely and repeatedly, so that the atherosclerotic process can be identified before the development of ischemic events; the same techniques may be used to follow the effects of interventions. As the carotid artery is easily imaged using available techniques, it may become one of the sites that is evaluated on a routine basis.

References

1. Shattock SG. A report on the pathological condition of the aorta of King Menephthah, traditionally regarded as the Pharaoh of the Exodus. Proc Royal Soc Med, Pathol Section 1909;2:122–127.
2. Holman RL, McGill HC, Strong JP, Geer JC. Arteriosclerosis—the lesion. Am J Clin Nutr 1960;8:85–94.
3. Enos WF, Holmes RH, Beyer J. Coronary disease among United States soldiers killed in action in Korea. JAMA 1953;152:1090–1093.
4. Rigal RD, Lovell FW, Townsend FM. Pathologic findings in the cardiovascular systems of military flying personnel. Am J Cardiol 1960;6:19–25.
5. Sternby NH. Atherosclerosis in a defined population. APMIS 1968;194(Suppl):5.
6. Tracey RE, Kissling GE. Comparisons of human populations for histologic features of atherosclerosis. Arch Pathol Lab Med 1988;112:1056–1065.
7. Ho KBJ, Biss K, Mikkelson B. The Masai of East Africa: some unique biological characteristics. Arch Pathol 1971; 91:387–410.
8. Wissler RW, Vesselinovitch D. Can atherosclerotic plaques regress? Anatomic and biochemical evidence from nonhuman models. Am J Cardiol 1990;65(Suppl):33F–40F.
9. Kritchevsky D, Tepper SA, Kim HK, et al. Experimental atherosclerosis in rabbits fed cholesterol-free diets. Comparison of peanut, corn, butter, and coconut oils. Exp Mol Pathol 1976;24:375–391.
10. Stehbens WE. Vascular complications in experimental atherosclerosis. Prog Cardiovasc Dis 1986;29:221–237.
11. Neufeld HN, Goldbourt U. Coronary heart disease: genetic aspects. Circulation 1983;67:943–954.
12. McCully KS. Atherosclerosis, serum cholesterol, and the homocysteine theory: a study of 194 consecutive autopsies. Am J Med Sci 1990;299:217–221.
13. Solberg LA, Strong JP. Risk factors and atherosclerotic lesions. A review of autopsy studies. Arteriosclerosis 1983;3:187–198.
14. Romm PA, Green CE, Reagan K, Rackley CE. Relation of serum lipoprotein cholesterol concentration levels to presence and severity of angiographic coronary artery disease. Am J Cardiol 1991;67:479–483.
15. Ginsburg GS, Safran C, Pasternak RC. Frequency of low serum high-density lipoprotein cholesterol levels in hospitalized patients with "desirable" total cholesterol levels. Am J Cardiol 1991;68:187–192.
16. Stary HC, Blankenhorn DH, Chandler AB, et al. A definition of the intima of human arteries and of its atherosclerosis prone regions. A report from the Committee on Vascular Lesions of the Council on Arteriosclerosis, American Heart Association. Circulation 1992;85:391–405.

17. Stary HC, Chandler AB, Glagov S, et al. A definition of initial, fatty streak, and intermediate lesions of atherosclerosis. A report from the Committee on Vascular Lesions of the Council on Arteriosclerosis, American Heart Association. Circulation 1994;89:2462–2478.

18. Stary HC, Chandler AB, Dinsmore RE, et al. A definition of advanced types of atherosclerotic lesions and a histological classification of atherosclerosis. A report from the Committee on Vascular Lesions of the Council of Atherosclerosis, American Heart Association. Arterioscler Thromb Vasc Biol 1995;15:1512–1531.

19. Mitchell JRA, Schwartz CJ (eds). Arterial Disease. Philadelphia: FA Davis, 1965.

20. Strong JP. Atherosclerotic lesions: natural history, risk factors, and topography. Arch Pathol Lab Med 1992;116:1268–1275.

21. Strong JP, Eggen DA, Tracy RE. The Geographic Pathology and Topography of Atherosclerosis and Risk Factors for Atherosclerotic Lesions. In AB Chandler, K Eurenius, GC McMillan, CB Nelson, CJ Schwartz, S Wessler (eds), The Thrombotic Process in Atherogenesis. New York: Plenum, 1978;11–31.

22. Glagov S, Ozoa AK. Significance of the relatively low incidence of atherosclerosis in the pulmonary, renal, and mesenteric arteries. Ann N Y Acad Sci 1968;149:940–955.

23. Duff GL, McMillan GC. Pathology of atherosclerosis. Am J Med 1951;11:92–108.

24. McGill HC, Arias-Stella J, Carbonell LM (eds). The Geographic Pathology of Atherosclerosis. Baltimore: Williams & Wilkins, 1968;38–42.

25. Strong JP, McGill HC. The pediatric aspects of atherosclerosis. J Atheroscl Res 1969;9:251–265.

26. Stary HC. Changes in the Cells of Atherosclerotic Lesions as Advanced Lesions Evolve in Coronary Arteries of Children and Young Adults. In S Glagov, WP Newman, SA Schaffer (eds), Pathobiology of the Human Atherosclerotic Plaque. New York: Springer, 1990;93–106.

27. Restrepo C, Tracey R. Variations in human aortic fatty streaks among geographic locations. Atherosclerosis 1975;21:179–193.

28. Bond MG, Adams MR, Bullock BC. Complicating factors in evaluating coronary artery atherosclerosis. Artery 1981;9:21–29.

29. Glagov S, Weisenberd E, Zarins C, et al. Compensatory enlargement of human atherosclerotic arteries. N Engl J Med 1987;316:1371–1375.

30. Stary HC. Evolution and progression of atherosclerotic lesions in coronary arteries of children and young adults. Arteriosclerosis 1989;9(Suppl II):19–32.

31. Stary HC. The sequence of cell and matrix changes in atherosclerotic lesions of coronary arteries in the first forty years of life. Eur Heart J 1990;11(Suppl E):3–9.

32. Stary HC. Composition and classification of human atherosclerotic lesions. Virchows Arch 1992;421:277–290.

33. Stary HC, Chandler AB, Dinsmore RE, et al. A definition of advanced types of atherosclerotic lesions and a histological classification of atherosclerosis. A report from the Committee on Vascular Lesions of the Council of Atherosclerosis, American Heart Association. Arterioscler Thromb Vasc Biol 1995;15:1512–1531.

34. Bell FP, Adamson IL, Schwartz CJ. Aortic endothelial permeability to albumin: focal and regional patterns of uptake and transmural distribution on 131 I-albumin in the young pig. Exp Mol Pathol 1974;20:57–68.

35. Packham MA, Rowsell HC, Jorgensen L, Mustard JF. Localized protein accumulation in the wall of the aorta. Exp Mol Pathol 1967;7:214–232.

36. Bell FP, Gallus AS, Schwartz CJ. Focal and regional patterns of uptake and the transmural distribution of 131 I-fibrinogen in the pig aorta. Exp Mol Pathol 1974;20:281–292.

37. Feldman DL, Hoff HF, Gerrity RG. Immunohistochemical localization of apolipoprotein B in aortas from hyperlipidemic swine demonstrates preferential accumulation in lesion prone areas. Arch Pathol Lab Med 1984;108:817–822.

38. Hoff HF, Lie JT, Titus JL, et al. Lipoproteins in atherosclerotic lesions. Localization by immunofluorescence of apo-density lipoproteins in human atherosclerotic arteries from normal and hyperlipoproteinemics. Arch Pathol 1975;99:252–258.

39. Gerrity RG, Richardson M, Bell FP, et al. Endothelial cell morphology in areas of in vivo Evans Blue uptake in the young pig aorta. II. Ultrastructure of the intima in areas of differing permeability to proteins. Am J Pathol 1977;89:313–323.

40. Caplan BA, Schwartz CJ. Increased endothelial cell turnover in areas of in vivo Evans Blue uptake in the pig aorta. Atherosclerosis 1973;17:401–417.

41. Gerrity RG, Naito KH. Alteration of endothelial cell surface morphology after experimental aortic coarctation. Artery 1980;8:267–274.

42. Gerrity RG, Goss JA, Soby L. Control of monocyte recruitment by chemotactic factor(s) in lesion-prone areas of swine aorta. Arteriosclerosis 1985;5:55–66.

43. Gerrity RG, Naito HK, Richardson M, Schwartz CJ. Dietary induced atherogenesis in swine. Morphology of the intima in prelesion stages. Am J Pathol 1979;95:775–792.

44. Gerrity RG. Arterial Endothelial Structure and Permeability as It Relates to Susceptibility to Atherogenesis. In S Glagov, WP Newman, SA Schafer (eds), Pathobiology of the Human Arteriosclerotic Plaque. New York: Springer, 1990;13–46.

45. Fajardo LF. The complexity of endothelial cells. Am J Clin Pathol 1989;92:241–250.

46. Jaffe EA. Cell biology of endothelial cells. Hum Pathol 1987;18:234–239.

47. Vane JR, Anggard EE, Boltingam R. Regulatory functions of the endothelium. N Engl J Med 1990;323:27–36.

48. Vanhoutte PM, Luscher TF, Graser T. Endothelium-dependent contractions. Blood Vessels 1991;28:74–83.

49. Loskutoff DJ, Curriden SA. The fibrinolytic system of the vessel wall and its role in the control of thrombosis. Ann N Y Acad Sci 1990;598:238–247.

50. Ware JA, Heistad DD. Seminars in medicine of the Beth Israel Hospital, Boston. Platelet-endothelium interactions. N Engl J Med 1993;328:628–635.

51. Thorgeirsson G, Robertson AL. The vascular endothelium—pathobiologic significance. Am J Pathol 1978;93:804–848.

52. Berliner JA, Territo MC, Sevanian A, et al. Minimally modified low-density lipoprotein stimulates monocyte endothelial interactions. J Clin Invest 1990;85:1260–1266.

53. Springer TA, Cybulsky ML. Traffic Signals on Endothelium for Leukocytes in Health, Inflammation, and Atherosclerosis. In Fuster V, Ross R, Topol EJ (eds), Atherosclerosis and Coronary Artery Disease. Philadelphia: Lippincott–Raven, 1996;511–537.

54. Ross R. The pathogenesis of atherosclerosis: a perspective for the 1990s. Nature 1993;362:801–809.

55. Thorin E, Shreeve SM. Heterogeneity of vascular endothelial cells in normal and disease states. Pharmacol Ther 1998;78:115–166.

56. Rosenberg RD, Aird WC. Vascular bed specific homeostasis and hypercoagulable states. New Engl J Med 1999;340:1555–1564.

57. Timpl R, Dziadek M. Structure, development, and molecular pathology of basement membranes. Int Rev Exp Pathol 1986;29:1–112.

58. Raines EW, Ross R. Smooth muscle cells and the pathogenesis of the lesions of atherosclerosis. Br Heart J 1993;69(Suppl):30–37.

59. Benditt EP, Benditt JM. Evidence for a monoclonal origin of human atherosclerotic plaques. Proc Natl Acad Sci U S A 1973;70:1753–1756.

60. Bini A, Fenoglio JJ, Mesa-Tejada R. Identification and distribution of fibrinogen, fibrin, and fibrin(ogen) degradation products in atherosclerosis. Use of monoclonal antibodies. Arteriosclerosis 1989;9:109–121.

61. Libby P, Ross R. Cytokines and Growth Regulatory Molecules in Atherosclerosis. In V Fuster, R Ross, EJ Topol (eds), Atherosclerosis and Coronary Artery Disease. Philadelphia: Lippincott–Raven, 1996:585–594.

62. Clinton SK, Libby P. Cytokines and growth factors in atherogenesis. Arch Pathol Lab Med 1992;116:1292–1300.

63. Klagsburn M, Edelman ER. Biological and biochemical properties of fibroblast growth factors. Arteriosclerosis 1989;9:269–278.

64. Ross R. Platelet derived growth factor. Lancet 1989;1:1179–1182.

65. Ross R. Atherosclerosis—an inflammatory disease. N Engl J Med 1999;340:115–126.

66. Libby P, Hansson GK. Involvement of the immune system in human atherogenesis: current knowledge and unanswered questions. Lab Invest 1991;64:5–15.

67. Poston RN, Haskard DO, Coucher JR, et al. Expression of intercellular adhesion molecule-1 in atherosclerotic plaques. Am J Pathol 1992;140:665–673.

68. Printeseva OY, Peclo MM, Gown AM. Various cell types in human atherosclerotic lesions express ICAM-1. Further immunocytochemical and immunochemical studies employing monoclonal antibody 10F3. Am J Pathol 1992;140:889–896.

69. O'Brien KD, Allen MD, McDonald TO, et al. Vascular cell adhesion molecule-1 is expressed in human coronary atherosclerotic plaques. Implications for the mode of progression of advanced coronary atherosclerosis. J Clin Invest 1993;92:945–951.

70. Navab M, Imes SS, Hama SY, et al. Monocyte transmigration induced by modification of low-density lipoprotein in cultures of human aortic wall cells is due to induction of monocyte chemotactic protein 1 synthesis and is abolished by high density lipoprotein. J Clin Invest 1991;88:2039–2046.

71. Valente AJ, Graves DT, Vialle-Valentin CE, et al. Purification of a monocyte chemotactic factor secreted by nonhuman primate vascular cells in culture. Biochemistry 1988; 27:4162–4168.

72. Yoshimura T, Robinson EA, Tanaka S, et al. Purification and amino acid analysis of two human monocyte chemoattractants produced by phytohemagglutinin-stimulated human blood mononuclear leukocytes. J Immunol 1989; 142:1956–1962.

73. Cybursky MI, Gimbrone MA. Endothelial expression of a mononuclear leukocyte adhesion molecule during atherogenesis. Science 1991;251:788–791.

74. Clinton SK, Underwood R, Hayes L. Macrophage colony-stimulating factor gene expression in vascular cells and in experimental and human atherosclerosis. Am J Pathol 1992;140:301–316.

75. Raines EW, Rosenfeld ME, Ross R. The Role of Macrophages. In V Fuster, R Ross, EJ Topol (eds), Atherosclerosis and Coronary Artery Disease. Philadelphia: Lippincott–Raven, 1996;539–555.

76. Schwartz CJ, Valente AJ, Sprague EA. A modern view of atherogenesis. Am J Cardiol 1993;71:9B–14B.

77. Libby P, Hansson GK. Involvement of the immune system in human atherogenesis: current knowledge and unanswered questions. Lab Invest 1991;64:5–15.

78. Hansson GK, Jonasson L, Seifert PS. Immune mechanism in atherosclerosis. Arteriosclerosis 1989;9:567–578.

79. Geng Y, Hansson GK. Interferon-gamma inhibits scavenger receptor expression and foam cell formation in human monocyte-derived macrophages. J Clin Invest 1992;89:1322–1330.

80. Wilson AC, Shaub RG, Goldstein RC, Kuo PT. Suppression of aortic atherosclerosis in cholesterol rabbits by purified rabbit interferon. Arteriosclerosis 1990;10:208–214.

81. Hansson GK, Holm J, Holm S, et al. T Lymphocytes inhibit the vascular response to injury. Proc Natl Acad Sci U S A 1991;88:10530–10534.

82. Hansson GK, Holm J. Interferon-gamma inhibits arterial stenosis after injury. Circulation 1991;84:1266–1272.

83. Markus HS, Mendall MA. *Helicobacter pylori* infection: a risk factor for ischemic cerebrovascular disease and carotid atheroma. J Neurol Neurosurg Psychiatry 1998; 64:104–107.

84. Hajjar DP. Viral pathogenesis of atherosclerosis. Am J Pathol 1991;139:1195–1211.

85. Adam E, Probtsfield JL, Burek J, et al. High levels of cytomegalovirus antibody in patients requiring vascular surgery for atherosclerosis. Lancet 1987;2:291–293.

86. Kuo C, Shor A, Campbell LA, et al. Demonstrations of *Chlamydia pneumoniae* in atherosclerotic lesions of the coronary arteries. J Infect Dis 1993;167:841–849.

87. Thom H, Grayston JT, Siscovik DS, et al. Association of prior infection with *Chlamydia pneumoniae* and angiographically documented coronary artery disease. JAMA 1992;268:68–72.

88. Hendrix MGR, Salimans MMM, van Boven CPA, Bruggeman CA. High prevalence of latently prevalent cytomega-

lovirus in arterial walls of patients suffering from grade III atherosclerosis. Am J Pathol 1990;136:23–28.

89. Grattan MT, Moreno-Cabral CE, Starnes VA, et al. Cytomegalovirus infection is associated with cardiac allograft rejection and atherosclerosis. JAMA 1989;261:3561–3566.

90. MacDonald K, Rector TS, Braunian EA, et al. Association of coronary artery disease in cardiac transplant recipients with cytomegalovirus infection. Am J Pathol 1989;64:359–362.

91. Wissler RW, Vesselinovitch D, Davis HR, et al. A new way to look at atherosclerotic involvement of the artery wall and the functional effects. Ann N Y Acad Sci 1985;454:9–22.

92. Stehbens WE. Focal intimal proliferation in the cerebral arteries. Am J Pathol 1960;36:289–301.

93. Stehbens WE. Pathology of the Cerebral Blood Vessels. St. Louis: Mosby, 1972.

94. Stehbens WE. Hemodynamics and the Blood Vessel Wall. Springfield, IL: Thomas, 1979.

95. Ku DN, Giddens DP, Zarins CK, Glagov S. Pulsatile flow and atherosclerosis in the human carotid bifurcation. Positive correlation between plaque location and low oscillatory shear stress. Arteriosclerosis 1985;5:293–302.

96. Glagov S, Zarins C, Giddens DP, Ku DN. Hemodynamics and atherosclerosis. Insights and perspectives gained from studies of human arteries. Arch Pathol Lab Med 1988;112:1018–1031.

97. Ginsberg HN. Lipoprotein metabolism and its relationship to atherosclerosis. Med Clin North Am 1994;78:1–20.

98. Kao V, Wissler RW. A study of the immunohistochemical localization of serum lipoproteins and other plasma proteins in human atherosclerotic lesions. Exp Mol Pathol 1965;4:465–479.

99. Bratzler RL, Chisolm GM, Colton CK, et al. The distribution of labeled low-density lipoproteins across the rabbit thoracic aorta in vivo. Atherosclerosis 1977;28:289–307.

100. Reichel D, Miller NE. Pathophysiology of reverse cholesterol transport. Insights from inherited disorders of lipoprotein metabolism. Arteriosclerosis 1989;9:785.

101. Yla-Herttuala S, Palinski W, Rosenfeld ME, et al. Evidence for the presence of oxidatively modified low-density lipoprotein in atherosclerotic lesions in rabbit and man. J Clin Invest 1989;84:1086–1095.

102. Steinberg D, Parthasarathy S, Carew TE, et al. Beyond cholesterol, modification of low-density lipoprotein that increase its atherogenicity. New Engl J Med 1989;320:915–924.

103. Steinberg D, Witztum JL. Lipoproteins and atherogenesis. Current concepts. JAMA 1990;264:3047–3052.

104. Lees AL, Lees RS, Schoen FJ, et al. Imaging human atherosclerosis with 99mTc–labeled low-density lipoproteins. Arteriosclerosis 1988;8:461–470.

105. Avogaro P, Bittolo Bon G, Cazzolato G. Presence of modified low-density lipoprotein in humans. Arteriosclerosis 1988;8:79–87.

106. Palinsky W, Rosenfeld ME, Yla-Herttuala S, et al. Low-density lipoprotein undergoes oxidative modification in vivo. Proc Natl Acad Sci U S A 1989;86:1372–1376.

107. Salonen JT, Yla-Herttuala S, Yamamoto R, et al. Autoantibody against oxidised LDL and progression of carotid atherosclerosis. Lancet 1992;339:883–887.

108. Eaton DL, Fless GM, Kohr WJ. Partial amino acid sequence of apolipoprotein(a) shows that it is homologous to plasminogen. Proc Natl Acad Sci U S A 1987;84:3228–3244.

109. Berg K. Genetics and clinical importance of Lp(a) lipoprotein. Atheroscl Rev 1991;23:63–75.

110. Schaefer EJ, Lamon–Fava S, Jenner JL, et al. Lipoprotein(a) levels and risk of coronary heart disease in men. JAMA 1994;271:999–1003.

111. Stehbens WE. The role of thrombosis and variants of the thrombogenic theory in the etiology and pathogenesis of atherosclerosis. Prog Cardiovasc Dis 1992;34:325–346.

112. Rabbini LE, Loscalzo J. Recent observations on the role of hemostatic determinants in the development of the atherothrombotic plaque. Atherosclerosis 1994;15:1–7.

113. Chandler AB, Hand RA. Phagocytized platelets: a source of lipids in human thrombi and atherosclerotic plaques. Science 1961;134:946–947.

114. Hand RA, Chandler AB. Atherosclerotic metamorphosis of autologous pulmonary thromboemboli in the rabbit. Am J Pathol 1962;40:469–486.

115. Mendelsohn ME, Loscalzo J. Role of platelets in cholesterol ester formation by U-937 cells. J Clin Invest 1988;81:62–68.

116. Maor I, Brook GJ, Aviram M. Platelet secreted lipoprotein-like particle is taken up by the macrophage scavenger receptor and enhances cellular cholesterol accumulation. Atherosclerosis 1991;88:163–174.

117. Sumiyoshi A, More RH, Weigensberg BI. Aortic fibrofatty atherosclerosis in thrombus from normolipidemic rabbits. Atherosclerosis 1973;18:43–57.

118. Chandler AB. An Overview of Thrombosis and Platelet Involvement in the Development of the Human Atherosclerotic Plaque. In SA Glagov, WP Newman, SA Schaffer (eds), Pathobiology of the Human Atherosclerotic Plaque. New York: Springer, 1990;359–377.

119. Schwartz CJ, Valente AJ, Kelley JL, et al. Thrombosis and the development of atherosclerosis: Rokitansky revisited. Semin Thromb Hemost 1988;14:189–195.

120. Falk E. Unstable angina with fatal outcome: dynamic coronary thrombosis leading to infarction and/or sudden death. Autopsy evidence of recurrent mural thrombosis with peripheral embolization culminating in total vascular occlusion. Circulation 1985;71:699–708.

121. Loscalzo J. The relation between atherosclerosis and thrombosis. Circulation 1992;86(Suppl III):95–99.

122. Zahavi J, Bitteridge JD, Jones NAG. Enhanced in vivo platelet release reaction and malondialdehyde formation in patients with hyperlipidemia. Am J Med 1981;70:59–64.

123. Carvalho ACA, Colman RW, Lees RS. Platelet function in hyperlipoproteinemia. N Engl J Med 1974;290:434–438.

124. Joist JH, Baker RK, Scholfeld G. Increased in vivo and in vitro platelet function in type II and type IV hyperlipoproteinemia. Thromb Res 1974;15:95–108.

125. Strano A, Davi G, Averna M, et al. Platelet sensitivity to prostacyclin and thromboxane production in hyperlipidemic patients. Thromb Haemost 1982;48:18–20.

126. Harker LA, Hazzard W. Platelet kinetic studies in patients with hyperlipoproteinemia: effects of clofibrate therapy. Circulation 1979;60:492–496.

127. Aviram M, Brook JG. Platelet activation by plasma lipoproteins. Prog Cardiovasc Dis 1987;30:61–72.

128. Muller JE, Toeffler GH, Stone PH. Circadian variation and triggers of onset of acute cardiovascular disease. Circulation 1989;79:733–743.

129. Badimon L, Badimon JJ, Galvez A, et al. Influence of arterial damage and wall shear rate on platelet deposition. Ex vivo study in a swine model. Arteriosclerosis 1986;6:312–320.

130. Solberg LA, Strong JP. Risk factors and atherosclerotic lesions. Arteriosclerosis 1983;3:187–198.

131. Hollander W, Prusty S, Kemper T, et al. The effects of hypertension on cerebral atherosclerosis in the cynomolgus monkey. Stroke 1993;24:1218–1227.

132. Hopkins PN, Williams RR. A survey of 246 suggested coronary risk factors. Atherosclerosis 1981;40:1–52.

133. Gordon T, Kannel WB. Multiple risk functions for predicting coronary artery disease: the concept, accuracy, and application. Am Heart J 1982;103:1031–1039.

134. Strong JP, Guzman MA. Decrease in coronary atherosclerosis in New Orleans. Lab Invest 1980;43:297–301.

135. Weber G, Bianciardi G, Bussani R, et al. Atherosclerosis and aging. A morphometric study on arterial lesions of elderly and very elderly necropsy subjects. Arch Pathol Lab Med 1988;112:1066–1070.

136. Chobanian AV, Lichtenstein AH, Nilakhe V, et al. Influence of hypertension on aortic atherosclerosis in the Watanabe rabbit. Hypertension 1989:14:203–209.

137. Robertson WB, Strong JP. Atherosclerosis in persons with hypertension and diabetes. Lab Invest 1968;18:538–551.

138. Solberg LA, McGarry PA. Cerebral atherosclerosis in Negroes and Caucasians. Atherosclerosis 1972;16:141–154.

139. Kramsch DM, Hollander W. Occlusive atherosclerosis of the coronary arteries in monkey (Macaca irus) induced by diet. Exp Mol Pathol 1968;9:1–22.

140. Bullock BC, Clarkson TB, Lehner NDM, et al. Atherosclerosis in Cebus albifrons monkeys. III. Clinical and pathologic studies. Exp Mol Pathol 1969;10:39–62.

141. Mann GV, Andrus SB. Xanthomatosis and atherosclerosis produced by diet in adult Rhesus monkey. J Lab Clin Med 1956;48:533–550.

142. Taylor CB, Cox GE, Manalo-Estrella P, et al. Atherosclerosis in Rhesus monkeys. II. Arterial lesions associated with hypercholesteremia induced by dietary fat and cholesterol. Arch Pathol 1962;74:16–34.

143. Summary of the second report of the National Cholesterol Education Program (NCEP) Expert Panel on Detection, Evaluation, and Treatment of High Blood Cholesterol in Adults. Expert Panel on Detection, Evaluation, and Treatment of High Blood Cholesterol in Adults. JAMA 1993: 269:3015–3023.

144. Groot PH, van Stiphout WA, Krauss XH, et al. Postprandial lipoprotein metabolism in normolipidemic men with and without coronary artery disease. Arterioscler Thromb 1992;11:653–662.

145. Austin MA. Plasma triglyceride and coronary heart disease. Arterioscler Thromb 1991;11:2–14.

146. Gianturco SH, Bradley WA. A Cellular Basis for the Potential Atherogenicity of Triglyceride Rich Lipoproteins. In S Glagov, WP Newman, SA Schaffer (eds), Pathobiology of the Human Atherosclerotic Plaque. New York: Springer, 1990;513–524.

147. Auerbach O, Hammond EC, Garfinkel L. Smoking in relation to atherosclerosis of the coronary arteries. N Engl J Med 1965;273:775–779.

148. Busacca M, Dejana E, Balconi G, et al. Reduced prostacyclin production by cultured endothelial cells from umbilical arteries of babies born to women who smoke. Lancet 1982;2:609–610.

149. Wilhelmson L, Svardsudd K, Koran-Bengtsen K, et al. Fibrinogen as a risk factor for stroke and myocardial infarction. N Engl J Med 1984;311:501–505.

150. Ernst E, Hammerscmidt DE, Bagge U, et al. Leukocytes and the risk of ischemic disease. JAMA 1987;257:2318–2324.

151. Sternby NH. Atherosclerosis, Smoking, and Other Risk Factors. In AM Gotto, LC Smith, B Allen (eds), Atherosclerosis V. Proceedings of the Fifth International Symposium on Atherosclerosis. New York: Springer, 1980;647–653.

152. Tell GS, Howard G, McKinney WM. Risk factors for site specific extracranial carotid artery plaque distribution as measured by B-mode ultrasound. J Clin Epidemiol 1989; 42:551–559.

153. Lyons TJ. Glycation and oxidation: a role in the pathogenesis of atherosclerosis. Am J Cardiol 1993;71(Suppl B): 26B–31B.

154. Chisolm GM, Irwin KC, Penn MS. Lipoprotein oxidation and lipoprotein-induced cell injury in diabetes. Diabetes 1992;41(Suppl 2):61–66.

155. Brattstrom L, Lindgren A, Israelsson B, et al. Hyperhomocystinemia in stroke: prevalence, cause, and relationships to type of stroke and stroke risk factors. Eur J Clin Invest 1992;22:214–221.

156. Malinow MR, Nieto F, Szklo M, et al. Carotid artery intimal-medial wall thickening and plasma homocyst(e)ine in asymptomatic adults. The Atherosclerosis Risk in Community Study. Circulation 1993;87:1107–1113.

157. Taylor LM, DeFrang RD, Harris EJ, Porter JM. The association of elevated plasma homocyst(e)ine with progression of symptomatic peripheral arterial disease. J Vasc Surg 1991;13:128–136.

158. Mudd SH, Levy HL, Skovby F. Disorders of Transsulfuration. In CR Scriver, AL Beaudet, WS Sly, D Valle (eds), The Metabolic Basis of Disease (6th ed). New York: McGraw-Hill, 1989;23:693–734.

159. Welch GM, Loscalzo J. Homocysteine and atherothrombosis. N Engl J Med 1998;338:1042–1050.

160. Ridker PM, Hennekens CH, Buring JE, Rifai N. C-reactive protein and other markers of inflammation in the prediction of cardiovascular disease in women. N Engl J Med 2000;342:836–843.

161. Ridker PM, Cushman M, Stampfer MJ, et al. Inflammation, aspirin, and the risk of cardiovascular disease in apparently healthy men. N Engl J Med 1997;336:973–979.

162. Hwang SJ, Ballantyne CM, Sharrett AR, et al. Circulating adhesion molecules VCAM-1, ICAM-1, and E-Selectin in carotid atherosclerosis and incident coronary heart disease

cases: the Atherosclerosis in Community (ARIC) study. Circulation 1997;96:4219–4225.

163. Hangartner JG, Charleston AJ, Davies MJ, Thomas AC. Morphological characteristics of clinically significant coronary stenosis in stable angina. Br Heart J 1986:56:501–508.

164. Davies MJ. A macro and micro view of coronary vascular insult in ischemic heart disease. Circulation 1990;82 (Suppl II):38–46.

165. van der Wal A, Becker AE, van der Loos CM, Das PK. Site of intimal rupture or erosion of thrombosed coronary atherosclerotic plaques is characterized by an inflammatory process irrespective of the dominant plaque morphology. Circulation 1994;89:36–44.

166. Tracy RE, Devaney K, Kissling G. Characteristics of the plaque under a coronary thrombus. Virchows Arch 1985; 405:411–427.

167. Lendon CL, Davies MJ, Born GVR, Richardson PD. Atherosclerotic plaque caps are locally weakened when macrophage density is increased. Atherosclerosis 1991;87: 87–90.

168. Born GVR, Richardson PD. Mechanical Properties of Human Atherosclerotic Plaque. In SA Glagov, WP Newman, SA Schaffer (eds), Pathobiology of the Human Atherosclerotic Plaque. New York: Springer, 1990:413–423.

169. Ogata J, Masuda J, Yutani C, Yamaguchi T. Rupture of atheromatous plaque as a cause of thrombotic occlusion of stenotic internal carotid artery. Stroke 1990;21:1740–1745.

170. Carr SC, Farb A, Pearce WH, et al. Activated inflammatory cells are associated with plaque rupture in carotid artery stenosis. Surgery 1997;122:757–763.

171. Lammie GA, Sandercock PA, Dennis MS. Recently occluded intracranial and extracranial carotid arteries. Relevance of the unstable atherosclerotic plaque. Stroke 1999;30:1319–1325.

172. McCarthy MJ, Loftus IM, Thompson MM, et al. Angiogenesis and the atherosclerotic carotid plaque: an association between symptomatology and plaque morphology. J Vasc Surg 1999;30:261–268.

173. Davies MJ, Thomas AC. Plaque fissuring—the cause of acute myocardial infarction, sudden ischemic death, and crescendo angina. Br Heart J 1985;53:363–373.

174. Constantinides P. Plaque Hemorrhages, Their Genesis and Their Role in Supra-Plaque Thrombosis and Atherogenesis. In SA Glagov, WP Newman, SA Schaffer (eds), Pathobiology of the Human Atherosclerotic Plaque. New York: Springer, 1990:394–411.

175. Fisher CM, Ojemann RG. A clinico-pathologic study of endarterectomy plaques. Rev Neurol (Paris) 1986;142: 573–589.

176. Davies MJ, Woolf N. Atherosclerosis: what is it and why does it occur? Br Heart J 1993;69:3–11.

177. Ip JH, Fuster V, Badimon L, et al. Syndromes of accelerated atherosclerosis: role of vascular injury and smooth muscle proliferation. J Am Coll Cardiol 1990;15:1667–1687.

178. Davies MJ, Bland JM, Hangartner JR, et al. Factors influencing the presence or absence of acute coronary thrombi in sudden ischemic death. Eur Heart J 1989;10:203–208.

179. Falk E. Plaque rupture with severe pre-existing precipitating coronary thrombosis: characteristics of coronary atherosclerotic plaques underlying fatal occlusive thrombi. Br Heart J 1983;50:127–134.

180. Richardson PD, Davies MJ, Born GVR. Influence of plaque configuration and stress distribution on fissuring of coronary atherosclerotic plaques. Lancet 1989;2:941–944.

181. MacIsaac AI, Thomas JD, Topol EJ. Toward the quiescent plaque. J Am Coll Cardiol 1993;22:1228–1241.

182. Badimon JJ, Fuster V, Badimon L. Role of high density lipoproteins in the regression of atherosclerosis. Circulation 1992;(Suppl III):86–94.

183. Multiple risk factor intervention trial. Risk factor changes and mortality results. Multiple Risk Factor Intervention Trial Research Group. JAMA 1982;248:1465–1477.

184. Malinow MR. Atherosclerosis Regression and Arterial Repair. In S Glagov, WP Newman, SA Schaffer (eds), Pathobiology of the Human Atherosclerotic Plaque. New York: Springer, 1990;433–468.

185. Crouse JR, Thompson CJ. An evaluation of methods for imaging and quantifying coronary and carotid lumen stenosis and atherosclerosis. Circulation 1993;87:(Suppl II):17–33.

186. de Feyter PJ, Serruys PW, Davies MJ, et al. Quantitative coronary angiography to measure progression and regression of coronary atherosclerosis. Value, limitations, and implications for clinical trials. Circulation 1991;84:412–423.

187. Waters D, Lesperance J, Craven TE, et al. Advantages and limitation of serial coronary arteriography for the assessment of progression and regression of coronary atherosclerosis. Implications for clinical trials. Circulation 1993; 87:(Suppl II):38–47.

188. Buchwald H, Matts JP, Fitch LL, et al. Changes in sequential coronary arteriograms and subsequent coronary events. Surgical Control of the Hyperlipidemias (POSCH) Group. JAMA 1992;268:1429–1433.

189. Zarins CK, Giddens DP, Bharadvaj BK, et al. Differential enlargement of artery segments in response to enlarging atherosclerotic plaque. J Vasc Surg 1988;7:386–394.

190. Thomas AC, Davies MJ, Dilly S, Francs F. Potential errors in the estimation of coronary arterial stenosis from clinical arteriography with reference to the shape of the coronary arterial lumen. Br Heart J 1986;55:129–139.

191. Pignoli P, Tremoli E, Poli A, et al. Intimal plus medial thickness of the arterial wall: a direct measurement with ultrasound imaging. Circulation 1986;74:1399–1406.

192. Craven TE, Ryu JE, Espeland MA, et al. Evaluation of the associations between carotid artery atherosclerosis and coronary artery stenosis. A case-control study. Circulation 1990;82:1230–1242.

193. Wofford JL, Kahl FR, Howard GR, et al. Relationship of extracranial carotid artery atherosclerosis as measured by B-mode ultrasound to the extent of coronary atherosclerosis. Arterioscler Thromb 1991;11:1786–1794.

194. Borhani NO, Mercuri M, Borhani PA, et al. Final outcome results of the Multicenter Isradipine Diuretic Atherosclerosis Study (MIDAS). A randomized controlled trial. JAMA 1996;276(10):785–791.

195. Simons PC, Algra A, Bots ML, et al. Common carotid intima-media thickness and arterial stiffness: indicators of cardiovascular risk in high-risk patients. The SMART

Study (Second Manifestations of ARTerial disease). Circulation 1999;100(9):951–957.

196. Mercuri M, Bond MG, Sirtori CR, et al. Pravastatin reduces carotid intima-media thickness progression in an asymptomatic hypercholesterolemic Mediterranean population: the Carotid Atherosclerosis Italian Ultrasound Study. Am J Med 1996;101(6):627–634.

197. Zanchetti A, Bond MG, Henning M, et al. Risk factors associated with alterations in carotid intima-media thickness in hypertension: baseline data from the European Lacidipine Study on Atherosclerosis. J Hypertens 1998; 16(7):949–961.

198. Kanters SD, Algra A, van Leeuwen MS, Banga JD. Reproducibility of in vivo carotid intima-media thickness measurements: a review. Stroke 1997;28(3):665–671.

199. Crouse JR, Harpold GH, Kahl FR, et al. Evaluation of a scoring system for extracranial carotid atherosclerosis extent with B-mode ultrasound. Stroke 1986;17:270–275.

200. High Resolution B-mode ultrasound scanning methods in the Atherosclerosis Risk in Communities Study (ARIC). The ARIC Study Group. J Neuroimaging 1991;1:68–73.

201. High resolution B-mode ultrasound reading methods in the Atherosclerosis Risk in Communities (ARIC) cohort. The ARIC Study Group. J Neuroimaging 1991;1:168–172.

202. O'Leary DH, Bryan FA, Goodison MW, et al. Measurement variability of carotid atherosclerosis: real time (B-mode) ultrasonography and angiography. Stroke 1987;18: 1011–1017.

203. Hennerici M, Rautenberg W, Trockel U, Kladetzky RG. Spontaneous progression and regression of small carotid atheroma. Lancet 1985;1:1415–1419.

204. von Birgelen C, van der Lugt A, Nicosia A, et al. Computerized assessment of coronary lumen and atherosclerotic plaque dimensions in three-dimensional intravascular ultrasound correlated with histomorphometry. Am J Cardiol 1996;78:1202–1209.

205. Gotsman MS, Mosseri M, Rozenman Y, et al. Atherosclerosis studies by intracoronary ultrasound. Adv Exp Med Biol 1997;430:197–212.

206. Slager CJ, Wentzel JJ, Oomen JA, et al. True reconstruction of vessel geometry from combined X-ray angiographic and intracoronary ultrasound data. Semin Interv Cardiol 1997;2:43–47.

207. Estes JM, Quist WC, Lo Gerfo FW, Costello P. Noninvasive characterization of plaque morphology using helical computed tomography. J Cardiovasc Surg (Torino) 1998; 39:527–534.

208. Zimmermann GG, Erhart P, Schneider J, et al. Intravascular MR imaging of atherosclerotic plaque: ex vivo analysis of human femoral arteries with histologic correlation. Radiology 1997;204:769–774.

209. Yuan C, Beach KW, Smith LH, Hatsukami TS. Measurement of atherosclerotic carotid plaque size in vivo using high-resolution magnetic resonance imaging. Circulation 1998;98:2666–2671.

210. Brown BG, Zhao XQ, Sacco DE, Albers JJ. Lipid lowering and plaque regression. New insights into prevention of plaque disruption and clinical events in coronary disease. Circulation 1993;87:1781–1791.

211. Paterson RW, Paat JJ, Steele GH, et al. Impact of intensive lipid modulation on angiographically defined coronary disease: clinical implications. South Med J 1994;87:236–242.

212. Brown BG, Fuster V. Impact of Management in Stabilization of Coronary Disease. In V Fuster, R Ross, EJ Topol (eds), Atherosclerosis and Coronary Artery Disease. Philadelphia: Lippincott–Raven, 1996:191–205.

213. Effects of Pravastatin in patients with serum total cholesterol levels from 5.2 to 7.8 mmol/liter (200–300 mg/dl) plus two additional atherosclerotic risk factors. The Pravastatin Multinational Study Group for Cardiac Risk Patients. Am J Cardiol 1993;72:1031–1037.

214. Wissler RW, Vesselinovitch D. Can atherosclerotic plaques regress? Anatomic and biochemical evidence from nonhuman primate models. Am J Cardiol 1990;65: 33–40.

215. Armstrong ML, Megan MB. Lipid depletion in atheromatous coronary arteries in rhesus monkeys after regression diets. Circ Res 1972;30:675–680.

216. Armstrong ML, Megan MB. Arterial fibrous protein in cynomolgus monkeys after atherogenic and regression diets. Circ Res 1975;36:256–261.

217. Clarkson TB, Bond MG, Bullock BC, Marzetta CA. A study of atherosclerosis regression in Macaca mulatta. IV. Changes in coronary arteries from animals with atherosclerosis induced for 19 months and then regressed for 24 or 48 months at plasma cholesterol concentrations of 300 or 200 mg/dl. Exp Mol Pathol 1981;34:345–368.

218. Small DM, Bond MG, Waugh D, et al. Physiochemical and histological changes in the arterial wall of nonhuman primates during progression and regression of atherosclerosis. J Clin Invest 1984;73:1590–1605.

219. Kane JP, Malloy MJ, Ports TA, et al. Regression of coronary atherosclerosis during treatment of familial hypercholesterolemia with combined drug regimens. JAMA 1990;264:3007–3012.

220. Brown G, Albers JJ, Fisher LD, et al. Regression of coronary artery disease as a result of intensive lipid-lowering therapy in men with high levels of apolipoprotein B. N Engl J Med 1990;323:1289–1298.

221. Ornish D, Brown SE, Scherwitz LW, et al. Can lifestyle changes reverse coronary artery disease? The Lifestyle Heart Trial. Lancet 1990;336:129–133.

222. Blankenhorn DH, Nessim SA, Johnson RL, et al. Beneficial effects of combined colestipol-niacin therapy on coronary atherosclerosis and coronary venous bypass grafts. JAMA 1987;257:3233–3240.

223. Blankenhorn DH, Johnson RI, Mack WJ, et al. The influence of diet on the appearance of new lesions in human coronary arteries. JAMA 1990;263:1646–1652.

224. Brensike JF, Levy RI, Kelsey SF, et al. Effects of therapy with cholestyramine on progression of coronary atherosclerosis: results of the NHLBI Type II Coronary Intervention Study. Circulation 1984;69:313–324.

225. Cashin-Hemphill L, Mack WJ, Pogoda JM, et al. Beneficial effects of colestipol-niacin on coronary atherosclerosis. JAMA 1990;264:3013–3017.

226. Buchwald H, Varco RI, Matts JP, et al. Effect of partial ileal bypass surgery on mortality and morbidity from cor-

onary heart disease in patients with hypercholesterolemia. Report of the Program on the Surgical Control of the Hyperlipidemias. N Engl J Med 1990;323:946–955.

227. Watts GF, Lewis B, Brunt JN, et al. Effects on coronary artery disease of lipid–lowering diet, or diet plus cholestyramine in the St. Thomas Atherosclerosis Regression Study (STARS). Lancet 1992;339:563–569.

228. The Lipid Research Clinics Coronary Primary Prevention Trial results. II. The relationship of reduction in incidence of coronary heart disease to cholesterol lowering. JAMA 1984;251:365–374.

229. Lipid Research Clinics Coronary Primary Prevention Trial results. I. Reduction in incidence of coronary heart disease. II. The relationship of reduction in incidence of coronary heart disease to cholesterol lowering. JAMA 1984; 251:351–364.

230. Frick MH, Elo O, Heinonen OP, et al. Helsinki Heart Study. Primary-prevention trial with gemfibrozil in middle-aged men with dyslipidemia. Safety of treatment, changes in risk factors, and incidence of coronary heart disease. N Engl J Med 1987;317:1237–1245.

231. Blankenhorn DH, Azen SP, Kramsch DM, et al. Coronary angiographic changes with lovastatin therapy. The Monitored Atherosclerosis Regression Study (MARS). The MARS Research Group. Ann Intern Med 1993;119:969–976.

232. Waters D, Higginson L, Gladstone P, et al. Effects of monotherapy with an HMG-CoA reductase inhibitor on the progression of coronary atherosclerosis as assessed by serial quantitative arteriography. The Canadian Atherosclerosis Intervention Trial. Circulation 1994;89:959–968.

233. Dumont JM. Effect of cholesterol reduction by simvastatin on progression of coronary atherosclerosis: design, baseline characteristics, and progress of the Multicenter Anti-Atheroma Study (MAAS). Control Clin Trials 1993; 14:209–228.

234. Badimon JJ, Badimon L, Fuster V. Regression of atherosclerotic lesions by high density lipoprotein plasma fraction in the cholesterol-fed rabbit. J Clin Invest 1990;85: 1234–1241.

235. Yatsu FM, Fisher M. Atherosclerosis: current concepts on pathogenesis and interventional therapies. Ann Neurol 1989;26:3–12.

236. Gordon DJ, Rifkin BM. High-density lipoprotein—the clinical implications of recent studies. N Engl J Med 1989;321:1311–1316.

237. Randomized trial of cholesterol lowering in 4,444 patients with coronary heart disease: the Scandinavian Simvastatin Survival Study (4S). Lancet 1994;344:1383–1389.

238. Pedersen TR, Kjekshus J, Pyorala K, et al. Effects of simvastatin on ischemic signs and symptoms in the Scandinavian Simvastatin Survival Study (4S). Am J Cardiol 1998; 81:333–335.

239. Sacks FM, Pfeffer MA, Moye LA, et al. The effect of pravastatin on coronary artery events after myocardial infarction in patients with average cholesterol levels. Cholesterol and Recurrent Events Trial investigators. N Engl J Med 1996;335:1001–1009.

240. Plehn JF, Davis BR, Sacks FM, et al. Reduction of stroke incidence following myocardial infarction with pravasta-

tin: the Cholesterol and Recurrent Events (CARE) study. The CARE investigators. Circulation 1999;99:216–223.

241. Prevention of cardiovascular events and death in patients with coronary heart disease and a broad range of initial cholesterol levels. The Long Term Intervention with Pravastatin in Ischemic Disease (LIPID) Study Group. N Engl J Med 1998;339:1349–1357.

242. Rosenson RS, Tangney CC. Antiatherothrombotic properties of statins: implications for cardiovascular event reduction. JAMA 1998;279:1643–1650.

243. Strandberg TE, Vanhanen H, Tikkanen MJ. Effects of statins on C-reactive proteins in patients with coronary artery disease. Lancet 1999;353:118–119.

244. Bellosta S, Bernini F, Ferri N, et al. Direct vascular effects of HMG-CoA reductase inhibitors. Arteriosclerosis 1998;137:S101–S109.

245. Vaughn CJ, Delaney N. Neuroprotective properties of statins in cerebral ischemia and stroke. Stroke 1999;30: 1969–1973.

246. Frei B, Stocker R, Ames BN. Antioxidant defenses and lipid peroxidation in human blood plasma. Proc Natl Acad Sci U S A 1988;85:9748–9752.

247. Carew TE, Schwenke DC, Steinberg D. Antiatherogenic effect of probucol unrelated to its hypocholesterolemic effect: evidence that antioxidants in vivo can selectively inhibit low density lipoprotein degradation in macrophage-rich fatty streaks and slow the progression of atherosclerosis in the Watanabe heritable hyperlipidemic rabbit. Proc Natl Acad Sci U S A 1987;84:7725–7729.

248. Kita T, Nagano Y, Yokode M, et al. Probucol prevents the progression of atherosclerosis in Watanabe heritable hyperlipidemic rabbit, an animal model for familial hypercholesterolemia. Proc Natl Acad Sci U S A 1987;84: 5928–5931.

249. Schneider JE, Berk BC, Gravanis MB, ct al. Probucol decreases neointimal formation in a swine model of coronary artery balloon injury: a possible role for antioxidants. Circulation 1993;88:628–637.

250. Kuzuya M, Kuzuya F. Probucol as an antioxidant and antiatherogenic drug. Free Radic Biol Med 1993;14:67–77.

251. Walldius G, Regnstrom J, Nilsson J, et al. The role of lipids and antioxidative factors for development of atherosclerosis: the Probucol Quantitative Regression Swedish Trial (PQRST). Am J Cardiol 1993;71(Suppl):15B–19B.

252. Walldius G, Erickson U, Olsson AG, et al. The effect of probucol on femoral atherosclerosis: the Probucol Quantitative Regression Swedish Trial (PQRST). Am J Cardiol 1994;74:875–883.

253. Johansson J, Olsson AG, Bergstrand L, et al. Lowering of HDL2b by probucol partly explains the failure of the drug to affect femoral atherosclerosis in subjects with hypercholesterolemia. A Probucol Quantitative Regression Swedish Trial (PQRST) Report. Arterioscler Thromb Vasc Biol 1995;15:1049–1056.

254. Verlangieri AJ, Bush MJ. Effects of d-alpha-tocopherol supplementation on experimentally induced primate atherosclerosis. J Am Coll Nutr 1992;11:131–138.

255. Upston JM, Terentis AC, Stocker R. Tocopherol mediated peroxidation of lipoproteins: implications for Vitamin E

as a potential antiatherogenic agent. FASEB J 1999;13: 977–994.

256. Keaney JF, Simon DL, Freedman JE. Vitamin E and vascular homeostasis: implications for atherosclerosis. FASEB J 1999;13:965–976.

257. Clowes AW, Karnovsky MJ. Suppression by heparin of smooth muscle cell proliferation in injured arteries. Nature 1979;265:625–627.

258. Jonasson L, Holm J, Hansson GK. Cyclosporin A inhibits smooth muscle proliferation in the vascular response to injury. Proc Natl Acad Sci U S A 1988;85:2303–2306.

259. Jackson CL, Bush RC, Bowyer DE. Inhibitory effect of calcium antagonists on balloon catheter induced arterial smooth muscle cell proliferation and lesion size. Atherosclerosis 1988;69:115–122.

260. Yatsu FM, Alam R, Alam S. Enhancement of cholesteryl ester metabolism in cultured human monocyte-derived macrophages by verapamil. Biochim Biophys Acta 1985;847:77–81.

261. Powell JS, Clozel J-P, Muller RK, et al. Inhibitors of angiotensin-converting enzyme prevent myointimal proliferation after vascular injury. Science 1989;245:186–188.

262. Chobanian AV, Haudenschild CC, Nickerson C, Hope S. Trandolapril inhibits atherosclerosis in the Watanabe heritable hyperlipidemic rabbit. Hypertension 1992;20:473–477.

263. Water D, Lesperance J, Francetich M, et al. A controlled clinical trial to assess the effect of a calcium channel blocker on the progression of coronary atherosclerosis. Circulation 1990;82:1940–1953.

264. Lichtlen PR, Hugenholtz PG, Rafflenbeul W, et al. Retardation of angiographic progression of coronary artery disease by nifedipine. Lancet 1990;335:1109–1113.

265. Goodnight SH. Fish oil and vascular disease. Trends Cardiovasc Med 1992;1:112–116.

266. Fisher M, Leaf A, Levine PH. N-3 fatty acids and cellular aspects of atherosclerosis. Arch Intern Med 1989;149: 1726–1728.

267. Weiner BH, Ockene IS, Levine PH. Inhibition of atherosclerosis by cod-liver oil in a hyperlipidemic swine model. N Engl J Med 1986;315:841–846.

268. Davis HR, Bridenstine RT, Vesselinovitch D, Wissler RW. Fish oil inhibits development of atherosclerosis in rhesus monkeys. Arteriosclerosis 1987;7:441–449.

269. Harker LA, Kelly AB, Hanson SR, et al. Dietary n-3 fatty acid interruption of vascular thrombus formation and vascular lesion formation in nonhuman primates. Circulation 1993;87:1017–1029.

270. Zhu B, Parmley WW. Modification of experimental and clinical atherosclerosis by dietary fish oil. Am Heart J 1990;119:168–178.

271. von Schacky C, Angerer P, Kothny W, et al. The effect of dietary omega-3 fatty acids on coronary atherosclerosis. A randomized, double blind, placebo controlled trial. Ann Intern Med 1999;130:554–562.

Chapter 9
Antiplatelet Aggregant Therapy to Prevent Stroke

Natan M. Bornstein

Stroke remains a major cause of worldwide morbidity and mortality, imposing an enormous economic burden that knows no borders. In most industrialized countries, it is the third leading cause of death and the primary cause of physical disability in people older than 60 years of age. Stroke is predicted to become an even larger burden over the next 25 years, given the aging of the population and the increase in other risk factors.[1] Recurrent stroke is also a major cause of mortality and morbidity among stroke survivors.[2] The high incidence and serious consequences of stroke make it one of the most important challenges faced by contemporary medicine. The limited effectiveness of current therapeutic approaches for acute stroke dictates that emphasis be placed on strategies for prevention. Large clinical trials conducted worldwide have enabled investigators to make significant progress in this area. In this chapter, current knowledge of antiaggregant strategies in stroke prevention is reviewed and how the results of some studies have impacted the conceptual approach to preventing stroke is examined.

Acetylsalicylic Acid (Aspirin)

History

Aspirin, or acetylsalicylic acid (ASA), is an old and widely used drug. Its antithrombotic role is the basis of its clinical use for prevention of stroke. The development of ASA as an active drug for stroke prevention involved some important milestones. Several cultures have known of the salutary effects of willow bark (saltix alba) for centuries. Salicin, its active ingredient, is a bitter glycoside, from which sodium salicylate was isolated in 1829 by Leroux, who demonstrated its antipyretic effects. The pharmaceutical chemist Hoffman found a way of acetylating the hydroxyl group on the benzene ring of salicylic acid to form ASA, which was shown to have anti-inflammatory and analgetic effects. ASA was introduced into clinical medicine at the turn of the twentieth century under the name "aspirin," which was given to the new drug by Bayer's chief pharmacologist, Heinrich Dreser.[3] In 1953, Craven suggested that ASA may act as an anticoagulant; in 1956, he suggested that it might prevent ischemic vascular disease.[4,5] In 1963, Blatrix[6] noted that ASA increases bleeding time. The inhibitory effect of this compound on the action of blood platelets was not discovered until the late 1960s.[7] In 1968, O'Brien[8] described a specific inhibitory effect of ASA on the aggregation response of blood. This property was linked to the irreversible inhibition of the cyclooxygenase enzyme responsible for the synthesis of eicosanoids (prostacyclin [PGI_2] and thromboxane A_2 [TxA_2]) and involved in arachidonic acid metabolism,[9] which is responsible for the conversion of arachidonic acid to TxA_2 in platelets and PGI_2 in the vascular wall.[10]

Mechanism of Action

Aspirin competes with arachidonic acid to bind with the hydroxyl group of a single amino acid residue (serine 529) in the polypeptide chain of platelet prostaglandin G/H synthase 1. As a result, aspirin completely and irreversibly inhibits the action of the enzyme cyclooxygenase, thereby suppressing the production of TxA_2 in platelets, which in turn induces platelet aggregation and vasoconstriction. This irreversible effect persists for the life span of the platelet. Aspirin also reduces the production of PGI_2 in the vessel wall, an effect that inhibits platelet aggregation and induces vasodilation, and, therefore, might have some antithrombogenic effect. Endothelial cells can rapidly recover from the inhibitory effect of aspirin on cyclooxygenase synthesis, however, in contrast to platelets.[11,12] In addition to its platelet antiaggregant effect, aspirin has other actions that may potentially play a role in stroke prevention, namely anti-inflammatory and antioxidant activities. Aspirin is rapidly absorbed in the stomach and upper intestine; peak plasma concentration occurs 15–20 minutes after ingestion, and the platelet antiaggregant activity is evident within 1 hour after administration.[12] Thus, the inhibitory effect is rapid and lasts for the life span of the platelet. Some effects of aspirin on hemostasis are cyclooxygenase-independent and should be taken into account. For example, aspirin may increase fibrinolytic activity for up to 4 hours after its administration[13] and may lower vitamin K–dependent clotting factors II, VII, IX, and X.[14] However, the dose-response relationship, duration, occurrence in clinical setting, and relevance to the antithrombotic effect of aspirin have not been established.

In summary, the two opposing actions of aspirin on blood platelets—blocking the proaggregatory and vasoconstrictive effects of TxA_2, and diminishing vasodilatation and antiaggregant activity of PGI_2—led to the coining of the term *aspirin dilemma*.[15] The aspirin dilemma refers mainly to the debate concerning the use of higher versus lower doses of aspirin in patients who are considered at high risk of cerebrovascular thrombosis.

Primary Prevention

Several trials aimed at investigating the use of aspirin for primary prevention of stroke yielded inconclusive results.

The Physicians' Health Study[16] was a double-blind, placebo-controlled trial conducted among 22,071 male physicians in the United States taking 325 mg ASA every other day with or without beta carotene. Participants ranged in age from 40 to 84 years; average follow-up was 5 years. The study revealed a 44% reduction in the incidence of myocardial infarction (MI)—a finding that resulted in the early termination of the study. Over the 5-year period, the incidence of cardiovascular death was similar in the ASA and placebo groups. A statistically insignificant increased risk of all stroke types, particularly for the small subgroup of hemorrhagic strokes (23 versus 12), was shown in the ASA-treated group compared with the placebo group. However, the number of events was too small to draw any firm conclusions.

The British Doctors' Trial[17] randomized 5,139 male physicians, age 50–78 years, in an open design, with one group taking 500 mg ASA per day (two-thirds of participants) and one group advised to avoid ASA (one-third of participants). This trial was unblinded, unbalanced, and smaller and less rigid than the Physicians' Health Study. After 6 years, there was no statistically significant difference between the two groups, either for the combined outcome event (vascular death, stroke, or MI), or for any of these events alone.[18] However, there was a slight increase in disabling strokes and a decrease in transient ischemic attacks (TIAs) among the ASA group. Limited data were available on which of the strokes were hemorrhagic and which were thrombotic, but these showed no excess of any particular type of stroke within the ASA group.

Barnett[19] suggested that any primary prevention studies designed to evaluate possible stroke reduction should be required to continue for 10 years longer or involve a population of subjects 10 years older than those in these two studies, because stroke incidence peaks 10 years later in life than MI.

An overview of these two trials of primary prevention[18,20] showed a 32% reduction in the odds of experiencing a nonfatal MI (SD ± 8%) and a 13% reduction of the combined vascular events (SD ± 6%), but a nonsignificant increase for nonfatal stroke (18% SD ± 13%). The results of these two studies led to the conclusion that routine use of ASA by healthy men may not be universally recommended when the side effects of ASA are compared with the reduction in risk of nonfatal MI.[18,21]

The Nurses' Health Study[22] included females taking one to six aspirin per week or placebo and was conducted in the United States. The analysis was based on 87,678 registered nurses, aged 34–65 years, and free of diagnosed coronary heart disease, stroke, and cancer at baseline. The study demonstrated that women who had taken ASA had a reduced risk of a first MI, but no alteration in the risk of stroke was observed. Cardiovascular death was slightly but not significantly reduced in the ASA group.

Several points should be emphasized regarding these studies. They included individuals who were engaged in health services and therefore could be considered as comprising an especially health-conscious group. This also may explain the rate of vascular events among study participants being lower than expected in the general population. Kronmal et al.[23] reported that aspirin use was associated with increased risk for ischemic stroke in women and hemorrhagic stroke in both men and women in a cohort of elderly people. The authors mentioned the possibility of there having been some confounding of results stemming from aspirin use per se, as opposed to cause and effect. In the Hypertension Optimal Treatment,[24] another randomized study in which 9,391 hypertensive patients were assigned to receive 75 mg aspirin per day and 9,391 patients received placebo, there was a significant beneficial effect of aspirin on MI (36% reduction) but there was no effect on stroke. In these studies, there was a small but definite chance of adverse events (i.e., bleeding), with approximately 1 in 1,000 cases of excessive bleeding due to aspirin.

Hart et al.[25] performed a meta-analysis to define the effect of aspirin use for primary prevention of stroke and other major vascular events. Five randomized trials were included, with 52,251 subjects randomized to aspirin doses ranging from 75 to 650 mg per day. There was no significant reduction of stroke by aspirin in persons without vascular risk factors (relative risk = 1.08; 95% confidence interval [CI], 0.95–1.24). Intracranial hemorrhage was increased by the regular use of aspirin (relative risk = 1.35; P = .03). In four large observational studies, self-selected use of aspirin was consistently associated with higher rates of stroke. However, aspirin was found to have a protective effect against stroke in patients with manifest vascular disease (P = .001). The authors concluded that when aspirin is given for primary prevention of vascular events, the dose should be 75–81 mg per day. The efficacy of ASA for stroke reduction in patients with asymptomatic carotid stenosis is

doubtful. In a double-blind, placebo-controlled trial, Cote et al.[26] demonstrated that ASA did not have a significant long-term protective effect in asymptomatic patients with high-grade (>50%) carotid stenosis. The median duration of follow-up was 2.3 years. The annual rate of all ischemic events and death from any cause was 12.3% for the placebo group and 11.0% for the ASA group (P = .61). The annual rates for vascular events only were 11% for the placebo group and 10.7% for the ASA group (P = .99).

The role of ASA in preventing initial stroke in patients with nonvalvular atrial fibrillation (NVAF) remains unclear. Only two placebo-controlled, randomized, primary prevention trials in patients with atrial fibrillation (AF) were performed, using warfarin and different doses of ASA. They were terminated early as monitoring of the results showed significant differences.[27]

The Atrial Fibrillation, Aspirin, Anticoagulation (AFASAK) study and the Stroke Prevention in Atrial Fibrillation (SPAF) study, conducted in Denmark[28] and the United States,[29] respectively, formally evaluated the use of ASA as an alternative treatment. The AFASAK study used 75 mg ASA per day and the SPAF trial used 325 mg ASA per day. Another study, the Boston Area Anticoagulation Trial for Atrial Fibrillation,[30] which was not specifically designed to evaluate the role of ASA, allowed patients in the placebo group to receive 325 mg ASA per day. The Boston Area Anticoagulation Trial for Atrial Fibrillation and AFASAK trial were not blinded, whereas the SPAF study was blinded for ASA but not for warfarin therapy.

In the AFASAK study,[28] 1,007 patients were randomly assigned to receive warfarin, ASA (75 mg/day), or placebo. After 2 years, the incidence of stroke, TIA, and systemic embolism was significantly lower in the warfarin group (1.5%) than in the ASA and placebo group (6% each). Analysis showed the risk of important vascular events was reduced by approximately 20% in the ASA group; however, the small number of vascular events that occurred during the trial resulted in a considerable amount of uncertainty about the results. The trial was reported as negative with respect to ASA. Its unblinded design and the fact that 38% of patients assigned to the warfarin group withdrew from this study, however, in addition to the efficacy analysis, necessitated confirmation of these findings by other trials.[27]

In the SPAF study,[29] 588 patients with NVAF were randomly selected to receive warfarin, ASA (325 mg/day), or placebo. In addition, 656 patients not eligible for treatment with warfarin received ASA or placebo in a double-blind design. After 1 year, the placebo arm of the study was terminated because active treatment (either warfarin or ASA) reduced the risk of stroke and systemic embolism by 81%. The study also revealed that ASA reduced the risk of stroke and embolism by 50%, but was not effective in patients older than 75 years of age. Various mechanisms of stroke may explain the lack of effectiveness of ASA in the AFASAK study compared to the SPAF study. The AFASAK study entered older patients who were probably at a higher risk of stroke than those in the SPAF study. This difference may be related to a higher prevalence of left atrial or ventricular stasis-related thrombi, which are anticoagulant sensitive, in the older patients in the AFASAK study, as indicated by the threefold to fourfold higher incidence of heart failure and the twofold higher incidence of previous MI in patients in that study. ASA reduced the occurrence of stroke categorized as noncardioembolic significantly more than it did in those categorized as cardioembolic ($P = .01$), an important finding of the SPAF investigation.[31] Another difference between the two studies was the lower dose of ASA used in the AFASAK study, compared to the dose used in the SPAF study. In addition, the Danish study included more females, which may be another confounder. Thus, ASA may have some stroke prevention benefit in patients with NVAF who tend to develop platelet-rich in situ thrombi or emboli. In these patients, AF is probably only a marker of vascular disease rather than a cause of left arterial thromboembolism.[32]

In light of these findings, there are no approved prescription indications for aspirin in the primary prevention of cerebrovascular disease at the time of this writing, and formal policy recommendations should await randomized trial results. In the meantime, the American Heart Association suggests that aspirin benefit may outweigh the harm in men with high risk for coronary disease, but no guidelines have been issued for women.

Secondary Prevention

Since the late 1970s, many clinical trials have been conducted to determine the value of aspirin in the prevention of ischemic stroke. The first placebo-controlled, randomized trial was done in Canada.[33] It involved almost 600 patients—290 patients assigned to the two groups that included aspirin treatment, compared with 295 patients assigned to one of two groups that did not take the drug—and showed that 1,300 mg aspirin per day reduced the incidence of stroke and death by 31%.

Another randomized, controlled study conducted in France on 604 patients with previous TIAs (16%) or completed stroke (84%) showed that 1,000 mg aspirin per day significantly reduced the risk of stroke (40%) in both sexes, but the mortality rate was not reduced.[34] In this study, co-treatment with dipyridamole (DP) did not offer additional benefits. Several other trials have been conducted with different doses of aspirin, ranging from 30 to 1,000 mg per day. The results of three trials were published in 1991. One was the final report of the United Kingdom Transient Ischemic Attack (UK-TIA) Aspirin Trial,[35] in which 2,435 patients with TIA or minor stroke were randomly assigned to receive "blind" treatment with 1,200 mg or 300 mg aspirin per day, or placebo. Mean patient follow-up was approximately 4 years. Outcomes (i.e., death, MI, and stroke) were similar in the two aspirin groups, and neither dose of aspirin was significantly better than placebo. It is noteworthy that the number of patients in each aspirin group was 815 and 806, respectively, which might be too small to rule out a type II error. In the final analysis, which combined both aspirin dose groups, the investigators found a significant reduction (15%) in the risk of death, MI, and stroke, but only a 7% reduction in disabling stroke and death, and 3% reduction in disabling stroke and vascular death. It is important to mention that the population of the UK-TIA study was somewhat different from other stroke studies, in that there was a relatively low annual rate of stroke (3.2%) in the placebo group, compared to 5.9–7.3% reported in other studies.[33,36]

A randomized double-blind Dutch TIA trial[36] compared the effectiveness of 30 mg aspirin per day to 283 mg aspirin per day on the occurrence of nonfatal stroke, MI, and vascular death in patients after TIA or minor stroke. A total of 3,131 patients were included and followed for an average of 2.6 years. No significant difference was found in vascular events between the 30 mg aspirin per day group (14.7%), compared with the group receiving 283 mg aspirin per day (15.2%). The Swedish

Aspirin Low-Dose Trial[37] was a double-blind, randomized trial that compared 75 mg aspirin per day with placebo for the prevention of stroke and death after TIA or minor stroke. The 1,360 study participants were followed for a mean of 32 months. There was a significant reduction (18%) in the primary outcome events (stroke or death).

In 1994, the Antiplatelet Trialists' Collaboration published the results of a meta-analysis,[20] in which they analyzed 18 placebo-controlled clinical trials involving 10,000 patients with TIAs or minor stroke. Allocation to a mean duration of 33 months of antiplatelet therapy produced a highly significant ($P <.00001$) reduction in risk of experiencing another vascular event, such as MI, stroke, or vascular death (37/1,000; SD = 8). The proportional reduction in important vascular events in these trials was 22% (SD = 5%).

Algra and Van Gijn[38] conducted a small meta-analysis on data from 10 randomized trials of aspirin only versus control treatment in 6,171 patients after TIA or minor stroke. They concluded that aspirin at any dose above 30 mg per day prevents 13% (95% CI, 4–12) of vascular events.

The data of meta-analyses are not free of criticism. In comparing the results of already published studies, difficulties are apparent due to the strikingly different methodologies that were used and diagnoses that were not determined under the same conditions. It should be asked whether the same therapy may be applied after TIA as well as after stroke. The criteria used to evaluate the effectiveness of the therapy varies, and little information concerning the compliance of the patients to criteria is given.

Comparisons can be direct or indirect, and the latter is not always acceptable. Dyken[39] warned that direct comparisons between clinical trials are difficult because of variations in the type of patients entered, duration of treatment, quality of follow-up, and endpoint definitions. He also warned that several variables other than the drug under investigation could influence the size of risk reduction between trials. There are other problems with making comparisons between studies that test high doses of ASA and those examining low doses. Many of the former studies were performed up to 15 years before the latter were carried out, and the changes in medical treatment of hypertension or heart disease may have altered the impact of ASA.

Dose of Aspirin

The issue of determining the optimal dose of aspirin is still controversial[38,40–44] and will remain unresolved until a proper trial comparing low doses (approximately 100 mg/day) to a high dose (1,000 mg/day) is conducted. In any event, a medium dose of aspirin (75–325 mg/day) is now the most widely used regimen as antiplatelet therapy for secondary stroke prevention.[45,46]

Adverse Effects

Regular use of aspirin increases the risk of gastrointestinal (GI) side effects, such as epigastric pain, peptic ulcer, gastritis, and GI bleeding. Administration of enteric-coated aspirin (but not the buffered type) may lessen the damage to the gastric mucosa.[47–49] In both the UK-TIA and the Dutch TIA trials, the bleeding complications were more frequent in the higher aspirin dose group. In the UK-TIA trial, GI bleeding occurred in 1.6% of patients on placebo, 2.6% of patients on 300 mg aspirin, and 4.7% of patients on 1,200 mg aspirin, and approximately one-half of the patients in each group required hospitalization. It is widely believed that all site bleeding with aspirin is not dose-related.[40] In the Dutch TIA, although major bleeding occurred only slightly less in the 30 mg aspirin group, minor bleeding occurred significantly less. Regarding aspirin and hemorrhagic stroke, in a meta-analysis of 16 randomized controlled trials involving 55,462 participants, aspirin use was associated with an absolute risk increase for hemorrhagic stroke of 12 events per 10,000 persons (95% CI, 5–20; $P <.001$).[50] In the Cardiovascular Health Study,[23] there was a fourfold increase (95% CI, 1.6–10.0) in risk of hemorrhagic stroke for both frequent and infrequent users of aspirin ($P = .003$).

Ticlopidine

Mechanism of Action

Ticlopidine hydrochloride is a potent inhibitor of platelet aggregation with a different mechanism of action than that of aspirin, although its mechanism of action is uncertain.[51] It appears that ticlopidine selectively inhibits adenosine diphosphate (ADP)–induced fibrinogen binding to platelets, but the exact molecular mechanism by which this is accomplished is unknown. Because ticlopidine is not a cyclooxygenase inhibitor, it has no effect on PGI_2 production. Ticlopidine is extensively metabolized by the liver, and, unlike aspirin, steady-state plasma concentrations are obtained only after a few days of repeated administration of 250 mg twice daily.

Secondary Prevention

Two major trials were conducted to determine the efficacy of ticlopidine in secondary stroke prevention. The Ticlopidine Aspirin Stroke Study (TASS)[52] was a triple-blind study comparing the effect of 1,300 mg aspirin per day and ticlopidine, 250 mg twice daily, in 3,069 patients with TIA (1,300) or minor stroke who were followed for up to 5.8 years. The primary analysis was an intent-to-treat assessment of death from all causes and nonfatal stroke. Ticlopidine effected a 13% greater reduction than aspirin in the primary endpoints (i.e., death and nonfatal stroke) and a 21% reduction in the 3-year event rate for fatal or nonfatal stroke. It is interesting to note that there was 42% relative risk reduction (RRR) for stroke and death in the first year. This reduction was largely maintained over the 2 years immediately after the study, but declined to 21% after 3 years. The superiority of ticlopidine over aspirin in the reduction of stroke was seen in both males and females.

The Canadian-American Ticlopidine Study (CATS)[53] was a randomized, double-blind, placebo-controlled trial involving 1,072 patients with a substantial completed stroke, rather than TIA or minor stroke, as in TASS. Patients were randomly assigned to receive ticlopidine, 250 mg twice daily, or placebo. The primary outcome events were a combination of recurrent nonfatal stroke, nonfatal MI, and vascular death. Follow-up lasted for an average of 2 years. This appears to be the largest trial to assess stroke recurrence in patients who experienced a major stroke. Using the efficacy approach, the cumulative events rate for the primary endpoints per year was 15.3% in the placebo group and 10.8% in the ticlopidine group (RRR, 30.2%; $P = .006$). Intent-to-treat analysis yielded an RRR of 23.3%

($P = .02$). Efficacy was found in both sexes. In addition, a Japanese TIA study[54] involving 170 patients assigned to receive 200 mg ticlopidine per day and 170 assigned to receive 500 mg aspirin per day found ticlopidine to be superior to aspirin, although the difference in this study was not statistically significant. Outcome events in this study included TIA, stroke, and MI.

Adverse Effects

The adverse effects of ticlopidine commonly described in both the CATS and TASS trials were mild GI complaints—mainly diarrhea (20.4%)—and skin rash (12%). The most important and threatening hematologic side effect was severe neutropenia (less than 0.45×10^9 /liter), which occurred within 3 months of treatment onset with a frequency of 0.8–0.9%. All adverse side effects were reversed with cessation of the study drug. Another severe side effect of ticlopidine, thrombotic thrombocytopenic purpura, with a mortality rate possibly as high as 33%, was more recently reported.[55] Due to these side effects, monitoring of complete blood cell counts and white cell differentials is required. In summary, TASS showed ticlopidine to be superior to aspirin in the prevention of all strokes and stroke plus death. CATS data provided strong evidence that ticlopidine conveys a clinically important reduction in the risk of stroke in patients with completed ischemic stroke. In general, it is assumed that ticlopidine reduces the relative risk of vascular events by an additional 10–20% more than the 15–20% risk reduction effect of aspirin, with only a small risk of reversible severe neutropenia (0.86%).

Clopidogrel

Clopidogrel is a thienopyridine derivative that is chemically related to ticlopidine.

Mechanism of Action

Clopidogrel blocks activation of platelets by ADP. This is achieved by selectively and irreversibly inhibiting the binding of ADP to its receptor on platelets, thereby affecting ADP-dependent activation of the glycoprotein IIb-IIIa (GPIIb-IIIa) complex platelet surface.[56]

Secondary Prevention

A large, randomized, blinded, international trial of clopidogrel versus aspirin in patients at risk of ischemic events (CAPRIE) was conducted and reported in 1996.[57] CAPRIE, which involved 19,185 patients, was the largest clinical trial of a secondary prevention strategy to prevent various vascular endpoints in a high-risk population. The trial was designed to assess the relative efficacy of 75 mg clopidogrel per day and 325 mg aspirin per day in reducing the risk of a composite outcome cluster of ischemic stroke, MI, or vascular death. Three clinical subgroups of patients at significant risk of vascular events—those with recent ischemic stroke (6,431), recent MI (6,302), or symptomatic peripheral arterial disease (PAD) (6,452)—were followed for up to 3 years. The result of the outcome cluster showed a significant RRR of 8.7% in favor of clopidogrel (95% CI, 0.3–16.5%; P = .043) and an absolute risk reduction of 0.51%. There were no significant differences in adverse events between the two regimens; specifically, there was no increased risk of neutropenia in the clopidogrel group. In a post hoc analysis, there were significant differences in the RRR for each of the three clinical subgroups, with the most striking effect appearing in patients with PAD (RRR, 23.8%; CI, 8.9–36.2). For stroke patients, there was a statistically insignificant benefit for clopidogrel over aspirin (RRR, 7.3%; 95% CI, 5.7–18.7). However, the trial was not powered to detect a realistic treatment effect in each of the three clinical subgroups. Moreover, an additional analysis of patients in the ischemic stroke and PAD subgroups with a previous history of MI demonstrated clear benefit for clopidogrel over aspirin. Hence, the conclusion of this study appears to strongly confirm and be consistent with the previous ticlopidine studies. When the absolute risk reduction of 0.5% is taken in consideration, it is calculated that 200 patients per year would need to be treated with clopidogrel rather than aspirin to prevent one adverse clinical event. Thus, it seems probable that clopidogrel will replace ticlopidine, but that it is less likely to replace aspirin as the first-line therapy for

secondary stroke prevention, given its only modest superiority and presumed higher cost.

Dipyridamole

Mechanism of Action

The principal mechanisms by which DP has been assumed to inhibit platelet function are[58]

- Inhibition of cyclic guanosine monophosphate-specific phosphodiesterase in platelets, resulting in an increase in intraplatelet cyclic guanosine monophosphate levels and a consequent potentiation of the platelet-inhibiting action of PGI_2.
- Direct stimulation of the release of PGI_2 by the vascular endothelium.
- Inhibition of the cellular uptake and metabolism of adenosine, thereby increasing its level at the platelet-vascular interface.

The absorption of DP from conventional formulations is variable and may result in low systemic bioavailability of the drug. A new modified-release formulation of DP with low-dose aspirin was developed with improved bioavailability and with a half-life of 10 hours (DP is eliminated by biliary excretion).

Secondary Prevention

The second European Stroke Prevention Study (ESPS-2) was a randomized, placebo-controlled, double-blind trial comparing the effect of low-dose aspirin (50 mg/day), modified-release DP (400 mg/day), and the combination of both drugs with the effects of placebo in 6,602 patients with a prior ischemic stroke or TIA.[59] The investigators reported that the combined therapy was more effective in preventing stroke (37% relative risk reduction) than aspirin alone (18.1% reduction) or DP alone (16.3% reduction). For the combination endpoint of stroke and death, the combined therapy was associated with a 24.4% relative risk reduction. The combination of aspirin and DP compared with aspirin alone was associated with a 12.9% (95% CI, 0–25%; P = .056) RRR in primary outcome event of stroke and death, and

22% (95% CI, 9–33%) relative event reduction for vascular death, nonfatal stroke, or nonfatal MI.[60,61]

None of the treatments significantly reduced the risk of death alone or fatal stroke. Before the ESPS-2, the four studies that had compared the combination of aspirin and DP with aspirin alone in TIA and stroke patients had collectively shown that the combination of the two drugs was associated with only a 3% (95% CI, –22% to 22%) reduction in the vascular events.[60]

These results are somewhat different from the result obtained by ESPS-2. A meta-analysis of all trials, including ESPS-2, indicates that among the 2,473 patients with prior stroke or TIA who were assigned to the combination of aspirin and DP, 356 (14.6%) experienced a vascular event, compared with 419 (17.2%) of the 2,436 patients assigned to receive aspirin—a RRR of 15% (P = .012).[61] In a review of all the DP trials, Wilterdink and Easton[62] concluded that DP plus aspirin reduces the odds of nonfatal stroke by approximately 25% over aspirin alone (99% CI, 0.09–0.42; P = .005), but surprisingly did not reduce MI and vascular death.

The results of ESPS-2 were criticized for several reasons:

1. There were ethical concerns regarding the use of a placebo arm when the efficacy of aspirin was proven.
2. Among the 25% of patients who withdrew from the study, most were in the DP and combination groups, and compliance was higher among patients assigned to DP (97%) than in those assigned to aspirin (84%).
3. The low dose of aspirin (50 mg/day) was considered to be inappropriate.

Adverse Effects

Headache is the most common adverse effect associated with DP. Bleeding was reported in 4.7% of the patients assigned to receive DP, and it occurred in 8.8% of combination regimen patients in the ESPS-2 trial. GI bleeding occurred in 1.6% of patients assigned to DP alone and 1.7% of those on placebo.

In summary, based on the current data, it seems that the combination of DP plus aspirin may be substantially better than aspirin, and according to the results of the meta-analysis, the combination of aspirin and DP prevents twice as many vascular events as does aspirin alone. However, some uncertainty regarding DP remains.

Atrial Fibrillation

Special attention has been paid to NVAF since the 1990s. The prevalence of AF increases with age, with a prevalence of approximately 5% of people older than 65 years of age and 10% of people older than 80 years of age. Also, approximately 30% of individuals with AF are unaware of their condition (NVAF). Approximately 15% of all ischemic strokes are associated with NVAF, with the frequency increasing with age. Approximately one-third of the patients with ischemic strokes older than 70 years have AF. On the other hand, the risk of stroke in people with NVAF increases fivefold, from 1% to 5% per year. Thus, AF has been accepted as an independent risk factor for stroke, and comprises approximately 45% of all cardioembolic strokes. Most ischemic strokes in patients with AF are likely due to embolism of thrombi from the left atrium and, in particular, its appendage. These thrombi are easily detected by transesophageal echocardiography.

In the 1990s, six clinical trials were conducted to test the efficacy of antithrombotic agents in reducing stroke in NVAF subjects.[63–66] Five were primary prevention studies and one was a secondary prevention study. Pooled data from all the primary prevention studies have shown that warfarin is highly efficacious in preventing stroke, reduces stroke risk by approximately two-thirds, and is relatively safe when the international normalized ratio is kept between 2.0 to 3.0.[63,64] Aspirin, on the other hand, offers much less benefit and should be used only in low-risk populations (e.g., young subjects with lone AF or no other vascular risk factors).[65]

Risk factors for stroke in AF include hypertension, prior TIA or stroke, left ventricular systolic dysfunction, diabetes, and coronary artery disease. One of the most worrisome aspects about treatment with warfarin is bleeding. However, the absolute increase in the rate of severe hemorrhage among the elderly, as reported in various studies, was 0.3–2.0% per year. It is known that the risk of major hemorrhage among elderly AF patients taking warfarin is related to the intensity of anticoagulation and age.

For secondary prevention in AF patients with TIA and stroke, the only study conducted was the European Atrial Fibrillation Trial.[66] Compared to placebo, the rate of recurrent stroke was nonsignificantly reduced by aspirin (15%), but was impressively reduced by warfarin (66%). The rate of major bleeding for patients on warfarin was 3% per year. The recommended international normalized ratio for secondary prevention is 3.0 (range, 2.0–3.9).[67]

Glycoprotein IIb/IIIa Antagonists

Although they are effective in preventing thromboembolic complications, the efficacy of antiplatelet drugs currently in use is limited, and a significant number of serious thromboembolic events still occur. GPIIb/IIIa has been identified as the final common pathway for all platelet agonists.[68] The binding of adhesive proteins, such as fibrinogen, to GPIIb/IIIa causes platelets to aggregate. Thus, many research groups have concentrated on developing small-molecule GPIIb/IIIa antagonists to find an agent that inhibits platelet activation in response to all agonists of platelet activators.[69] In cardiology, the combination of aspirin and a parenteral GPIIb/IIIa blocker was proven to be significantly more effective than aspirin alone in reducing the 30-day rate of death or nonfatal MI for patients with unstable angina or non-Q wave MI, or those undergoing percutaneous coronary intervention.[70] These agents are in the early stages of clinical trials. In the future, clinicians may have a potent and more efficacious antiplatelet drug for preventing ischemic thromboembolic events.

Conclusions

Primary Prevention

There is no substantial evidence to recommend aspirin for primary stroke prevention in high-risk groups. Aspirin could even be harmful considering its adverse side effects. However, in certain patients with nonvascular AF who are considered at low-risk (i.e., age <65 years, no high-risk features) for embolic stroke (approximately 1% per year) or when warfarin is contraindicated, 325 mg aspirin per day is recommended.

Secondary Prevention

Antiplatelets are the pivotal drugs in preventing recurrent stroke or other major vascular events in patients who have undergone TIA or stroke.

Aspirin

Aspirin is the most widely used secondary prevention therapy, although its effect is modest (RRR = 20%), and, despite the fact that the optimal dose has not been determined, most physicians use between 100 to 325 mg per day as a maintenance dose. For patients who develop stroke on aspirin treatment, the options are either to increase the dose of aspirin or to administer another platelet antiaggregant. No study has yet been performed to provide conclusive evidence for these approaches.

Clopidogrel and Dipyridamole

In patients who can not tolerate aspirin, or have had a stroke while on aspirin ("aspirin failure"), the options are clopidogrel, 75 mg per day, or sustained-release DP, 200 mg, combined with low-dose aspirin (25 mg twice daily).

Combined Aspirin/Clopidogrel

An approach that is appealing, but not yet proven, is to combine aspirin and clopidogrel with different modes of action to achieve a better and more effective antithrombotic effect. Further controlled trials are needed to justify the use of the aspirin-clopidogrel combination.

References

1. Kaste M, Fogelholm R, Rissanen A. Economic burden of stroke and the evaluation of new therapies. Public Health 1998;112:103–112.
2. Bornstein NM, Korczyn AD. Prevention of Recurrent Stroke. In JW Norris, V Hachinski (eds), Prevention of Stroke. New York: Springer, 1985;261–268.
3. Flower RJ, Moncada S, Vane JR. Analgetic-Antipyretics and Anti-Inflammatory Agents: Drugs Employed in the Treatment of Gout. In AG Gilman, IS Goodman, TW Rall, F Murad (eds), Goodman and Gilman's The Pharmaco-

logical Basis of Therapeutics (7th ed). New York: Macmillan, 1985;674–675.

4. Craven LL. Experience with aspirin (acetylsalicylic acid) in the non-specific prophylaxis of coronary thrombosis. Mississippi Valley Med J 1953;75:38–44.

5. Craven LL. Prevention of coronary and cerebral thrombosis. Mississippi Valley Med J 1956;78:213.

6. Blatrix C. Allongement du temps de saignement sous l'influence de certains medicaments. Nouv Rev Franc Hemat 1963;3:346.

7. Weiss HJ, Aledort LM. Impaired platelet-connective-tissue reaction in man after aspirin ingestion. Lancet 1967; 2:495–497.

8. O'Brien JR. Effects of salicylates on human platelets. Lancet 1968;1:779–783.

9. Majerus PW. Arachidonate metabolism in vascular disorders. J Clin Invest 1983;72:1521–1525.

10. Weksler BB, Pett SB, Alonso D, et al. Differential inhibition by aspirin of vascular and platelet prostaglandin synthesis in atherosclerotic patients. N Engl J Med 1983;308: 800–805.

11. Jaffe EA, Weksler BB. Recovery of endothelial cell prostacyclin production after inhibition by low doses of aspirin. J Clin Invest 1979;63:532–535.

12. Patrono C. Aspirin as an antiplatelet drug. N Engl J Med 1994;330:1287–1294.

13. Bjornsson TD, Scheider DE, Berger H. Aspirin acetylates fibrinogen and enhances fibrinolysis. J Pharmacol Exp Ther 1989;250:154–161.

14. Lekstrom JA, Bell WR. Aspirin in the prevention of thrombosis. Medicine (Baltimore) 1991;70:161–178.

15. van Gijn J. Aspirin: Dose and Indications in Modern Stroke Prevention. In HJ Barnett, VC Hachinski (eds), Cerebral Ischemia: Treatment and Prevention. Philadelphia: Saunders, 1992;193–208.

16. Final report on the aspirin component of the ongoing Physicians' Health Study. Steering Committee of the Physicians' Health Study Research Group. N Engl J Med 1989; 321:129–135.

17. Peto R, Gray R, Collins R, et al. Randomised trial of prophylactic daily aspirin in British male doctors. BMJ 1988;296:313–316.

18. Hennekens CH, Buring JE, Sandercock P, et al. Aspirin and other antiplatelet agents in the secondary and primary prevention of cardiovascular disease. Circulation 1989; 80:749–756.

19. Barnett HJ. 35 years of stroke prevention: challenges, disappointments and successes. Cerebrovasc Dis 1991;1:61–70.

20. Collaborative overview of randomised trials of antiplatelet therapy. I. Prevention of death, myocardial infarction, and stroke by prolonged antiplatelet therapy in various categories of patients. Antiplatelet Trialists' Collaboration. BMJ 1994;308:71–106.

21. Herbert P, Fuster V, Hennekens CH. Antiplatelet and Anticoagulant Therapy in Evolving Myocardial Infarction and Primary Prevention. In V Fuster, M Verstraete (eds), Thrombosis in Cardiovascular Disorders. Philadelphia: Saunders, 1992;261–273.

22. Manson JE, Stampfer MJ, Colditz GA, et al. A prospective study of aspirin use and primary prevention of cardiovascular disease in women. JAMA 1991;266:521–527.

23. Kronmal RA, Hart RG, Manolio TA, et al. Aspirin use and incident stroke in the cardiovascular health study. CHS Collaborative Research Group. Stroke 1998;29:887–894.

24. Hansson L, Zanchetti A, Carruthers SG. Effects of intensive blood-pressure lowering and low-dose aspirin in patients with hypertension: principal results of the Hypertension Optimal Treatment (HOT) randomised trial. The HOT Study Group. Lancet 1998;351:1755–1762.

25. Hart RG, Halperin JL, McBride R, et al. Aspirin for the primary prevention of stroke and other major vascular events: meta-analysis and hypotheses. Arch Neurol 2000; 57:326–332.

26. Cote R, Battista RN, Abrahamowicz M, et al. Lack of effect of aspirin in asymptomatic patients with carotid bruits and substantial carotid narrowing. The Asymptomatic Cervical Bruit Study Group. Ann Intern Med 1995; 123:649–655.

27. Ezekowitz MD, Cohen IS, Gornick CC, et al. Atrial Fibrillation. In WG Daniel, I Kronson, A Mugge (eds), Cardiogenic Embolism. Baltimore: Williams & Wilkins, 1996;27–44.

28. Petersen P, Boysen G, Godtfredsen J, et al. Placebo-controlled, randomized trial of warfarin and aspirin for prevention of thromboembolic complications in chronic atrial fibrillation. The Copenhagen AFASAK Study. Lancet 1989;1:175–179.

29. Stroke Prevention in Atrial Fibrillation Study. Final results. Circulation 1991;84:527–539.

30. The effect of low-dose warfarin on the risk of stroke in nonrheumatic atrial fibrillation. Boston Area Anticoagulation Trial for Atrial Fibrillation Investigators. N Engl J Med 1990;323:1505–1511.

31. Miller VT, Rothrock JF, Pearce LA, et al. Ischemic stroke in patients with atrial fibrillation: effect of aspirin according to stroke mechanism. Stroke Prevention in Atrial Fibrillation Investigators. Neurology 1993;43:32–36.

32. Chesebro JH, Fuster V, Halperin JL. Atrial fibrillation—risk marker for stroke. N Engl J Med 1990;323:392–394.

33. A randomized trial of aspirin and sulfinpyrazone in threatened stroke. The Canadian Cooperative Study Group. N Engl J Med 1978;299:53–59.

34. Bousser MG, Eschwege E, Haguemau M, et al. "AICLA" controlled trial of ASA and dipyridamole in the secondary prevention of atherothrombotic cerebral ischemia. Stroke 1983;15:5–14.

35. Farrell B, Godwin J, Richards S, Warlow C. The United Kingdom Transient Ischemic Attack (UK-TIA) Aspirin Trial. Final results. J Neurol Neurosurg Psychiatry 1991; 54:1044–1054.

36. A comparison of two doses of aspirin (30 mg vs. 283 mg a day) in patients after a transient ischemic attack of minor ischemic stroke. The Dutch TIA Study Group. N Engl J Med 1991;325:1261–1266.

37. Swedish Aspirin Low-Dose Trial (SALT) of 75 mg aspirin as secondary prophylaxis after cerebrovascular ischemic events. The SALT Collaborative Group. Lancet 1991;338: 1345–1349.

38. Algra A, van Gijn J. Aspirin at any dose above 30 mg offers only modest protection after cerebral ischaemia. J Neurol Neurosurg Psychiatry 1996;60:197–199.

39. Dyken ML. Meta-analysis in the assessment of therapy for stroke prevention. Cerebrovasc Dis 1992;2(Suppl):35–40.

40. Adams HP, Bendixen BH. Low- versus high-dose aspirin in prevention of ischemic stroke. Clin Neuropharmacol 1993;16:485–500.
41. Dyken ML, Barnet HJ, Easton DJ, et al. Low-dose aspirin and stroke. "It ain't necessarily so." Stroke 1992;23:1395–1399.
42. Hart RG, Harrison MJ. Aspirin wars: the optimal dose of aspirin to prevent stroke. Stroke 1996;27:585–587.
43. Barnett HJ, Kaste M, Meldrum H, Eliasziw M. Aspirin dose in stroke prevention; beautiful hypotheses slain by ugly facts. Stroke 1996;27:588–592.
44. Patrono C, Roth GJ. Aspirin in ischemic cerebrovascular disease. How strong is the case for a different dosing regimen? Stroke 1996;27:756–760.
45. Hennerici MG. Aspirin dosage—a never-ending story? Cerebrovasc Dis 1995;5:308–309.
46. Goldstein LB, Farmer A, Matchar DB. Primary care physician-reported secondary and tertiary stroke prevention practices. A comparison between the United States and the United Kingdom. Stroke 1997;28:746–751.
47. Robbins DC, Schwartz RS, Kutny K, et al. Comparative effects of aspirin and enteric-coated aspirin on loss of chromium 51-labeled erythrocytes from the gastrointestinal tract. Clin Ther 1984;6:461–466.
48. Lanza FL, Rover GL, Nelson RS. Endoscopic evaluation of the effects of aspirin, buffered aspirin, and enteric-coated aspirin on gastric and duodenal mucosa. N Engl J Med 1990;303:136–138.
49. Kelly JP, Kaufman DW, Jurgelon JM, et al. Risk of aspirin-associated major upper-gastrointestinal bleeding with enteric-coated or buffered product. Lancet 1996;348:1413–1416.
50. He J, Whelton PK, Vu B, Klag MJ. Aspirin and risk of hemorrhagic stroke: a meta-analysis of randomized controlled trials. JAMA 1998;280:1930–1935.
51. Kent RA. Ticlopidine. Lancet 1991;337:459–460.
52. Hass WK, Easton JD, Adams HP, et al. A randomized trial comparing ticlopidine hydrochloride with aspirin for the prevention of stroke in high-risk patients. Ticlopidine Aspirin Stroke Study Group. N Engl J Med 1989;321:501–507.
53. Gent M, Blakely JA, Easton JD, et al. The Canadian American Ticlopidine Study (CATS) in thromboembolic stroke. Lancet 1989;1:1215–1220.
54. Tohgi H, Murakami M. The effect of ticlopidine on TIA compared with aspirin. A double-blind, 12-month and open 24-month follow-up study. Jpn J Med 1987;26:49–51.
55. Bennett CL, Weinberg PD, Rozenberg-Ben-Dror K, et al. Thrombotic thrombocytopenic purpura associated with ticlopidine. A review of 60 cases. Ann Intern Med 1998;128:541–544.
56. Herber JM, Frehel D, Vallee E, et al. Clopidogrel, a novel antiplatelet and antithrombotic agent. Cardiovasc Drug Rev 1993;11:180–198.
57. A randomised, blinded trial of clopidogrel versus aspirin in patients at risk of ischaemic events (CAPRIE). CAPRIE Steering Committee. Lancet 1996;348:1329–1339.
58. Kappelle LJ, Adams HP, Bendixen BH. Antiaggregant Therapy for Stroke Prevention. In MD Ginsberg, J Bogousslavsky (eds), Cerebrovascular Disease: Pathophysiology, Diagnosis, and Management. Malden, MA: Blackwell Science, 1998;1826–1838.
59. Diener H, Cunha L, Forbes C, et al. European Stroke Prevention Study. 2. Dipyridamole and acetylsalicylic acid in the secondary prevention of stroke. J Neurol Sci 1996;143:1–13.
60. van Gijn J, Algra A. Secondary stroke prevention with antithrombotic drugs: what to do next? Cerebrovasc Dis 1997;7(Suppl 6):30–32.
61. Hankey GJ. One year after CAPRIE, IST and ESPS 2. Any changes in concepts? Cerebrovasc Dis 1998;8(Suppl 5):1–7.
62. Wilterding JL, Easton JD. Dipyridamole plus aspirin in cerebrovascular disease. Arch Neurol 1999;56:1087–1092.
63. Risk factors for stroke and efficacy of antithrombotic therapy in atrial fibrillation. Analysis of pooled data from five randomized controlled trials. Atrial Fibrillation Investigators. Arch Intern Med 1994;154:1449–1457.
64. Hylek EM, Skates SJ, Sheehan MA, Singer DE. An analysis of the lowest effective intensity of prophylactic anticoagulation for patients with nonrheumatic atrial fibrillation. N Engl J Med 1996;335:540–546.
65. The efficacy of aspirin in patients with atrial fibrillation. Analysis of pooled data from 3 randomized trials. The Atrial Fibrillation Investigators. Arch Intern Med 1997;157:1237–1240.
66. Secondary prevention in non-rheumatic atrial fibrillation after transient ischaemic attack or minor stroke. EAFT (European Atrial Fibrillation Trial) Study Group. Lancet 1993;342:1255–1262.
67. Optimal oral anticoagulant therapy in patients with non-rheumatic atrial fibrillation and recent cerebral ischemia. The European Atrial Fibrillation Trial Study Group. N Engl J Med 1995;333:5–10.
68. Philips DR, Charo IF, Scarborough RM. GPIIb-IIIa: the responsive integrin. Cell 1991;65:359–362.
69. Mousa SA, DeGrado WF, Mu D-X, et al. Oral antiplatelet, antithrombotic efficacy of DMP 728, a novel platelet GPIIb/IIIa antagonist. Circulation 1996;93:537–543.
70. Topol EJ. Toward a new frontier in myocardial reperfusion therapy. Emerging platelet prominence. Circulation 1998;97:211–218.

Chapter 10
Medical Therapy for Cardioembolic Stroke

David C. Tong and Gregory W. Albers

It is estimated that cardiac sources of embolization (SOE) are responsible for approximately 20% (range, 15–45%) of all ischemic strokes.[1,2] Recently, there has been increasing awareness of a variety of additional cardiac and proximal aortic SOE that may be responsible for a significant percentage of strokes of previously unknown origin. The discovery of these newer causes of cerebral embolization has led to increased interest in obtaining a more thorough evaluation of potential proximal embolic sources, although the most appropriate treatment for many of these conditions remains unclear.

Principles of Management

When deciding on the management of a patient with a presumed cardiac or aortic source of embolization, the clinician is frequently faced with the problem of estimating the risk versus the benefit of specific therapies. Three important issues should be considered:

1. What is the risk of embolic events associated with the condition in question?
2. How effective is the proposed therapy in reducing the risk of recurrent events?
3. What are the risks of the treatment?

A fourth factor of increasing importance is the question of whether the chosen approach is cost-effective. Not surprisingly, these decisions are difficult in many patients because limited data are available for many conditions. Moreover, even when clinical trial data on the risks and benefits of

a particular treatment are available, it may be difficult to extrapolate these results to an individual patient. Nevertheless, focusing on these questions helps organize the decision-making process.

Treatment Options

For most patients with a cardiac or proximal aortic SOE, the primary treatment decision involves whether to institute oral anticoagulant therapy. The clinician is frequently faced with balancing the effectiveness of anticoagulation for stroke prevention with the potential risk of hemorrhagic complications. The goal is to assess the absolute risk/benefit ratio for the individual patient being considered for therapy.

This problem is particularly well illustrated by patients with such cardioembolic risk factors as a patent foramen ovale (PFO) or atrial septal aneurysm (ASA). For these conditions, the risks and benefits of different treatments have not been adequately established. In these situations, clinician judgment, rather than objective data, plays a substantially greater role in the decision-making process.

Risks of Anticoagulation

The only major complication of oral anticoagulant treatment is bleeding. This risk is increased in many anticoagulation candidates due to concomitant bleeding risk factors, such as a history of prior bleeding. In addition, there is the added cost and inconvenience

Table 10-1. Relative Embolic Risk of Various
Cardiac Conditions

High-risk embolic sources
  Prosthetic cardiac valves
  Atrial fibrillation
  Aortic arch atheroma
  Recent myocardial infarction
  Dilated cardiomyopathy
  Left ventricular thrombus
  Mitral stenosis
  Infective endocarditis
  Marantic endocarditis
  Rheumatic valvular disease
  Atrial myxoma
Low-risk embolic sources
  Mitral valve prolapse
  Mitral annular calcification
Embolic sources of uncertain significance
  Patent foramen ovale
  Atrial septal aneurysm

of laboratory monitoring. Controversy exists regarding the true risk of anticoagulant-associated bleeding in community practice compared with the controlled setting of randomized clinical trials. For example, most clinical trials of atrial fibrillation (AF) patients report a major hemorrhage rate of between 1% to 2% per year in patients receiving dose-adjusted anticoagulation. In contrast, some community-based outpatient studies have reported significantly higher major bleeding rates of up to 6% per year,[3–7] although others have reported rates similar to those seen in clinical trials.[8,9] The most important factor associated with bleeding complications is the degree of anticoagulation. Increasing age has also been a significant factor in several studies.[10]

If an individual patient's estimated bleeding risk is high, the benefit of anticoagulant treatment is reduced, making the decision to institute anticoagulant therapy more difficult. However, many patients still benefit from anticoagulant therapy, despite the increased bleeding risk.

Cardiac and Aortic Sources of Embolization: Overview

Cardioembolic sources of stroke can be divided into major and minor types. Major cardioembolic

risk factors include a variety of high-risk conditions, such as prosthetic mechanical heart valves (MHVs) (Table 10-1). In general, these cardiac sources require aggressive treatment with anticoagulation because of the substantial risk of both primary and recurrent ischemic events. In some conditions, such as AF, for example, absolute stroke risk has been stratified, and in a minority of cases anticoagulation may not be necessary at all. Minor embolic sources are believed to have a much lower, but still elevated, risk of embolization. In addition, there are a number of newly discovered conditions for which the risk of embolization is uncertain. These conditions are among the most problematic to treat because the risk of recurrence is uncertain.

Major Cardioembolic Etiologies

Prosthetic Cardiac Valves

The role of anticoagulation in patients with MHVs is well established. Patients possessing MHVs have a substantially increased risk of both cerebral and systemic embolization. Although few data are available on the risk of stroke in untreated patients with MHVs, the annualized risk (extrapolated from follow-up studies of 3 or 4 months' duration) has been reported to be between 12% to 22%, depending on valve location and type.[11] This risk can be reduced to approximately 0.5–4.0% per year with anticoagulation.[12,13] Patients with multiple valves or a valve in the mitral position, as well as other cardiac risk factors, such as AF, are at higher risk.[13] Older style cage-ball heart valves (e.g., Starr-Edwards) have a higher embolic potential than modern tilting disk (e.g., Björk-Shiley) or bi-leaflet (e.g., St. Jude Medical) valves.[12] The frequency of embolization with bi-leaflet and tilting disk valves on anticoagulation ranges from 0.5–0.7% per year.[12]

Although higher levels of anticoagulation (international normalized ratio [INR] 3.5–4.5) have been advocated, some studies have suggested that lower levels of anticoagulation cause less bleeding and do not increase the risk of systemic embolization. An INR of 2.0–3.0 for bi-leaflet aortic valves and 2.5–3.5 for most other valve types has been recommended.[12] Older cage-ball–type valves are believed to require higher intensities of anticoagulation, although the optimum level is unknown. Fortunately, few such valves are currently in use.

Combining oral anticoagulation with either aspirin or dipyridamole (DP) treatment has also been investigated. In these studies, aspirin doses of 100–660 mg per day in combination with anticoagulation (INR, 2.0–4.5) were associated with a similar or lower rate of subsequent ischemic events compared with anticoagulation alone.[14–17] However, combination therapy has also been associated with an increased risk of bleeding complications in some,[14] but not all,[17] studies. An INR of 2.0–3.0 plus aspirin (330 mg b.i.d.) and DP (75 mg t.i.d.),[17] as well as fixed-dose warfarin plus aspirin (100 mg) and DP (75 mg t.i.d.),[18] have also been reported to be safe and effective. Thus, anticoagulant therapy in conjunction with antiplatelet therapy may be more effective than anticoagulation alone. Nevertheless, at present, combination treatment is generally reserved for high-risk patients because of the potential increase in the risk of bleeding. High-risk patients include individuals who have developed thromboembolic complications while therapeutically anticoagulated and patients with a particularly high risk of embolization, including those with multiple MHVs or other associated risk factors, such as AF, that substantially increase their thromboembolic potential.[12]

Patients with bioprosthetic heart valves do not require long-term anticoagulation.[12] During the first 3 months after valve implantation, however, anticoagulation is indicated because of an increased risk of stroke during the initial perioperative time period, particularly in patients receiving a mitral valve replacement. The frequency of embolic events is particularly high in the first 10 days after surgery.[19] An INR of 2.0–3.0 is recommended.[12] The long-term rate of thromboembolism in these patients is between 0.2% to 2.9% per year.[20–23] Aspirin therapy is generally recommended after the first 3 months to reduce this long-term risk. In clinical trials, the dose of aspirin used has generally been between 500 mg to 1 g per day. However, it is likely that lower doses have similar effectiveness and doses as low as 160 mg have been advocated.[12] In patients with additional risk factors, such as AF, treatment should be modified to address the highest risk condition.

Atrial Fibrillation

AF is the most common cardiac cause of stroke. It has been estimated that between 11% to 29% of all ischemic strokes are associated with this arrhythmia.[1]

No condition better illustrates the important balance between the risks and benefits of anticoagulant therapy than AF. A meta-analysis of 16 AF trials indicates that the overall risk of stroke can be reduced by an average of 62% with anticoagulation (68% for ischemic stroke alone).[24] Aspirin is estimated to reduce ischemic stroke by approximately 20% and appears to have the greatest effect on non-cardioembolic events. Noncardioembolic strokes are estimated to account for approximately one-third of the strokes that occur in AF patients. Anticoagulation appears to produce the same relative risk reduction in both primary and secondary stroke prevention.[25–32] The risk of stroke associated with AF varies greatly, however, ranging from 0.5% to 17% per year.[27–29,33,34] Thus, individualization of therapy is of great importance in this condition, due to the wide variation in the absolute benefit of therapy depending on the patient's individual risk profile.

For example, AF patients younger than 65 years old with no additional stroke risk factors (i.e., lone AF), have an annual stroke rate of only 0.5–1.0% per year. Thus, although such a patient still experiences a 60–70% relative risk reduction in stroke incidence with anticoagulation, the absolute degree of stroke risk reduction is less than 1%. In this situation, the small absolute benefit of anticoagulation does not appear to justify routine anticoagulation. This example clearly illustrates that appropriate risk stratification can have a major impact on the management of individual AF patients.

Several major risk stratification schemes have emerged. They are remarkably consistent, identifying a history of hypertension, diabetes, prior stroke or transient ischemic attack (TIA), and older age (age >65 years in one study,[35] women >75 years in another[36]) as risk factors. These studies also indicate that evidence of heart failure (recent heart failure,[37] impaired left ventricular [LV] function, or cardiomegaly on chest x-ray) are additional risk factors.[35,37,38] These results are summarized in Table 10-2. In general, AF patients younger than 75 years old with no identifiable additional risk factors have a low risk of cerebral embolization

Table 10-2. Risk Stratification for Patients with Atrial Fibrillation

Risk Factors*	Recommended Therapy
Any high risk factor *or* >1 moderate risk factor	Warfarin (target INR 2.5; range, 2.0–3.0)
One moderate risk factor	Aspirin, 80–325 mg q.d., or warfarin (target INR 2.5; range, 2.0–3.0)
No high risk factors *and* no moderate risk factors	Aspirin, 80–325 mg q.d.

INR = international normalized ratio.
*High risk factors: Prior transient ischemic attack, systemic embolus or stroke; history of hypertension; poor left ventricular function; age >75 years; rheumatic mitral valve disease; prosthetic heart valve. Moderate risk factors: Age 65–75 years, diabetes mellitus, coronary artery disease.

and do not require anticoagulant therapy. The vast majority of AF patients possess at least one risk factor, however, and are therefore appropriate candidates for anticoagulation.

The risk of anticoagulant-related hemorrhage in AF patients has been extensively studied. In clinical trials, the risk of major hemorrhage has been reported to be between 0.6% to 4.2% per year. Higher hemorrhage rates have been associated with higher intensities of anticoagulation and increasing age.[39] In fact, most hemorrhages have been reported to occur when the INR was >3.0.[40]

Aspirin reduces the risk of recurrent stroke in AF patients by approximately 20%.[41] Aspirin should be considered in AF patients who are not candidates for anticoagulation or who are at low risk of stroke. Combination therapy with fixed-dose warfarin and low-dose aspirin has been evaluated, and is ineffective.[29] Lower intensities of anticoagulation (INRs 1.5–2.0) are substantially less effective for stroke prevention compared with INRs ≥2.[29,42] There is no clear evidence of a difference in relative risk of stroke associated with chronic versus intermittent AF, although patients with intermittent AF tend to have fewer associated risk factors and, therefore, generally have lower stroke rates.[35,37,43]

Patients with sick-sinus syndrome (SSS) and atrial flutter may also be candidates for anticoagulation. These arrhythmias are often seen in conjunction with AF, and thus it is not surprising that there may be an increased risk of stroke associated with these conditions. In one long-term follow-up study, SSS was associated with a 2.3% annual thromboembolic risk.[44,45] However, the absolute rate of stroke is difficult to accurately determine because of the common coexistence of AF. The rate of embolization is lower in patients with dual-chamber pacemakers compared with ventricular pacemakers.[44,46] All patients with SSS who experience thromboembolic events should be considered for anticoagulation, however, regardless of pacer type, especially if their risk of hemorrhagic complications is low.

Acute Myocardial Infarction

Patients experiencing an acute myocardial infarction (MI) have a stroke risk of approximately 2% (range, 1–5%) within 2–4 weeks.[1] This risk is particularly high in patients experiencing an anterior wall MI (2–6%), probably because these infarctions are associated with an increased incidence of LV thrombi.[47] Up to 40% of acute MI patients develop LV thrombi.[47] Although anticoagulation reduces the risk of stroke in these patients by approximately 50–70%, the absolute risk reduction is only approximately 0.5 per 100 patient years.[48,49] Thus, for most MI patients this degree of small risk reduction does not justify long-term anticoagulation, and antiplatelet treatment is recommended unless another high-risk condition is present, such as LV thrombus, severe LV dysfunction, or AF. Similarly, in patients with an MI and a mural thrombus, anticoagulation is frequently recommended. The optimal duration of anticoagulant therapy in these patients is uncertain. Treatment for 3 months is typically advocated, because most thrombi resolve within this interval, and the recurrent embolization risk is generally agreed to drop significantly after the acute phase unless another high-risk source is present.[1,12]

Other High-Risk Cardioembolic Sources

Other potential high-risk embolic sources are listed in Table 10-1. In general, the appropriate treatment of these conditions is long-term anticoagulation with warfarin due to the high risk of systemic embolization.

One exception is bacterial endocarditis. Anticoagulation is generally not indicated due to the presumed increased risk of hemorrhagic complications, including rupture of mycotic aneurysms and hemorrhage from septic emboli. Although anticoagulation is generally recommended in prosthetic valve endocarditis, one study suggests that even in this situation anticoagulation should be withheld, at least until the infection is under control.[50] In all cases of bacterial endocarditis, appropriate antibiotic treatment remains the mainstay of management.

Patients with cardiac tumors are another exception, because they generally require surgery rather than anticoagulation for definitive management. Atrial myxoma is the most common tumor, although other tumors, such as fibroelastomas, can rarely occur.[1] Patients usually present with nonspecific constitutional symptoms and systemic embolization. In these patients, surgical resection is necessary for cure. The role of acute anticoagulation while awaiting surgical management in these patients is unclear.

Another possible exception is marantic endocarditis. Also known as *nonbacterial thrombotic endocarditis*, it is believed to be caused by noninfectious vegetations on cardiac valves that are frequently too small to appreciate on either transthoracic (TTE) or transesophageal echocardiography (TEE). There is an association between NBTE and malignancy, sepsis, systemic lupus, erythematosus, the antiphospholipid antibody syndrome, as well as disseminated intravascular coagulation.[51,52] In contrast to other embolic sources, nonbacterial thrombotic endocarditis has been reported to have a greater response to heparin than warfarin therapy, although data substantiating this observation are sparse.[53]

Cardiac Conditions of Low or No Risk

Previously, mitral valve prolapse was believed to be a significant cardiac source of cerebral embolization based on several case control studies. When larger, population-based studies were performed, however, the relationship between mitral valve prolapse and stroke was found to be minimal to nonexistent. Similarly, although mitral annular calcification has also been associated with stroke,[54] the absolute risk is low, and prophylaxis is generally not indicated unless the patient is symptomatic and other SOE have been completely excluded.[55]

Cardiac Conditions of Uncertain Significance

Patent Foramen Ovale and Atrial Septal Aneurysm

The risk of recurrent stroke associated with either PFO or ASA is unknown and has varied widely, ranging from 1.0% to 14.5% per year in reported small series.[56–59] It is likely that the risk associated with PFO is quite variable and probably depends on both the specific morphologic features of the cardiac abnormality as well as the presence of other stroke risk factors. One major problem with attributing an individual patient's stroke to a PFO is the high prevalence of PFO in the general population: It is estimated that the prevalence of PFO in the general population is between 10% to 35%.[60–65] Thus, differentiating symptomatic versus coincidental PFOs is problematic. The proportion of PFOs is higher in younger patients with strokes, however, and in patients without another identifiable cardiac cause.[63,65–67] In addition, because PFO and ASA are frequently present in the same person, it is difficult to determine the relative risk related to each abnormality individually. In fact, the combination of the two conditions has been associated with a higher risk of stroke than either abnormality alone in some studies.[67,68]

Several PFO characteristics have been associated with an increased risk of stroke. Increasing PFO size, as determined by a greater right-to-left shunt and a larger PFO aperture on TEE, has been associated with an increased risk of recurrent cerebral ischemic events.[65,68,69] It has also been suggested that clinically relevant PFOs are generally so large that they can be identified by TTE alone.[65] However, TEE remains the study of choice for identifying this condition.[70] Strokes involving the posterior cerebral artery distribution, as well as strokes associated with migraine, have also been reported to be more common in patients with PFOs, although these observations are based on small numbers and require confirmation.[56] In addition, larger infarcts and multiple infarcts in superficial territories have been reported to be more frequent in patients with large (≥4 mm) PFOs.[69]

A number of unanswered questions remain regarding PFO and stroke risk. First, there are technical concerns regarding identification and morphologic characterization of PFOs. For example, the echocardiographic technique (i.e., bi-plane versus multi-plane) and the diagnostic criteria used to define large versus small cardiac shunts have both varied substantially between different case series. In addition, the methods used for quantifying the degree of shunting have varied among different investigators. For example, the number of bubbles crossing the intra-atrial septum has been used in some series, whereas the relative percentage of contrast in the left atrium within the first few cardiac cycles after injection has been used in others. Clearly, more uniform standards would be helpful. However, it appears that some patients at high risk for stroke recurrence can be identified, probably those with a larger PFO opening (≥4–5 mm), substantial shunting (various criteria), and perhaps the presence of an ASA.

ASAs are far less common than PFOs. Some studies report a prevalence of between 1.9% to 10.0% in the general population, although some series with more rigid inclusion criteria estimate a prevalence of approximately 2%.[60,67,71,72] Several studies have shown a significant relationship between ASAs and stroke, particularly if associated with a PFO.[72,73]

It is difficult to estimate the recurrent stroke risk associated with these two conditions. The small number of patients in reported series and the paucity of natural history studies limit any estimates of stroke recurrence rates. In addition, the recurrent stroke rate is generally assessed while the patient is receiving a stroke prevention therapy, making determination of the natural history of these conditions even more difficult.

One study, for example, found a recurrent stroke rate of 1.9%, but more than one-half the patients received either anticoagulation or surgical closure of their PFOs.[56] In contrast, another study reported a 25% stroke recurrence rate at a mean follow-up of 22 months in patients with "large" PFOs, for an average rate of 14% per year.[57] However, 25% of the patients in this study had other cardiac embolic sources, such as AF and LV thrombus, making an estimate of risk attributable to the PFO alone more difficult. In this study, the use of anticoagulant versus antiplatelet therapy had no significant effect on the rate of recurrence. In contrast, others have reported a benefit of warfarin or surgery compared with ASA or no treatment.[58] These conflicting reports reflect the difficulty in obtaining accurate data upon which to make treatment decisions.

Overall, however, current data suggest at least some benefit to preventive therapy, although the absolute risk/benefit ratio remains unclear.

Because data from prospective randomized clinical trials are lacking, decision modeling has been used to aid in assessing the risks and benefits of various treatments. In one analysis, a Markov model was used to assess the risk/benefit ratio of aspirin versus warfarin versus surgery for PFOs over a wide range of risk-recurrent stroke rates.[74] This analysis found that if the recurrent stroke rate was ≥0.8% per year, both warfarin and surgery had similar benefit, resulting in an increase of 0.4–0.6 quality-adjusted life years compared with antiplatelet or no treatment. Surgery was slightly superior to warfarin therapy. It should be noted that the model was strongly dependent on the estimated stroke rate, as well as the anticoagulation-associated hemorrhage risk and the surgical complication rate. In addition, it assumed that all risks are constant over a 5-year period. Furthermore, the efficacy of the three therapies was estimated, and as noted previously in this section, adequate data are not available to provide reliable estimates of these treatment effects. In addition, the model requires acceptance of an early increased surgical morbidity to achieve long-term benefit, just as in surgical treatment of other stroke conditions, such as endarterectomy for asymptomatic carotid stenosis. In contrast to carotid endarterectomy, however, sensitivity analysis found that even if the surgical procedure reduced the recurrent stroke rate by just 50%, the model would still favor surgical intervention.

Based on these data, surgery may be a reasonable option, particularly if the individual is unwilling or unable to tolerate anticoagulant therapy or has a high estimated risk of recurrent stroke. Surgical management also may be considered in patients who have recurrent symptoms despite antithrombotic therapy.

However, although surgery is often believed to be a permanent cure, this may not always be the case. In one reported surgical series, for example, the rate of recurrent stroke or TIAs in patients with PFO who were treated with surgical ablation was reported to be as high as 35%. It is noteworthy that the recurrent events were observed exclusively in patients ≥45 years old.[75] This observation suggests that in these particular cases the etiology of the patients' symptoms was not related to the PFO.

Table 10-3. Prevalence of Complex Aortic Plaques in Patients with Cryptogenic Strokes in Studies of Consecutive Stroke Patients

Study	Protruding Plaque (≥4–5 mm, Complex, or Mobile)	Complex Plaque	Mobile Plaque
Amarenco[82]	28% (22/78)	—	—
Jones[84]	20% (14/69)	20% (14/69)	5% (11/215)
Tunick[88]	27% (33/122)	—	9% (11/122)
Mean	26% (69/269)	—	—

Thus, caution should be exercised when attributing cerebrovascular symptoms to a PFO, particularly in older patients being considered for surgical management.

There has also been renewed interest in the use of transcatheter devices to close PFOs. These devices, originally designed for ablation of atrial septal defects, have also been used for PFO closure.[76–81] Initial studies reported an unacceptably high rate of device failure, but newer devices are under development. If successful, these devices could provide a less invasive and potentially lower-risk method of preventing recurrent embolization. However, their use must be considered investigational at this time.

Aortic Atheroma

Atheromatous plaques affecting the aortic arch have also been associated with an increased risk of stroke (Table 10-3).[82–84] The prevalence of aortic atheroma in unselected patients receiving TEE has varied from 2% to 13% in different series, depending on the patient population studied.[82,85,86] In contrast, the prevalence of protruding aortic plaque in stroke patients has been reported to range from 22% to 82%.[82,84,87,88] The prevalence of significant (≥4–5 mm, complex or mobile) plaque in patients with cryptogenic stroke has been reported to be from 26% to 44%.[89] The stroke risk associated with significant aortic plaque appears to be similar in white, Hispanic, and possibly also black populations, but the prevalence of more complex (mobile or ulcerated) lesions may be higher in white patients.[85]

In prospective studies, atheromas of ≥4–5 mm in thickness affecting the ascending aortic arch were associated with an annual recurrent stroke rate of 12–16% per year.[83,90] A similar stroke risk of 9–14% per year has been reported in unselected patients with large aortic plaques who were referred for echocardiography.[91–93] Several plaque characteristics have been associated with increased stroke risk. Although plaque thickness ≥4–5 mm alone was originally reported to be most strongly associated with stroke risk,[82,84,89,90,94] some studies have implicated other plaque characteristics as being potentially more important. Compared with calcified plaques, for example, noncalcified, echogenic plaques appear to be associated with a higher rate of recurrent risk for ischemic events, presumably because noncalcified plaques frequently contain fresh thrombi.[95] The presence of such thrombi on the surface of noncalcified plaques has been confirmed on pathologic examination.[96,97] Mobile or ulcerated plaques may convey the highest risk of stroke recurrence.[85,98] One case series reported that the annualized risk of systemic vascular events or death in patients with mobile atheroma was 50%.[86] The stroke rate alone was 30% per year. Risk was unrelated to the size of the mobile component. Similarly, plaque ulceration has been associated with increased stroke risk in many,[88,98–101] but not all, studies.[95]

The most appropriate therapy for patients with significant atheroma (≥4 mm, complex or mobile) remains uncertain. Although anticoagulant, antiplatelet, and cholesterol-lowering therapies have all been advocated, there are few data regarding the efficacy of specific therapies. However, several small studies of patients with mobile or complex ulcerated atheroma have suggested that the risk of recurrent ischemic events can be significantly reduced by anticoagulant therapy.[86,93,102,103]

In addition, data from the Stroke Prevention in Atrial Fibrillation III trial (SPAF III), in which the prevalence of complex aortic atheroma was high, reported a low incidence of embolic complications on warfarin (INR, 2.0–3.0) treatment (0.7%/year).[105,106] On the other hand, a few case reports have suggested an association between anticoagulation therapy and cholesterol embolization in these patients.[104] In addition, some series have reported continued thromboembolic events despite anticoagulant therapy.[88,101] However, because the prevalence of aortic atheroma is high and anticoagulation is common in the general medical population, it would be expected that there would be a high reported rate of cholesterol embolization in anticoagulated patients if this were a frequent occurrence. Because such reports are quite rare, the rate of cholesterol embolization related to anticoagulation is probably quite low.[107]

Atheromatous plaques are also reported to be quite dynamic, with formation and resolution of mobile components reported in up to 70% of patients.[108] Whether resolution of mobile components reduces subsequent stroke risk is unclear. Nevertheless, in light of the reported high rate of embolization associated with complex plaque ≥4–5 mm, particularly with a mobile component, anticoagulant therapy may be a consideration. The optimal management of arch atheroma remains unclear, however, particularly for noncomplex lesions.

Diagnosis: The Role of Transthoracic versus Transesophageal Echocardiography

Echocardiography is the diagnostic test of choice for identifying most cardiac and aortic causes of cerebral embolization. TTE yields reliable information regarding the anterior portions of the heart, including the left ventricle, mitral, and aortic valves. TEE permits better evaluation of the posterior portions of the heart, particularly the left atrial appendage, interatrial septum, and the aortic arch. In addition, TEE provides better visualization of the atrial septum, making it the superior for diagnosing ASA and PFO. A bubble study should be performed in either case to assess for a right-to-left shunt, particularly after a Valsalva maneuver.

The appropriate use of echocardiography in stroke and TIA patients remains controversial. TTE has low yield potential for cardiac SOE in patients with a normal cardiac history and examination, chest x-ray, and electrocardiogram (0–5%).

In contrast, many TEE studies have reported a high yield of potential cardiac SOE in stroke patients with a negative TTE. Although the number of high-risk embolic sources missed by TTE and detected by TEE is low (0–3%), minor-risk embolic sources are frequently missed by TTE (8–24%).[1] These minor-risk sources include PFO and minor valvular abnormalities, such as mitral annular calcification or mitral valve prolapse, particularly in younger patients (<45 years old). In addition, many of the positive TEE studies occur in individuals for whom anticoagulation is already indicated, such as an atrial thrombus in a patient with preexisting AF. Few data are available on the yield of TEE in individuals without preexisting indications for anticoagulation. Moreover, the most appropriate management of many of these conditions, such as PFO and aortic atheroma, is unknown.

A cost-benefit analysis has suggested that both initial use of TEE in all stroke patients as well as selective TEE based on a clinical risk profile is more cost-effective than other diagnostic strategies.[109] In addition, because some studies suggest that several more recently identified conditions may respond better to anticoagulant (e.g., aortic atheroma) or surgical treatment (e.g., PFOs, ASAs) than antiplatelet therapy, more frequent use of TEE may eventually be justified. Nevertheless, unselected use of either TEE or TTE in stroke patients does not appear to be warranted at present.

In the future, new neuroimaging techniques such as DWI (diffusion-weighted imaging) may help in identifying the most appropriate patients for TEE. Several studies have reported that particular DWI-detected patterns of cerebral infarction may be associated with an embolic etiology.[110–113] This suggests that DWI may be helpful in increasing the yield of TEE. However, further studies are needed to clarify the reliability of the association between individual DWI patterns and specific stroke etiologies.

Echocardiography Recommendations

At our institution, we advocate performing TEE in patients in whom the detection of cardiac or aortic arch abnormalities would significantly alter the clinician's treatment plan. For example, if the clinician believes that the finding of a PFO might alter his or her management of a patient with an otherwise cryptogenic stroke, then TEE may be appropriate. For routine stroke patients with clinically identifiable cardioembolic risk factors that require anticoagulation, however, the added value of either TTE or TEE is too low to warrant performing the procedure on a routine basis. In addition, if the finding of an additional risk factor would significantly influence subsequent patient management, TEE might also be indicated. For example, if an AF patient with recent cerebral ischemic symptoms has relative contraindications to anticoagulation, such as recent bleeding, a TEE finding of a left atrial thrombus might influence the clinician on the timing of anticoagulation. Ultimately, the decision to perform echocardiography depends heavily on the individual patient situation, and clinical judgment regarding the risks and benefits of different treatments.

Conclusion

The number of potential cardiac and aortic causes of stroke is progressively increasing. Although the appropriate diagnostic approach and the ideal management for many of these conditions has not been fully elucidated, it is clear that a greater appreciation and understanding of the wide spectrum of potential proximal embolic sources is necessary. It appears that many of these conditions may respond to specific management strategies, including surgery or anticoagulation. Future studies are needed to provide better risk stratification and identify the most appropriate therapy for individual patients.

References

1. Hart RG, Albers GW, Koudstall PJ. Cardioembolic Stroke. In: M Ginsberg, J Bogousslavsky (eds), Cerebrovascular Disease. Pathophysiology, Diagnosis and Management. Malden, MA: Blackwell, 1998;1392–1429.
2. Cardiogenic brain embolism. Cerebral Embolism Task Force. Arch Neurol 1986;43:71–84.
3. Steffensen FH, Kristensen K, Ejlersen E, et al. Major haemorrhagic complications during oral anticoagulant therapy in a Danish population-based cohort. J Intern Med 1997;242:497–503.
4. Petty GW, Brown RD Jr., Whisnant JP, et al. Frequency of major complications of aspirin, warfarin, and intravenous heparin for secondary stroke prevention. A population-based study. Ann Intern Med 1999;130:14–22.
5. McMahan DA, Smith DM, Carey MA, Zhou XH. Risk of major hemorrhage for outpatients treated with warfarin. J Gen Intern Med 1998;13:311–316.
6. Gitter MJ, Jaeger TM, Petterson TM, et al. Bleeding and thromboembolism during anticoagulant therapy: a population-based study in Rochester, Minnesota. Mayo Clin Proc 1995;70:725–733.
7. Beyth RJ, Quinn LM, Landefeld CS. Prospective evaluation of an index for predicting the risk of major bleeding in outpatients treated with warfarin. Am J Med 1998;105:91–99.
8. Gottlieb LK, Salem-Schatz S. Anticoagulation in atrial fibrillation. Does efficacy in clinical trials translate into effectiveness in practice? Arch Intern Med 1994;154:1945–1953.
9. Radford MJ, Smith K, Lewis J, Brass LM. Anticoagulation for stroke prevention is underutilized for elderly patients with atrial fibrillation. Annu Meet Int Soc Technol Assess Health Care 1997;13(abstract):87.
10. Levine MN, Raskob G, Landefeld S, Kearon C. Hemorrhagic complications of anticoagulant treatment. Chest 1998;114(Suppl 5):511S–523S.
11. Baudet EM, Oca CC, Roques XF, et al. A 5 1/2 year experience with the St. Jude Medical cardiac valve prosthesis. Early and late results of 737 valve replacements in 671 patients. J Thorac Cardiovasc Surg 1985;90:137–144.
12. Stein PD, Alpert JS, Dalen JE, et al. Antithrombotic therapy in patients with mechanical and biological prosthetic heart valves. Chest 1998;114(Suppl 5):602S–610S.
13. Cannegieter SC, Rosendaal FR, Wintzen AR, et al. Optimal oral anticoagulant therapy in patients with mechanical heart valves. N Engl J Med 1995;333:11–17.
14. Turpie AG, Gent M, Laupacis A, et al. A comparison of aspirin with placebo in patients treated with warfarin after heart-valve replacement. N Engl J Med 1993;329:524–529.
15. Cappelleri JC, Fiore LD, Brophy MT, et al. Efficacy and safety of combined anticoagulant and antiplatelet therapy versus anticoagulant monotherapy after mechanical heart-valve replacement: a meta-analysis. Am Heart J 1995;130(3 Pt 1):547–552.
16. Altman R, Rouvier J, Gurfinkel E, et al. Comparison of high-dose with low-dose aspirin in patients with mechanical heart valve replacement treated with oral anticoagulant. Circulation 1996;94:2113–2116.
17. Altman R, Rouvier J, Gurfinkel E, et al. Comparison of two levels of anticoagulant therapy in patients with substitute heart valves. J Thorac Cardiovasc Surg 1991;101:427–431.
18. Yamak B, Iscan Z, Mavitas B, et al. Low-dose oral anticoagulation and antiplatelet therapy with St. Jude Medical heart valve prosthesis. J Heart Valve Dis 1999;8:665–673.
19. Heras M, Chesebro JH, Fuster V, et al. High risk of thromboembolia early after bioprosthetic cardiac valve replacement. J Am Coll Cardiol 1995;25:1111–1119.
20. Bolooki H, Kaiser GA, Mallon SM, Palatianos GM. Comparison of long-term results of Carpentier-Edwards and Hancock bioprosthetic valves. Ann Thorac Surg 1986;42:494–499.
21. Bloomfield P, Kitchin AH, Wheatley DJ, et al. A prospective evaluation of the Björk-Shiley, Hancock, and Carpentier-

Edwards heart valve prostheses. Circulation 1986;73: 1213–1222.

22. Cohn LH, Allred EN, Cohn LA, et al. Early and late risk of mitral valve replacement. A 12 year concomitant comparison of the porcine bioprosthetic and prosthetic disc mitral valves. J Thorac Cardiovasc Surg 1985;90:872–881.

23. Cohn LH, Allred EN, DiSesa VJ, et al. Early and late risk of aortic valve replacement. A 12 year concomitant comparison of the porcine bioprosthetic and tilting disc prosthetic aortic valves. J Thorac Cardiovasc Surg 1984;88: 695–705.

24. Hart RG, Benavente O, McBride R, Pearce LA. Antithrombotic therapy to prevent stroke in patients with atrial fibrillation: a meta-analysis. Ann Intern Med 1999;131: 492–501.

25. The effect of low-dose warfarin on the risk of stroke in patients with nonrheumatic atrial fibrillation. The Boston Area Anticoagulation Trial for Atrial Fibrillation Investigators. N Engl J Med 1990;323:1505–1511.

26. Stroke Prevention in Atrial Fibrillation Study. Final results. Circulation 1991;84:527–539.

27. Secondary prevention in non-rheumatic atrial fibrillation after transient ischaemic attack or minor stroke. European Atrial Fibrillation Trial (EAFT) Study Group. Lancet 1993;342:1255–1262.

28. Warfarin versus aspirin for prevention of thromboembolism in atrial fibrillation: Stroke Prevention in Atrial Fibrillation II Study. Lancet 1994;343:687–691.

29. Adjusted-dose warfarin versus low-intensity, fixed-dose warfarin plus aspirin for high-risk patients with atrial fibrillation: Stroke Prevention in Atrial Fibrillation III randomized clinical trial. Lancet 1996;348:633–638.

30. Petersen P, Boysen G, Godtfredsen J, et al. Placebo-controlled, randomized trial of warfarin and aspirin for prevention of thromboembolic complications in chronic atrial fibrillation. The Copenhagen AFASAK study. Lancet 1989;1:175–179.

31. Kistler JP, Singer DE, Millenson MM, et al. Effect of low-intensity warfarin anticoagulation on level of activity of the hemostatic system in patients with atrial fibrillation. BAATAF Investigators. Stroke 1993;24:1360–1365.

32. Connolly SJ, Laupacis A, Gent M, et al. Canadian Atrial Fibrillation Anticoagulation (CAFA) Study. J Am Coll Cardiol 1991;18:349–355.

33. Zabalgoitia M, Halperin JL, Pearce LA, et al. Transesophageal echocardiographic correlates of clinical risk of thromboembolism in nonvalvular atrial fibrillation. Stroke Prevention in Atrial Fibrillation III Investigators. J Am Coll Cardiol 1998;31:1622–1666.

34. The efficacy of aspirin in patients with atrial fibrillation. Analysis of pooled data from 3 randomized trials. The Atrial Fibrillation Investigators. Arch Intern Med 1997; 157:1237–1240.

35. Risk factors for stroke and efficacy of antithrombotic therapy in atrial fibrillation. Analysis of pooled data from five randomized controlled trials. Arch Intern Med 1994; 154:1449–1457.

36. The Stroke Prevention in Atrial Fibrillation Investigators. Risk factors for thromboembolism during aspirin therapy in atrial fibrillation. J Stroke Cerebrovasc Dis 1995;5:147–157.

37. Predictors of thromboembolism in atrial fibrillation: I. Clinical features of patients at risk. The Stroke Prevention in Atrial Fibrillation Investigators. Ann Intern Med 1992; 116:1–5.

38. van Latum JC, Koudstaal PJ, Venables GS, et al. Predictors of major vascular events in patients with a transient ischemic attack or minor ischemic stroke and with nonrheumatic atrial fibrillation. European Atrial Fibrillation Trial (EAFT) Study Group. Stroke 1995;26:801–806.

39. Bleeding during antithrombotic therapy in patients with atrial fibrillation. The Stroke Prevention in Atrial Fibrillation Investigators. Arch Intern Med 1996;156:409–416.

40. Albers GW. Atrial fibrillation and stroke. Three new studies, three remaining questions. Arch Intern Med 1994; 154:1443–1448.

41. Hart RG, Pearce LA, Miller VT, et al. Cardioembolic vs. noncardioembolic strokes in atrial fibrillation: frequency and effect of antithrombotic agents in the stroke prevention in atrial fibrillation studies. Cerebrovasc Dis 2000;10:39–43.

42. Hart RG. Intensity of anticoagulation to prevent stroke in patients with atrial fibrillation. Ann Intern Med 1998; 128:408.

43. Hart RG, Pearce LA, Rothbart RM, et al. Stroke with intermittent atrial fibrillation: incidence and predictors during aspirin therapy. Stroke Prevention in Atrial Fibrillation Investigators. J Am Coll Cardiol 2000;35:183–187.

44. Andersen HR, Nielsen JC, Thomsen PE, et al. Long-term follow-up of patients from a randomised trial of atrial versus ventricular pacing for sick-sinus syndrome. Lancet 1997;350:1210–1216.

45. Andersen HR, Nielsen JC, Thomsen PE, et al. Arterial thromboembolism in patients with sick sinus syndrome: prediction from pacing mode, atrial fibrillation, and echocardiographic findings. Heart 1999;81:412–418.

46. McComb JM, Gribbin GM. Effect of pacing mode on morbidity and mortality: update of clinical pacing trials. Am J Cardiol 1999;83:211D–213D.

47. Cairns JA, Theroux P, Lewis HD Jr., et al. Antithrombotic agents in coronary artery disease. Chest 1998;114(Suppl 5):611S–633S.

48. Anand SS, Yusuf S. Oral anticoagulant therapy in patients with coronary artery disease: a meta-analysis. JAMA 1999;282:2058–2067.

49. Azar AJ, Koudstaal PJ, Wintzen AR, et al. Risk of stroke during long-term anticoagulant therapy in patients after myocardial infarction. Ann Neurol 1996;39:301–307.

50. Tornos P, Almirante B, Mirabet S, et al. Infective endocarditis due to Staphylococcus aureus: deleterious effect of anticoagulant therapy. Arch Intern Med 1999; 159:473–475.

51. Lopez JA, Ross RS, Fishbein MC, Siegel RJ. Nonbacterial thrombotic endocarditis: a review. Am Heart J 1987;113: 773–784.

52. Hojnik M, George J, Ziporen L, Shoenfeld Y. Heart valve involvement (Libman-Sacks endocarditis) in the antiphospholipid syndrome. Circulation 1996;93:1579–1587.

53. Rogers LR, Cho ES, Kempin S, Posner JB. Cerebral infarction from non-bacterial thrombotic endocarditis. Clinical and pathological study including the effects of anticoagulation. Am J Med 1987;83:746–756.

54. Benjamin EJ, Plehn JF, D'Agostino RB, et al. Mitral annular calcification and the risk of stroke in an elderly cohort. N Engl J Med 1992;327:374–379.

55. Hart RG. Cardiogenic stroke. Am Fam Physician 1989;40(Suppl 5):35S–38S.

56. Bogousslavsky J, Garazi S, Jeanrenaud X, et al. Stroke recurrence in patients with patent foramen ovale: the Lausanne Study. Lausanne Stroke with Paradoxal Embolism Study Group. Neurology 1996;46:1301–1305.

57. Stone DA, Godard J, Corretti MC, et al. Patent foramen ovale: association between the degree of shunt by contrast transesophageal echocardiography and the risk of future ischemic neurologic events. Am Heart J 1996;131:158–161.

58. Cujec B, Mainra R, Johnson DH. Prevention of recurrent cerebral ischemic events in patients with patent foramen ovale and cryptogenic strokes or transient ischemic attacks. Can J Cardiol 1999;15:57–64.

59. Mas JL, Zuber M. Recurrent cerebrovascular events in patients with patent foramen ovale, atrial septal aneurysm, or both and cryptogenic stroke or transient ischemic attack. French Study Group on Patent Foramen Ovale and Atrial Septal Aneurysm. Am Heart J 1995;130: 1083–1088.

60. Meissner I, Whisnant JP, Khandheria BK, et al. Prevalence of potential risk factors for stroke assessed by transesophageal echocardiography and carotid ultrasonography: the SPARC study. Stroke Prevention: Assessment of Risk in a Community. Mayo Clin Proc 1999;74:862–869.

61. Lechat P, Mas JL, Lascault G, et al. Prevalence of patent foramen ovale in patients with stroke. N Engl J Med 1988;318:1148–1152.

62. Webster MW, Chancellor AM, Smith HJ, et al. Patent foramen ovale in young stroke patients. Lancet 1988; 2:11–12.

63. de Belder MA, Tourikis L, Leech G, Camm AJ. Risk of patent foramen ovale for thromboembolic events in all age groups. Am J Cardiol 1992;69:1316–1320.

64. Hagen PT, Scholz DG, Edwards WD. Incidence and size of patent foramen ovale during the first 10 decades of life: an autopsy study of 965 normal hearts. Mayo Clin Proc 1984;59:17–20.

65. Hausmann D, Mugge A, Becht I, Daniel WG. Diagnosis of patent foramen ovale by transesophageal echocardiography and association with cerebral and peripheral embolic events. Am J Cardiol 1992;70:668–672.

66. Di Tullio M, Sacco RL, Gopal A, et al. Patent foramen ovale as a risk factor for cryptogenic stroke. Ann Intern Med 1992;117:461–465.

67. Cabanes L, Mas JL, Cohen A, et al. Atrial septal aneurysm and patent foramen ovale as risk factors for cryptogenic stroke in patients less than 55 years of age. A study using transesophageal echocardiography. Stroke 1993;24: 1865–1873.

68. Hanna JP, Sun JP, Furlan AJ, et al. Patent foramen ovale and brain infarct. Echocardiographic predictors, recurrence, and prevention. Stroke 1994;25:782–786.

69. Homma S, Di Tullio MR, Sacco RL, et al. Characteristics of patent foramen ovale associated with cryptogenic stroke. A biplane transesophageal echocardiographic study. Stroke 1994;25:582–586.

70. Pearson AC, Labovitz AJ, Tatineni S, Gomez CR. Superiority of transesophageal echocardiography in detecting cardiac source of embolism in patients with cerebral ischemia of uncertain etiology. J Am Coll Cardiol 1991; 17:66–72.

71. Olivares-Reyes A, Chan S, Lazar EJ, et al. Atrial septal aneurysm: a new classification in two hundred five adults. J Am Soc Echocardiogr 1997;10:644–656.

72. Pearson AC, Nagelhout D, Castello R, et al. Atrial septal aneurysm and stroke: a transesophageal echocardiographic study. J Am Coll Cardiol 1991;18:1223–1229.

73. Schneider B, Hanrath P, Vogel P, Meinertz T. Improved morphologic characterization of atrial septal aneurysm by transesophageal echocardiography: relation to cerebrovascular events. J Am Coll Cardiol 1990;16:1000–1009.

74. Nendaz MR, Sarasin FP, Junod AF, Bogousslavsky J. Preventing stroke recurrence in patients with patent foramen ovale: antithrombotic therapy, foramen closure, or therapeutic abstention? A decision analytic perspective. Am Heart J 1998;135:532–541.

75. Homma S, Di Tullio MR, Sacco RL, et al. Surgical closure of patent foramen ovale in cryptogenic stroke patients. Stroke 1997;28:2376–2381.

76. Bridges ND, Hellenbrand W, Latson L, et al. Transcatheter closure of patent foramen ovale after presumed paradoxical embolism. Circulation 1992;86:1902–1908.

77. Ende DJ, Chopra PS, Rao PS. Transcatheter closure of atrial septal defect or patent foramen ovale with the buttoned device for prevention of recurrence of paradoxic embolism. Am J Cardiol 1996;78:233–236.

78. Chan KC, Godman MJ, Walsh K, et al. Transcatheter closure of atrial septal defect and interatrial communications with a new self expanding nitinol double disc device (Amplatzer septal occluder): multicentre UK experience. Heart 1999;82:300–306.

79. Sievert H, Babic UU, Hausdorf G, et al. Transcatheter closure of atrial septal defect and patent foramen ovale with ASDOS device (a multi-institutional European trial). Am J Cardiol 1998;82:1405–1413.

80. Rao PS, Wilson AD, Chopra PS. Transcatheter closure of atrial septal defect by "buttoned" devices. Am J Cardiol 1992;69:1056–1061.

81. Hung J, Landzberg MJ, Jenkins KJ, et al. Closure of patent foramen ovale for paradoxical emboli: intermediate-term risk of recurrent neurological events following transcatheter device placement. J Am Coll Cardiol 2000; 35:1311–1316.

82. Amarenco P, Cohen A, Tzourio C, et al. Atherosclerotic disease of the aortic arch and the risk of ischemic stroke. N Engl J Med 1994;331:1474–1479.

83. Tunick PA, Rosenzweig BP, Katz ES, et al. High risk for vascular events in patients with protruding aortic atheromas: a prospective study. J Am Coll Cardiol 1994;23: 1085–1090.

84. Jones EF, Kalman JM, Calafiore P, et al. Proximal aortic atheroma. An independent risk factor for cerebral ischemia. Stroke 1995;26:218–224.

85. Di Tullio MR, Sacco RL, Savoia MT, et al. Aortic atheroma morphology and the risk of ischemic stroke in a multiethnic population. Am Heart J 2000;139:329–336.

86. Dressler FA, Craig WR, Castello R, Labovitz AJ. Mobile aortic atheroma and systemic emboli: efficacy of anticoagulation and influence of plaque morphology on recurrent stroke. J Am Coll Cardiol 1998;31:134–138.

87. Amarenco P, Duyckaerts C, Tzourio C, et al. The prevalence of ulcerated plaques in the aortic arch in patients with stroke. N Engl J Med 1992;326:221–225.

88. Tunick PA, Perez JL, Kronzon I. Protruding atheromas in the thoracic aorta and systemic embolization. Ann Intern Med 1991;115:423–427.

89. Di Tullio MR, Sacco RL, Gersony D, et al. Aortic atheromas and acute ischemic stroke: a transesophageal echocardiographic study in an ethnically mixed population. Neurology 1996;46:1560–1566.

90. Atherosclerotic disease of the aortic arch as a risk factor for recurrent ischemic stroke. The French Study of Aortic Plaques in Stroke Group. N Engl J Med 1996;334: 1216–1221.

91. Davila-Roman VG, Barzilai B, Wareing TH, et al. Atherosclerosis of the ascending aorta. Prevalence and role as an independent predictor of cerebrovascular events in cardiac patients. Stroke 1994;25:2010–2016.

92. Mitusch R, Doherty C, Wucherpfennig H, et al. Vascular events during follow-up in patients with aortic arch atherosclerosis. Stroke 1997;28:36–39.

93. Ferrari E, Vidal R, Chevallier T, Baudouy M. Atherosclerosis of the thoracic aorta and aortic debris as a marker of poor prognosis: benefit of oral anticoagulants. J Am Coll Cardiol 1999;33:1317–1322.

94. Amarenco P, Cohen A, Baudrimont M, Bousser MG. Transesophageal echocardiographic detection of aortic arch disease in patients with cerebral infarction. Stroke 1992;23:1005–1009.

95. Cohen A, Tzourio C, Bertrand B, et al. Aortic plaque morphology and vascular events: a follow-up study in patients with ischemic stroke. FAPS Investigators. French Study of Aortic Plaques in Stroke. Circulation 1997;96:3838–3841.

96. Vaduganathan P, Ewton A, Nagueh SF, et al. Pathologic correlates of aortic plaques, thrombi and mobile "aortic debris" imaged in vivo with transesophageal echocardiography. J Am Coll Cardiol 1997;30:357–363.

97. Khatibzadeh M, Mitusch R, Stierle U, et al. Aortic atherosclerotic plaques as a source of systemic embolism. J Am Coll Cardiol 1996;27:664–669.

98. Stone DA, Hawke MW, LaMonte M, et al. Ulcerated atherosclerotic plaques in the thoracic aorta are associated with cryptogenic stroke: a multiplane transesophageal echocardiographic study. Am Heart J 1995;130:105–108.

99. Rubin DC, Burch C, Plotnick GD, Hawke MW. Complex intraaortic debris in the absence of carotid disease in patients with embolic stroke. Am Heart J 1993;126:233–234.

100. Nihoyannopoulos P, Joshi J, Athanasopoulos G, Oakley CM. Detection of atherosclerotic lesions in the aorta by transesophageal echocardiography. Am J Cardiol 1993;71: 1208–1212.

101. Karalis DG, Chandrasekaran K, Victor MF, et al. Recognition and embolic potential of intraaortic atherosclerotic debris. J Am Coll Cardiol 1991;17:73–78.

102. Arko F, Buckley C, Baisden C, Manning L. Mobile atheroma of the aortic arch is an underestimated source of embolization. Am J Surg 1997;174:737–739; discussion 739–740.

103. Arko FR, Fritcher S, Mettauer M, et al. Mobile atheroma of the aortic arch and the risk of carotid artery disease. Am J Surg 1999;178:206–208.

104. Applebaum RM, Kronzon I. Evaluation and management of cholesterol embolization and the blue toe syndrome. Curr Opin Cardiol 1996;11:533–542.

105. Transesophageal echocardiographic correlates of thromboembolism in high-risk patients with nonvalvular atrial fibrillation. The Stroke Prevention in Atrial Fibrillation Investigators Committee on Echocardiography. Ann Intern Med 1998;128:639–647.

106. Blackshear JL, Zabalgoitia M, Pennock G, et al. Warfarin safety and efficacy in patients with thoracic aortic plaque and atrial fibrillation. SPAF TEE Investigators. Stroke Prevention and Atrial Fibrillation. Transesophageal echocardiography. Am J Cardiol 1999;83:453–455,A9.

107. Amerencis P, Mommel M, Bousser MG. Atherosclerotic disease of the aortic arch and the risk of ischemic stroke (letter). N Engl J Med 1995;332:1237.

108. Montgomery DH, Ververis JJ, McGorisk G, et al. Natural history of severe atheromatous disease of the thoracic aorta: a transesophageal echocardiographic study. J Am Coll Cardiol 1996;27:95–101.

109. McNamara RL, Lima JA, Whelton PK, Powe NR. Echocardiographic identification of cardiovascular sources of emboli to guide clinical management of stroke: a cost-effectiveness analysis. Ann Intern Med 1997;127:775–787.

110. Lee L, Kidwell CS, Alger J, et al. Impact on stroke subtype diagnosis of early diffusion-weighted magnetic resonance imaging and magnetic resonance angiography. Stroke 2000;31:1081–1089.

111. Baird AE, Lovblad KO, Schlaug G, et al. Multiple acute stroke syndrome: marker of embolic disease? Neurology 2000;54:674–678.

112. Roh JK, Kang DW, Lee SH, et al. Significance of acute multiple brain infarction on diffusion-weighted imaging. Stroke 2000;31:688–694.

113. Albers GW, Lansberg MG , Norbash A, et al. Yield of diffusion-weighted MRI for detection of potentially relevant findings in stroke patients. Neurology 2000;54:1562–1567.

Chapter 11
Surgical Therapy to Prevent Stroke

Markku Kaste

Stroke is a major cause of death in all societies. The care of stroke patients consumes more days in acute hospitals and institutional care than any other neurologic illness in most countries. Surgery for the prevention of a disorder as common and devastating as stroke is of utmost importance, but the decision for or against surgery has to be based on scientific evidence, not on an impression of benefit or anecdotal evidence.

Since its introduction in the 1960s,[1] the value of carotid endarterectomy (CEA) in stroke prevention has been controversial. In the 1980s, CEA was the most commonly performed arterial vascular surgery, but the medical profession and the public became increasingly concerned about perioperative morbidity and mortality and its use declined.[2] Finally, there is definitive information about the indications and benefits of CEA in appropriately symptomatic patients with tight or moderate ipsilateral carotid stenosis, although its role in asymptomatic patients remains less clear.[3–13]

Extracranial-Intracranial Bypass Surgery

The rise and fall of extracranial-intracranial (EC-IC) bypass surgery was a short but unhappy episode in the history of modern surgery for stroke prevention. The definitive trial, which showed that EC-IC was not beneficial, is an example of a well-designed, randomized trial that clearly answered the question it was designed to address (i.e., whether EC-IC bypass surgery had a role in threatened stroke caused by intracranial atherosclerotic disease or proximal carotid artery occlusion). The answer was unequivocally, no.[14]

Carotid Endarterectomy in Symptomatic Patients

Not long ago, clinicians did not know which patients with atherosclerotic lesions detected by a variety of tests should be operated on and with what surgical therapies.[15] The nihilistic attitude toward the surgical management of stroke prevention changed on February 21, 1991, when Dr. H. J. M. Barnett, the principal investigator of the North American Symptomatic Carotid Endarterectomy Trial (NASCET), announced the results of the interim analysis of approximately 600 patients at the International Joint Conference on Stroke and Cerebral Circulation in San Francisco. The results unequivocally demonstrated that patients with hemispheric transient ischemic attack (TIA) or mild nondisabling stroke ipsilateral to tight stenosis of the internal carotid artery (70–99%) were best treated by surgical therapy (Figure 11-1).

Simultaneously, with the cessation of the randomization of NASCET patients with severe stenosis, a similar conclusion was reached by the European Carotid Surgery Trialists' (ECST) Collaborative Group headed by Dr. C. Warlow (Figure 11-2). NASCET and ECST published the results of their interim analyses in 1991,[3,4] both reporting the superiority of surgery over medical therapy in patients with symptomatic carotid artery stenosis of greater than 70% for stroke prevention.

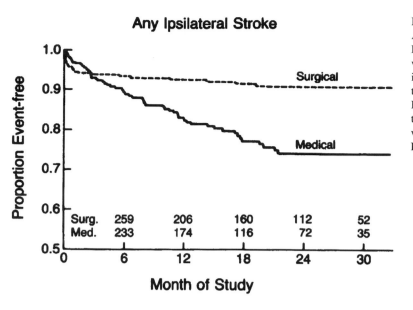

Figure 11-1. Results of North American Symptomatic Carotid Endarterectomy Trial. (Reproduced with permission from North American Symptomatic Carotid Endarterectomy Trial Collaborators. Beneficial effect of carotid endarterectomy in symptomatic patients with high-grade carotid stenosis. N Engl J Med 1991;325:445–453.)

The cumulative ipsilateral stroke rate at 2 years was 26% for those in the medical group of NASCET, but only 9% for those in the surgical group. This 17% absolute reduction in the surgical group means that six CEAs need to be performed to prevent one ipsilateral stroke over 2 years. For the most significant outcomes of CEA—major or fatal stroke—there was a 10.6% absolute risk reduction, which means that 10 CEAs need to be performed to prevent one of these events. The benefits from surgery were somewhat lower in ECST, but the variance between NASCET and ECST may be explained by differences in trial design.

Among these differences was the measurement method used to determine the percent of carotid stenosis. The ECST measurement method estimated the degree of stenosis to be higher than the NASCET method. An 82% stenosis in ECST is approximately equivalent to a 70% stenosis in NASCET.[16] ECST did not preselect surgeons, whereas NASCET did. The perioperative stroke and death rates were 7.5% in ECST and 5.8% in NASCET, which also contributes to the difference of overall absolute risk reduction in the trials. NASCET included patients within a span of 120 days after symptoms, whereas ECST had a

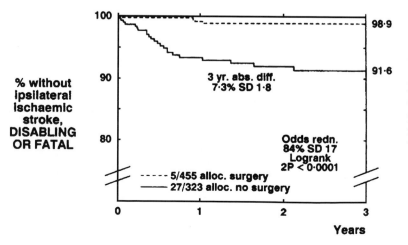

Figure 11-2. Results of European Carotid Surgery Trialists' group. (abs. diff. = absolute difference; odds redn. = odds reduction.) (Reproduced with permission from European Carotid Surgery Trialists' Collaborative Group. MRC European Carotid Surgery Trial: interim results for symptomatic patients with severe [70–99%] or with mild [0–29%] carotid stenosis. Lancet 1991;337:1235–1243.)

6-month enrollment window. The inclusion in ECST of patients with more remote symptoms than in NASCET may have contributed to their overall lower subsequent event rate. There were also many other differences. For instance, patients enrolled in ECST were only randomized when the local neurologist and surgeon were "substantially uncertain" whether to recommend CEA for the relevant artery. Other patients for whom physicians were "reasonably certain" that surgery was indicated or not indicated were treated accordingly. Despite these differences, both trials proved the superiority of surgery in stroke prevention in symptomatic patients with high-grade carotid stenosis.

The early disadvantages of employing surgical treatment (perioperative stroke and death) were rapidly overcome with event-free survival curves for the medical and surgical patients, crossing approximately 3 months after randomization. There was no evidence of convergence of the two curves during continuing follow-up, demonstrating that the benefits of surgery persisted (see Figures 11-1 and 11-2).

A finer division of the degree of stenosis correlated with the risk reduction after surgery in NASCET. The absolute risk reduction favoring surgery at 2 years was 26% for those with 90–99% stenosis, 18% for those with 80–89% stenosis, and 12% for those with 70–79% stenosis. Patients with less severe stenosis had a lower risk of stroke, and their gains from surgery were smaller than those of patients with more severe stenosis.

The cumulative stroke rate of 26% in the medical group, in spite of the best medical therapy at 2 years, and the stroke plus death rate of 3.3% in the medical group during the first month after randomization, in spite of optimal medical therapy, underline the grave natural history of the disease. Nearly all (95%) strokes that occurred during follow-up in the medical group were ipsilateral to the symptomatic artery, leading to randomization of the patient. This observation suggests that the stenosis was causative and not coincidental. The outcome of patients treated conservatively in the medical group again underlines the efficacy of surgery in tight symptomatic carotid stenosis, provided that the surgeon is as capable as those in NASCET and ECST.

Which Type of Preoperative Evaluation?

Standard angiography should be considered when it is necessary to answer clinically relevant questions that cannot be answered satisfactorily by less invasive means.[17] If CEA is considered, conventional angiography is needed, because the methods it uses to measure stenosis are standardized, and the NASCET results can only be applied to the NASCET method of measuring stenosis. The formula to obtain the percentage of stenosis uses the diameter of the narrowest, diseased portion of the artery as the numerator and the diameter of the normal carotid artery beyond the bulb as the denominator (Figure 11-3). The ECST investigators measured the lumen diameter at the most stenotic portion of the vessel and compared that to the presumed and unseen original diameter at this region of maximal arterial stenosis (see Figure 11-3). Because the tightest stenosis is generally in the carotid bulb, a wider portion of the artery than the distally located normal artery, the ECST method consistently estimates the degree of stenosis to be higher than the NASCET method. For example, a 70% stenosis in ECST is approximately a 45% stenosis in NASCET.[16]

In the typical clinical routine evaluation of carotid angiograms, it is common to use as the denominator the widest part of the carotid bulb or a speculative estimation about its location, as in the ECST method. Such a measurement often overestimates the tightness of the carotid stenosis and may result in surgery being recommended when the stenosis is not really severe enough for surgery to be appropriate.[18] This is a particular possibility for patients with a stenosis below 50%, and it may lead to performance of CEA in some patients for whom CEA has not yet been shown to be of value. The stricter NASCET method of measuring carotid stenosis is recommended and should be adopted as a universal standard.[19] If stenosis is underestimated, the patient may be denied the benefit of surgery.

It is especially dangerous to use "casual carotid eyeball" methods to measure the percentage of carotid stenosis on carotid angiograms.[16] The patient being selected for CEA deserves an objective method of evaluation, which an experienced neuroradiologist can provide. Whatever method is used, it

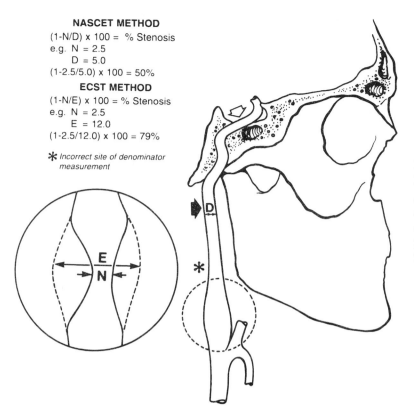

NASCET METHOD

$(1-N/D) \times 100 = \%$ Stenosis

e.g. N = 2.5

     D = 5.0

$(1-2.5/5.0) \times 100 = 50\%$

ECST METHOD

$(1-N/E) \times 100 = \%$ Stenosis

e.g. N = 2.5

     E = 12.0

$(1-2.5/12.0) \times 100 = 79\%$

* *Incorrect site of denominator measurement*

Figure 11-3. Two ways (North American Symptomatic Carotid Endarterectomy Trial [NASCET] and European Carotid Surgery Trialists [ECST]) to measure tightness of carotid stenosis. (N = numerator; D = North American Symptomatic Carotid Endarterectomy Trial denominator; E = European Carotid Surgery Trial denominator.) (Reproduced with permission from HJM Barnett, HE Meldrum, M Eliasziw. The North American Symptomatic Carotid Endarterectomy Trial: Further Observations. In EJ Veith [ed], Current Critical Problems in Vascular Surgery. St. Louis: Quality Medical Publishing, 1994.)

is imperative to employ it carefully, to understand its limitations, and to compare the results with the results of a trial using the same method. It is also important to study the vessel supplying the territory of ischemic event first. This increases the likelihood that clinically relevant and important questions can be answered, even if complications may occur.[17] The benefit of surgery persists even if angiography itself involves a risk as high as 1% of permanent stroke.[20] The risk of angiography to induce permanent neurologic complications in patients with cerebrovascular disease, including TIA, is typically less than 1% in the literature.[21] It has been suggested that cerebral angiography should be performed solely by a neuroradiologist and should be requested by neurologists, neurosurgeons, or vascular or cardiac surgeons after a neurologic consultation,[17] although internists specializing in stroke care[22,23] could probably request cerebral angiography as well.

Magnetic resonance angiography does not yet have the spatial resolution, selectivity, or dynamic character of conventional angiography. The use of combined Doppler and magnetic resonance angiography may replace conventional angiography in the future, however, although it may be premature at the time of this writing and should not lead to elimination of conventional angiography in the evaluation of carotid stenosis in patients with threatened stroke.[19]

Which Patients Should Be Evaluated?

CEA is a prophylactic operation. Restoration of blood flow has not been shown to improve a persistent neurologic deficit. For this reason, CEA is only indicated in patients without substantial neurologic deficits, such as those with TIA or mild completed stroke and with ipsilateral atherosclerotic moderate or high-grade stenosis localized to the common carotid bifurcation. Whisnant and others estimated that approximately 35,000 new patients each year in the United States with TIA or recovered stroke with carotid stenosis would be candidates for CEA.[24] If these figures are correct, the annual number of CEAs performed in symptomatic patients is far too high. Because of NASCET and ECST, clinicians know the indications for CEA in a large proportion of potential candidates for the procedure. These guidelines include the following:

1. *Symptomatic patients.* A patient with a tight (>70%) or moderate (50–69%) carotid stenosis must have symptoms appropriate to the diseased artery.

2. *Hemispheric TIAs or mild strokes.* CEA is a prophylactic operation and is not indicated in patients with nothing to lose in that hemisphere. Patients with fixed severe deficits are not candidates for CEA,[25] although the noninvasive evaluation of ipsilateral carotid bifurcation has revealed a tight stenosis.

3. *Tight ipsilateral carotid stenosis.* CEA is clearly beneficial in patients with ipsilateral high-grade stenosis (70–99%) with a recent carotid distribution, TIA, or minor stroke. The patients will have a 17% absolute and a 65% relative risk reduction for ipsilateral stroke and stroke death if CEA is added to the best medical care. This means that for every 100 patients treated surgically, 17 will be spared an ipsilateral stroke or stroke death (i.e., two-thirds of the risk of having an ipsilateral stroke or stroke death is eliminated by CEA). The benefit is related to the severity of stenosis. The benefit from surgery decreases as the percentage of stenosis diminishes.

4. *Moderate ipsilateral carotid stenosis.* In patients with moderate ipsilateral stenosis (50–69%), the absolute risk reduction over 5 years is 6.5% when CEA is added to the best medical care.[12] This means that for every 100 patients treated surgically, six to seven will be spared an ipsilateral stroke or stroke death. The number needed to treat (NNT) to prevent one stroke or stroke death is 15. Exceptional surgical competence is obligatory for performing CEA in this category. A 30-day rate of surgical death and disabling stroke should not exceed 2%. The decision on CEA and evaluation for it must take risk factors into account. Patients with high risk of stroke during the next 2–3 years when treated medically can be expected to benefit from CEA. Male sex, recent stroke, or recent hemispheric TIA support surgery.[12] The risk of perioperative stroke or death is increased in patients with diabetes, elevated blood pressure, contralateral occlusion of the carotid artery, or left side involvement of the lesion on computed tomography (CT)

Table 11-1. Risk Factors for Stroke in the North American Symptomatic Carotid Endarterectomy Trial

Age older than 70 years
Male sex
Blood pressure >160/90
Recency of ischemic event <31 days
Type of the event stroke, not transient ischemic attack
Degree of stenosis >80%
Ulceration on the arteriogram
History of smoking, hypertension, myocardial infarction, congestive heart failure, intermittent claudication, diabetes, or high blood lipids

or magnetic resonance imaging. Patients with a stenosis less than 50% do not benefit from CEA.[12]

5. *Time window of 4–6 months after the ischemic event.* The longest time periods from the onset of symptoms to CEA were 4 and 6 months in NASCET and ECST, respectively. The benefit of surgery in patients having survived without stroke for longer than 4–6 months after their index TIA or minor stroke is not known with certainty, but NASCET patients with TIAs during the first 6 months after randomization had a higher stroke risk than those without, whereas patients free of TIAs for 12–18 months after randomization had a relatively low risk.[16]

6. *Age criteria.* The risk of stroke increases with age, but age is not a contraindication for CEA in symptomatic patients with an ipsilateral high-grade carotid stenosis. The NASCET trial demonstrated that surgery not only is beneficial for younger patients but also for elderly patients up to 80 years of age.[3,12]

7. *Multiple risk factors.* The likelihood of stroke increases with the number of risk factors (Table 11-1), and patients with multiple risk factors are those most likely to benefit from surgery. In NASCET, the overall risk of stroke was much greater in patients with multiple risk factors than in those without them or with only a few risk factors. This untoward effect of multiple risk factors was eliminated by CEA.[12] After successful surgery, there was no difference between the cumulative risk after 2 years of ipsilateral stroke in patients with multiple risk factors and in those with no or a few risk factors. Accordingly, those who most benefited from surgery were those at the highest risk.[20]

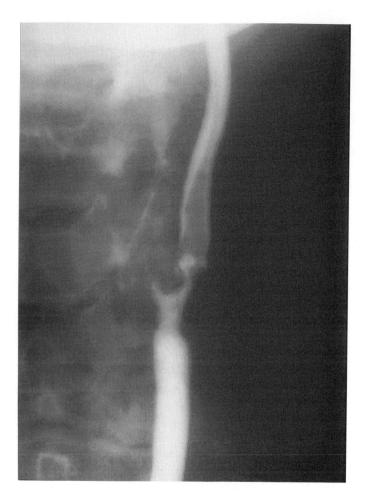

Figure 11-4. Intraluminal thrombus in tight internal carotid artery stenosis.

8. *TIA versus amaurosis fugax.* Patients with hemispheric TIAs have a higher risk of ipsilateral stroke than patients with amaurosis fugax. The risk of any ipsilateral stroke at 2 years is 44% for patients with hemispheric TIAs, compared to 17% for those with a transient monocular blindness. When weighing the risks and benefits of CEA in an individual patient, the symptom type needs appropriate attention. This holds true particularly for patients with a moderate stenosis (50–69%).[12]

9. *Ulceration of the carotid lesion.* Ulceration on the symptomatic stenotic carotid artery increased the risk of nonfatal stroke or any vascular death in the medical group of NASCET. Irregular or ulcerated plaques increase perioperative complication rates, but CEA is ultimately beneficial compared with patients treated only with the best medical care.[26]

10. *Intraluminal thrombus.* Intraluminal thrombus visualized on the angiogram (Figure 11-4) increases the risk of stroke within a few days after detection; however, it also increases perioperative risk. The stroke-free survival at 5 years of these patients was not increased by carotid surgery. Contrary to other subgroups with factors that individually increase the perioperative risks, the patients with intraluminal thrombus did not benefit from surgery. Other risk factors that increased the perioperative risks were an occlusion of the contralateral carotid artery, the presence of lesions on CT compatible with ischemia in the territory of the brain supplied by the symptomatic diseased artery, a history of diabetes, a diastolic blood pressure higher than 90 mm Hg, an ulcerated plaque, and a left side lesion, but these patients benefited from CEA compared with patients treated only with the best medical care.[26]

11. *Occlusion of the contralateral carotid artery.* Occlusion or tight stenosis of the contralateral carotid artery is often considered a contraindication for CEA of the symptomatic ipsilateral tight carotid stenosis, but it also means a grave natural history without surgery. Thirty-four percent of such individuals have a stroke or die within 2 years without surgery, whereas surgery improved equally the outcome in patients with and without contralateral tight stenosis or occlusion at 2 years in NASCET.[12] The situation in patients with moderate stenosis (50–69%) differs. These individuals have a better natural history without surgery than those with tight stenosis, whereas CEA in patients with moderate stenosis and contralateral occlusion doubles the operative risks.[27] Special attention should be paid to the state of the contralateral carotid artery. Expertise in surgical technique, anesthesia, and postoperative care is mandatory.[26]

12. *Concomitant intracranial carotid artery stenosis.* Intracranial atherosclerotic disease is an independent risk factor for subsequent stroke in patients with symptomatic internal carotid stenosis treated with the best medical care, but not in patients treated with CEA.[28] Unexpectedly, patients who had evidence of concomitant intracranial carotid artery stenosis rather than normal intracranial arteries benefit more from surgery. The presence of mild or moderate intracranial atherosclerotic disease is not a reason to abandon carotid surgery in patients with severe symptomatic carotid stenosis.[28]

13. *Silent brain infarctions.* Silent brain infarctions are common in patients with TIA and high-grade stenosis. They may locate ipsilaterally or in other vascular territories. If located in an appropriate brain region for the stenotic vessel, they seem to increase the risk of ipsilateral stroke in medically treated patients as compared to patients with nonappropriate localization. In patients with moderate stenosis, ipsilateral lesion on CT or magnetic resonance imaging increases the perioperative risks[12] but surgery also is beneficial for these patients.[26]

Which Surgeon Should Perform the Carotid Endarterectomy?

Not all surgeons are equal. The beneficial results detected in NASCET and ECST only apply to surgeons and institutions with as low a perioperative morbidity and mortality as was characteristic for the surgeons and centers in NASCET.[3,12] Patient selection plays a role, but selection of the surgeon and hospital team is equally important. In NASCET, there was a rate of 5.8% for all perioperative strokes and deaths, and 2.1% for major strokes or deaths with a fatality rate of 0.6%. However, during the perioperative time there was a 3.3% event rate in the medical group despite optimal medical therapy, a rate of 1.2% for major strokes or deaths, and a fatality rate of 0.3%. This means that there was only 2.5% overall excess of morbidity, 1.2% excess of major strokes and deaths, and 0.3% excess of deaths attributable to CEA.[3] In patients with moderate stenosis enrolled in NASCET, the rate of perioperative strokes and deaths was 6.7%, the rate of disabling strokes or deaths was 2.8%, and there was a fatality rate of 1.2%. In the NASCET medical group during the perioperative time, the rate of stroke and deaths was 2.4% despite best medical therapy, and the rate of disabling stroke or deaths was 1.4%. The net increase in risk at 30 days was 4.3% for stroke or deaths and 1.4% for disabling stroke or deaths. These figures are impressive, but they also underscore the fact that preventive surgery is only indicated when it can be performed with exceptionally low complication rates. A "break-even" analysis demonstrates that in the tight stenosis group, if only 11 more perioperative strokes or deaths had occurred in the surgical group, the benefit would no longer have been statistically significant.[16] This implies that the referring physician and the patient consenting to CEA should know the perioperative complication rate of the surgeon and the institution. It also highlights the importance of vigorous quality control for surgeons and institutions and the responsibility of hospital audit committees. The benefits of CEA in moderate and tight symptomatic carotid stenoses only apply to institutions and surgeons who have a low perioperative morbidity and mortality rate, as characterized by the NASCET institutions and surgeons. The greatest misunderstanding of the results from NASCET and ECST is to assume that the beneficial effects of CEA apply in an equal way locally if one does not know the local surgical complication rate.

Best Medical Therapy

A successfully performed CEA for threatened stroke does not imply that all patient care needs have been addressed. The best medical therapy is as important for each surgical patient as it is for patients without surgery. One-half to two-thirds of all deaths among patients in the six randomized CEA trials were due to heart disease that cannot be prevented by CEA, and a much smaller proportion was due to stroke.[3–8] The great majority of strokes were ipsilateral. This observation again emphasizes the need for optimal atherosclerotic risk factor management and antiplatelet or anticoagulant therapy.

The event rates in the medical groups were high, especially in the tight stenosis group of NASCET, in which one out of four medically treated patients experienced ipsilateral stroke within the next 2 years. In contrast, in the moderate stenosis group of NASCET, one out of six medically treated patients experienced a stroke within the next 5 years, despite the best medical therapy. This reinforces the severity of the disorder and implies that energetic risk factor treatment together with antiplatelet therapy is necessary for cases in which surgery is contraindicated.

Asymptomatic Patients

The Asymptomatic Carotid Artery Study, the largest and most recent of the trials studying the benefits of prophylactic CEA in asymptomatic patients, showed that surgical treatment of asymptomatic stenosis of carotid artery bifurcation increases the chance of being alive and stroke-free for 5 years.[9] The trial enrolled four times as many patients as any of the earlier asymptomatic trials. After a median follow-up of 2.7 years, the aggregate risk over 5 years for ipsilateral stroke and any perioperative stroke or death was estimated to be 5.1% for surgical patients and 11.0% for patients treated medically—an absolute risk reduction of 5.9% and relative risk reduction of 53% (95% confidence; 22%, 72%). The perioperative stroke and death rate was 2.3%, again underscoring that exceptional surgical competence is a prerequisite for CEA in asymptomatic patients. One meta-analysis confirmed that CEA reduces the incidence of ipsilateral stroke. The odds of ipsilateral stroke plus perioperative stroke or death were 0.62 (95% confidence lim-

its, 0.44–0.86), corresponding to a 2% absolute risk reduction over approximately 3.1 years.[13] A meta-analysis showed that CEA in patients with asymptomatic carotid stenosis unequivocally reduces the incidence of ipsilateral stroke, although the absolute benefit is relatively small. The NNT to prevent one stroke was 50 during a 3-year follow-up. Benavente and colleagues came to the conclusion that CEA cannot be routinely recommended for patients with asymptomatic carotid stenosis, but a reliable means to identify high-risk patients is needed.[13]

Stenting and Angioplasty

In the future, carotid angioplasty and stenting may be good alternatives for CEA. At the time of this writing, however, with few exceptions, the use of carotid angioplasty and stenting should be limited to well-designed, well-conducted, randomized studies with careful dispassionate overview according to the statement of the American Heart Association Expert Group.[29]

Health Economics of Carotid Endarterectomy

In their review, Hankey and Warlow came to the conclusion that CEA among TIA and stroke patients with carotid stenosis does not seem cost-effective for preventing stroke, but if ways could be found to focus the procedure on those patients at especially high risk, it would become more affordable.[30] They did not weigh the human suffering involved in stroke. According to the World Bank, stroke causes greater loss of quality-adjusted life years than any other disease.[31] The cost of CEA differs in different countries. Hankey and Warlow estimated that it costs 182,000 Australian dollars to avoid one stroke per year for 3 years if the costs per patient are 7,000 Australian dollars for preoperative investigations, the surgery itself, and postoperative management. They concluded such a strategy did not seem an affordable way to prevent stroke, and determined that if high-risk subgroups could be identified, the cost-effectiveness could be vastly improved. In Finland, the lifetime cost of stroke was U.S. $60,000 in 1991,[32] which at the time of this writing equals approximately $72,000, based on a 2% annual cost increase. The estimated cost of CEA offered by Hankey and

Warlow—7,000 Australian dollars—equals approximately U.S. $4,500 and corresponds to the present costs of CEA in Finland. For symptomatic tight stenosis, the NNT is 6 (i.e., it only costs $27,000 to prevent one stroke and saves society $72,000 in associated health care costs, resulting in net savings of $45,000). Hankey and Warlow also accounted for the costs involved in screening patients who never were operated on, yet CEA in patients with symptomatic tight stenosis seems a fair preventive procedure from the health economic point of view. The break-even point for surgery for symptomatic moderate stenosis may be near when the NNT is 15. However, even in such cases, the human aspect of treatment should be kept in mind. In one survey, stroke was feared more than death by lay people at risk of stroke.[33] For asymptomatic patients with carotid stenosis, the NNT is 50, which implies that CEA among these patients is hardly economically justified.

Conclusion

CEA for ipsilateral tight carotid stenosis (70% or more) in a symptomatic patient is highly beneficial in the hands of a surgeon with as low perioperative mortality and morbidity as the surgeons involved in NASCET and ECST. The natural history of this disease without surgery, and even with the best medical therapy, is grave, and the more risk factors for stroke a patient has, the worse the potential outcome without CEA. The effect of multiple risk factors on ipsilateral stroke can be eliminated by successful surgery. This does not mean, however, that surgery is the only treatment patients need. Management of risk factors and antiplatelet therapy are of vital importance, because patients die more often as a result of a coronary disease than stroke, and carotid surgery does not decrease the risk of cardiac death. Surgery is equally beneficial for elderly symptomatic patients and younger patients. Contralateral occlusion of the carotid artery is not a contraindication for surgery, but actually helps to identify a particularly high-risk subgroup. Postponing surgery does not reduce perioperative mortality or morbidity, but if the symptomatic patient survives without stroke for 1 or 2 years, the annual risk of stroke is markedly reduced even without surgery.

The way to measure the degree of carotid stenosis is important. Surgery has only been shown to be effective in patients with tight (70% or more) or moderate (50–69%) stenosis as measured by the NASCET method. The benefits of surgery decrease when stenosis becomes less severe or if the perioperative complication rate increases. In patients with moderate symptomatic stenosis, surgery is beneficial, but the NNT to prevent one stroke or death is 15, whereas in case of tight stenosis the NNT is six. It is important for the patient and his or her physician to know the complication rate of the surgeon and the surgical team performing the CEA. There is scientific evidence that asymptomatic patients with greater than 60% carotid stenosis benefit from CEA, although the NNT to prevent one stroke is 50. Surgery in patients with symptomatic tight stenosis is cost-effective and can be economically justified. For patients with moderate symptomatic stenosis, however, this is not so clear, and conclusions cannot be drawn from patients with asymptomatic stenosis. For most patients with moderate symptomatic or asymptomatic stenosis, medical therapy is probably the best alternative, but if surgery is preferred, exceptional surgical competence is required to justify the procedure in these patients.

References

1. Eascott JD, Pickering GW, Rob CG. Reconstruction of internal carotid artery in a patient with intermittent attacks of hemiplegia. Lancet 1954;2:994–996.
2. Pokras R, Dyken ML. Dramatic changes in the performance of endarterectomy for the disease of the external arteries of the head. Stroke 1988;19:1289–1290.
3. Beneficial effect of carotid endarterectomy in symptomatic patients with high-grade carotid stenosis. North American Symptomatic Carotid Endarterectomy Trial Collaborators. N Engl J Med 1991;325:445–453.
4. MRC European Carotid Surgery Trial: interim results for symptomatic patients with severe (70–99%) or with mild (0–29%) carotid stenosis. European Carotid Surgery Trialists' Collaborative Group. Lancet 1991;337:1235–1243.
5. Mayberg MR, Wilson E, Yatsu F, et al. Carotid endarterectomy and prevention of cerebral ischemia in symptomatic carotid stenosis. Veterans Affairs Cooperative Studies Program 309 Trialist Group. JAMA 1991;226;3289–3294.
6. Carotid surgery versus medical therapy in asymptomatic carotid stenosis. The CASANOVA Study Group. Stroke 1991;22:1229–1235.
7. Results of a randomized controlled trial of carotid endarterectomy for asymptomatic carotid stenosis. Mayo Asymptomatic Carotid Endarterectomy Study Group. Mayo Clin Proc 1992;67:513–518.

8. Hobson RW, Weiss DG, Fields WS, et al. Efficacy of carotid endarterectomy for asymptomatic atherosclerosis. The Veterans Affairs Cooperative Study Group. N Engl J Med 1993;328:221–227.

9. Endarterectomy for asymptomatic carotid artery stenosis. The Asymptomatic Carotid Atherosclerosis Study Group. JAMA 1995;273:1421–1428.

10. Risk of stroke in the distribution of an asymptomatic carotid artery. European Carotid Surgery Trialists' Collaborative Group. Lancet 1995;345:209–212.

11. Randomised trial of endarterectomy for recently symptomatic carotid stenosis: final results of the MRC European Carotid Surgery Trial. Lancet 1998;351:1379–1387.

12. Barnett HJ, Taylor DW, Eliasziw M, et al. Benefit of carotid endarterectomy in patients with symptomatic moderate or severe stenosis. North American Symptomatic Carotid Endarterectomy Trial Collaborators. New Engl J Med 1998;339:1415–1425.

13. Benavente O, Moher D, Pham BA. Carotid endarterectomy for asymptomatic carotid stenosis: a meta-analysis. BMJ 1999;317:1477–1480.

14. Failure of extracranial-intracranial arterial bypass to reduce the risk of ischemic stroke. Results of an international randomized trial. The EC/IC Bypass Study Group. N Engl J Med 1985;313:1191–1200.

15. Caplan RL. Carotid artery disease. N Engl J Med 1986; 315:886–888.

16. Easton JD, Wilterdink JL. Carotid endarterectomy: trials and tribulations. Ann Neurol 1994;35:5–17.

17. Caplan LR, Wolpert SM. Angiography in patients with occlusive cerebrovascular disease: views of a stroke neurologist and neuroradiologist. AJNR Am J Neuroradiol 1991;12:593–601.

18. Ranval TJ, Bailey T, Slis ME, et al. Overestimation of carotid stenosis: implications for carotid endarterectomy. Stroke 1992;23:142.

19. Fox AJ. How to measure carotid stenosis. Radiology 1993;186:316–318.

20. Barnett HJ. Stroke prevention by surgery for symptomatic disease in carotid territory. Neurol Clin 1992;10: 281–292.

21. Dion JE, Gates PC, Fox AJ, et al. Clinical events following neuroangiography: a prospective study. Stroke 1987; 18:997–1004.

22. Strand T, Asplund K, Erikson S, et al. A non-invasive stroke unit reduces functional disability and the need for long-term hospitalization. Stroke 1985;16:29–34.

23. Indredavik B, Bakke F, Solberg R, et al. Benefit of a stroke unit: a randomized controlled trial. Stroke 1991;22: 1026–1031.

24. Whisnant JP, Fisher L, Robertson JT, Scheinberg P. Carotid endarterectomy decreased stroke and death in patients with transient ischemic attacks. Ann Neurol 1987;22:72.

25. Easton JD, Hart RG, Sherman DG, Kaste M. Diagnosis and management of ischemic stroke. Part I. Threatened stroke and its management. Curr Probl Cardiol 1983;7:6–76.

26. Barnett HJM, Meldrum HE. Carotid endarterectomy. A neurotherapeutic advance. Arch Neurol 2000;57:40–45.

27. Barnett HJM, Eliasziw M, Meldrum HE. Prevention of ischaemic stroke. BMJ 999;318:1539–1543.

28. Kappelle LJ, Eliasziw M, Fox AJ, et al. Importance of intracranial atherosclerotic disease in patients with symptomatic stenosis of the internal carotid artery. The North American Symptomatic Carotid Endarterectomy Trial Group. Stroke 1999;30:282–286.

29. Bettmann MA, Katzen BT, Whisnant J, et al. Carotid Stenting and Angioplasty: a statement for healthcare professionals from the Councils on Cardiovascular Radiology, Stroke, Cardio-Thoracic and Vascular Surgery, Epidemiology and Prevention, and Clinical Cardiology, American Heart Association. Stroke 1998;29:336–348.

30. Hankey GJ, Warlow CP. Treatment and secondary prevention of stroke: evidence, costs, and effects on individuals and population. Lancet 1999;354:1457–1463.

31. World Bank. World Development Report: Investing in Health. New York: Oxford University Press, 1993.

32. Kaste M, Fogelholm R, Rissanen A. Economic burden of stroke and the evaluation of new therapies. Public Health 1998;112:103–112.

33. Samsa GP, Matchar DB, Goldstein L, et al. Utilities for major stroke: results from a survey of preferences among persons at increased risk for stroke. Am Heart J 1998;136:703–713.

Chapter 12

Angioplasty and Stenting of the Cerebral Vasculature

Camilo R. Gomez

The value of carotid endarterectomy (CEA) for the prevention of stroke in patients with symptomatic and asymptomatic carotid artery lesions has been clearly established by the results of prospective randomized trials.[1-4] Although there are limitations for this technique in the treatment of extracranial carotid artery pathology, there are no comparable surgical procedures to prevent stroke in patients with lesions in other regions of the cerebral vasculature. Since 1980, the technology used for endovascular therapy has also improved the capability to treat stenotic lesions of different arterial systems, and the brain circulation is not an exception to its application. Thus, endovascular techniques (i.e., angioplasty and stenting) are being actively studied in the treatment of lesions in the extracranial carotid artery,[5-11] the vertebrobasilar circulation, and the intracranial brain arteries. The trend is to perform stenting whenever possible, because it appears that the durability and periprocedural safety of this technique are better than those of simple balloon angioplasty. Nevertheless, stents cannot always be deployed in the cerebral arteries, particularly in the intracranial segments; therefore, balloon angioplasty should be considered in this discussion. This chapter provides an update on the topic of angioplasty and stenting of the cerebral arteries, their applications, progress, data available, comparability with alternative treatments, and future outlook.

General Considerations

The discussion of neurovascular angioplasty and stenting must include a consideration of the following issues:

1. Variability of cerebrovascular pathology, both in location and type, and its impact on the risk of stroke
2. Benefits and shortcomings of alternative forms of treatment (e.g., medical therapy, CEA)
3. Candidacy of patients for intervention of any type (i.e., feasibility vs. reasonableness)

Variability of Cerebrovascular Pathology

Although atherosclerotic plaques represent the most common and best-studied lesion affecting the cerebral arteries, other pathologic conditions are also capable of causing stenosis of these vessels and carry their own inherent risk for stroke. Furthermore, the location of the stenotic lesion greatly determines the potential for symptom formation, the likelihood of severe symptoms, and the candidacy of the patient for one or another form of intervention. For example, in the carotid system, the incidence of stroke in patients with intracranial plaques is believed to be higher than that in patients with extracranial lesions. In addition, the latter is the only type of pathology that, when located in a surgically accessible site, has been the subject of randomized prospective controlled studies of the potential benefit of surgical intervention. The problem, as demonstrated in this chapter, becomes compounded further when lesions in the vertebrobasilar system are considered, particularly due to the anatomic peculiarities of these vessels.

In contrast to atherosclerotic plaques, nonatherosclerotic lesions have not been as widely studied because the populations affected are smaller and treatment has been limited. In many of these patients, surgical intervention is not as simple or effective, or is not available, whereas the efficacy of medical treatment is unpredictable at best. From this viewpoint, in fact, the only form of cerebrovascular pathology for which specific surgical intervention has been convincingly shown to benefit patients is atherosclerotic narrowing of the extracranial carotid system, particularly at the point of bifurcation of the common carotid artery (CCA). As also discussed, however, even in this subpopulation there are circumstances that make the application of surgical intervention unwarranted.

Benefits and Shortcomings of Other Treatment Methods

The treatment of patients at risk for stroke from stenotic lesions of the cerebral arteries can be categorized as *medical*, *surgical*, or *endovascular*. Medical and surgical treatments have been the only types traditionally available, and their effectiveness (and limitations) provide perspective to discussion of endovascular treatments. The use of antithrombotic agents (i.e., antiplatelet therapies and anticoagulants) has been the subject of considerable study. At the time of this writing, the antiplatelet agents available for stroke prevention include aspirin (acetylsalicylic acid [ASA]), ticlopidine (Ticlid), clopidogrel (Plavix), and ASA/dipyridamole (Aggrenox). Aspirin, the oldest of these agents, has been shown to reduce the risk of stroke by approximately 20–25% in the general population, without specifically addressing the stroke subtype being prevented. Both ticlopidine and clopidogrel have been shown to be somewhat more effective than ASA in overall stroke prevention but, again, without specifically targeting a subpopulation of stroke victims. Finally, the combination of low-dose ASA and extended-release dipyridamole has also been shown to reduce stroke in a heterogeneous population. Thus, it is impossible to draw any conclusions from the studies cited about how specific cerebrovascular lesions differentially respond to these agents. In regard to oral anticoagulation, warfarin (Coumadin) has been tested mainly in the context of cardiogenic brain embolism, and the results apply only in part to this discussion. For extracranial carotid atherosclerotic lesions, the studies cited tested CEA against "best medical therapy," largely showing the lack of efficacy of treatment with ASA in nonsurgical patients. For intracranial atherosclerotic lesions, the only data available are retrospective and suggest that warfarin may be better than antiplatelet agents for stroke prevention; the results of an ongoing randomized, prospective trial are unavailable. Finally, data addressing the efficacy of medical treatment for vertebrobasilar lesions, or nonatherosclerotic pathology, is largely anecdotal or derived from small retrospective series.

The benefit of CEA over medical therapy alone for the prevention of ischemic stroke in patients with atherosclerotic lesions of the extracranial carotid artery has been demonstrated in several randomized, prospective, controlled trials encompassing both symptomatic[2] and asymptomatic patients.[3] This benefit holds true only if the risk of stroke and death from the procedure is kept below 6% in symptomatic patients[2,12] and 3% in asymptomatic patients. Both of these numbers are widely quoted as a benchmark for what clinicians should demand of their surgeons before to referring patients for CEA. These same numbers also have been used as a point of comparison to judge the potential viability of newer, alternative, interventional procedures. These figures do not convey the entire experience with CEA, however, as well as some of its limitations. For example, in the North American Symptomatic Carotid Endarterectomy Trial (NASCET), the incidence of cranial nerve injuries resulting from CEA was approximately 7%, creating another subgroup of patients with neurologic deficits related to surgery.[2] Furthermore, the results of the European Carotid Surgery Trial are somewhat different. Despite having a slightly different methodology than NASCET, the procedural major stroke and death rates in the European Carotid Surgery Trial were approximately 7%—three times the

2.1% major stroke and death rate of NASCET.[1] Furthermore, in a review of the use of CEA to treat Medicare patients, the mortality from CEA varied from 1.7% to 2.5%, with the highest rate occurring in situations in which the surgeon did not perform CEAs on a regular basis. There is also evidence that the rate of complications reported after CEA depends in part on the medical specialties of the authors of the study being published. Thus, having a neurologist among the authors of CEA studies results in a higher rate of complications reported, which may be due to the difficulty experienced by other specialists in recognizing subtle neurologic complications.[13,14]

The surgical treatment of patients with extracranial vertebrobasilar pathology has been the subject of some study, but has not been as rigorously investigated as surgical treatment of extracranial carotid pathology. One such technique involves transection of the vessel above the stenosis with reimplantation in either the ipsilateral carotid or subclavian arteries.[15,16] In addition to the risk of stroke, such procedures have significant limitations, including an overall 10–20% risk of injury to the sympathetic fibers, the phrenic nerve, the recurrent laryngeal nerve, the vagus nerve, or the thoracic nerve, and the potential for pulmonary complications from the thoracotomy.[15,16] In the largest reported series of vertebral operations, the Joint Study of Extracranial Arterial Occlusion, vertebral arteries were treated in 165 patients with a mortality rate of 4.2% and a 6% incidence of perioperative vertebral artery occlusion.[17] In a large series, 109 vertebral operations were performed, with a 3% mortality rate and a 2% rate of immediate thrombosis.[16] These facts underscore the need for a minimally invasive, low-morbidity technique with good short- and long-term patency to treat extracranial arterial occlusion.

Candidacy for Surgical or Endovascular Intervention

Patient candidacy for surgical or endovascular intervention involves two different issues: feasibility versus reasonableness. The former relates to whether a procedure *can be performed* as the treatment of a specific lesion, whereas the latter relates to whether such a procedure *should be performed* in a specific patient, even if feasible. For example, in some instances, surgery is simply a technical impossibility (e.g., petrous internal carotid stenoses), whereas in others, it represents a more complicated and risky operation (e.g., intrathoracic common carotid stenoses). In other cases, patients have perfectly accessible lesions that are not atherosclerotic. Finally, there is the group of patients comprised by the truly "high-risk" surgical candidates, whose severe comorbidities confer on them an inordinate risk for surgical intervention.

A fundamental principle of statistics is that the sample population in a trial must be representative of the overall population to which the results of a study are applied. Keeping this principle in mind, a review of the clinical characteristics of patients who participated in NASCET indicates that they comprised an extremely healthy, low-risk group and are somewhat different than most stroke patients treated by clinicians on a daily basis.[18] The overwhelming majority of NASCET patients were younger than the age of 80 years and lacked clinically significant coronary artery disease, as evidenced by only 19% of them having had a previous myocardial infarction and 23% experiencing preexisting angina. Also, few NASCET patients had congestive heart failure (2.6%), cardiac arrhythmias (5%), or valvular heart disease (2%), and by exclusion, none experienced renal failure, hepatic insufficiency, or cancer.[18] In addition, less than two-thirds of the NASCET patients had hypertension, less than one-fifth had diabetes and hyperlipidemia, and only one-third smoked. The Asymptomatic Carotid Artery Study (ACAS) showed that CEA is effective as long as the procedural risk is less than 3%. However, the ACAS patients also comprised an extremely healthy, handpicked, low-risk population.[3] Therefore, it is fair to say that it is uncertain whether the benefit of CEA holds true to the same degree in higher risk patient populations.

In fact, there is evidence in the literature that the application of CEA does not carry the same low risk as has been reported by some clinical trials, even in tertiary care centers.[19,20] For example, the mortality from CEA in hospitals that participated in the prospective trials cited is approximately 1.4% for treatment of Medicare patients. This figure is more than twice that of the trial in which the same surgeons participated, and, therefore, underscores the importance of the characteristics of the treatment population. Even in NASCET, the existence of certain comorbidities significantly increased the risk of CEA, particularly contralateral carotid occlusion (14%) and tandem siphon lesions (9%).[21]

Accumulated Experience in Neurovascular Stenting

Extracranial Carotid Angioplasty and Stenting

The use of percutaneous endovascular techniques to treat carotid artery lesions dates back to the early 1980s. In one of the first reports found in the literature, four attempts were made to treat four patients with carotid artery atheromatous lesions.[22] Only three of the patients could be treated, one of whom developed a transient neurologic deficit. In the fourth patient, the procedure was not successful. Also in 1983, reports by Tievsky et al. and Wiggli and Gratzl described three successful percutaneous balloon angioplasties (PTAs) of the carotid artery, one of which was performed in a patient with postsurgical stenosis.[23,24]

The late 1980s witnessed many reports about the use of PTA to treat fibromuscular dysplasia of the carotid.[25,26] In general, success was reported by all authors, although at least two patients were noted to have experienced transient neurologic deficits and one had a dissection that healed completely. Concurrently, other groups began to report their successful use of PTA in the treatment of various forms of carotid artery pathology, both atheromatous and nonatheromatous.[27,28] In 1987, Theron et al. reported the first large series of carotid PTA, including six patients with atheromatous lesions and five with postsurgical stenoses.[29]

In 1990, Brown et al. described their experience in seven patients with symptomatic carotid artery stenosis.[30] They were successful in only five patients, two of whom had TIA during the procedures. That same year, Theron et al. described an additional group of 13 patients treated with a new technique for PTA, which included occlusion of the distal internal carotid artery (ICA) for protection against distal cerebral embolization.[31] This group has continued to report no complications using this original methodology. By the early 1990s, larger series began to appear in the literature, including those by Munari et al. and Kachel et al.[32–34] One of

these groups reported only one TIA in a series of 65 carotid PTAs, with no deaths and no restenoses.[34] In addition, the results of the Carotid and Vertebral Artery Transluminal Angioplasty Study (CAVATAS) were presented. This was a prospective study, in which patients were assigned to have either PTA or CEA, with stenting used only as a bailout maneuver (22% of all patients treated with PTA had stents placed). The overall results and complication rates were similar between the two groups and underscore the need for further study.[35]

It was not until 1995, however, that the first series of carotid artery stenting (CAS) was published. The series of Bergeron et al. included patients treated using angioplasty with and without stents.[5] Thirteen of the patients in this series had balloon-expandable stents placed, nine of which were placed in the ICA. Complications included one death due to hyperperfusion syndrome, one minor stroke, one TIA, and reported instances of spasm, transient hyperperfusion, acute occlusion, and silent stroke. It is interesting to note that all of the complications occurred in the patients treated with PTA alone. In a large series that included more than 600 patients treated for supra-aortic stenoses, Mathias et al. reported the implantation of 42 self-expandable stents among 305 cases of carotid PTA.[36] The use of stents by these authors was guided by lesion characteristics, such as degree of complexity, degree of stenosis after predilatation, and severity of plaque fracture. Their long-term results showed no restenosis, no neurologic events, and increased wall thickness within the stent.[36] Our group at the University of Alabama at Birmingham (UAB) has shown that CAS is technically effective and considerably safe, even in a high-risk population of patients with carotid lesions (Figure 12-1).[6,37,38] Other series have also shown similarly good results.[39] In addition, the European Carotid Stent Trial has demonstrated a competitive low rate of complications, even though in this trial investigators favored a direct cervical puncture approach to the procedure instead of the more widely used femoral access.[40]

Finally, an international registry of extracranial CAS has allowed the experience of the most active centers around the world to be compiled.[41] The most recent update includes data from 33 institutions from North and South America (including UAB), Asia, and Europe. A total of 4,865 carotid PTAs were reported, with a technical success rate of

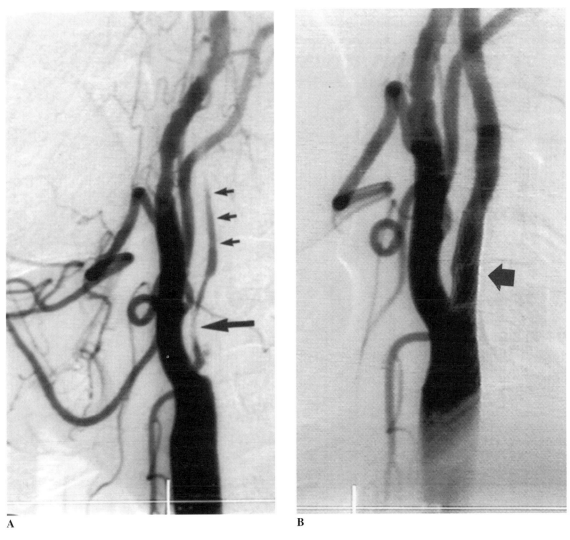

A   **B**

Figure 12-1. Elective stenting of a critically stenotic extracranial internal carotid artery (ICA) lesion (lateral views). **(A)** The ICA is severely stenotic at its origin (*large arrow*) and distal flow stagnation is evident (*small arrows*). **(B)** Final result shows how stent deployment results in restoration of the vessel's lumen (*arrow*).

98.6%. The overall safety statistics include a 30-day mortality of 0.84% and an all-stroke rate of 3.94%, which seem competitive with those of CEA (M.H. Wholey, personal communication, 1999).

In regard to the durability of CAS, available data from the international CAS registry show stroke occurrence of 3% over a follow-up period of 24–36 months and a restenosis (i.e., greater than 50% stenosis of the treated vessel) rate of 4.5% over the same period. These results are also competitive, considering that the stroke rate in the surgical arm of NASCET was 14% over 3 years and 10% in ACAS over 5 years.[41] An analysis of the

data collected by the group at UAB and Lenox Hill Hospital over a period of several years shows a preliminary 3-year stroke-free rate of more than 95% (G.S. Roubin, unpublished data, 2000).

Extracranial Vertebral Artery Stenting

In regard to the extracranial vertebral arteries, balloon angioplasty alone has been performed safely and is widely reported to benefit symptomatic patients. However, one of the largest series of extracranial vertebral artery angioplasties reported

34 patients who, as a result of the procedure, had an 8.8% incidence of transient neurologic complications and no permanent neurologic complications. In addition, investigators noted a rate of restenosis of 8.8% in those patients studied 2–5 months after PTA, with an undisclosed angiographic follow-up rate.[42] In fact, a review of the illustrations in previous vertebral angioplasty reports demonstrates significant residual postprocedure stenoses, probably underscoring the problem of elastic recoil. Finally, the studies reviewed do not include routine follow-up angiography in their protocol.[42–45] Our group at UAB reported the feasibility, safety, and outcome of elective extracranial vertebral artery stenting in 50 patients (55 vessels) (Figures 12-2 and 12-3).[46] Technical success was achieved in 54 of 55 patients (98%) with no procedure-related complications. However, one patient died of non-neurologic causes (2%), and one patient had a stroke (2%) related to a complicated coronary intervention occurring within the 30-day postprocedural period. Clinical follow-up at a mean of 25 ± 10 months revealed two patients with recurrence of vertebrobasilar symptoms (4%). Six-month angiographic follow-up was carried out in 90% of eligible patients, with a 10% incidence of restenosis (defined by >50% luminal narrowing).[46] The 30-day morbidity and mortality rate of 4% in our series compared well with previously published data, particularly when the details of the two perioperative events are considered, because neither occurred as a direct result of the vertebral endovascular procedure. The rate of restenosis also appeared rather low, even considering the inherent limitations of a short-term (6-month) follow-up.

Intracranial Carotid and Vertebrobasilar Stenting

Balloon angioplasty of the intracranial arteries has been applied for a number of years and, with the existing technology, the results have been considerably encouraging. As noted, however, there is significant interest in the use of stents whenever possible. Yet the feasibility of treating intracranial carotid artery lesions with stents is a less explored, although certainly feasible, procedure. The main limiting factor has been the availability of stents that could be tracked and deployed within the intracranial cavity. However, several case reports have been published, demonstrating the possibility of undertaking such a

treatment.[47–53] From the interventional point of view, the intracranial carotid artery is an interesting vessel with characteristics that vary according to its different segments. The petrous segment, the most proximal, involves an artery that is completely surrounded by a bony canal (Figure 12-4). As it exits through the foramen lacerum, the ICA is surrounded by a venous sinus in its cavernous portion. Finally, it enters the subarachnoid space shortly after forming the carotid siphon and constitutes its clinoid segment. Each of these three portions has different mechanical and anatomic characteristics, and these must be taken into consideration when planning therapy. At present, the bulk of the experience involves stenting of lesions in the petrous and cavernous portions, the two areas most accessible for treatment with available technology. In the experience at UAB, the incidence of dissection of the petrous carotid artery after balloon angioplasty is so high that the author was reluctant to treat these vessels without stenting them.

Stenting of the intracranial portions of the vertebrobasilar system, namely the V3 and V4 portions of the vertebral artery and the basilar artery, has also been shown to be feasible and relatively safe. In fact, it has proven to be an easier system in which to work, compared to the carotid system. At the time of this writing, the author has electively treated a total of 50 intracranial arteries with stenting, with only one death and one major stroke occurring as a result of the procedures (C. R. Gomez et al., unpublished data, 2000). Although encouraging, the results require wider demonstration and further prospective confirmation, and a pilot trial of a dedicated cerebral stent is going to be launched.

Basic Principles of Elective Neurovascular Angioplasty and Stenting

General Principles

The performance of endovascular therapy of the carotid artery involves the introduction of coaxial systems of catheters, microcatheters, balloons, and other devices into the cerebral blood vessels. Most commonly, the vasculature is first accessed via the femoral artery, from which catheterization is most comfortable, convenient, and practical, both for the operator and for the patient. A vascular sheath (6–7 Fr in diameter) is usually introduced into the femoral vessels and left in place, assuring repeated

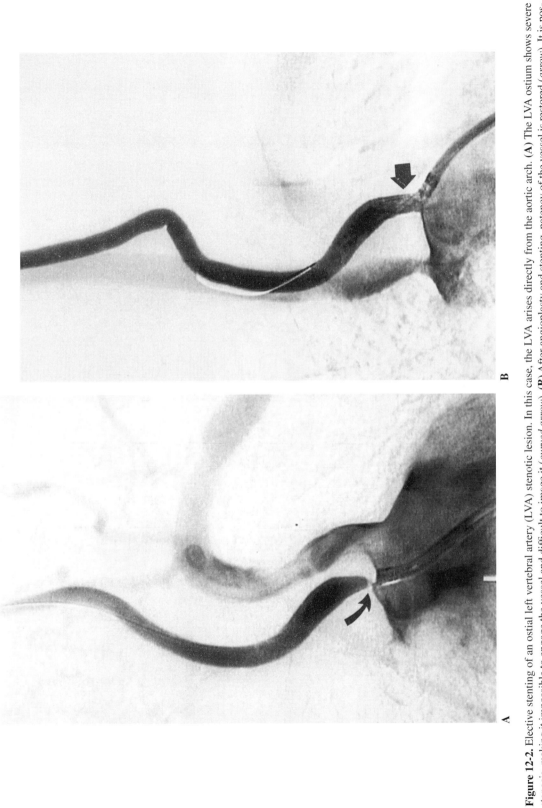

Figure 12-2. Elective stenting of an ostial left vertebral artery (LVA) stenotic lesion. In this case, the LVA arises directly from the aortic arch. (**A**) The LVA ostium shows severe stenosis, making it impossible to engage the vessel and difficult to image it (*curved arrow*). (**B**) After angioplasty and stenting, patency of the vessel is restored (*arrow*). It is possible to see a mild to moderate lesion of the left common carotid artery ostium.

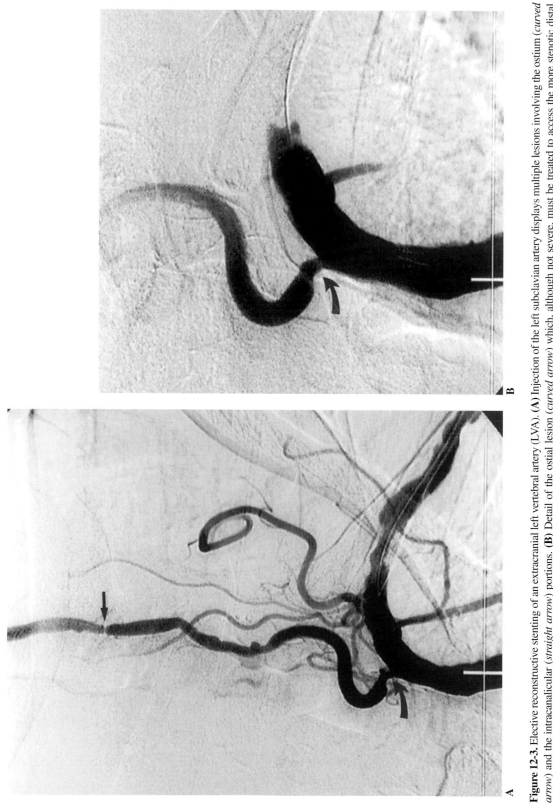

Figure 12-3. Elective reconstructive stenting of an extracranial left vertebral artery (LVA). (**A**) Injection of the left subclavian artery displays multiple lesions involving the ostium (*curved arrow*) and the intracanalicular (*straight arrow*) portions. (**B**) Detail of the ostial lesion (*curved arrow*) which, although not severe, must be treated to access the more stenotic distal lesions. (**C**) After stent deployment, the lumen of the LVA ostium is much improved (*arrow*). (**D**) The distal lesion is slightly more complex and shows significant stenosis (*arrow*).

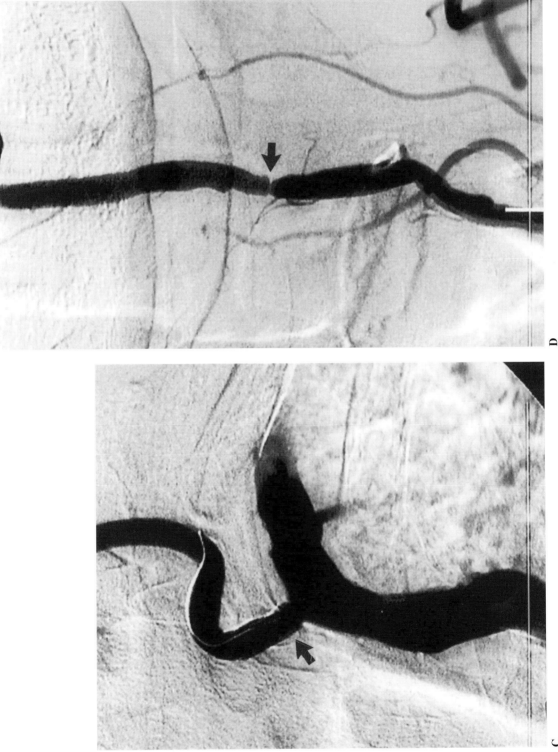

D

C

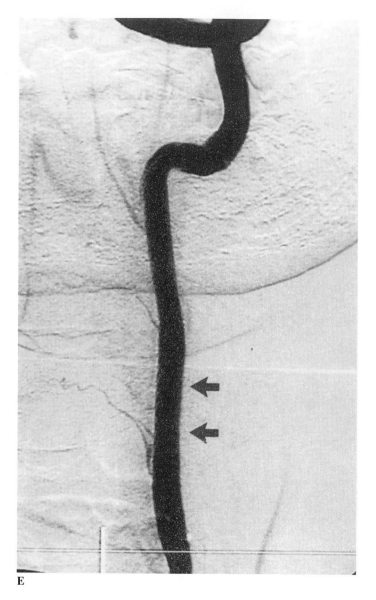

E

Figure 12-3. (*Continued*) (**E**) Deployment of self-expanding stents normalizes the vessel's anatomy (*arrows*).

access by means of different types of catheters throughout the procedure. Typically, a conventional diagnostic cerebral catheter is used to engage the carotid arteries. Once in place, the diagnostic catheter allows the acquisition of scout images used to plan the procedure.

Extracranial Carotid Angioplasty and Stenting

The technique of angioplasty and stenting of the extracranial carotid artery is similar in principle to

that used in coronary and peripheral circulation. Patients are premedicated with aspirin (325 mg/day) and clopidogrel (75 mg/day) for at least 2 days before the procedure. A 90-cm-long, 7-Fr sheath (Cook Endovascular, Bloomington, IN), which has the inner lumen equivalent to a 9-Fr guiding catheter, is placed in the femoral artery. The CCA is catheterized with a 125-cm-long 5-Fr Newton No. 5 catheter over a 0.038-in., hydrophilic-coated wire (e.g., Glidewire, Terumo Medical Corporation, Somerset, NJ). Heparin (100 U/kg) is administered intra-arterially via the diagnostic catheter. Throughout the procedure, addi-

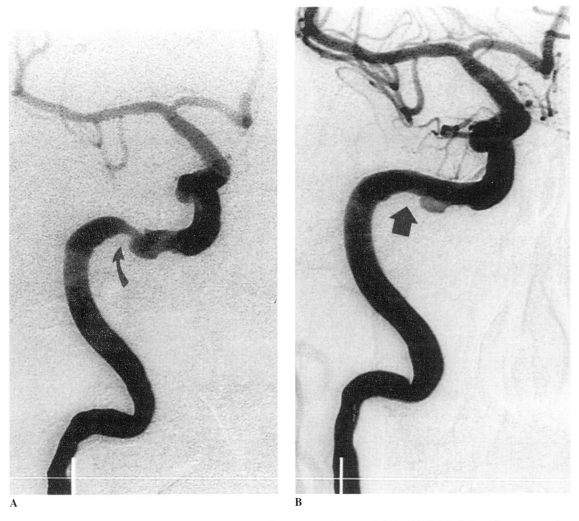

A   **B**

Figure 12-4. Elective stenting of a symptomatic petrous internal carotid artery (ICA). (**A**) Original view shows a complex stenotic segment of the petrous portion of the ICA (*curved arrow*). (**B**) Final result of the vessel after deployment of a self-expandable coronary stent (*arrow*). The crater in the plaque is covered by the stent, preventing distal embolization.

tional doses of heparin are given as needed to maintain the activated clotting time between 200 to 250 seconds. The 0.038-in. wire is anchored in the external carotid artery, the diagnostic catheter is advanced over the wire and used as an introducer for the sheath, and the sheath is advanced into the distal CCA (see Figure 12-1A). Online quantitative angiography of the lesion and the adjacent arterial segments is performed, using the contrast-filled sheath for calibration. With the use of a standard coaxial system, the lesion is crossed using a floppy-tipped, 0.014-in. guidewire (e.g., Traverse, Advanced Cardiovascular Systems, Santa Clara, CA) and predilated with low-profile compliant coronary balloons (e.g., Cobra,

Scimed Life Systems, Maple Grove, MN). The floppy-tipped wire is then exchanged for an extra-support, 0.018-in., 300-cm-long wire (Roadrunner, Cook Cardiology, Bloomington, IN). One or more stents are then deployed across the lesion as necessary (see Figure 12-lB). The stents are further dilated at high pressure (i.e., 12 atm) to firmly embed them into the vessel wall. Clopidogrel is continued for 4 weeks, and aspirin is continued indefinitely. The procedure typically lasts 20–40 minutes and it is performed with the patient fully awake and without sedation. Constant neurologic monitoring is an intrinsic part of the technique,[54] and the results are typically satisfactory.

Intracranial Carotid Artery Stenting

The technique of intracranial angioplasty is slightly different (see Figure 12-4). The author uses a 6-Fr multipurpose guiding catheter instead of the long sheath described in the preceding section. The tip of the guide catheter is placed in the distal cervical ICA, before its entrance into the petrous bone. Patients are premedicated with antiplatelet agents in the same fashion as described. We then approach these lesions with a hydrophilic-coated, floppy-tipped, 0.014-in. microwire (e.g., Transend, Meditech, Natick, MA) and a moderately compliant coronary balloon (Ninja, Cordis, Miami Lakes, FL) (see Figure 12-2B). An alternative approach involves the use of a microcatheter (e.g., Turbo Tracker-18, Target Therapeutics, Boston, MA), particularly in vessels that are unusually tortuous and difficult to access. Once the lesion is crossed with the microwire and the microcatheter, these are advanced distally to one of the branches of the ipsilateral middle cerebral artery. At this point, the microwire is substituted for a more supportive exchange wire (e.g., Luge, Scimed Life Systems, Maple Grove, MN). The microcatheter is removed and the balloons and stents are introduced over the exchange microwire, which remains anchored in the distal arterial circulation.

Technical Issues Relevant to Carotid Artery Stenting

One of the important aspects to discuss about technical issues relevant to CAS is the type of stent used. At present, there are two major categories of stents available: balloon-expandable and self-expandable. These are further categorized based on their structure and material. These variables give each stent a particular set of characteristics that makes it more or less suitable for use in different circumstances. It is important to mention that none of the stents available has been designed or approved for use in the carotid artery system. Each type of stent has advantages and disadvantages and, as with any other interventional instrumentation, any gain in flexibility is balanced by decreased pushability and possibly radial strength.

The technique of extracranial CAS is the product of an evolution that encompasses a variety of changes in strategy and materials (i.e., wires, balloons) used during the procedure. Among the changes introduced since 1995, perhaps the most important to note is that of the choice of stent to be used. At present, the author almost exclusively uses self-expandable stents (Wallstent, Schneider, Plymouth, MN, or Smart, Cordis, Miami Lakes, FL) due to their superior durability in this location. In our experience, 14 patients were found to have deformed Palmaz stents during routine 6-month angiographic follow-up, some requiring repeat treatment with additional balloon inflations, and raising the concern of applicability of these devices for the treatment of CCA bifurcation lesions.[55] The most likely reason for this problem is the superficial location of the deployed stent with respect to the surface of the neck, making it susceptible to the effect of external compression. When choosing stents, it is important to consider the fact that nitinol stents do not have as much foreshortening as stainless steel stents, allowing for more precise placement (see Figure 12-1). Stainless steel stents undergo significant foreshortening and, thus, are commonly used when a precise deployment is not necessary.

For intracranial carotid artery lesions, the author also favors self-expandable stents (e.g., Radius, Scimed Life Systems, Maple Grove, MN) whenever possible (see Figure 12-4). This stent has been useful when treating petrous and proximal cavernous carotid artery lesions. However, it is slightly bulkier than the existing balloon-expandable coronary stents and not as trackable through tortuous vessels. More distal lesions can be easily treated using small balloon-expandable stents (e.g., Multilink Duet, Guidant Corp., Temecula, CA).

Issue of Cerebral Protection

Perhaps one of the most important controversial topics related to carotid PTAs is the use of a protection device to decrease the risk of distal embolization to the brain tissue. The most widely used CAS technique is that described in the preceding sections, and it does not involve any specific steps for protection against distal embolism. Essentially, it is analogous to that used in the coronary and peripheral circulations. However, Theron et al. have introduced and championed a technique that involves the use of a distally placed protection balloon designed to catch and help remove any embolic material.[11,29,31,56] This protection balloon technique is rather clumsy, however, and could use significant improvement. The future is likely to bring improved techniques for cerebral protection from distal embolism, including the use of microwire-based balloons[57] and umbrella filters that allow entrapment of debris without occluding flow in the vessel being treated.

Clinical Applications of Elective Neurovascular Stenting

The application of extracranial CAS is the most controversial topic in neuroendovascular therapy. Its introduction as an alternative mode of therapy to CEA has met with considerable resistance from the surgical community.[58,59] Despite this resistance, the considerations noted earlier support the notions of (1) applicability in specific subpopulations, and (2) clinical equipoise to justify randomized trials. In regards to the former point, it is the author's opinion that CAS should be considered in the following circumstances:

1. Patients whose stenotic lesion is relatively inaccessible, including proximal common carotid lesions (intrathoracic) and distal internal carotid pathology (distal cervical or intracranial) (see Figure 12-4)
2. Patients with nonatherosclerotic pathology (e.g., dissection, postradiation angiitis, dysplasia, restenosis after CEA) (Figures 12-5 and 12-6)[25,26,60,61]
3. Patients with higher than average risk for CEA (e.g., class IV cardiomyopathy or contralateral carotid occlusion)[10,62]

What remains is the unanswered question of which of the two techniques is better for the treatment of uncomplicated focal carotid lesions in patients with low operative risk. However, the existing experience with CAS supports the notion of clinical equipoise and the need for further randomized trials.

Equipoise for Carotid Revascularization: Randomized Trials

It is clear that extracranial CAS offers a potentially exciting alternative to CEA. Undoubtedly, further randomized prospective studies are necessary to illustrate the role and applications of CAS in relation to patients who can otherwise be safely treated with CEA. However, there is controversy about the timeliness of such a trial. I believe the following prerequisites must be met for a prospective trial of CAS versus CEA to be fair:

- *The procedure of CAS must be mature and standardized.* Based on discussions with different groups of interventionists, the author has found that the use of different materials (i.e., catheters, balloons, and stents) is variable. Procedural details continue to evolve, and they should be more homogeneous before study of CAS in a prospective fashion. Among other concerns, the issue of cerebral protection should be solved before trials (e.g., Is it necessary? How should it be carried out?).
- *There must be enough experienced endovascular therapists to carry out the study.* If the experience of the surgeon has an impact on the outcome of CEA,[63] shouldn't a similar logic apply to PTAs? The fact remains that experience in performing carotid PTAs is limited. Regardless of the background of the interventionist, a minimal number of procedures as well as evidence of proficiency and safety must be shown before acceptance into groups of investigators. This is analogous to the audits that were conducted on the surgeons that participated in the CEA trials.[2]
- *Patient care must be entrusted to expert clinicians.* This is not a small point. It has been the author's experience that the care of patients before and after the procedure has a significant impact on their outcome. The great majority of interventionists who are capable of performing carotid CAS do not have sufficient experience in the care of neurologic patients, patients at risk for stroke, and patients who have had a stroke. Simple issues, such as how to manage fluids, blood pressure, and anticoagulation, become relevant when caring for these patients, and underscore the necessity for involving experienced vascular neurologists.
- *The technology of stents must have evolved to the point of using devices ideally suited for the carotid artery.* Stent technology is advancing rapidly. It would be ideal to wait for the most suitable stent before testing the procedure. In fact, a point may be reached at which different lesions may require different stents. These considerations must be

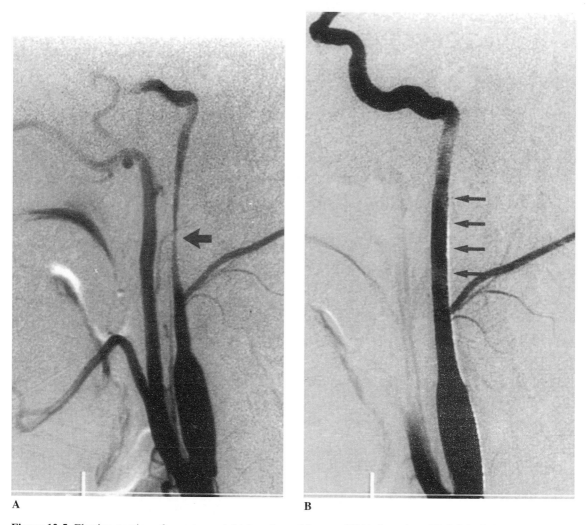

A   B

Figure 12-5. Elective stenting of an extracranial internal carotid artery (ICA) dissection. **(A)** Original view demonstrates severe stenosis of an extensive segment of the cervical ICA, all the way to the base of the skull (*arrow*). **(B)** After treatment with stainless steel self-expandable stents, the true vessel lumen is restored (*arrows*).

developed after sufficient experience with the technique has been acquired.

Issues Relative to Intracranial Stenting

With regard to intracranial stenting, there simply is no surgical alternative and, thus, the only conceivable randomization would have to be between endovascular treatment and medical treatment. However, there is no consensus about what constitutes optimal medical therapy. The literature suggests that long-term anticoagulation with warfarin is superior to antiplatelet agents in prevention of stroke[64]; however, a prospective, randomized, controlled trial comparing both forms of treatment is ongoing. Needless to say, the prerequisites noted in the preceding section about the organization of a randomized trial for extracranial CAS also apply to intracranial stenting. In fact, such prerequisites may be more critical for intracranial stenting because it is technically more challenging, and there is less experience with it (Figure 12-7; see Figure 12-4). In any case, the risk of stroke as a result of intracranial cerebral lesions is sufficiently high to warrant further study of this subject.

Figure 12-6. Elective stenting of an innominate artery. (**A**) Original view displays the stenosis, the guide catheter, and the guidewire already across the lesion (*curved arrow*). (**B**) Final image displays normalization of the vessel lumen (*thick arrow*). Note that the patient has previously required stenting of the left vertebral and left common carotid arteries' ostia (*thin arrows*).

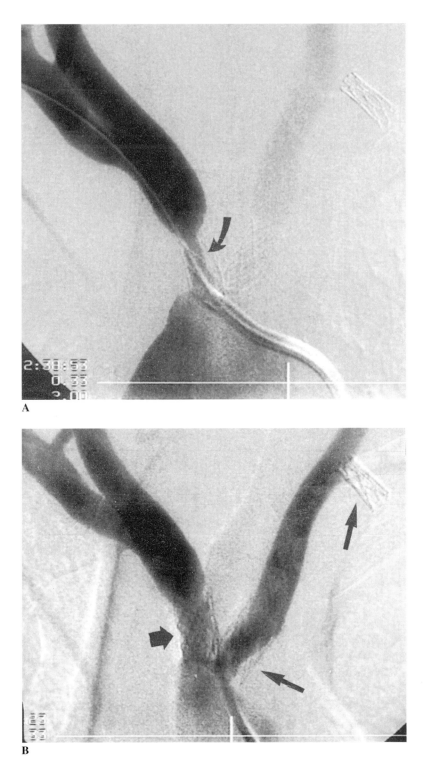

A

B

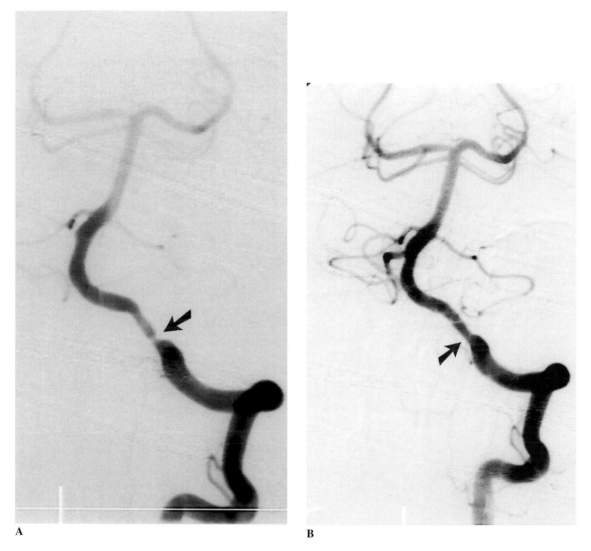

A   B

Figure 12-7. Elective stenting of an intracranial left vertebral artery (LVA). (**A**) Original image shows significant stenosis of the distal LVA (*arrow*). The patient also has severe contralateral vertebral artery stenosis. (**B**) After deployment of a balloon-expandable coronary stent, the lumen is restored (*arrow*).

Conclusion

The prevention of stroke, the third leading cause of death and the most important cause of disability, is the responsibility of everyone involved in the care of neurologic patients. Therefore, the availability, development, maturation, and proliferation of endovascular techniques for the correction of carotid artery pathology should be a welcome addition to the therapeutic armamentarium in the fight against stroke. Further study of these techniques and their application should be fostered to help determine the right approach to each type of patient with each type of carotid pathology. The study of extracranial CAS as it compares with CEA should be carried out under optimal conditions to assure the most realistic and applicable results. The study of extracranial vertebrobasilar and intracranial stenting requires further technical advances and better therapeutic medical outcome data.

References

1. MRC European Carotid Surgery Trial: interim results for symptomatic patients with severe (70–99%) or with mild (0–29%) carotid stenosis. European Carotid Surgery Trialists' Collaborative Group. Lancet 1991;337: 1235–1243.
2. Beneficial effect of carotid endarterectomy in symptomatic patients with high-grade carotid stenosis. North American Symptomatic Carotid Endarterectomy Trial Collaborators. N Engl J Med 1991;325:445–453.
3. Endarterectomy for asymptomatic carotid artery stenosis. Executive Committee for the Asymptomatic Carotid Atherosclerosis Study. JAMA 1995;273:1421–1428.
4. Barnett HJ, Taylor DW, Eliasziw M, et al. Benefit of carotid endarterectomy in patients with symptomatic moderate or severe stenosis. North American Symptomatic Carotid Endarterectomy Trial Collaborators. N Engl J Med 1998;339:1415–1425.
5. Bergeron P, Rudondy P, Benichou H, et al. Transluminal angioplasty for recurrent stenosis after carotid endarterectomy. Prognostic factors and indications. Int Angiol 1993;12:256–259.
6. Yadav JS, Roubin GS, King P, et al. Angioplasty and stenting for restenosis after carotid endarterectomy. Initial experience. Stroke 1996;27:2075–2079.
7. Courtheoux P, Theron J, Tournade A, et al. Percutaneous endoluminal angioplasty of post endarterectomy carotid stenoses. Neuroradiology 1987;29:186–189.
8. Atar E, Garniek A, Rabi I, et al. [Angioplasty and stenting of the carotid artery]. Harefuah 1997;132:388–391,448.
9. Ferguson RD, Ferguson JG. Carotid angioplasty. In search of a worthy alternative to endarterectomy. Arch Neurol 1996;53:696–698.
10. Babatasi G, Theron J, Massetti M, et al. [Value of percutaneous carotid angioplasty before cardiac surgery]. Ann Cardiol Angeiol (Paris) 1996;45:24 29.
11. Theron J. [Protected carotid angioplasty and carotid stents]. J Mal Vasc 1996;21(Suppl A):113–122.
12. Moore WS, Barnett HJ, Beebe HG, et al. Guidelines for carotid endarterectomy. A multidisciplinary consensus statement from the ad hoc Committee, American Heart Association. Stroke 1995;26:188–201.
13. Rothwell PM, Slattery J, Warlow CP. A systematic comparison of the risks of stroke and death due to carotid endarterectomy for symptomatic and asymptomatic stenosis. Stroke 1996;27:266–269.
14. Rothwell PM, Slattery J, Warlow CP. A systematic review of the risks of stroke and death due to endarterectomy for symptomatic carotid stenosis. Stroke 1996;27:260–265.
15. Spetzler RF, Hadley MN, Martin NA, et al. Vertebrobasilar insufficiency. Part 1. Microsurgical treatment of extracranial vertebrobasilar disease. J Neurosurg 1987;66:648–661.
16. Imparato AM. Vertebral arterial reconstruction: a nineteen-year experience. J Vasc Surg 1985;2:626–634.
17. Hass WK, Fields WS, North RR, et al. Joint Study of Extracranial Arterial Occlusion. II. Arteriography, techniques, sites, and complications. JAMA 1968;203:159–166.
18. North American Symptomatic Carotid Endarterectomy Trial. Methods, patient characteristics, and progress. Stroke 1991;22:711–720.
19. Goldstein LB, McCrory DC, Landsman PB, et al. Multicenter review of preoperative risk factors for carotid endarterectomy in patients with ipsilateral symptoms. Stroke 1994;25:1116–1121.
20. McCrory DC, Goldstein LB, Samsa GP, et al. Predicting complications of carotid endarterectomy. Stroke 1993;24:1285–1291.
21. Gasecki AP, Eliasziw M, Ferguson GG, et al. Long-term prognosis and effect of endarterectomy in patients with symptomatic severe carotid stenosis and contralateral carotid stenosis or occlusion: results from NASCET. North American Symptomatic Carotid Endarterectomy Trial (NASCET) Group. J Neurosurg 1995;83:778–782.
22. Bockenheimer SA, Mathias K. Percutaneous transluminal angioplasty in arteriosclerotic internal carotid artery stenosis. AJNR Am J Neuroradiol 1983;4:791–792.
23. Tievsky AL, Druy EM, Mardiat JG. Transluminal angioplasty in postsurgical stenosis of the extracranial carotid artery. AJNR Am J Neuroradiol 1983;4:800–802.
24. Wiggli U, Gratzl O. Transluminal angioplasty of stenotic carotid arteries: case reports and protocol. AJNR Am J Neuroradiol 1983;4:793–795.
25. Dublin AB, Baltaxe HA, Cobb CA III. Percutaneous transluminal carotid angioplasty in fibromuscular dysplasia. Case report. J Neurosurg 1983;591:162–165.
26. Dublin AB, Baltaxe HA, Cobb CA 3d. Percutaneous transluminal carotid angioplasty and detachable balloon embolization in fibromuscular dysplasia. AJNR Am J Neuroradiol 1984;5:646–648.
27. Tsai FY, Matovich V, Hieshima G, et al. Percutaneous transluminal angioplasty of the carotid artery. AJNR Am J Neuroradiol 1986;7:349–358.
28. Tsai FY, Matovich VB, Hieshima GB, et al. Practical aspects of percutaneous transluminal angioplasty of the carotid artery. Acta Radiol Suppl 1986;369:127–130.
29. Theron J, Raymond J, Casasco A, et al. Percutaneous angioplasty of atherosclerotic and postsurgical stenosis of carotid arteries. AJNR Am J Neuroradiol 1987;8:495–500.
30. Brown MM, Butler P, Gibbs J, et al. Feasibility of percutaneous transluminal angioplasty for carotid artery stenosis. J Neurol Neurosurg Psychiatry 1990;53:238–243.
31. Theron J, Courtheoux P, Alachkar F, et al. New triple coaxial catheter system for carotid angioplasty with cerebral protection. AJNR Am J Neuroradiol 1990;11:869–874; discussion 875–877.
32. Munari LM, Belloni G, Perretti A, et al. Carotid percutaneous angioplasty. Neurol Res 1992;14(Suppl 2):156–158.
33. Kachel R, Basche S, Heerklotz I, et al. Percutaneous transluminal angioplasty (PTA) of supra-aortic arteries especially the internal carotid artery. Neuroradiology 1991;33:191–194.
34. Kachel R. Results of balloon angioplasty in the carotid arteries. J Endovasc Surg 1996;3:22–30.
35. Brown M. Results of the Carotid and Vertebral Artery Transluminal Angioplasty Study (CAVATAS). Cerebrovasc Dis 1998;8(Suppl 4):21.

36. Mathias K. [Catheter treatment of arterial occlusive disease of supra-aortic vessels]. Radiology 1987;27:547–554.

37. Yadav JS, Roubin GS, Iyer S, et al. Elective stenting of the extracranial carotid arteries. Circulation 1997;95:376–381.

38. Roubin GS, Yadav S, Iyer SS, Vitek J. Carotid stent-supported angioplasty: a neurovascular intervention to prevent stroke. Am J Cardiol 1996;78:8–12.

39. Lanzino G, Mericle RA, Lopes D, et al. Percutaneous transluminal angioplasty and stent placement for recurrent carotid artery stenosis. J Neurosurg 1999;90:688–694.

40. Bergeron P, Becquemin JP, Jausseran JM, et al. Percutaneous stenting of the internal carotid artery: the European CAST I Study. Carotid Artery Stent Trial. J Endovasc Surg 1999;6:155–159.

41. Wholey M, Wholey M, Eles G, et al. Current international status of carotid artery stenting. J Endovasc Surg 1998;5(Suppl I):38–39.

42. Higashida RT, Tsai FY, Halbach VV, et al. Transluminal angioplasty for atherosclerotic disease of the vertebral and basilar arteries. J Neurosurg 1993;78:192–198.

43. Mortarjeme A, Keifer JW, Zuska AJ. Percutaneous transluminal angioplasty of the vertebral arteries. Radiology 1981;139:715–717.

44. Theron J, Courtheoux P, Henriet JP, et al. Angioplasty of supra-aortic arteries. J Neuroradiol 1984;11:187–200.

45. Courtheoux P, Tournade A, Theron J, et al. Transcutaneous angioplasty of vertebral artery atheromatous ostial stricture. Neuroradiology 1985;27:259–264.

46. Chastain HD, Campbell MS, Iyer S, et al. Extracranial vertebral artery stent placement: in-hospital and follow-up results. J Neurosurg 1999;91:547–552.

47. Al-Mubarak N, Gomez CR, Vitek JJ, Roubin GS. Stenting of symptomatic intracranial internal carotid artery stenosis: a case report. AJNR Am J Neuroradiol 1998;19:1949–1951.

48. Dorros G, Cohn JM, Palmer LE. Stent deployment resolves a petrous carotid artery angioplasty dissection. AJNR Am J Neuroradiol 1998;19:392–394.

49. Mori T, Kazita K, Mori K. Cerebral angioplasty and stenting for intracranial vertebral atherosclerotic stenosis. AJNR Am J Neuroradiol 1999;20:787–789.

50. Mori T, Kazita K, Seike M, et al. Successful cerebral stent placement for total occlusion of the vertebrobasilar artery in a patient experiencing from acute stroke. Case report. J Neurosurg 1999;90:955–958.

51. Lanzino G, Wakhloo AK, Fessler RD, et al. Efficacy and current limitations of intravascular stents for intracranial internal carotid, vertebral, and basilar artery aneurysms. J Neurosurg 1999;91:538–546.

52. Lanzino G, Fessler RD, Miletich RS, et al. Angioplasty and stenting of basilar artery stenosis: technical case report. Neurosurgery 1999;45:404–408.

53. Malek AM, Higashida RT, Halbach VV, et al. Tandem intracranial stent deployment for treatment of an iatrogenic, flow-limiting, basilar artery dissection: technical case report. Neurosurgery 1999;45:919–924.

54. Gomez CR, Roubin GS, Dean LS, et al. Neurological monitoring during carotid artery stenting: the Duck Squeezing Test. J Endovasc Surg 1999;6:332–336.

55. Mathur A, Dorros G, Iyer SS, et al. Palmaz stent compression in patients following carotid artery stenting. Cathet Cardiovasc Design 1997;41:137–140.

56. Theron JG, Payelle GG, Coskun O, et al. Carotid artery stenosis: treatment with protected balloon angioplasty and stent placement. Radiology 1996;201:627–636.

57. Henry M, Amor M, Henry I, et al. Carotid stenting with cerebral protection: first clinical experience using the PercuSurge GuardWire system. J Endovasc Surg 1999;66:321–331.

58. Beebe HG, Archie JP, Baker WH, et al. Concern about safety of carotid angioplasty. Stroke 1996;27:197–198.

59. Statement regarding carotid angioplasty and stenting. Society for Vascular Surgery. International Society for Cardiovascular Surgery, North American Chapter. J Vasc Surg 1996;24:900.

60. Miyachi S, Ishiguchi T, Taniguchi K, et al. Endovascular stenting of a traumatic dissecting aneurysm of the extracranial internal carotid artery—case report. Neurol Med Chirur (Tokyo) 1997;37:270–274.

61. DeOcampo J, Brillman J, Levy DI. Stenting: a new approach to carotid dissection. J Neuroimaging 1997;7:187–190.

62. Mathur A, Roubin GS, Gomez CR, et al. Elective carotid artery stenting in the presence of contralateral occlusion. Am J Cardiol 1998;81:1315–1317.

63. Ruby ST, Robinson D, Lynch JT, Mark H. Outcome analysis of carotid endarterectomy in Connecticut: the impact of volume and specialty. Ann Vasc Surg 1996;10:22–26.

64. Chimowitz MI, Kokkinos J, Strong J, et al. The Warfarin-Aspirin Symptomatic Intracranial Disease Study. Neurology 1995;45:1488–1493.

Chapter 13
General Management of Acute Stroke

Serge A. Blecic and Gérald Devuyst

Despite medical progress leading to a decline in incidence and mortality, stroke remains the third leading cause of death in developed countries after cardiovascular diseases and cancer.[1] The control of risk factors, such as arterial hypertension, diabetes, or hypercholesterolemia, is a major contributor to the decrease of stroke incidence. There is also increasing interest in the management of physiologic variables after acute stroke, particularly blood pressure (BP) (to treat or not to treat?), glucose, and body temperature, with growing evidence that modification of these parameters could result in a reduction of stroke severity and improved long-term functional outcome. However, stroke occurs in approximately 170 per 100,000 people annually, corresponding to a prevalence of 5% of the population older than age 65 years.[2–4] The estimated yearly direct cost of stroke disability is approximately $16.8 billion in the United States.[4]

Recently, special attention has been given to the pathophysiology of stroke, the development of sophisticated diagnostic devices, and new treatments resulting from specific drugs.[5–8] No specific therapy aside from recombinant tissue plasminogen activator has proven to be effective in the treatment of acute ischemic stroke, however, partly because of major differences between animal models and human stroke. Other reasons for this probably also include the heterogeneity of stroke pathogenesis, the difference between stroke subtypes, and the lack of consensus in stroke management.

Stroke management does not concern only acute treatment but also patient management. The lack of efficacy of acute treatments may be related to the fact that many patients are referred and treated too late after the onset of stroke symptoms.[8,9] The ideal management of stroke patients implies a quick evaluation of the neurologic condition, performance of selected investigations, and management of the patient in a special stroke care unit.[10,11] The importance of clinical evaluation, which is the basis for the choice and timing of investigations as well as for evaluating the efficacy of treatment, will be emphasized here.

Investigations in Acute Ischemic Stroke

The choice and timing of investigations is fundamental, but it is difficult to establish a standard protocol because it depends on patient characteristics, stroke topography, and the existence of other medical problems. Investigations in acute stroke include two steps: (1) confirmation of stroke, and (2) the determination of the most likely etiology of stroke.

Investigations to Confirm the Diagnosis of Stroke

Computed Tomography

Computed tomography (CT) is the key for diagnosis and the pursuit of future investigations, and is usually necessary before treatment.[12] CT on an emergency basis is available at most medical centers. It is safe, noninvasive, and commonly performed without contrast administration. CT usually excludes intracranial hemorrhage or a space-occupying lesion, such as tumor or abscess.[13,14] When CT is performed within the first 6 hours of stroke onset, an ischemic lesion can be missed; however, in this particular situation, indirect infarct signs, such as a spontaneous hyperdense middle artery or obscuration of the cortico–subcortical gradient, are useful as general indicators of large infarctions leading to poor prognosis.[15] CT has other limitations, however (e.g., brain stem and posterior inferior cerebellar artery territory infarcts are not often seen even after stroke, and small cortical or subcortical infarcts can sometimes only be seen after contrast enhancement). When the baseline CT is normal, a repeat study a week after stroke onset is commonly recommended.

Magnetic Resonance Imaging

Magnetic resonance imaging (MRI) is the best examination tool for diagnosis and localization of ischemic stroke. Compared to CT, MRI is more sensitive and is better able to detect recent stroke.[16] The high sensitivity of MRI allows detection of the infarct hours after stroke, mainly with the appearance of T2 hyperintensity.[17] Because there is usually no problem with bone artifacts, MRI is the first choice for the detection of brain stem or cerebellar infarcts.[16,17] MRI can improve stroke localization and detect small infarcts.[18] The use of gadolinium-diethylenetriamine pentaacetic acid for contrast enhancement can improve the early detection of stroke and define the age of ischemic lesions.[19] Vascular occlusion or low flow can be seen on MRI, especially in large vessels, and the differentiation between thrombus and embolus can sometimes be made.[20] MRI also allows early detection of hemorrhagic transformation of ischemic stroke. Disadvantages of MRI include difficulties in ultra-early diagnosis of hemorrhage, high cost, and a long acquisition time, necessitating cooperation of the patient, which may not always occur in stroke patients. In addition, the specificity of MRI may lead to the detection of minor changes in brain water content without any clinical correlations.[12,17]

Investigations to Determine the Etiology of Stroke

Because the differential diagnosis of the cause of ischemic stroke is broad and the complete evaluation is potentially extensive and expensive, the rationale for etiologic investigations must be tailored to the individual patient.[21,22] An exhaustive search for less common causes of stroke should be reserved mainly for children, adults younger than age 45 years, and patients without an obvious risk of stroke.[12,22,23] In some cases, however, despite extensive investigations, the etiology of stroke remains uncertain.

Hematologic Investigations

Hematologic investigations are usually the first investigations prescribed and typically are obtained in the emergency room. Initial tests generally include a sedimentation rate, red and white blood cell count, platelet count, serum enzymes, cholesterol and lipids count, and routine coagulation profile.[24,25] Careful attention should be given to coagulation studies. In most cases, a routine coagulation profile, including serum fibrinogen, prothrombin time, and partial thromboplastin time is sufficient. In stroke patients without obvious risk factors for stroke, however, a coagulation disorder with a congenital defect in protein C, protein S, or antithrombin III can be present.[25–27] In some studies, antiphospholipid antibodies were suspected to be the cause of stroke.[28] To rule these out as possible causes of stroke, the levels of these proteins or antibodies should be obtained in the absence of anticoagulant therapy.[27–29] These analyses should be done as soon as possible in selected patients. The significance of abnormal findings for these proteins or antibodies has yet to be clarified, however, and the ischemic event or associated conditions can themselves induce coagulation changes.[29–33] We recommend interpreting these results cautiously and, when in doubt, reconfirming them with additional tests several weeks after stroke onset.

Noninvasive Studies

Noninvasive studies to confirm the diagnosis of stroke include echocardiography to examine the heart and ultrasound studies of the cervical and intracranial arteries. In cases of suspected cardioembolism, the investigation should include at least 24-hour, three-lead electrocardiographic monitoring and exercise electrocardiography (ECG) in selected patients.[12,24]

Echocardiography. The role of echocardiography is crucial in stroke investigation because cardioembolism is the cause of approximately 25–30% of ischemic strokes.[34] The neurologic presentation is often suggestive of cardioembolism.[34–37] Two-dimensional transthoracic echocardiography (TTE) is widely available and gives reliable information about ventricular walls as well as the aortic and mitral valves. TTE can exclude a left ventricular thrombus, and, when performed with contrast, can demonstrate intracardiac shunts,[35,36] which are frequent in young adults with stroke. However, the clinical significance of these abnormalities remains controversial in several instances.[36] One disadvantage of TTE is that most abnormalities are not as well demonstrated as with transesophageal echocardiography (TEE). In addition, TTE findings in obese patients are not reliable.[12]

Transesophageal Echocardiography. TEE represents an important advance in stroke diagnosis. It is critical for investigation of the posterior part of the heart, particularly the left atrium and its appendage.[37,38] TEE can also provide information on atheromatosis and ulcerated plaques located in the aortic arch.[39] Because it is semi-invasive, it should be considered primarily for patients suspected of having cardioembolism, in whom TTE is normal or unreliable. The disadvantages of TEE are largely due to the endoscopic procedure that necessitates cooperation from the patient. Rarely, electrophysiologic studies or exercise ECG may contribute to the determination of stroke etiology.[39,40]

Duplex Investigations. Duplex imaging of the extracranial carotid and vertebral arteries is easy, safe, and noninvasive. It can provide information on a possible arterial source of emboli and on arterial occlusion. Duplex imaging is performed as a screening procedure before more invasive investigations (i.e., cerebral angiography).[41] It is not likely to replace cerebral angiography before carotid surgery, however, because it does not evaluate the carotid siphon and the cerebral vessels. Duplex imaging can be combined with transcranial Doppler ultrasonography, which provides information on the cerebral circulation.[42] Its role in the detection of asymptomatic cerebral emboli has been emphasized.[43]

Electroencephalography. The use of electroencephalography in acute stroke is not essential, but it can provide information on stroke localization (deep vs. superficial) and sometimes may differentiate migraine from stroke.[44]

Magnetic Resonance Angiography. Magnetic resonance angiography gives information on blood vessels and blood flow,[45] and ultimately may replace conventional arteriography. Magnetic resonance angiography has the advantage of being noninvasive and giving technical resolution comparable to conventional angiography, with the possibility of having three-dimensional images.[46] This technique is only available in some centers, however, and its cost and reduced availability usually reserves it for selected patients.

Invasive Studies

Conventional Angiography. Conventional angiography is used to determine the presence of abnormalities in both intracranial and extracranial vessels.[12] In the first hours after stroke, small cerebral artery occlusions can be demonstrated, but in the management of acute stroke, the role of conventional angiography remains controversial.[47] In central nervous system vasculitis, abnormalities of cerebral vessels can be demonstrated on angiography, but the probability is only approximately 50%.[48] Finally, complications of this technique are not rare, though permanent complications are below 0.5%.[49] At the time of this writing, angiography is performed in the acute setting only in selected cases.

Cerebrospinal Fluid Investigations. Cerebrospinal fluid examination is rarely required for a patient with acute ischemic stroke. It can provide information in cases of cerebral venous thrombosis by the presence of red blood cells and high cerebrospinal fluid pressure, and in cases of vasculitis.

Neurochemical Monitoring. Microdialysis has been used to monitor neurochemical levels in basic science research. In a case report of Berger et al.,[50] microdialysis was used to monitor a severe middle cerebral artery (MCA) infarction. Investigators found a correlation between the early increase in the excitatory amino acid glutamate and glycerine levels, as well as a correlation between the lactate-pyruvate ratio and the neurologic evolution. This technique remains experimental but could be promising for future monitoring of patients with severe brain infarction.[50]

Other Investigations. Other investigations are rarely performed in acute stroke. Skin biopsy can be done when a cutaneovascular syndrome, a vasculitis, or collagen abnormalities are suspected.[51,52] Urine tests can also be performed in young stroke patients without well-known risk factors to exclude heterozygote homocystinuria[53] or the presence of drugs, such as cocaine, amphetamine-like substances, or cannabinoid in addicted patients.

Treatment of Stroke

Treatment of patients with acute stroke can be divided into the following aspects:

- Treatment of the stroke itself
- Management of physiologic variables after stroke, particularly BP, glucose, and body temperature
- Management of medical problems, including cardiac and respiratory care, fluid and metabolic maintenance, prevention of decubitus sores, prevention of phlebitis, and, sometimes, treatment of elevated intracranial pressure (ICP)[8,54,55]

Treatment of stroke also includes rehabilitation, which must start early in the course of patient care.[56,57]

Stroke Units

An important contribution to stroke management was the advent of stroke units (SUs). The initial concept was established in the late 1960s and modeled on coronary units, in the hope that patients with acute stroke could benefit from intensive care. SUs are organized similarly to coronary units.[9] Generally, they have monitoring facilities, including 24-hour heart rate, BP, and electroencephalogram recording. Artificially ventilated patients are usually not admitted, but patients with other acute neurologic conditions, such as myasthenia gravis or status epilepticus, can be admitted. Thus, such units may be more accurately called *neurologic acute care units*.[9,10] The aim of SUs was to decrease mortality related to stroke and offer a more secure place for patients receiving experimental treatment.[58] However, neither prospective nor retrospective studies showed a convincing modification in the death rate in SUs compared to conventional neurologic wards.[9,59] The early mortality rate in SUs is largely related to major brain damage due to severe strokes, which remains beyond therapeutic means, whereas late death primarily is due to secondary complications in disabled patients.[9,10,59–62] Patients in an SU can benefit from a specialized team, and monitoring of main vital functions helps detect potential complications early.

General Management, Prevention, and Treatment of Medical Complications after Acute Stroke

Treatment of acute stroke focuses on the management of general conditions, such as cardiac, pulmonary, or metabolic function, and treatment of medical complications associated with acute stroke, rather than on specific stroke treatment, such as reperfusion or prevention of extension of ischemic brain damage. A better prognosis of stroke is more often the consequence of good general management than of a specific therapy. Some authors also include treatment of elevated ICP.[8,63] Although it is well established that careful monitoring of vital functions may be the basis of successful treatment, several areas of treatment, such as arterial hypertension or cardiac arrhythmias, remain controversial.

Pulmonary Function and Prevention of Respiratory Complications

Maintenance of good blood oxygenation is appropriate in stroke patients and attention must be paid to respiratory status, although blood oxygenation has little effect on the damaged ischemic region of the brain. In addition to optimal oxygenation, some authors recommend a decrease in $Paco_2$ to between 25 mm Hg and 30 mm Hg to reduce ICP.[8,64] Oxygenation can be delivered either by nasal tube or mask; the oxygen concentration should be related to the result of blood arterial gas samples.[64] Artificial ventilation, which requires intubation, is sometimes necessary in brain stem stroke patients or in patients with large MCA territory infarct. Under these conditions, which are associated with a poor prognosis, patients are usually treated in a traditional intensive care unit rather than an SU. Respiratory tract infections are among the most serious complications of stroke, and pneumonia may account for 20–40% of deaths after stroke.[64,65] Large-spectrum antibiotic therapy must be started empirically when pneumonia is suspected and must be adapted to the results of cultures. Aspiration is a serious consequence of acute stroke and is most often encountered after brain stem infarct, with a prevalence of approximately 60–70%. It can remain undetected despite the presence of signs, such as absence of gag reflex or dysphagia.[63–65] In brain stem stroke, gastrostomy may be indicated in some instances. Pulmonary embolism after deep vein thrombosis is frequent.

The incidence of deep vein thrombosis is approximately 50–70%, and clinical pulmonary emboli occur in approximately 10–30% of patients.[66] The majority of patients experiencing deep venous thrombosis are asymptomatic, and clinical signs are often absent. The initial signs are commonly those related to pulmonary embolism, such as acute chest pain and respiratory distress syndrome. Diagnosis of deep vein thrombosis is difficult and can be missed on phlebography.[63,67] Diagnosis depends mainly on plethysmography, Doppler ultrasonography, and Duplex scanning.[66] In addition, diagnosis of pulmonary embolism may be difficult. Chest x-rays and ECGs may not be able to rule out embolism, but they can reveal other diseases, such as pneumonia or myocardial infarction. Alkalosis, hypoxemia, and hypocapnia on blood gas samples can be helpful, but normal blood gas findings are not sufficient to rule out embolism. Apart from pulmonary angiography, the best investigation method is lung perfusion scintigraphy compared to ventilation, but it requires a fully cooperative patient, at least for the ventilation test. Once the diagnosis of embolism is established, the best treatment is anticoagulation with continuous heparin infusion. The doses must be adjusted to the activated partial thromboplastin time, which must be maintained between 1.5 and 2.0 times the control values. There is no evidence

that low-molecular-weight heparin is more effective or safer than heparin, but its administration may be easier. Warfarin should be started approximately 3–7 days after the first dose of heparin and should be maintained for at least 3 months in case of major deep venous thrombosis.[66,67] Some studies have shown a reduction of 15–20% in the risk of deep vein thrombosis when preventive therapy for deep vein thrombosis is used. It should be initiated immediately after stroke by leg compression and with low doses of subcutaneous heparin (5,000–10,000 units twice daily) or with low-molecular-weight heparin subcutaneously.[67]

Cardiovascular Management

The optimization of the cardiac parameters is essential in stroke management.[8] Indeed, acute stroke is often associated with cardiovascular disturbances, and cerebral ischemia itself can induce ECG changes, paroxysmal arrhythmia, and even raise transaminase enzymes. More often, stroke is the consequence of cardiac dysfunction, such as myocardial infarct, cardiac arrhythmia, or right-to-left shunt.

Atrial arrhythmias are the most common cardiac abnormalities seen in stroke patients. Sudden death attributable to cardiac rhythm disturbances may account for approximately 5% of stroke deaths.[63,68] Atrial arrhythmia is the reason why cardiovascular monitoring is recommended in most cases. Other ECG abnormalities can be found in stroke patients, including repolarization abnormalities (abnormalities in U or T waves or S-T segments). These abnormalities are the consequence of coronary disease, with increased stress caused by stroke or by myocytolysis induced by marked sympathetic hyperactivity after acute brain injury. In 20% of stroke patients, elevated myocardial band enzymes of creatine phosphokinase are found.[69] Treatment of acute transient cardiac arrhythmia is not codified, contrary to known atrial fibrillation (AF), which necessitates anticoagulation or antiarrhythmic drugs, or both.[68,69]

Blood Pressure in Acute Ischemic Stroke:
To Treat or Not to Treat?

Despite the conclusive benefits of antihypertensive therapy in stroke prevention, BP reduction in acute stroke remains potentially hazardous. Arterial hypertension is common in acute stroke in both previously normotensive and hypertensive patients, and although it may be severe the first day, it usually decreases over the following 2 weeks. Several conditions lead to arterial hypertension, but the increase of vascular resistances and the Cushing phenomenon are commonly incriminated.[70] The management of arterial hypertension in acute stroke remains controversial because cerebral perfusion is directly related to systemic arterial BP and ICP. Secondary to cerebral autoregulation, cerebral blood flow (CBF) remains constant in healthy patients, with a mean arterial pressure between 80 mm Hg and 150 mm Hg. In chronic arterial hypertension patients, however, the lowest mean arterial pressure that maintains cerebral perfusion is increased to approximately 120 mm Hg or 150 mm Hg. In cerebral ischemia, the zone surrounding infarction is highly dependent on CBF, and, as autoregulation is impaired, a decrease in mean arterial pressure can lead to the extension of the ischemic zone. On the contrary, an increase in arterial pressure can raise CBF and lead to cerebral edema. The treatment of arterial hypertension remains controversial and depends on clinical factors. Patients with evidence for acute systemic disorders, such as cardiac failure or renal insufficiency due to hypertension or hypertensive encephalopathy, require urgent therapy. In other conditions, stroke guidelines are different, and patients with systolic BP >220 mm Hg, or mean BP >160 mm Hg may be cautiously treated with an acute antihypertensive therapy (unless tissue plasminogen activator [t-PA] is being administered), because a gradual decrease in BP is preferred.[71] One study using single-photon emission CT recommended careful attention to the choice of therapy in arterial hypertension and emphasized potential harmful effects of calcium channel blockers due to decreased blood flow in the penumbra.[70] It is well established that infarct size depends on perfusion within the ischemic penumbra, which is critically hypoperfused "at risk" tissue surrounding the infarct core. The blood vessels maximally dilate in this region, and with the paralysis of cerebral autoregulation, hypotension can be hazardous.[72] It generally has been concluded that acute treatment of hypertension in acute stroke may do more harm than good, and some authors have emphasized the uncertainties concerning manage-

ment of hypertension in acute stroke.[73] One clinical study conducted by Chamorro et al.[74] reported that it was unclear whether typical poststroke hypertension was a pathophysiologic response to maintain perfusion in the penumbral tissue, or a marker of stroke severity or progressive stroke. In this prospective study,[74] in which one-half of ischemic stroke patients received oral antihypertensive treatment within 24 hours of stroke onset, a 20–30% drop in mean arterial BP on the second day after stroke almost tripled the odds of recovery, and this reduction of BP was not associated with deteriorating stroke.[74] Britton et al.[75] also concluded that high BP in acute stroke was correlated with a worse outcome, whereas controlled hypertension in acute stroke may reduce the risk of hemorrhagic transformation.[72] Conversely, Jorgensen et al.[76] found an inverse relationship between high systolic BP and the risk of further stroke progression. However, the weight of evidence concerning the management of BP after stroke suggests the need for caution, except in hypertensive encephalopathy. There is still considerable uncertainty, and some literature[74,75] suggests that a modest BP reduction may improve functional outcome. This hypothesis is expected to be tested on a greater number of acute ischemic stroke patients in the near future. Intravenous administration is preferred because the treatment is infused continuously and can be removed when mean arterial pressure falls. Appropriate antihypertensive drugs should also be selected after the evaluation of concomitant conditions in individual patients. As mentioned before, calcium channels blockers should be avoided.

Adrenoceptor antagonists such as labetalol are often used because they have a short half-life, are relatively cardioprotective, and induce a relatively slight fall in arterial pressure; however, they must be cautiously used in patients with asthma, diabetes, or congestive heart failure. Angiotensin-converting enzyme inhibitors can be used in such patients, but intravenous forms are still in trials. Clonidine, a presynaptic adrenoreceptor agonist, can also be used but can sometimes induce a sharp drop in arterial pressure values.

Elevated Intracranial Pressure and Brain Edema

Management of increased ICP in acute stroke remains controversial.[77] Progressive clinical deterioration due to massive hemispheric edema occurs in 10% of patients and is also called *malignant MCA syndrome*. Cerebral edema due to ischemic stroke occurs within hours after stroke onset and is associated with an 80% mortality rate.[77] It is not common to have invasive monitoring of ICP in stroke patients, and, thus, its value is often difficult to appreciate. However, indirect clinical signs, such as stupor or coma, can indicate high ICP. Hyperventilation is considered a potential therapy, with maintenance of $PaCO_2$ at approximately 25–35 mm Hg and a slightly increased (30-degree) position of the head to decrease high ICP. When drugs are considered necessary, mannitol is used in the acute phase with an initial dose of 25–50 g over 30 minutes, followed by repeated 25-g doses every 6 hours, according to the clinical response and serum osmolarity.[77] Glycerol is also used and may be preferred for longer treatment.[78] In rare cases, such as large MCA territory infarct with cerebral edema or cerebellar infarct with obstructive hydrocephalus, decompressive surgery with craniotomy (and removing of the infarct zone in cerebellar stroke) is recommended.[79,80]

Blood Glucose in Acute Ischemic Stroke

Diabetes mellitus is often encountered in stroke patients, in whom it constitutes a well-known risk factor and is associated with a two- to threefold increased risk of ischemic stroke.[81] Pre-existing diabetes may worsen during acute stroke and necessitate an increase in insulin treatment. Hyperglycemia accompanying acute stroke in nondiabetic patients is due to elevation in serum levels of cortisol, catecholamines, growth hormone, and glucagon secondary to stress. The release of these hormones is directly related to the size of infarct, and because they stimulate neoglycogenesis, hyperglycemia may occur, especially in patients with pre-existing glucose intolerance. The elevated glucose level is correlated to lactic acidosis (lactate accumulation, intracellular acidosis) and contributes to the extension of brain damage.[82] It is debated whether hyperglycemia is merely a reflection of a more severe stroke, however, rather than having a casual relationship, and there is evidence that hyperglycemia in acute stroke might be a secondary stress response.[83,84] In some nondiabetic acute stroke patients, insulin can temporarily be prescribed when the blood glucose level exceeds 12 mmol per 100 ml.

Body Temperature

There is substantial observational and experimental evidence to indicate that elevated body temperature after stroke is associated with worse outcome. In animal models, the histologic effects of ischemia can be related to brain temperature, and reduced intraischemic temperature is associated with a range of effects, including an attenuation of glutamate release.[85,86] Multiple mechanisms are likely associated with worsened ischemic injury due to hyperthermia, such as enhanced release of neurotransmitters and excitotoxic amino acids, exaggerated oxygen free radical production, more extensive blood-brain barrier breakdown, increased number of potentially damaging postischemic depolarizations in the penumbral region, impaired recovery of energy metabolism, worsening of cytoskeleton proteolysis, and increased lactic acidosis. Increase in body temperature is common after focal and global ischemia. Experimental studies suggested that moderate degrees of brain cooling could protect against global ischemic neuronal injury, as in cardiac arrest.[87] Mild degrees of hypothermia (e.g., brain temperature of 35°C, optimized at 32°C) have been applied in neurosurgical procedures, brain trauma, and open heart surgery. Severe hypothermia of less than 27°C commonly produces cardiac arrhythmias, such as AF, myocardial depression, hypotension, bleeding disorders, and adverse metabolic effects.[87] Several studies in rat models of MCA occlusion have demonstrated infarct size reduction with transient hypothermia.[88–90] The study of Maier et al.[89] showed that mild hypothermia of 33°C or 30°C was neuroprotective (33°C was better tolerated), and that hypothermia had to be maintained for 1–2 hours to reach optimal neuroprotection. In acute stroke patients, body temperature has been associated with initial stroke severity, infarct size, mortality, and functional outcome.[91,92] Reith et al.[91] found that an elevated body temperature was independently related to initial stroke severity, infarct size, mortality, and outcome in survivors. In stroke patients studied within 6 hours of stroke onset, Reith et al.[91] found that for each 1°C increase in body temperature, the relative risk of poor outcome (death or disability) was increased by an odds ratio of 2.2 (95% confidence interval, 1.4–3.5). A study conducted by Schwab et al.[93] showed that moderate hypothermia (e.g., maintaining a body core temperature of 33°C for 48–72 hours with cooling blankets, cold infusions, and cold washing) in 25 stroke patients with severe MCA infarction within 48 hours of stroke onset was associated with a reduction in elevated ICP, the most common cause of death in this group. Forty percent of these patients developed pneumonia, and there was no control group. Schwab et al.[93] concluded that moderate hypothermia could decrease ICP and potentially reduce mortality in stroke patients with space-occupying MCA infarct. Even if there is compelling evidence that hyperthermia is associated with worse outcome after stroke, the use of induced moderate hypothermia should await results from further randomized and controlled clinical trials. Recommendations are to detect and correct early hyperthermia even if the increase in temperature is mild to moderate.[91,94,95]

Water and Electrolyte Balance

The maintenance of fluid and electrolyte balance is fundamental in stroke patients. It is important to avoid dehydration and impairment of blood viscosity. Some authors suggest that in cases of raised ICP, a slightly negative fluid balance should be considered.[8,78] Syndrome of inappropriate secretion of antidiuretic hormone is seen in approximately 10% of stroke patients and should be differentiated from other causes of hyponatremia, which can be ruled out by assessment of serum and urine osmolarity. Management of this syndrome should be conservative because most cases recover spontaneously. In refractory cases, the first therapy is an increase in sodium intake and a slight decrease in water balance. If this approach fails, specific treatments, such as fluorocortisone or furosemide, may be introduced.[63]

Urinary Tract Infections

Urinary tract infections are a frequent cause of morbidity and mortality in stroke patients. The presence of a urinary catheter is frequently implicated in the development of infection.[65] Diagnosis is usually easy; treatment consists of removing the catheter and starting appropriate antibiotic therapy.

Prevention of Seizures

Stroke can be accompanied by generalized or focal seizures.[96,97] When seizures occur, treatment should be started with diphenyl-hydantoin, 1 g intravenously, over 30–60 minutes with cardiac rhythm monitoring, or with clonazepam or diazepam, 10–20 mg injected slowly, followed by 3–4 mg per hour administered continuously. For single seizures, oral diphenylhydantoin loading is preferred.

Bedsore Prevention

Bedsores are frequent in disabled and bedridden patients. They are responsible for a marked increase in morbidity and mortality and the risk of sepsis. Treatment requires careful nursing attention, alternate side positioning in bed, local treatment, and reconstructive surgery in cases of severe ulceration. Attention must be paid to diet, which should include adequate protein to avoid hypoproteinemia, a condition commonly associated with bedsores.

Specific Treatment of Ischemic Stroke

Acute ischemic stroke therapy includes three main aspects: (1) reperfusion of the occluded artery territory, (2) prevention of extension or increase in the ischemic areas, and (3) immediate prevention of stroke recurrence. The importance for patients to be referred early for evaluation is reemphasized. Animal studies have demonstrated that focal ischemic insults require several hours to progress after artery occlusion and are complete after approximately 6 hours. In humans, the time window depends on several factors, such as stroke localization or other medical conditions; however, 6 hours after the onset of stroke has been arbitrarily defined as the limit to initiate reperfusion.[98,99]

Thrombolytic Therapy

The aim of thrombolytic therapy is to induce early artery recanalization.[99] The efficacy of thrombolysis in acute ischemic coronary diseases led to use in cerebral infarction. Several reports demonstrated significant neurologic improvement after thrombolysis initiated within the first hours after stroke, with better outcomes when recanalization was demonstrated.[99–104] The European Cooperative Acute Stroke Study used 1.1 mg/kg t-PA infused intravenously with a window of up to 6 hours after symptom onset. Patients showing early infarct signs

(>33% of the MCA territory) on CT were excluded.[102] There was a nonsignificant difference in the 30-day mortality rate, although the incidence of major hemorrhagic transformation was 19.8% for patients receiving t-PA, compared with 6.5% for patients in the control group. At 3 months, 41% of t-PA patients were symptomatic or had minimal disability, compared with 29% in the placebo group, although there was only a slight difference between the two groups in Barthel Index and Rankin Scale scores. In the National Institute of Neurological Disorders and Stroke trial, intravenous t-PA was given to patients earlier than in the European Cooperative Acute Stroke Study (e.g., 0.9 mg/kg within 3 hours of symptom onset). Investigators found significant improvement in the National Institutes of Health Stroke Scale at 24 hours (8 vs. 12 for the control group), and significant improvement in the National Institutes of Health Stroke Scale, Barthel Index, Rankin Scale, and Glasgow Outcome Scale at 3 months.[103,104] Although 6.4% of intravenous t-PA patients had symptomatic intracerebral hemorrhage (compared with 0.6% of control patients), the mortality rate at 3 months was slightly better for patients treated with intravenous t-PA (death was observed in 21% of placebo patients vs. 17% of intravenous t-PA patients).[104] Several authors reported on reperfusion after local thrombolysis.[105–107] This technique requires emergency angiography and expertise in vessel catheterization; thus, it is reserved for selected centers. Intra-arterial thrombolysis may be delivered systemically or not. Advantages of local delivery include faster recanalization, with a reduction in the total dose of drug administered. The Prolyse in Acute Cerebral Thromboembolism study used 6 mg of recombinant prourokinase (rpro-UK) given intra-arterially plus intravenous heparin within 6 hours of a proximal MCA (M1 or M2) stroke.[108] The recanalization rate was 66% for the rpro-UK group and 27% for the control group. At 3 months, 40% of the rpro-UK patients had slight or no neurologic disability compared with 25% of placebo patients. Although the rate of intracerebral hemorrhage with neurologic deterioration was 10% for the rpro-UK patients, compared with 2% for the control group, there was no statistically significant difference in overall mortality (25% for the treatment group vs. 27% for the control group). Observations on thrombolysis-induced recanalization should be tempered by the fact that artery recanalization is also observed spontaneously in approximately one-fifth of patients during the first hours after stroke and in more than one-half of the population after 18 hours.[109]

Anticoagulation and Antiaggregant Therapy

In comparison to thrombolysis, anticoagulation with heparin cannot dissolve thrombi. The rationale for anticoagulation in acute stroke is to impair thrombogenesis resulting from the clotting cascade and prevent thrombus extension and early recurrence of embolism.[110–112] Heparin is mainly used to prevent recurrence of stroke in patients with cardiac arrhythmia or ventricular dysfunction.[110–119] Its role in the treatment of "stroke in evolution" or in the prevention of occlusion in carotid stenosis remains controversial.[115–118] Non–contrast-enhanced CT is sufficient to exclude primary hemorrhage before anticoagulation. CT is controlled in case of neurologic worsening; if hemorrhagic transformation is demonstrated, heparin is usually stopped, although one study showed the absence of neurologic worsening in patients with hemorrhagic stroke.[119] Optimal anticoagulation requires daily monitoring of the activated partial thromboplastin time, which should be between 1.5 and 2.0 times the control value. Heparin is maintained for no more than 10 days to avoid thrombocytopenia, a frequently overlooked side effect.[120] The use of the anticoagulant treatment with warfarin is recommended in cases of cardioembolism. Although it is clear that anticoagulation is beneficial in patients with a definite cardiac source of embolism, no study has demonstrated a beneficial role of early anticoagulation in the general stroke population. The large randomized International Stroke Trial (IST) divided patients into several groups: those who received aspirin (300 mg/day) and those who were treated either with subcutaneous heparin (5,000 units twice daily or 12,500 units twice daily) or without.[121] There was no difference in mortality at 14 days (9% of heparin recipients and 9.3% for those without heparin) or at 6 months (62.9% for both). At 14 days, the recurrence rate of stroke was only slightly reduced for the heparin group compared with the nonheparin group (2.9% vs. 3.8%), but hemorrhagic stroke increased from 0.4% for the nonheparin group to 1.2% in the heparin group. The group receiving the higher dose of heparin was associated with an increase in hemorrhagic transformation, systemic bleeding, and an increase in death at 14 days, compared with the lower dose group. The lower dose of heparin reduced the risk of early death or nonfatal stroke, with only a small increase in the risk of hemorrhage. Overall, the IST showed subcutaneous heparin reduced the risk of stroke recurrence, but the benefit was counterbalanced by the increase in overall hemorrhage. In this study, however, coagulation monitoring was not systematically performed, and therapy could be started before a CT scan was obtained to verify that the stroke was not hemorrhagic. This might slightly impact the negative results of this study. In addition, patients who could benefit the most from heparin treatment (i.e., patients with a possible cardiac source of embolism) were not always included. In the IST study, patients with AF accounted for only 14% of the total, which is less than in a general stroke population. This was explained by the fact that inclusions were dependent on medical opinion, and patients who required treatment with heparin were excluded.[121] The Trial of ORG 10172 in Acute Stroke Treatment evaluated danaparoid given within 24 hours of stroke onset. A nonsignificant difference in the proportion of patients with a favorable outcome at 3 months (75.2% vs. 73.7% for the placebo group) was observed.[122]

Platelet antiaggregant therapy is based on three main principles: (1) reduction of platelet adhesivity, (2) reduction in platelet aggregation, and (3) a decrease in the release of active platelet substances. Three antiplatelet agents have proven efficacy in stroke recurrence prevention: aspirin, an inhibitor of cyclooxygenase (the crucial enzyme in the pathway of arachidonic acid), and ticlopidine and clopidogrel, which act on the adenosine diphosphate pathway of platelet activation. Aspirin is easier to handle, and ticlopidine or clopidogrel is used as an alternative therapy. The exact dose of aspirin remains controversial; in Europe and the United States, 300 mg per day is commonly prescribed, whereas more than 1,000 mg is recommended in Canada, and 30 mg is recommended in the Netherlands.[99] Inhibitors of the glycoprotein IIb-IIIa platelet receptor are promising but are still under investigation.[123] Preliminary studies of cardiac and experimental occlusion models have shown early vascular repermeability after intravenous infusion of glycoprotein IIb-IIIa platelet receptor inhibitors.[123]

Hemodilution

Hemodilution has been shown to increase blood flow in the ischemic brain in experimental and clinical trials. Several studies using different techniques of hemodilution failed to show improvement of neurologic status[124–126]; moreover, one study was stopped early because of increased death attributed to brain edema.[126] However, hemodilution remains indicated in acute stroke with high hematocrit or in systemic disease with hyperviscosity state. This treatment requires careful monitoring in patients with heart disease or cerebral edema.[8]

Calcium Channel Antagonists

The pathologic role of calcium in the development of ischemia is well established. Calcium intake is mediated by different calcium channels. Nimodipine and other calcium blockers, such as flunarizine or nifedipine, are antagonists of voltage-dependent calcium channels. Also, ischemia leads to the release of excitatory neurotransmitters, such as glutamate or aspartate, which induce entry of calcium into cells via receptor-mediated membrane channels (receptors include kainate, alpha-amino-3-hydroxy-5-methyl-4-isoxazolepropionic acid, or N-methyl-D-aspartate). These receptors have several different sites linked to neurotransmitters. The N-methyl-D-aspartate receptor has six different sites that can be occupied by different antagonists. Several experimental animal model trials have shown a beneficial role of calcium channel antagonists, but these findings were not replicated in several human studies.[127–133] Calcium antagonists are not used in clinical practice.

Management of Cerebral Hemorrhage

Hemorrhages can be distinguished by their localization (e.g., epidural or subdural, subarachnoidal or intraparenchymatous). This distinction is fundamental because management and treatment are different, and subarachnoidal hemorrhage as well as epidural or subdural hematomas necessitate a prompt neurosurgical assessment.

Intraparenchymatous hemorrhage is characterized by bleeding into the brain. It primarily results in rupture of Charcot-Bouchard microaneurysms located on the small penetrator arteries; arterial hypertension is often the related risk factor.[133-136]

In elderly patients without hypertension, lobar hemorrhage can also occur and is usually due to amyloid angiopathy. Special attention should be paid to treatment of arterial hypertension, because although acutely elevated BP can favor bleeding, cerebral hemorrhage is a space-occupying lesion and induces intracranial hypertension. In that condition, an increase in arterial BP is the sole means to preserve cerebral perfusion, and treatment is recommended only when mean arterial BP rises to more than 130–150 mm Hg. There is no specific treatment for cerebral hemorrhage, but in case of cerebellar hemorrhage when vital prognosis is compromised, surgery is commonly proposed. Surgery is also performed at several centers in patients with large, nondominant hemispheric hemorrhage, but benefit remains unproved.[79,80]

References

1. Mas JL, Zuber M. Epidemiology of ischemic stroke. Cerebrovasc Dis 1991;1(Suppl 1):36–44.
2. Homer D, Whisnant JP, Schoenberg BS. Trends in the incidence rates of stroke. Ann Neurol 1983;14:1–7.
3. Wolf PA, Cobb JL, D'Agostino RB. Epidemiology of Stroke. In Barnett HJM, Mohr JP, Stein BM, Yatsu FM (eds), Stroke: Pathophysiology, Diagnosis, and Management. (2nd ed). New York: Churchill Livingstone, 1992;3–27.
4. World Health Organization. Cerebrovascular diseases: prevention, treatment and rehabilitation. World Health Organ Tech Rep Ser 1971;469:469–570.
5. American Heart Association. The National Health and Nutrition Examination Survey II, 1976–1980. In Heart and Stroke Facts, 1992. Dallas, 1991.
6. Recommendations on stroke prevention, diagnosis, and therapy. Report of the WHO Task Force on Stroke and Other Cerebrovascular Disorders. Stroke 1989;20:1407–1431.
7. Bogousslavsky J. Topographic patterns of cerebral infarcts. Cerebrovasc Dis 1991;1(Suppl 1):61–68.
8. Hacke W, Krieger D, Hirschberg M. General principles in the treatment of ischemic stroke. Cerebrovasc Dis 1991;1(Suppl 1):93–99.
9. Modan B, Wagener DK. Some epidemiological aspects of stroke: mortality and morbidity trends, age, sex, race, socioeconomic status. Stroke 1992;23:1230–1236.
10. Hommel M, Memin B, Besson G, Perret J. Hospital admission and acute stroke units. Cerebrovasc Dis 1991;1(Suppl 1):50–53.
11. Norris JW, Hachinski VC. Stroke units or stroke centers? Stroke 1986;17:360–362.
12. Adams H Jr. Investigation of the patient with ischemic stroke. Cerebrovasc Dis 1991;1(Suppl 1):54–56.
13. Shinar D, Gross C, Hier D, et al. Interobserver reliability in the interpretation of computed tomographic scans of stroke patients. Arch Neurol 1987;44;149–155.
14. Wang A-M, Lin JCT, Rumbaugh CL. What is expected of CT in the evaluation of Stroke? Neuroradiology 1988;30:50–58.
15. Launes J, Ketonen L. Dense middle cerebral artery sign: an indicator of poor outcome in middle cerebral artery area infarction. J Neurol Neurosurg Psychiatry 1987;50:1550–1552.
16. De Witt LD. Clinical use of nuclear magnetic resonance imaging in stroke. Stroke 1986;17:328–332.
17. Kertesz A, Black SE, Nicholson L, Carr T. The sensitivity and specificity of MRI in stroke. Neurology 1987;37:1580–1587.
18. Hommel M, Besson G, Le-Bas JF, et al. Prospective study of lacunar infarction using magnetic resonance imaging. Stroke 1990;21:546–554.
19. Viraponge C, Manusco A, Quisling R. Human brain infarcts. Gd-DTPA enhanced MR imaging. Radiology 1986;161:785–794.
20. Mills CM, Brant-Zawadzki M, Crooks LE, et al. Nuclear magnetic resonance: principles of blood flow imaging. AJR Am J Roentgenol 1983;4:1161–1166.
21. Bogousslavsky J, Van Melle G, Regli F. The Lausanne Stroke Registry: analysis of 1,000 consecutive patients with first stroke. Stroke 1988;19:1083–1092.
22. Hankey GJ, Warlow CP. Cost-effective investigation of patients with suspected transient ischemic attacks. J Neurol Neurosurg Psychiatry 1993;55:171–176.
23. Hart RG, Miller VT. Cerebral infarction in young adults: a practical approach. Stroke 1983;14:110–114.
24. Norris JW, Hachinski VC, Meyers MG, et al. Serum cardiac enzymes in stroke. Stroke 1979;10:548–552.
25. Martinez HR, Rangel-Guerra RA, Marfil RJ. Ischemic stroke due to deficiency of coagulation inhibitors. Report of 10 young adults. Stroke 1993;24:19–25.
26. D'Angelo A, Landi G, D'Angelo SV, et al. Protein C in acute stroke. Stroke 1988;19:579–583.
27. Camerlingo M, Finazzi G, Casto L, et al. Inherited protein C deficiency and nonhemorrhagic arterial stroke in young adults. Neurology 1991;41:1371–1373.
28. Montalban J, Codina A, Ordi J, et al. Antiphospholipid antibodies in cerebral ischemia. Stroke 1991;22:750–753.
29. Miletich J, Sherman L, Broze G Jr. Absence of thrombosis in subjects with heterozygous protein C deficiency. N Engl J Med 1987;317:991–996.
30. Broekmans AW. Hereditary protein C deficiency. Haemostasis 1985;15:233–240.
31. Griffin JH, Evatt B, Zimmerman TS, et al. Deficiency of protein C in congenital thrombotic disease. J Clin Invest 1981;68:1370–1373.
32. Esmon CT. Protein C: biochemistry, physiology, and clinical implications. Blood 1983;62:1155–1168.
33. Kloczko J, Wojtukiewicz M, Bielawiec M, Borowska M. Reduced protein C levels in patients with essential hypertension. Thromb Haemost 1987;58:793.
34. Bogousslavsky J, Cachin C, Regli F, et al. Cardiac sources of embolism and cerebral infarction—clinical conse-

quences and vascular concomitants: the Lausanne Stroke Registry. Neurology 1991;41:855–859.

35. Biller J, Johnson MR, Adams HP Jr, et al. Echocardiographic evaluation of young adults with nonhemorrhagic cerebral infarction. Stroke 1986;17:608–612.

36. Lechat P, Mas JL, Mas PD, et al. Prevalence of patient foramen ovale in patients with strokes. N Engl J Med 1988;318:1148–1152.

37. Biller J, Adams HP Jr, Johnson MR, et al. Paradoxical cerebral embolism: eight cases. Neurology 1986;36:1356–1360.

38. Fisher EA, Goldman ME. Transesophageal echocardiography: a new view of the heart. Ann Intern Med 1990;113;91–93.

39. Amarenco P, Duyckaerts C, Tzourio C, et al. The prevalence of ulcerated plaques in the aortic arch in patients with stroke. N Engl J Med 1992;326:221–225.

40. Di Pasquale G, Andreoli A, Pinelli G, et al. Cerebral ischemia and asymptomatic coronary artery disease: a prospective study of 83 patients. Stroke 1986;17:1098–1101.

41. Steinke W, Hennerici M, Rautenberg W, Mohr JP. Symptomatic and asymptomatic high-grade carotid stenoses in Doppler color-flow imaging. Neurology 1992;42:131–138.

42. De Witt LD, Weschler LR. Transcranial Doppler. Stroke 1988;19:915–921.

43. Markus H, Loh A, Brown MM. Computerized detection of cerebral emboli and discrimination from artifact using Doppler ultrasound. Stroke 1993;24:1667–1672.

44. Niedermeyer E. Cerebrovascular Disorder and EEG. In E Niedermeyer, F Lopes da Silva (eds), Electroencephalography. Basic Principles, Clinical Applications and Related Fields (2nd ed). New York: Urban & Schwarzengerg, 275–299.

45. Anderson CM. What is MRA? In CM Anderson, RR Edelman, PA Turski (eds), Clinical Magnetic Resonance Angiography. New York: Raven Press, 1993;1–12.

46. Turski PA. Intracranial Magnetic Resonance Angiography and Stroke. In CM Anderson, RR Edelman, PA Turski. Clinical Magnetic Resonance Angiography. New York: Raven Press, 1993;181–216.

47. Bozzao L, Fantozi LM, Bastianello S, et al. Ischaemic supratentorial stroke: angiographic findings in patients examined in the very early phase. J Neurol 1989;236:340–342.

48. Beyer R, Paden P, Sobel D, Flynn FG. Moyamoya patterns of vascular occlusion after radiotherapy for glioma of the optic chiasm. Neurology 1986;36:1173–1178.

49. Theodotu BC, Whaley R, Mahaley MS. Complications following transfemoral cerebral angiography for cerebral ischemia. Report of 159 angiograms and correlation with surgical risk. Surg Neurol 1987;28:90–92.

50. Berger C, Annecke A, Aschoff A, et al. Neurochemical monitoring of fatal middle cerebral artery infarction. Stroke 1999;30:460–463.

51. Doutre MS, Beylot C, Bioulac P, et al. Skin lesion resembling malignant atrophic papulosis in lupus erythematosus. Dermatologica 1987;182:45–46.

52. Bruyn RP, van der Veen JP, Donker AJ, et al. Sneddon's syndrome. Case report and literature review. J Neurol Sci 1987;79:243–253.

53. Mudd SH. Vascular disease and homocysteine metabolism. N Engl J Med 1985;313:751–753.

54. Levine SR, Welch KM. Cocaine and stroke. Stroke 1988;19:779–783.

55. Whisnant JP. The role of the neurologist in the decline of stroke. Ann Neurol 1983;14:1–7.

56. Forster A, Young J. Stroke rehabilitation: can we do better? BMJ 1992;305:1146–1147.

57. Redding MJ, McDowell FH. Focused stroke rehabilitation programs improve outcome. Arch Neurol 1989;46:700–703.

58. Norris JW, Hachinski VC. Intensive care management of stroke patients. Stroke 1976;7:573–577.

59. Cooper SW, Olivet JA, Woolsey FM Jr. Establishment and operation of combined intensive care units. N Y State J Med 1972;72:2215–2220.

60. Strand T, Asplund K, Eriksson S, et al. Stroke unit care: who benefits? Comparisons with general medical care in relation to prognostic indicators on admission. Stroke 1986;17:377–381.

61. Grotta JC. Medical and surgical therapy for cerebrovascular diseases. N Engl J Med 1987;315:1505–1516.

62. Brott T, Reed RL. Intensive care for acute stroke in a community hospital setting: the first 24 hours. Stroke 1989;20:694–697.

63. Arron MJ, McDermott MM, Dolan N, Lefevre F. Management of medical complications associated with stroke. Heart Dis Stroke 1994;3:103–109.

64. Kennedy SF. Airway management and respiratory support. In AH Ropper, SF Kennedy (eds), Neurological and Neurosurgical Intensive Care (2nd ed). Rockville, MD: Aspen, 1988;57–79.

65. Silver FL, Norris JW, Lewis AJ, Hachinski VC. Early mortality following stroke: a prospective review. Stroke 1984;15:492–496.

66. Swann KW, Black PM, Baker MA. Management of symptomatic deep venous thrombosis and pulmonary emboli in a neurosurgical service. J Neurosurg 1986;64:563–567.

67. Brandstater ME, Roth EJ, Siebens HC. Venous thromboembolism in stroke: literature review and implications for clinical practice. Arch Phys Med Rehabil 1992;73:379–391.

68. Cardiogenic brain embolism. The second report of the Cerebral Embolism Task Force. Arch Neurol 1989;46:727–743.

69. Oppenheimer SM, Hachinski VC. The cardiac consequence of stroke. Neurol Clin 1992;10:167–176.

70. Lisk DR, Grotta JC, Lamki LM, et al. Should hypertension be treated after acute stroke? A randomized controlled trial using single photon emission computed tomography. Arch Neurol 1993;50:855–862.

71. Adams HP Jr, Brott TG, Crowell RM, et al. Guidelines for the management of patients with acute ischemic stroke. A statement for healthcare professionals from a special writing group of the Stroke Council, American Heart Association. Stroke 1994;25:1901–1914.

72. Lees KR, Dyker AG. Blood pressure control after stroke. J Hypertens 1996;14:S35–S38.

73. Spence JD, Del Maestro RF. Hypertension in acute ischemic strokes. Arch Neurol 1986;42:1000–1002.

74. Chamorro A, Vila N, Ascaso C, et al. Blood pressure and functional recovery in acute ischemic stroke. Stroke 1998;29:1850–1853.

75. Britton M, Carlsson A. Very high blood pressure in acute stroke. J Intern Med 1990;228:611–615.

76. Jorgensen HS, Nakayama H, Raaschou HO, Olsen TS. Effect of blood pressure and diabetes on stroke in progression. Lancet 1994;344:156–159.
77. Ropper AH, Rockoff MA. Treatment of Intracranial Hypertension. In AH Ropper, Kennedy SF (eds), Neurological and Neurosurgical Intensive Care (2nd ed). Rockville, MD: Aspen, 1988;23–42.
78. Rogvi-Hansen B, Boysen G. Intravenous glycerol treatment in acute stroke: a statistical review. Cerebrovasc Dis 1992;2:11–13.
79. Kondziolka D, Fazi M. Functional recovery after decompressive craniectomy for cerebral infarction. Neurosurgery 1988;23:143–147.
80. Heros RC. Cerebellar hemorrhage and infarction. Stroke 1982;13:106–108.
81. Kannel WB, McGee DL. Diabetes and cardiovascular disease. The Framingham study. JAMA 1979;241:2035–2038.
82. Pulsinelli WA, Levy DE, Sigsbee B, et al. Increased damage after ischemic stroke in patients with hyperglycemia with or without established diabetes mellitus. Am J Med 1983;74:540–544.
83. Tracey F, Crawford VL, Lawson JT, et al. Hyperglycemia and mortality from acute stroke. QJM 1993;86:439–446.
84. Woo J, Lam CW, Kay R, et al. The influence of hyperglycemia and diabetes mellitus on immediate and 3-month morbidity and mortality after acute stroke. Arch Neurol 1990;47:1174–1177.
85. Ginsberg MD, Busto R. Rodent models of cerebral ischemia. Stroke 1989;20:1627–1642.
86. Ginsberg MD, Busto R. Combating hyperthermia in acute stroke: a significant clinical concern. Stroke 1998;29:529–534.
87. Milde LN. Clinical use of mild hypothermia for brain protection: a dream revisited. J Neurosurg Anesthesiol 1992;4:211–215.
88. Onesti ST, Baker CJ, Sun PP, Solomon RA. Transient hypothermia reduces focal ischemic brain injury in the rat. Neurosurgery 1991;29:369–373.
89. Maier CM, Ahern KVB, Cheng ML, et al. Optimal depth and duration of mild hypothermia in a focal model of transient cerebral ischemia. Stroke 1998;29:2171–2180.
90. Ridenour TR, Warner DS, Todd MM, McAllister AC. Mild hypothermia reduces infarct size resulting from temporary but not permanent focal ischemia in rats. Stroke 1992;23:733–738.
91. Reith J, Jorgensen HS, Perdersen PM, et al. Body temperature in acute stroke: relation to stroke severity, infarct size, mortality and outcome. Lancet 1996;347:422–425.
92. Azzimondi G, Bassein L, Nonino F, et al. Fever in acute stroke worsens prognosis: a prospective study. Stroke 1995;26:2040–2043.
93. Schwab S, Scharz S, Spranger M, et al. Moderate hypothermia in the treatment of patients with severe middle cerebral artery infarction. Stroke 1998;29:2461–2466.
94. Chen H, Chopp M, Welch KM. Effect of mild hyperthermia on the ischemic infarct volume after middle cerebral artery occlusion in the rat. Neurology 1991;41:1133–1135.
95. Sulter G, De Keyser J. From stroke unit care to stroke care unit. J Neurol Sci 1999;162:1–5.

96. Davalos A, Cendra E, Genis D, Lopez-Pousa S. The frequency, characteristics, and prognosis of epileptic seizures at the onset of stroke. J Neurol Neurosurg Psychiatry 1988;51:1464–1467.
97. Kilpatrick CJ, Davis SM, Hopper JL, Rossiter SC. Early seizures after acute stroke. Risk of late seizures. Arch Neurol 1992;49:509–511.
98. Takizawa S, Hakim AM. Animal models of cerebral ischemia. 2. Rat models. Cerebrovasc Dis 1991;1(Suppl 1):16–21.
99. Marshall RS, Mohr JP. Current management of ischaemic stroke. J Neurol Neurosurg Psychiatry 1993;56:6–16.
100. Pessin MS, del Zoppo GJ, Estol CJ. Thrombolitic agents in the treatment of stroke. Clin Neuropharmacol 1990;13:271–289.
101. Hacke W, Zeumer H, Ferbert A, et al. Intra-arterial thrombolytic therapy improves outcome in patients with acute vertebrobasilar occlusive disease. Stroke 1988;19:1216–1222.
102. Hacke W, Kaste M, Fieschi C, et al. Intravenous thrombolysis with recombinant tissue plasminogen activator for acute hemispheric stroke. The European Cooperative Acute Stroke Study. JAMA 1995;274:1017–1025.
103. Generalized efficacy of t-PA for acute stroke. Subgroup analysis of the NINDS t-PA Stroke Trial. Stroke 1997;28:2119–2125.
104. Intracerebral hemorrhage after intravenous t-PA for ischemic stroke. The NINDS t-PA Stroke Study Group. Stroke 1997;28:2109–2118.
105. del Zoppo GJ, Poeck K, Pessin MS, et al. Recombinant tissue plasminogen activator in acute thrombotic and embolic stroke. Ann Neurol 1992;32:78–86.
106. del Zoppo GJ. An open multicenter trial of recombinant tissue plasminogen activator in acute stroke: a progress report. Stroke 1990;21:174–175.
107. Von Kummer R, Hacke W. Safety and efficacy of intravenous tissue plasminogen activator and heparin in acute middle cerebral artery stroke. Stroke 1992;23:646–652.
108. Furlan A, Higashida R, Wechsler L, et al. Intra-arterial prourokinase for acute ischemic stroke. The PROACT study: a randomized controlled trial. Prolyse in Acute Cerebral Thromboembolism. JAMA 1999;282:2003–2011.
109. Biller J, Love BB, Marsh EE. Spontaneous improvement after acute ischemic stroke. Stroke 1990;21:1008–1012.
110. Marsh EE, Adams HP, Biller J, et al. Use of antithrombotic drugs in the treatment of acute ischemic stroke: a survey of neurologists in practice in the United States. Neurology 1989;39:1631–1634.
111. Fisher CM. Anticoagulant therapy in cerebral thrombosis and cerebral embolism. Neurology 1961;11:119–131.
112. Miller VT, Hart RG. Heparin anticoagulation in acute brain ischemia. Stroke 1988;19:403–406.
113. Keith DS, Phillips SJ, Whisnant JP, et al. Heparin therapy for recent transient focal cerebral ischemia. Mayo Clin Proc 1987;62:1101–1106.
114. Van Merwijk G, Lodder J. Presumed basilar artery thrombosis and anticoagulation. Cerebrovasc Dis 1991;1:227–230.
115. Carter AB. Anticoagulant treatment in progressing stroke. BMJ 1961;2:70–73.

116. Haley EC, Kasel NF, Torner JC. Failure of heparin to prevent progression in progressing ischemic infarction. Stroke 1988;19:10–14.

117. Hart RG. Anticoagulants are underused in cerebrovascular diseases. Controversies and Consensus in Neurology. Am Acad Neurol Ann Meet 1990;42:1–7.

118. Sandercock PA, van den Belt AG, Lindley RI, Slattery J. Antithrombotic therapy in acute ischaemic stroke: an overview of the completed randomized trials. J Neurol Neurosurg Psychiatry 1993;56:17–25.

119. Pessin MS, Estol CJ, Lafranchise F, Caplan LR. Safety of anticoagulation after hemorrhagic infarction. Neurology 1993;43:1298–1303.

120. Kelton JG. Heparin-induced thrombocytopenia. Haemostasis 1986;16:173–186.

121. The International Stroke Trial (IST): a randomized trial of aspirin, subcutaneous heparin, both, or neither among 19,435 patients with acute ischaemic stroke. International Stroke Trial Collaborative Group. Lancet 1997;349:1569–1581.

122. Low molecular weight heparinoid, ORG 10172 (danaparoid), and outcome after acute ischemic stroke: a randomized controlled trial. The Publications Committee for the Trial of ORG 10172 in Acute Stroke Treatment (TOAST) Investigators. JAMA 1998;279:1265–1272.

123. Choudhri TF, Hoh BL, Zerwes HG, et al. Reduced microvascular thrombosis and improved outcome in acute murine stroke by inhibiting GP IIb/IIIa receptor-mediated platelet aggregation. J Clin Invest 1998;102:1301–1310.

124. Asplund K. Hemodilution in acute stroke. Cerebrovasc Dis 1991;1(Suppl 1):129–138.

125. Koller M, Haenny P, Hess K, et al. Adjusted hypervolemic hemodilution in acute ischemic stroke. Stroke 1990;21: 1429–1434.

126. Haemodilution in acute stroke: results of the Italian haemodilution trial. Italian Acute Stroke Study Group. Lancet 1988;1:318–321.

127. Multicenter trial of hemodilution in acute ischemic stroke. I. Results in the total patient population. Scandinavian Stroke Study Group. Stroke 1987;18:691–699.

128. Gelmers HJ, Gorter K, de Weerdt CJ, Wiezer HJ. A controlled trial of nimodipine in acute ischemic stroke. N Engl J Med 1988;318:203–207.

129. Martinez-Vila E, Guillen F, Villanueva JA, et al. Placebo-controlled trial of nimodipine in the treatment of acute ischemic cerebral infarction. Stroke 1990;21: 1023–1028.

130. Teasdale G, Sokard PJ, Shawn D. Treatment of subarachnoidal hemorrhage with calcium antagonist: a large randomized control trial. International Symposium on Cerebral Ischemia and Calcium. Chiemese, Germany. 12–15 June 1988;9.

131. Clinical trial of nimodipine in acute stroke. The American Nimodipine Study Group. Stroke 1992;23:3–9.

132. Scatton B, Carter C, Benavides J, Giroux C. N-methyl-D-aspartate receptor antagonists. A novel therapeutic perspective for the treatment of ischemic brain injury. Cerebrovasc Dis 1991;1:121–135.

133. Park CK, Nelhs DJ, Graham DI, et al. The glutamate antagonist MK 801 reduces focal ischemic brain damage in the rats. Ann Neurol 1988;24:543–551.

134. Trouillat R, Bogousslavsky J, Regli F, Uske A. [Supratentorial intracerebral hemorrhage]. Schweiz Med Wochenschr 1990;120:1056–1063.

135. Omae T, Ueda K, Ogata J, Yamaguchi T. Parenchymatous Hemorrhage: Etiology, Pathology, and Clinical Aspects. In PJ Vinken, GW Bruyn, HL Klawans (eds), Handbook of Clinical Neurology. (Vol 10 [54]). Vascular Diseases. Part II. JF Toole (ed). Amsterdam: Elsevier, 1989;287–331.

136. Kalyan-Raman UP, Kalyan-Raman K. Cerebral amyloid angiopathy causing intracranial hemorrhage. Ann Neurol 1984;16:321–329.

Chapter 14

Critical Care of Cerebrovascular Disease

Stefan Schwab, Markus Bertram, and Werner Hacke

General Principles in the Management of Neurologic Critical Care Patients

Airway Management and Pulmonary Function

Although respiratory problems are rare in the first few hours after an acute stroke, pulmonary complications constitute a major cause of morbidity and mortality in intensive care unit (ICU) patients with cerebrovascular disease.[1] Maintenance of adequate ventilation and oxygenation is an important prerequisite for the preservation of metabolic turnover in the marginal zone of an ischemic stroke, the so-called penumbra. Therefore, oxygen saturation should be measured, at least transcutaneously, in the emergency room, stroke unit, and ICU.

Respiratory Dysfunction in Stroke Patients

Respiratory dysfunction may develop as the result of a reduction in alveolar gas exchange due to atelectases or pneumonia in immobilized patients, hypoventilation due to impaired central respiratory drive or critical care neuropathy, or upper airway obstruction due to oropharyngeal muscular dysfunction. Patients with an extensive supratentorial infarction, vertebrobasilar infarction, seizure activity, or massive intracranial or subarachnoid hemorrhage (SAH) are generally unconscious and at particular risk of aspiration.

One phenomenon seen in stroke patients is neurogenic pulmonary edema or neurogenic heart disease, which leads to respiratory distress. Neurogenic pulmonary edema may develop rapidly after SAH

and epileptic seizures, and in pandysautonomia. It is characterized by a protein-rich alveolar fluid. The pathophysiologic mechanisms are unclear, but a combination of factors may contribute to it, such as left atrial hypertension, systemic hypertension, and increased sympathetic activity.[2] Furthermore, lesions of the central nervous system may induce arrhythmias, and repolarization disturbances with increased cardiac enzyme levels may occur after SAH, head trauma, or epileptic seizures.[3] As in neurogenic pulmonary edema, an increased sympathetic drive with elevated catecholamine levels leads to excitotoxicity with consequent cell death and leakage of cardiac enzymes into serum. For prevention and treatment, the administration of benzodiazepines, barbiturates, beta-blockers, calcium channel blockers, and free radical scavengers, which intervene in the described cascade, may be favorable, especially when given early in the clinical course, although there are no prospective studies supporting this hypothesis.

Intubation and Ventilation

The indications for endotracheal intubation and artificial ventilation are summarized in Table 14-1. Initially, orotracheal intubation is preferred to nasotracheal intubation because of the high incidence of paranasal sinusitis, common technical problems during intubation, tube contamination during nasal passage, and the smaller diameters of nasal tubes.

Anesthesia in a neurocritically ill patient presents a variety of specific problems. In general, it should be assumed that all patients have a full stomach.

Table 14-1. Indications for Endotracheal Intubation and Ventilation

PO_2 <50–60 mm Hg, despite O_2 administration via nasal probe or mask
PCO_2 >50–60 mm Hg
Vital capacity <500–800 ml
Risk of aspiration due to loss of protective airway reflexes
Tachypnea >35/min
Dyspnea with use of accessory muscles
Severe respiratory acidosis

Additionally, laryngoscopy and intubation often affect the hemodynamics to a significant degree, which, in the case of hemodynamically relevant carotid artery stenosis, can be deleterious. Some drugs may exacerbate already elevated intracranial pressure (ICP). Therefore, short-acting agents are recommended, such as sufentanil (70 μg) followed by etomidate (0.3–0.5 mg/kg), or propofol (1.5–3.0 mg/kg) in conjugation with a depolarizing neuromuscular blocking agent, such as succinylcholine (1.2 mg/kg) given in rapid sequence. For further sedation, the use of analgesic or sedative drugs is recommended (e.g., fentanyl, 0.05 mg/ml, and midazolam, 1.8 mg/ml, via infusion pump). Most intubated patients with acute cerebrovascular diseases require ventilatory support (Table 14-2).

In long-term patients, it is often necessary to apply positive end-expiratory pressure to treat various lung injuries (pneumonia, pulmonary edema, or adult respiratory distress syndrome). However, it is important to note that positive end-expiratory pressure may increase ICP.[4] In general, early intubation and vigorous physical chest therapy can help prevent pulmonary complications and improve the outcome of patients with cerebrovascular diseases.

Table 14-2. Initial Ventilator Setting

Intermittent of continuous mandatory ventilator mode model
Tidal volume: 12 ml/kg
Respiratory rate: PCO_2 <40 mm Hg (8–12 breaths/min)
FIO_2 = 1.0
I:E = 1:2–3
Inspiratory flow: 30 liters/min

FIO_2 = fraction of inspired oxygen; I:E = inspiratory/expiratory ratio.

Table 14-3. Indications for Tracheotomy

Coma and need for ventilatory support for >14 days
Bronchial cleansing/protection
Swallowing disturbances with risk of aspiration
Laryngeal obstruction
Prolonged weaning

Tracheotomy

With the development of high-volume, low-pressure cuffs, the risk of tracheal stenosis has markedly decreased. Nevertheless, prolonged orotracheal or nasotracheal intubation may cause laryngeal damage and a phonation disability. When the benefits of better patient mobility and care outweigh the risks and complications, tracheotomy should be performed regardless of the duration of orotracheal intubation (Table 14-3). In general, tracheotomy has to be performed 2–3 weeks after orotracheal intubation because of sores in the mouth and laryngeal damage.

Fluids and Nutrition

Fluid Balance

Fluid and electrolyte disturbances are frequently observed in patients treated in neurocritical care units (NCCUs). They may occur as a result of sympathetic responses to ischemic or hemorrhagic neuronal injury or may be the effect of fluid and electrolyte substitution, the nutritional regimen, or the administration of diuretics and other drugs. Sympathetic nervous system stimulation induces adrenal release of aldosterone, which causes sodium retention and kaliuresis and activates the renin-angiotensin system, affecting renal function. Antidiuretic hormone secretion may also be affected by central nervous system lesions, which results in sodium and water retention and decreased urine output (syndrome of inappropriate secretion of antidiuretic hormone) or diabetes insipidus.

Fluid disturbances can be assessed by (1) clinical observation (e.g., signs of exsiccation, edema), (2) evaluation of fluid intake and output in respect of calculated fluid requirements (Table 14-4), (3) measurement of central venous pressure

Table 14-4. Assessment of the Daily Fluid Requirement

Physiologic Parameters	Values Required
Basal requirement	30 ml/kg body weight
Output	Urine output the day before
	Stool water: 100 ml (more in diarrhea)
	Loss via enteral probes or drainages
Insensible loss (skin and airway)	800 ml (ventilated patients: 400 ml) 500 ml/°C >37°C

Table 14-5. Serum Osmolarity Evaluation Approach

Measurement of osmolarity, including serum sodium, glucose, and urea

Calculation of osmolarity: mOs/liter H_2O = 2 × glucose + urea (mmol/liter)

Calculation of the osmotic gap (measured by calculated osmolarity)

Causes for increased osmotic gap >10 mOs/liter H_2O

  Reduced serum water

    Hyperlipidemia

    Hyperproteinemia

    Additional low-molecular-weight substances:

      Mannitol, ethanol, methanol, ethylenglycol, and other toxins <150 kd

Laboratory failure

(CVP) (n 2–12 cm H_2O) via a central venous line or measurement of pulmonary capillary wedge pressure via pulmonal catheter to detect hypovolemic states, and (4) measurement of serum osmolarity (Table 14-5), urine osmolarity, and sodium concentration. Urine osmolarity is of particular interest for differential diagnosis of polyuric states (Figure 14-1).

Sodium salts are the main electrolytes of extracellular fluid and account for more than 90% of its osmolarity. There is a close relationship between sodium and water shifts. Sodium concentrations and the hydration state of the patient provide the main guidelines for the treatment of fluid imbalances. Table 14-6 gives an overview of the common causes of isotonic volume depletion. The treatment of choice is to immediately administer standard fluids via an enteral or parenteral route. If fluid and electrolyte losses continue, careful fluid balancing and monitoring of CVP are necessary to determine the amount of fluids needed, especially in nonresponsive patients. In patients with concomitant left ventricular failure, chest x-rays, echocardiographic (ECG) findings, or pulmonal catheterization may help avoid fluid overload.

For hypernatriemic or hyponatriemic states, the therapeutic regimen depends on the hydration of the patient, as summarized in Figures 14-2 and 14-3. In the case of a central diabetes insipidus (see Figures 14-1 through 14-3) as one cause for fluid and electrolyte imbalance, subcutaneous or intravenous (i.v.) administration of 2–5 units of aqueous vasopressin or 1–5 µg of its analogue desmopressin effectively reduces water diuresis. For further details concerning fluid management in critically ill patients, see Robertson et al.[5] and Brown.[6]

Nutrition

Patients admitted to an NCCU for treatment of ischemic or hemorrhagic stroke normally are unlikely to have any nutritional deficit and vitamin or mineral deficiencies, so that, in general, accepted guidelines can be applied.

The caloric requirements should be estimated individually to avoid malnutrition or overfeeding. As a rule, a proportion of 1-part lipids, 1-part protein, and 3-parts carbohydrates should be chosen. Malnutrition predisposes patients to infections and weaning problems and may cause catabolism, whereas overfeeding may lead to hyperglycemia, hypertriglyceridemia, steatosis hepatis, cholestasis, and respiratory stress by increasing CO_2 production. The basal energy expenditure (BEE) is generally assumed to be approximately 25 kcal/kg body weight, which is increased by 40% in severe illness. Calorie requirements can be determined more precisely by indirect calorimetry, by which the respiratory quotient (RQ) can be calculated, thus providing a measure of the resting energy expenditure (Table 14-7). An RQ close to 0.7 may reflect inadequate feeding, whereas an RQ of more than 1.0 may indicate overfeeding.

Because this technique is not available on a daily basis in most cases, the calorie requirement should be estimated using the Harris-Benedict equation (see Table 14-7) for calculation of the BEE. Total calorie requirements in ICU patients can be approximated by multiplying the BEE by a stress factor, depending on underlying conditions and illness (see Table 14-7).

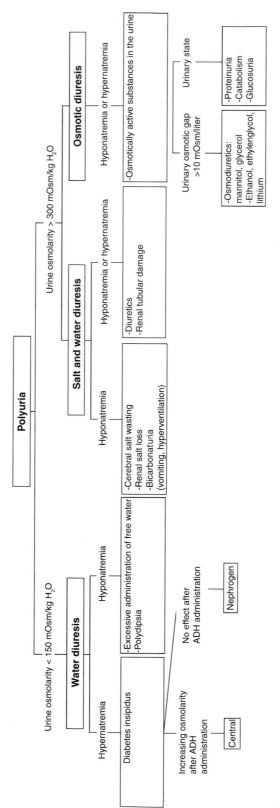

Figure 14-1. Flow sheet for the differential diagnosis of polyuria. (ADH = antidiuretic hormone.)

Table 14-6. Common Causes of Isotonic Volume Depletion

Inadequate fluid intake
    Impaired thirst mechanisms (hypothalamic lesions, old age)
    Impaired ability to maintain adequate fluid intake (altered consciousness, altered mentation, dysphagia, pareses)
    Inadequate fluid administration during critical care
Renal loss
    Polyuric kidney diseases (see Figure 14-1)
    Diuretics
    Osmotic diuresis (mannitol, sorbitol, diabetic glucosuria)
    Endocrine (adrenal or anterior pituitary insufficiency)
Extrarenal loss
    Gastrointestinal (diarrhea, vomiting, gastric suction, fistulas, abdominal sequestration)
    Pulmonary (hyperventilation, mechanical ventilation without warming and humidification)
    Cutaneous (sweating, fever, high ambient temperature, wounds, burns)

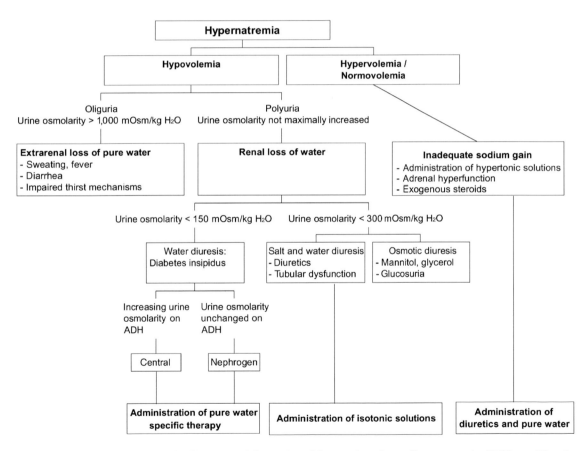

Figure 14-2. Flow sheet for differential diagnosis and diagnostic and therapeutic regimen of hypernatremia. (ADH = antidiuretic hormone.)

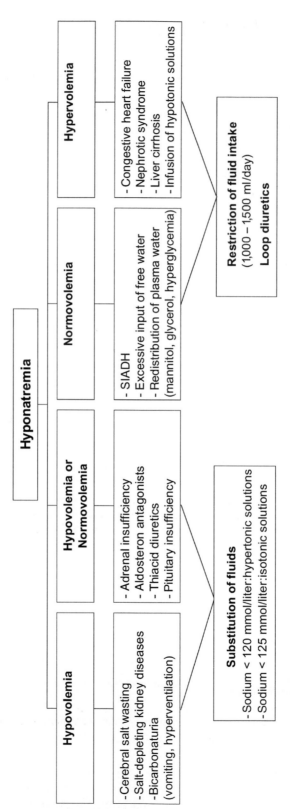

Figure 14-3. Flow sheet for differential diagnosis and diagnostic and therapeutic regimen of hyponatremia. (SIADH = syndrome of inappropriate secretion of antidiuretic hormone.)

Table 14-7. Determination of Calorie Requirements and Monitoring of Protein Intake

Resting energy expenditure

Respiratory quotient (RQ) (oxygen consumption/CO_2 production): RQ = $\dot{V}CO_2/\dot{V}O_2$

RQ = 0.7	Fat utilization
RQ = 0.85	Mixed fuel oxidation
RQ = 1.0	Carbohydrate oxidation
RQ > 1.0	Lipogenesis

Basal energy expenditure (BEE) and total energy expenditure

Harris-Benedict equation (W = weight in kg, H = height in cm, A = age in years):

BEE (men) = 66.47 + 13.75 × W + 5.0 × H – 6.76 × A [kcal/day]

BEE (women) = 655.1 + 9.56 × W + 1.85 × H – 4.68 × A [kcal/day]

Stress factors (to be multiplied with BEE for estimated total calorie requirement)

Critical care:	F = 1.25
Pneumonia:	F = 1.5
Large hemispheric infarction, MOV:	F = 1.75
Fever:	F = 1.13 / 1°C

Nitrogen balance

^{N}balance = ^{N}intake – (^{N}output + 0.4 g)

(^{N}intake = daily protein intake [g] divided by 6.25; ^{N}output = 24-hr urea nitrogen [g])

^{N}balance = 0–1 g/day:	Nitrogen equilibrium
^{N}balance > 1 g/day:	Net increase in body protein
^{N}balance < 0 g/day:	Loss of body protein, catabolism

F = factor; MOV = multi-organ failure; $\dot{V}CO_2$ = volume of carbon dioxide; $\dot{V}O_2$ = oxygen consumption per unit time.

Protein requirements in critically ill patients are almost always higher (1.2–1.5 g/kg body weight) than in nonstressed healthy persons (0.8 g/kg body weight). Protein intakes have to be adjusted as needed according to the urine urea nitrogen (N_2) test results (see Table 14-7). If N_2 excretion exceeds the protein equivalent of 2.5 g/kg, higher protein intakes usually do not promote N_2 retention, but drive ureagenesis instead. For further details concerning the assessment of nutrition requirements in critically ill patients, see Long et al.[7] or Ott et al.[8]

Feeding Routes and Strategies

Although an adequate fluid and electrolyte supply should be initiated at the beginning of ICU treatment, institution of complete, optimized nutrition, including controversial lipid administration, should be guaranteed by day 3 of ICU treatment. Vitamin and mineral supplements may be added after 1 week, but must be given sooner if pre-existent malnutrition is suspected.

If possible, oral feeding should be allowed and carefully monitored to ensure adequate intake. If intake is consistently below 50–75% of the nutritional goals for 1 week, supplemental nutritional support should be initiated. This is the case in most patients treated on an NCCU because of depressed levels of consciousness, impaired swallowing function, or mechanical ventilation.

For nutritional support, enteral nutrition using a nasogastric probe is preferred. The enteral route has the advantages of lower cost, simpler application, and a lower risk of sepsis than parenteral nutrition, and also utilizes the normal physiologic functions of digestion and absorption, which maintains the intestinal mucosa. Intestinal function and motility must be monitored regularly (bowel sounds, aspiration of gastric residuals) and may be supported by motility stimulants, such as metoclopramide or cisapride. However, there are pharmacologic interactions with risk of ventricular arrhythmias. Continuous pump-assisted infusion is better tolerated than bolus administration of food. Patients who require long-term enteral nutritional

Table 14-8. Indications for Central Venous Catheterization

Measurement of the central venous pressure
Parenteral nutrition
Administration of hyperoncotic or locally aggressive substances
Dialysis, hemofiltration
Guide for transvenous pacemakers, pulmonary catheters, and bulb catheters
Lack of adequate veins for peripheral lines

support should be scheduled early for percutaneous endoscopic gastrostomy, which is better tolerated and causes fewer local complications. A common complication of enteral feeding is diarrhea resulting from the hyperosmolar electrolyte solutions or quickly advanced enteral feeding after an extended period of fasting or parenteral nutrition. Another complication may be gastric retention due to multiple medical conditions and their pharmacologic treatments, with the risk of regurgitation and pulmonary aspiration. If motility stimulants do not work, postpyloric feeding (endoscopically placed nasoduodenal or nasojejunal probe) or parenteral nutrition are required.

Parenteral nutrition is indicated in cases of imminent intubation or operation, gastrointestinal leakage, ileus, pancreatitis, or other conditions in which the patient's gastrointestinal tract is unable to tolerate oral or enteral feeding for at least 5–7 days. For short-term parenteral nutrition, a peripheral venous line is suggested, using formulas of not more than 1,000 mOs/kg, which may be combined with lipid solutions. Long-term parenteral nutrition, which meets patients' full calorie and protein requirements without giving an excess fluid volume, requires hyperosmolar formulas of up to 1,800 mOs/kg H_2O. Because they are irritating to the venous endothelium, they have to be administered via central venous lines (see under Central Venous Lines). Complications of parenteral feeding include central, catheter-associated risks (arterial puncture, pneumothorax, central venous thrombosis, catheter sepsis) and metabolic problems. Hyperglycemia, a common side effect, often requires continuous insulin infusion; hypoglycemia after discontinuation of parenteral nutrition may be prevented by tapering off the formula slowly. Liver function abnormalities with mild to moderate elevation of serum liver enzyme activity

and bilirubin are also common and are usually benign and self-limiting.

Central Venous Lines

A central venous catheter provides direct information about the intravascular volume and is a safe route of administration for fluids, parenteral nutrition, and medication. Indications for central venous catheterization are summarized in Table 14-8. The safest approach is via the cubital vein; in patients who need multilumen catheters, the subclavian or internal jugular vein approach is recommended. In patients with elevated ICP, positioning of internal jugular vein catheters and the catheters themselves can impede central venous drainage and further increase ICP. Thus, subclavian catheters are preferred in these patients.

In some cases, a pulmonary artery catheter may help monitor and guide fluid and cardiocirculatory therapy in patients with severe heart failure and distinguish the type of cardiocirculatory insufficiency (e.g., cardiogenic shock, characterized by low output and high filling pressure; or sepsis, characterized by high output and low filling pressure). The effectiveness of pulmonary catheterization remains controversial, however, and its application should be limited to centers with technical expertise and experience in interpreting the data.

Agitation and Pain

Agitation and Sedation

Patients treated in an ICU or NCCU are exposed to a number of environmental, medical, and psychological factors that can cause excessive stress and anxiety. Environmental factors include unpleasant and unfamiliar visual and auditory stimuli or low temperature. Psychologically induced stress may be due to the awareness of severe and disabling illness, sleep disturbances and deprivation, or anxiety, confusion, and other psychiatric disorders that may be pre-existent or associated with the treated neurologic disorder or the therapy (drugs, mechanical ventilation, weaning). Medical factors include respiratory failure, pain, endocrine disorders, infection, sepsis, cardiovascular impairment, hypoxemia, and drug effects. It is also important to treat agitation because it may increase morbidity and mortality.[9] Inadequate sedation and analgesia may cause postaggression syndrome, thereby increasing the metabolic rate and oxygen consumption and promoting hemodynamic instability. In patients with pulmonary failure, postaggression syndrome may make effective ventilation difficult or even impossible. Furthermore, agitation may lead to problems in nursing care and risk of self-injury.

There is no clear-cut, ideal strategy for therapy of agitation. In some cases, nonmedical measures may be sufficient, such as special nursing and psychological care and treatment of pain or other underlying causes. Pharmacologic treatment includes administration of benzodiazepines, neuroleptics, barbiturates, and other drugs. Commonly administered substances, their route of administration, and important advantages and disadvantages or side effects are summarized in Table 14-9.

Pain Relief

Anxiety, stress, and behavioral disturbances may be due to pain. Some form of pain is experienced by almost every patient during some stage of stroke and may have cardiocirculatory and metabolic effects. Sedation is never an appropriate substitute for adequate analgesia. Prostaglandin inhibitors, such as paracetamol or salicylates, primarily should be used for pain relief, but often prove not to be sufficient. In such cases, opioids should be given, such as fentanyl (0.1 mg i.v.) or buprenorphine (0.2–0.4 mg according to rules, intramuscularly or i.v.), which are widely used analgetic substances during ICU treatment. Alfentanil has the advantage of a short redistribution half-life (approximately 11 minutes) and a short elimination half-life (approximately 94 minutes); however, it is expensive and should therefore not be used for prolonged anesthesia. The principal advantages of opioids are their potent analgetic properties without relevant hemodynamic side effects, even in high-risk patients. The sedating side effect and suppression of cough reflexes are only desired in ventilated patients; thus, tramadol (50–100 mg oral or subcutaneous, rectally intramuscular or i.v.) or tilidine (50–100 mg oral) should be preferred in awake, spontaneously breathing patients.

Elevated Intracranial Pressure

The assessment and treatment of ICP is fundamental to the management of any central nervous sys-

tem trauma. Intracranial hypertension affects an injured brain in several ways: elevation of ICP may ultimately result in herniation of the brain through the incisura, the foramen magnum, or subfalcine, resulting in distortion and further injury to vital brain structures. A continuous rise of ICP may also cause secondary ischemic insults. Additional ischemia is a major factor for further clinical deterioration after any neuronal injury. The main goal of ICP treatment is to minimize or, if possible, eliminate secondary ischemic insults resulting from ischemia. With regard to critical care of patients with head injuries, the focus of ICP therapy has shifted from purely pressure-oriented management to a cerebral perfusion pressure (CPP)–oriented regimen.

Definition of Intracranial Hypertension

Thresholds of intracranial hypertension have never been conclusively established, and the critical thresholds may vary among individuals. However, ICP readings of 20 mm Hg or more are usually considered the cutoff point of intracranial hypertension.

Intracranial Pressure Monitoring

ICP monitoring provides the physician with additional data for rational ICP management. ICP devices can be positioned at epidural, subdural, intraparenchymal, or intraventricular sites. The ICP can be obtained using fluid-coupled (ventricular catheter, subarachnoid bolt) or nonfluid-coupled (fiberoptic, pneumatic devices) systems (Table 14-10). However, no system works satisfactorily to date. The main disadvantages are unreliable measurements and risk of infections. Intraparenchymatous ICP probes, which are easy to handle and give exact measurements, are used most widely. Invasive monitoring of ICP may be suggested if

- The patient is suspected to be at risk for elevated ICP
- The patient is comatose and has an intracranial pathologic condition
- The prognosis of the disease calls for aggressive therapy

Table 14-9. Sedational Pharmacologic Treatment: Commonly Administered Substances, Route of Administration, Important Advantages, and Disadvantages or Side Effects

Generic Name	Single Dose	Continuous Perfusion	Properties/Advantages	Side Effects	Remarks
Midazolam	2.5–5.0 mg	3.6–36.0 mg/hr	Mild hypotension Double effectivity and less half-life compared to diazepam	Ventilatory depression	Drug of choice for sedation in long-term mandatory ventilation
Lorazepam	1.0–2.5 mg s.l. i.v.		Long half-life but little accumulation Potent antiepileptic		
Thiopental	3–7 mg/kg	4–200 (–900) mg/hr	No ceiling effect or accumulation	Hypotension Respiratory depression Liver dysfunction Agranulocytosis	Decreases ICP (n.b. CPP reduction by hypotension)
Methohexital			Shorter half-life Non-hepatic metabolism		
Clonidine	0.075–0.300 mg i.v. or s.c.	9–45 μg/hr	Reduces sympathetic tone	Initial hypertensive effect	Rebound phenomena after abrupt discontinuation
Dihydrobenzperidol	5–15 mg i.v.	2.5–15.0 mg/hr		Extrapyramidal symptoms Paradoxic effects Hypotension Distributive shock	Stepwise discontinuation
Disoprivane	2–4 mg/kg	Initial bolus of 100 mg 100–600 mg/hr	Short half-life Minimal accumulation Nutritional effect (lipids)	Respiratory depression Hypotension Seizures Tachyphylaxis	Should be preferred for short-term analgosedation during mechanical ventilation, weaning
GABA	50 mg/kg	Initial bolus of 50 mg/kg 10–20 mg/kg/hr	Less ventilatory suppression	Seizures Hypernatremia	
Ketamine	1–2 mg/kg i.v. 5–10 mg/kg i.m.	0.5–4.0 mg/kg/hr	Bronchodilation Minimal ventilatory suppression Anesthesia in higher dosage	Tachycardia Hypertension Hallucination End-of-dose excitation	Advantageous in asthmatic patients ICP elevation (?)
Etomidate	0.15–0.30 mg/kg	Repetitive injections up to maximum 80 mg	No hemodynamic effects No histamine delivery	Myoclonias Dyskinesias Locally painful injection	Short sedation for painful diagnostic or therapeutic measures

s.l. = according to rules; ICP = intracranial pressure; CPP = cerebral perfusion pressure; GABA = γ-aminobutyric acid; n.b. = note well.

Table 14-10. Intracranial Pressure Monitoring Devices

Monitor	Advantage	Disadvantage
Ventricular catheter	Drainage and exact measures	Major surgery, high infection rate
Subarachnoid bolt	Low infection rate, noninvasive	Unreliable, obstruction of device possible
Pneumatic device	Accurate measures	Expensive, dislocation possible
Fiberoptic device	Accurate measures, subdural, intraparenchymal, and intraventricular location	No further calibration possible, breakage risk

Intracranial Pressure and Cerebral Perfusion Pressure

CPP is defined as mean arterial pressure minus ICP. One of the primary goals of medical management for stroke is maintaining a sufficient CPP. This is of particular importance because cerebral autoregulation may be impaired in and around the ischemic lesion, and blood flow changes passively in these regions as the perfusion pressure changes. In addition, the lower limit of autoregulation may be shifted toward a higher level in patients with long-standing arterial hypertension. Although there is a large body of evidence proving that lowering blood pressure (BP) in the acute phase can be deleterious, it is less certain whether normal BP should be raised. In analogy to patients with head trauma, it seems prudent to raise the CPP above 70 mm Hg in patients with arterial hypotension, although the

effects of this strategy have not been determined. BP should only be lowered if marked hypertension is present (systolic BP >220 mm Hg or diastolic BP >120 mm Hg), and this should be done carefully to avoid a sudden drop in BP or hypotensive values (Figures 14-4 and 14-5).

All treatment modalities that lower ICP at the expense of BP must be considered dangerous. Hypovolemia should be strictly avoided. Adequate volumes of crystalloid, colloid, and, if necessary, blood products should be given. A CVP of 8 mm Hg might reflect isovolemia. In patients with decreased systemic vascular resistance, pressors, such as dopamine and epinephrine, may be required. In patients with impaired cardiac output, dobutamine can be used. Taking all this into account, it is important to be aware of the fact that the optimal CPP is not known. Recommendations from the literature differ, giving values between 50 mm Hg and 70 mm Hg.

Figure 14-4. Autoregulation of cerebral blood flow (CBF). The cerebral vascular bed is capable of maintaining a constant CBF between a mean arterial blood pressure of approximately 60–50 mm Hg. This phenomenon of "autoregulation" is achieved either through a reduction (vasodilatation) or an increase (vasoconstriction) of arterial resistances when the cerebral perfusion pressure (CPP) decreases or increases. If the autoregulation is impaired (dotted line), the CBF passively changes with the CPP. (MAP = mean arterial pressure; ICP = intracranial pressure.)

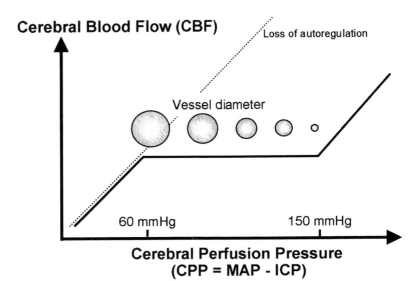

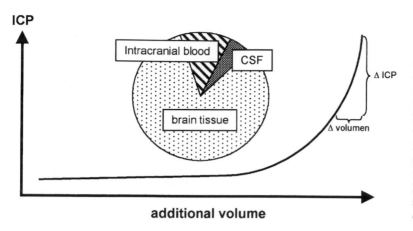

Figure 14-5. Cerebral compliance. An increase of edematous brain tissue requires a compensatory decrease of the other two physiologic compartments contained in the skull, intracranial blood and cerebrospinal fluid (CSF). After the failure of these limited compensatory mechanisms, the intracranial pressure (ICP) rapidly rises, and a small increase in the intracranial volume (Δ volumen) may substantially raise the ICP (Δ ICP). In this situation, however, a small reduction of brain edema can dramatically lower the ICP.

Treatment of Elevated Intracranial Pressure

Neurologic deterioration subsequent to increasing brain edema is a common phenomenon in patients with large infarcts or intracerebral hemorrhage (ICH). Several treatment options for brain space–occupying edema are used. Traditionally, the mainstay of conventional therapy included ventilation, sedation, BP control, hyperventilation, osmotic agents, and barbiturates. Recommendations for these therapies are based on small case series, evidence from animal experiments, or theoretical observations.[10] None has been evaluated in a randomized study.

Whether ICP monitoring should be included in the routine management of patients with large ischemic strokes remains a matter of controversy.[11] However, without knowledge of the ICP, CPP- or ICP-targeted therapies appear to be impossible.

As a basic procedure, the head should be positioned upright at approximately 20 degrees. Euvolemia should be established before elevating the head because of the risk of mean arterial pressure and CPP drop in hypovolemic patients. Fever has detrimental effects in cerebral schema and edema formation and should be rigorously treated. Electrolyte imbalance should be avoided, especially hyponatremia, which potentially aggravates the developing cerebral edema. Late reperfusion, extreme arterial hypertension, and the combination of both may increase brain edema significantly and should be prevented. An overview of conventional therapy for elevated ICP is provided in Table 14-11.

Table 14-11. Conventional Therapy of Raised Intracranial Pressure

Osmotherapy
   Glycerol 10%: 4 × 125 or 250 ml/24hr
   Mannitol 15%: 4–6 × 100 ml
   Hypertonic saline (NaCl 7.5%, peak serum sodium of
      170 mol)

Controlled hyperventilation
   Controlled mandatory ventilation
   No PEEP (if possible)
   Paco₂: 30–35 mm Hg

Barbiturates
   Pentobarbital administration of 3–5 mg/kg/hr
   Continuous infusion
   EEG (burst-suppression pattern) monitoring
   Hemodynamic monitoring with Swan-Ganz catheter

THAM-buffer solution
   Continuous infusion 1 mmol/kg/hr via central venous line

PEEP = positive end-expiratory pressure; EEG = electroencephalograph; THAM = tris-hydroxy-methyl-aminomethane or tromethamine.

Osmotherapy

Hypertonic, low-molecular-weight solutions, such as mannitol, sorbitol, glycerol, or hypertonic saline, are used to reduce the brain water content by creating an osmotic gradient between brain and plasma, drawing water into the plasma. An intact blood-brain barrier is essential for establishing an osmotic gradient. It has been assumed that brain tissue dehydration is more pronounced on the side contralateral to the lesion, where the brain tissue is preserved. Hypertonic solutions decrease an elevated

ICP and, therefore, may be beneficial in emergency situations in an acutely deteriorating patient before therapies, such as hematoma evacuation or decompressive surgery, can be initiated. However, their effect is not sustained. The long-term effects of repeated treatments with hypertonic solutions are still unknown. Repeated infusion of mannitol may aggravate cerebral edema by allowing the osmotic substances to migrate through a damaged blood-brain barrier into the brain tissue, thereby reversing the osmotic gradient. Furthermore, osmotic agents predominantly lead to dehydration and shrinkage of normal brain tissue and may facilitate displacement of brain tissue and increase the risk of herniation. However, these largely theoretical considerations have not been substantiated in clinical studies. Other complications of osmotic agents are electrolyte imbalances, hypervolemia with cardiac failure, and renal dysfunction. Serum osmolarity should be closely monitored.

Alternative Therapies to Treat
Elevated Intracranial Pressure

In principle, the same dilemma encountered with osmotic agents applies to all other treatment strategies: All of these therapies can transiently decrease elevated ICP; however, the long-term effects are less clear or even potentially noxious.

Hyperventilation. Hyperventilation causes serum and cerebrospinal fluid (CSF) alkalosis-induced cerebral vasoconstriction, and reduces cerebral blood volume and ICP. The effects of hyperventilation are short-lived because of rapid compensation of CSF alkalosis and rebound vasodilatation. A rebound increase in ICP occurs if normoventilation is resumed too rapidly. Deep hyperventilation may reduce the cerebral blood flow (CBF), leading to additional ischemic damage. Therefore, the CO_2 levels should not fall below 30 mm Hg.

Steroids. Steroids continue to be administered in patients with ischemic stroke and ICH. Several studies showed no benefit of this therapy; to the contrary, they demonstrated a higher risk of infection and gastrointestinal hemorrhage. There is no indication for the routine administration of steroids in severe postischemic brain edema or after ICH.

Drainage of Cerebrospinal Fluid. Drainage of CSF is an effective method of lowering ICP, especially when the ventricular size is not compromised. This is true, for instance, in patients with acute hydrocephalus after SAH or space-occupying cerebellar infarction. The drawback of this method is a relatively high infection rate (2–10%), which increases when drainage is maintained for more than 10 days.

Short-Acting Barbiturates. Short-acting barbiturates are frequently used in patients with elevated ICP. Barbiturates promptly and significantly reduce CBF and ICP. In addition to their action as a sedative, barbiturates reduce the cerebral metabolic rate of oxygen ($CMRO_2$), induce vasoconstriction and inhibit free radical-induced lipid peroxidation. Barbiturate treatment is initiated with a loading dose of 10 mg/kg of pentobarbital over 30 minutes. The maintenance dose is usually 3–5 mg/kg per hour. Suppression of electroencephalography is usually seen at serum barbiturate levels of 30–40 mg/dl. However, the use of barbiturates is limited due to various side effects, such as hypotension, cardiac depression, hepatotoxicity, and predisposition to infection, and two studies failed to demonstrate any long-term beneficial effects of prolonged barbiturate coma in patients with elevated ICP.

Alternative Agents to Treat
Elevated Intracranial Pressure

Intravenous administration of tris-hydroxy-methyl-aminomethane (THAM) or tromethamine induces vasoconstriction and thereby decreases ICP. The mode of action is not clearly understood. THAM increases the capacity of CSF to buffer pH changes and neutralizes acidosis-mediated vasodilatation. THAM, 60 mmol, in 100 ml in 5% dextrose, may be infused over 45 minutes as a test dose. ICP should fall by 10–15 mm Hg. A central venous line should be used for continuous intravenous infusion (1 mmol/kg/hour), because the substance may cause severe tissue necrosis. At high doses it can impair ventilation, which typically is not a problem because patients requiring THAM are usually ventilated. However, THAM is also nephrotoxic, and therefore, it is used only when all other conservative therapies have failed.[12]

Propofol is a hypnotic drug with a rapid onset and a short duration of action. It depresses $CMRO_2$, and reduces ICP in patients with head injuries. Side effects include a drop in systemic BP, which may impair CPP, thus limiting its use for ICP control.

Lidocaine decreases synaptic transmission either directly or through blockade of sodium channels. It also reduces $CMRO_2$ and acts as a vasoconstrictive. Lidocaine may lower ICP, but its efficacy over time is not established yet.

Intensive Care Unit Management of Severe Ischemic Stroke

Acute Middle Cerebral Artery Stroke

Clinical Course of Severe Middle Cerebral Artery Infarction

The clinical course of severe middle cerebral artery (MCA) infarction follows a predictable pattern in most patients.[13–15] At the time of initial clinical assessment within the first few hours after onset of symptoms, patients with large supratentorial infarcts are typically fully awake. Mild drowsiness may occasionally be present. Unresponsiveness due to aphasia or hemineglect should not be misinterpreted as loss of consciousness. Patients usually show a severe contralateral hemiparesis or hemiplegia and hemi-hypesthesia. Pyramidal tract signs, such as Babinski's sign, may also be found. Hemianopia is another frequent finding if the posterior cerebral artery territory or the dorsal portion of the MCA territory is affected. Patients with infarcts of the speech-dominant hemisphere present with global aphasia, although some residual speech comprehension may be preserved. Fixed conjugate eye and head deviation toward the affected side are typical findings in patients with large supratentorial strokes, although this clinical sign is neither highly sensitive nor specific.[13,16]

Bilateral motor signs, coma, posturing, or pupillary abnormalities are usually not present in the early phase of large supratentorial infarcts.

Neurologic deterioration occurs during the first 24 hours in most patients with large supratentorial infarcts, corresponding to the development of brain edema. The patient loses consciousness to varying degrees from drowsiness to coma, and the neurologic deficit that already exists may worsen, if possible. Pupillary enlargement and nonreactivity to light, at first unilaterally on the side of the infarction and later bilaterally, nausea, vomiting, posturing, and abnormal breathing patterns are signs of secondary brain stem dysfunction due to impending herniation.

In uncal herniation syndrome, as extensively described by Plum and Posner,[17] reaction of the pupil unilateral to the lesion first becomes sluggish, then the pupil gradually enlarges, accompanied by progressive loss of consciousness. If the opposite cerebral peduncle is compressed, hemiparesis develops ipsilaterally to the lesion. The progression of clinical signs reflects brain stem damage in a cranio-caudal direction from the midbrain to the medulla, manifesting as loss of oculomotor responses, contralateral pupillary enlargement, loss of corneal reflexes, posturing, and ultimately leading to respiratory arrest and cardiac arrhythmias. Central herniation syndrome is characterized by loss of consciousness and bilaterally small, reactive pupils in the initial phase.

If ICP is being monitored, it is typically only moderately elevated (approximately 20 mm Hg) at the onset of deterioration. ICP values will subsequently rise over the next 24–48 hours. Elevated ICP is a reliable prognostic sign, and an ICP exceeding 30 mm Hg is usually associated with fatal outcome.[11]

Prognosis

With medical therapy only, the outcome in patients with large supratentorial infarcts is generally poor, and mortality rates from 55% to 80% have been reported.[13–15] Most patients who deteriorate neurologically after the first few hours will die as a result of the infarct. Various predictors for deterioration and poor clinical outcome have been identified. Regarding vascular pathology, distal internal carotid artery (ICA) occlusion almost uniformly indicates fatal outcome. Proximal occlusion of the MCA stem is also an unfavorable radiologic finding. This typically leads to a complete MCA infarction, including the basal ganglia, which are often spared in patients with a more distal MCA occlusion. It seems plausible that the extent of the infarcted area closely correlates with mortality. Complete MCA and anterior cerebral artery infarcts and panhemispheric infarcts are usually lethal. The prognostic importance of collateral blood supply, which shows considerable interindividual variation, has been mentioned. With regard to clinical signs, progressive loss of consciousness during the first few hours after onset of symptoms is probably the most reliable predictor of a poor outcome.[13] Rapid onset of neurologic deterioration with loss of consciousness during the first 6 hours indicates an aggressive course of disease and is associated with high mortality. Once coma, pupillary abnormalities, or abnormal breathing patterns are observed, the anticipated outcome is death in most patients.

The extent of brain edema depends largely on the infarct size and location, but also shows substantial individual variability. As a general rule, young and middle-aged patients have less compensation capacity for space-occupying intracranial lesions than older patients with cerebral atrophy. As a consequence, younger patients tend to develop elevated ICP more often, and an infarct of the same size may result in higher mortality in these patients compared with older stroke victims.

General Management

Large hemispheric infarcts must be recognized in the emergency department as a life-threatening condition that requires prompt and massive intervention.[10] After stabilization of the airway, breathing, and circulation, the initial diagnostic workup and transfer to a neurointensive care unit should not be delayed. If indicated, early reperfusion therapies can be initiated in the emergency room.

Venous access, continuous monitoring of BP, ECG, and pulse oxygenation are part of routine intensive care measures. Continuous ECG monitoring is especially important because neurogenic cardiac arrhythmias are frequently observed, particularly in patients with large right-hemispheric infarcts.

Although respiratory problems are uncommon on presentation, their frequency sharply increases within the first 24 hours, reflecting increasing brain edema and brain stem dysfunction. Most patients with large infarcts require ventilatory support. To achieve sufficient cerebral oxygenation, oxygen should be insufflated via a face mask to reach arterial Po_2 values greater than 90 mm Hg. Indications for intubation and mechanical ventilation are hypoventilation with either hypercapnia or hypoxia, or maintenance of stable airways in patients with reduced consciousness and a high risk of aspiration. Both hypercapnia and hypoxia lead to vasodilatation, resulting in an increase of intracranial blood volume and thereby raising ICP. Approximately 60% of patients with large infarcts who have to be intubated eventually die, despite maximum conservative therapy. However, some have a chance of a satisfactory outcome. If the decision for full medical management has been made, elective intubation should not be delayed to the point at which additional complications from hypoxia or aspiration have already developed.[18] During intubation, arterial hypotension should be meticulously avoided.

Patients with large strokes have an increased risk of secondary hemorrhage into the infarcted area. This is one reason why intravenous heparin, which has been advocated for many years despite the lack of evidence supporting its use, should be restricted to patients with a clear indication for anticoagulant therapy (e.g., patients with prosthetic heart valves). However, stroke patients in general are at high risk for venous thrombosis and pulmonary embolism and should be prophylactically treated with low-dose heparin.

Intravenous or intra-arterial thrombolysis with tissue plasminogen activator (t-PA) as a revascularizing therapy are treatment options that can only be used in the early course of cerebral ischemia before a large infarction has resulted. If baseline radiologic findings demonstrate changes suggestive of a large infarction, thrombolytic therapy is contraindicated because of a high risk of intracranial hemorrhage.[19] The use of thrombolytic therapy is also questionable in the presence of distal ICA occlusion because revascularization rarely occurs in these patients.

Neuroradiologic Findings

Whereas cranial computed tomography (CT) was previously believed to be of limited use in the detection of an ischemic lesion in the early phase of the disease, it is now known that early parenchymatous signs of infarctions (i.e., parenchymal hypoattenuation, loss of differentiation between gray and white matter, and hemispheric sulcus effacement) are present within the first 6 hours in almost all patients with large infarctions.[20–22] Hypodensity of more than

50% of the MCA territory in the early stages is a predictor of poor clinical outcome and mortality in such patients reaches 85% if only medical treatment is provided. After 24 hours, compression of the ipsilateral ventricle and the extent of midline shift are markers of the extent and progression of postischemic brain edema. The early development of perifocal brain swelling within the first 24 hours is probably an indicator of an aggressive course and poor clinical outcome. Doppler ultrasound, CT angiography, and magnetic resonance angiography (MRA) are used as supplementary techniques to study the underlying vascular pathology. A unilateral hyperdense MCA sign on the baseline CT scan indicates the occlusion of the MCA trunk, although the sensitivity of this radiologic sign is not high.[23] The bilateral presence of the hyperdense MCA sign is a frequent finding in asymptomatic subjects and is of no diagnostic value. Occlusion of the distal ICA or proximal (M1 segment) MCA is associated with the development of complete MCA infarctions and is an ominous prognostic finding.[13] This is particularly true for patients with distal ICA occlusion, in whom mortality has consistently been shown to be high (Figure 14-6).

Residual perfusion of the ischemic penumbra can be preserved by leptomeningeal collateral blood supply, which may reduce infarct size. In patients with proximal MCA occlusion, survivors typically have a good collateral blood supply, whereas most patients with no or little collateral blood flow die.

Rapid new magnetic resonance imaging techniques (e.g., diffusion-weighted imaging [DWI] and perfusion-weighted imaging [PWI]) have been developed.[24–26] These techniques offer new insights into the pathophysiology and ultra-early diagnostic criteria of cerebral ischemia. In animal models, DWI has been shown to detect an increased diffusion of fluid into brain tissue as a marker of potentially irreversible cytotoxic cell damage within minutes after occlusion of the supplying blood vessel, and the first clinical studies confirming these results have been published.[25] It is assumed that DWI shows the area of irreversible ischemic damage (i.e., the infarct core), whereas the size and extent of the tissue with reduced perfusion that is still viable can be measured with PWI. The discrepancy between these areas, with the PWI abnormality being larger than the DWI abnormality, may represent the ischemic penumbra, which may be saved if early reperfusion can be achieved.[26] In the future, a complete set of DWI and PWI scans and MRA may be implemented into the routine evaluation of the most acute phase of ischemia, replacing CT examinations and providing more information about the underlying vascular pathology, extent of the already infarcted tissue, and the tissue at risk that could be saved by a tailored therapeutic approach.

New and Experimental Therapies of Severe Postischemic Brain Edema

Recognition of the high mortality in patients with large hemispheric infarcts and the obvious ineffectiveness of medical therapy alone has prompted innovative therapeutic approaches. Although the effects of these therapies have not been proven in randomized trials, the results of pilot studies are promising.

Decompressive Surgery. Space-occupying hemispheric infarction, the so-called malignant MCA infarction, has a high mortality and morbidity, even with optimal conservative treatment. More than 80% of these patients die, despite maximal conservative treatment. Since the 1980s, several studies have shown that decompressive surgery is a possible treatment strategy for otherwise uncontrollable, increased ICP after severe hemispheric stroke. Surgical decompression seems to be effective in lowering increased ICP and preventing transtentorial herniation and has been tested extensively in head trauma patients with varying results, as well as in patients with space-occupying cerebellar infarctions, with a significant decrease in mortality and morbidity in comatose patients. Several cohorts of patients with large MCA infarction showed that decompressive surgery could reduce mortality to less than 50%. Previously reported initial results revealed a mortality rate of 34%, with the majority of survivors only mildly to moderately disabled.[27] This is particularly important because 75% of patients in this series already showed clinical signs of uncal herniation. Because the clinical course of patients with severe MCA stroke is highly predictable, waiting for pupillary dilation causes an unnecessary delay, as allowing mesencephalic ischemia to occur potentially worsens prognosis. Therefore, surgery is recommended within the first 24 hours after stroke onset, on clinical and neuroradiologic grounds. Surgery is advocated within 24 hours

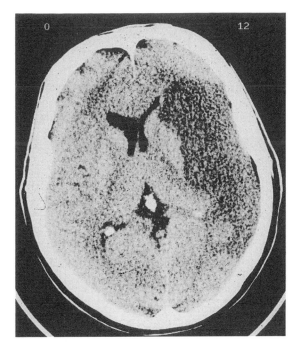

Day 2

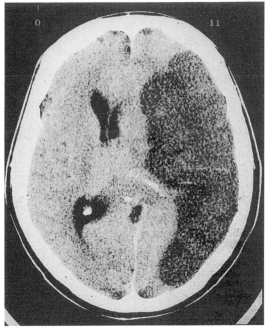

Day 3

Figure 14-6. Course of edema development in malignant middle cerebral artery infarction.

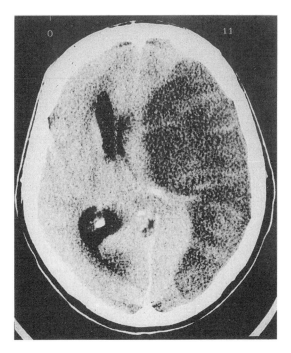

Day 4

when patients show the early neuroradiologic criteria of complete MCA infarction coupled with further clinical deterioration. Considering these two major points together, without surgical intervention the subsequent clinical course in these patients is highly predictable. With these criteria for early selection of patients for decompressive surgery, mortality could be reduced to only 16%.[27] The clinical rating of functional performance, as measured with the Barthel Index, also tended to be better.

Further support for earlier intervention comes from the fact that the duration of the need for critical care is significantly reduced in the group of patients treated early after severe stroke. Clearly, patients with anisocoria as a sign of an impending herniation syndrome require more (and more advanced) critical care support than those patients treated before mesencephalic ischemia can occur. This may also account for the relatively better outcome in the patient group treated early. In the future, integration of the clinical examination with early CT findings and new imaging techniques, such as PWI and DWI, might make it possible to determine the clinical significance of brain edema early after onset, thereby allowing clinicians to indicate decompressive craniectomy before life-threatening brain swelling and herniation occur (Figures 14-7 and 14-8).

Induced Hypothermia in Severe Ischemic Stroke. Normal body temperature is 37°C, although there is a significant diurnal variation of ± 0.6°C. Core body temperature can be measured at varying sites; the shell temperatures are measured either sublingually, axillary, or on the skin. Core temperatures reflect tympanic membrane, esophageal, rectal, bladder, and pulmonary artery temperature measurements. Hypothermia is defined as mild (–33°C), moderate (–29°C), and deep (below 28°C).
PHYSIOLOGY AND EXPERIMENTAL BASIS OF HYPOTHERMIA. The systemic oxygen demand decreases when the core body temperatures drop. Correspondingly, a drop in CO_2 production, plasma potassium levels, and carbohydrate metabolism is also seen. Hypothermia reduces both the cerebral demand for neuronal activity and the energy requirements necessary for intrinsic cellular support and membrane homeostasis. Additional mechanisms of cerebral protection include decreased glutamate and dopamine release, lowering of ICP,

and altered expression of the genes involved in programmed cell death (apoptosis).

There is a considerable body of experimental evidence that shows hypothermia is protective after global hypoxic injury to the brain. In addition, in experimental focal ischemia, a significant hypothermia-associated reduction of postischemic brain edema and a reduction of ICP have been shown. Hypothermia decreases metabolism and reduces global CBF. Furthermore, hypothermia reduces cerebral blood volume. Other mechanisms under investigation are protection against free radicals, reduction of heat-shock protein expression after ischemia, and blockade of adenosine triphosphate depletion. The response of calcium channels and excitatory receptors seems to be lowered during hypothermia, as are the concentrations of glutamate and other excitatory amino acids.
CLINICAL APPLICATION. Deep hypothermia is used routinely during open heart surgery and occasionally for cerebral protection during neurosurgical operations. Solomon has reported a series of patients with giant aneurysms operated on under deep hypothermic circulatory arrest. Arrest periods of up to 50 minutes were tolerated. Several neurosurgical studies showed a positive effect of mild hypothermia on uncontrollable intracranial hypertension after severe head trauma. Patients with head injuries treated with mild hypothermia of between 32°C and 34°C core temperature showed a significant reduction in ICP and CBF compared to a normothermic control group. All studies indicated better outcome with hypothermia and a beneficial effect in limiting secondary brain injury.[28] In most of these studies, hypothermia was delivered within the first 6 to 16 hours after head injury. The duration of hypothermia varied from 24 to 48 hours, but neither the optimal duration of hypothermia nor the optimal time after the trauma for therapy in these patients could be identified.

The results of the first clinical trial on the use of moderate hypothermia in severe MCA infarction were published by Schwab et al. in 1998.[29] Hypothermia was induced at a mean of 14 hours after ischemic injury and maintained for more than 72 hours to overcome the maximum brain swelling, which is known to occur between 2 and 5 days after ischemia. In this trial, all patients fulfilled the criteria for diagnosis of a "malignant" MCA infarction. However, the mortality rate was only

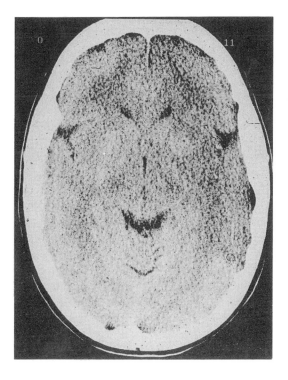

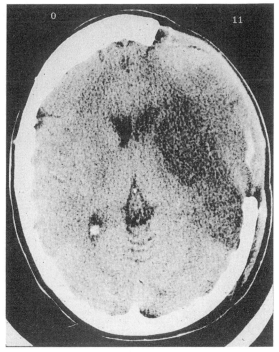

Day 1

Day 4

Figure 14-7. Decompressive surgery after malignant middle cerebral artery infarction.

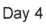

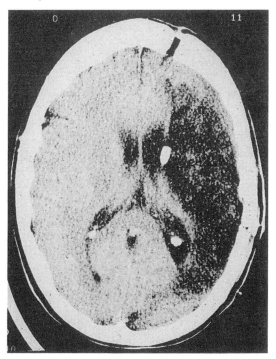

After 3 months

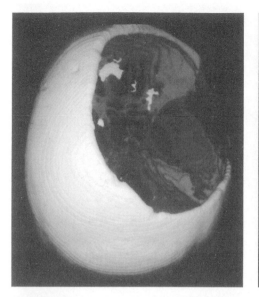

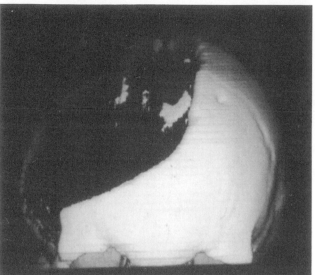

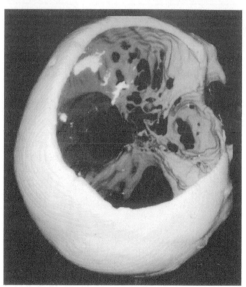

Figure 14-8. Three-dimensional computed tomography reconstruction of extension of bone flap after decompressive surgery in a patient with malignant middle cerebral artery infarction.

44%, and survivors reached a favorable outcome, with a mean Barthel Index score of 70.

Hypothermia significantly reduced ICP, a finding similar to the results of Marion and Shiozaki, who used hypothermic therapy in traumatic brain injuries.[28] However, rewarming patients constantly led to a secondary rise of ICP, which required additional ICP therapy with mannitol. In some cases, it exaggerated the initial ICP levels. It is known that the rewarming period is a high-risk time in brain injury, because metabolic needs may outstrip oxygen delivery at various temperatures. Hence, rewarming is considered the "critical phase" of hypothermic therapy. This rebound after rewarming might be due to a proposed hypermetabolic response after induced hypothermia, as it was described after cardiopulmonary bypass surgery.

SIDE EFFECTS. Hypothermia affects virtually every organ system. Ventricular ectopy and fibrillation limit the extent of hypothermia, but this is only known to occur at temperatures below 30°C. In the study mentioned previously, pneumonia was the only severe side effect of moderate hypothermia. Other side effects of hypothermia, which have been shown in animal studies, are clotting abnormalities and coagulopathy. In baboons, systemic hypothermia led to an increase in bleeding times. In men, the enzymatic reactions of the coagulation cascade were shown to be strongly inhibited by hypothermia. Pancreatitis with high serum amylase and lipase levels was also observed after hypothermic therapy; however, the association between hypothermia and pancreatitis is poorly understood.

Moderate hypothermia can decrease ICP and lower mortality in patients with severe postischemic brain edema. Important side effects are reduction of platelet count, increased rate of pneumonia, and elevation of serum amylase and lipase levels. Results suggest a beneficial effect of moderate hypothermia in the treatment of severe space-occupying MCA infarction.[29]

Acute Basilar Occlusion

The introduction of local intra-arterial fibrinolytic therapy in the early 1980s marked a change in the prognosis for acute basilar artery occlusion. If recanalization is achieved, mortality drops from approximately 90% (without recanalization) to 40–50%. Factors that predict poor outcome are clot localization, neurologic status on admission, and duration of occlusion. Patients with acute basilar occlusion should be treated in an ICU. Diagnosis is made according to the clinical signs and confirmed with Doppler ultrasound or either MRA, CT angiography, or conventional angiography. In cases of impaired consciousness, immediate endotracheal intubation and analgosedation are necessary. Patients who are comatose on admission and in whom somatosensory cortical-evoked potentials are lost have a poor prognosis despite rapid treatment, and no further interventional procedures should be undertaken. Patients with favorable predictors of outcome (young age, presumed embolic occlusion, distal clot location, and responsiveness at the time of presentation) should receive local thrombolysis with intra-arterial urokinase, 1.000.000 IU per hour,[30] under general anesthesia. These patients receive full-dose heparin after thrombolysis. Repeated CT scans after angiography are necessary to exclude ICH.

As stated previously, recanalization after thrombolysis can often be achieved if a thrombus is of embolic origin, distally located in the basilar artery, and if there is a good collateral blood flow and no underlying arteriosclerotic vasculopathy.[30,31]

Cerebellar Infarction

Cerebellar infarction constitutes 1.9–10.5% of cases in clinicopathologic series of patients with cerebral infarctions. A subgroup of patients with large cerebellar infarctions deteriorates after a variable interval. The main cause of this is probably infarct size, even though other factors, such as underlying vascular lesion, hemorrhagic transformation, and poor collateral blood flow, play a role as well. Neurologic deterioration occurs as a result of progression of concurrent brain stem infarction or an increasing mass effect of the infarcted cerebellum in the posterior fossa, leading to compression of the brain stem and associated occlusive hydrocephalus. Cerebellar infarction due to occlusion of basilar artery branches generally has a good clinical outcome even without aggressive treatment. In some cases, however, postischemic edema causes occlusive hydrocephalus or brain stem compression with rapid deterioration of brain stem functions. Therefore, close clinical monitoring and frequent CT scans to estimate the grade of obstructive hydrocephalus are mandatory. Neurocritical care is required if the CT scan reveals signs of increased pressure in the posterior fossa. In patients with rapid decline of consciousness, decompressive surgery of the posterior fossa—with or without removal of infarcted cerebellar tissue—is significantly better than ventriculostomy.[32–34] Ventriculostomy alone may be a temporary measure, but great care should be taken because it may promote ascending herniation. As stated previously, this approach is not used in patients with additional basilar thrombosis and large brain stem infarcts. Because it is often difficult to clearly distinguish the mechanisms leading to further clinical deterioration, median sensory-evoked potentials (MSEP) and brain stem auditory-evoked potential (BAEP) give further information for deciding about treatment in those patients. Patients with normal BAEP and somatosensory-evoked potential are treated with osmotherapeutics. Prolonged interpeak latencies in BAEP and altered amplitudes in somatosensory-evoked potential indicate decompressive surgery, and ventriculostomy alone is performed if CT only shows signs of hydrocephalus.

Spontaneous Intracerebral Hemorrhage

Most patients admitted with stroke symptoms due to ICH require neurologic or neurosurgical intensive care or treatment on a stroke unit. Clinical presentation depends on both the location and the size of the hematoma. Management of patients with ICH includes (1) general medical management, which is intended to stabilize vital parameters and prevent rebleeding and complications, and (2) surgical removal in subgroups.

General Management and Treatment of Complications

Besides the neurologic assessment and determining the cause of hemorrhage, medical therapy is the mainstay of the initial management of patients with ICH. Immediate monitoring and stabilization of vital parameters is mandatory. Patients with large, space-occupying or infratentorial bleeding are at particularly high-risk for upper airway obstruction and aspiration because of weakness of upper airway muscles, impaired airway and swallowing reflexes, and vomiting. Adequate airway protection, including early endotracheal intubation to ensure oxygenation, is essential in these patients, because hypoxia increases CBF, which may increase ICP.[35] If endotracheal intubation is necessary, an increase in ICP during tracheal stimulation can be counteracted with short-acting barbiturates, such as thiopental (1.0–1.5 mg/kg i.v.), during the procedure.

Many patients with ICH experience various central vegetative disturbances, such as bradycardia, tachycardia, hypotension, and hypertension; therefore, constant monitoring of these parameters and readiness for cardiopulmonary resuscitation is recommended. In particular, severe hypertension is commonly observed in patients with acute ICH. On one hand, this type of stroke is often caused by chronic or acute hypertension, whereas on the other hand, hypertension can be the result of the ICH, particularly in the presence of elevated ICP (Cushing's phenomenon). Reduction of ICP may be sufficient to control BP, but more rapid-action pharmacologic treatment often is needed. BP lowering should not be too drastic because of the risk of lowering the CPP in hypertensive patients with impaired cerebrovascular autoregulation. There are no specific guidelines for the treatment of hypertension in ICH based on randomized, controlled studies, but there is agreement on treating diastolic BPs of more than 120 mm Hg and mean BPs of more than 125–135 mm Hg.[35,36] Pharmacologic agents that cause cerebral vasodilation, such as hydralazine, nitroglycerin, and nitroprusside, should be avoided because of the risk of further ICP increase. Appropriate agents are labetalol, captopril, clonidine, or urapidil.

During laboratory analysis in patients with ICH, early assessment and correction of the coagulation status is of particular importance, because it may affect the progression of cerebral bleeding and the rate of early rebleeding. Patients with prolonged, activated partial thromboplastin time due to heparin use should be treated with protamine sulfate, 1 mg/100 IU heparin. Prolonged prothrombin time due to phenprocoumon or warfarin therapy should be reversed with as much intravenous vitamin K and fresh frozen plasma as needed. If available, a prothrombin complex concentrate (prothrombin, proconvertin, Stuart-Prower factor, antihemophilic globulin B), which acts more rapidly than vitamin K and fresh frozen plasma, should be administered[37]; however, this involves a potential risk of generalized thromboembolism. A special therapeutic dilemma arises when a patient with acute spontaneous ICH is admitted who requires high-intensity anticoagulation for high risk of thromboembolism (e.g., prosthetic heart valve replacement). Favorable outcome is frequent in patients with small anticoagulation-associated ICH; however, outcomes may be worsened by continuing anticoagulation, which may prevent severe, disabling thromboembolic events. Some authors favor discontinuation of any anticoagulation during acute hospital treatment of ICH,[38] whereas others point out the risk of early thromboembolism and suggest treatment with intravenous heparin (activated partial thromboplastin time, 1.5–2.0 times baseline value) after normalization of the international normalized ratio (Figure 14-9).[39] ICH associated with thrombolytic therapy (streptokinase more frequently than urokinase and t-PA) should be treated with alpha-epsilon-aminocaproic acid (5 g over 15–30 minutes) and cryoprecipitate.[35]

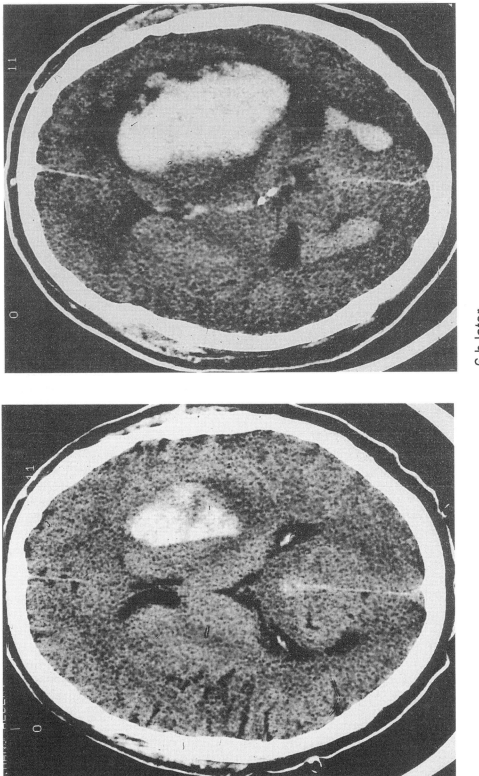

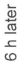

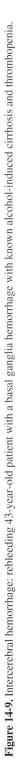

On admission

6 h later

Figure 14-9. Intercerebral hemorrhage: rebleeding 43-year-old patient with a basal ganglia hemorrhage with known alcohol-induced cirrhosis and thrombopenia.

Headache can be primarily treated with mild analgetics, such as paracetamol. However, substances with high thrombocyte antiaggregatory activity, such as aspirin, should be avoided. Frequently, opioids are needed for proper pain control (see Agitation and Pain). Distressing anxiety can be alleviated with short-acting benzodiazepines. Stools should be kept soft with oral laxatives and an adequate intake of fluids. Acute management of patients with ICH should also include close monitoring and correction of glucose levels and body temperature, because these parameters affect long-term outcome in these patients.[40] ICH patients can be mobilized early, as in ischemic stroke, but care should be taken with special monitoring of BP to avoid abrupt and excessive BP elevations.

An important component of general medical treatment is the prevention and treatment of the following complications associated with ICH:

Hydrocephalus: Patients with ICH are at risk for hydrocephalus due to mass effects (blockade of the foramen of Monro, compression of the aqueduct or fourth ventricle; intraventricular blood). A decline in the level of consciousness is the major symptom of developing hydrocephalus, at which time a CT scan should be performed. External ventricular device (EVD) is advantageous, even prophylactically, when the amount of intraventricular blood makes the development of hydrocephalus likely (see also Treatment of Intraventricular Hemorrhage). Catheters should be removed or replaced after 7 days, because the rate of infection increases rapidly afterwards. A definite ventriculoperitoneal shunt should be implanted only if the CSF is free of blood and occlusion of the external drainage increases ICP.

Seizures: During the first 3 days, 10–15% of all patients with ICH and 15–35% of patients with lobar hemorrhages develop seizures,[41] which may lead to severe elevations in ICP. Seizures are initially treated with benzodiazepines, such as clonazepam or lorazepam, and should be followed by secondary prophylaxis with phenytoin (intravenous loading with a bolus of 250 mg, followed by an infusion of 750 mg over 4–6 hours). If a second agent is needed, phenobarbital may be used, although side effects, such as somnolence and respiratory suppression, should be considered. If seizures are not controlled with these two agents, thiopental may be used (n.b.: be aware of severe hypotension with lowering of CPP).

Elevated ICP: The sudden development of an intracranial mass compressing and displacing brain tissue is often associated with an increase in ICP. Secondarily, intracranial volume may further increase during development of parenchymal edema or hydrocephalus. Management of elevated ICP consists of specific measures to treat the ICP itself and factors that contribute to increasing ICP. The guidelines for ICP treatment are similar to those for ischemic stroke presented in Treatment of Elevated Intracranial Pressure.

Surgical Evacuation of Hemorrhage

Early hematoma evacuation seems to be indicated because it may reduce perihematoma ischemia and toxic effects of blood components. Furthermore, it may prevent hematoma progression, because some studies found hematoma expansion in 38% of ICH patients within 20 hours of ictus (Figure 14-10).[42]

Supratentorial Hematomas

The indication for surgery in supratentorial cerebral hematoma remains under dispute. Most of the information on this subject has been derived from clinical series with several types of biases. There is no proof that evacuation of a hematoma by conventional surgery reduces residual deficits or expedites recovery. Randomized controlled surgical trials for spontaneous supratentorial ICH have been performed by McKissok et al.,[43] Juvela et al.,[44] Auer et al.,[45] Batjer et al.,[46] Morgenstern et al.,[47] and Zuccarello et al.[48] The essential data from these studies are summarized in Table 14-12.

Treatment strategies depend largely (1) on the size and location of the hemorrhage, and (2) on clinical impairment and course. A small hemorrhage with mild to moderate focal deficit only requires careful observation and conservative treatment to reduce cerebral edema. Surgery may be indicated in patients with increasing ICP and secondary deterioration of consciousness. It should be restricted to easily accessible putaminal or lobar hematomas,

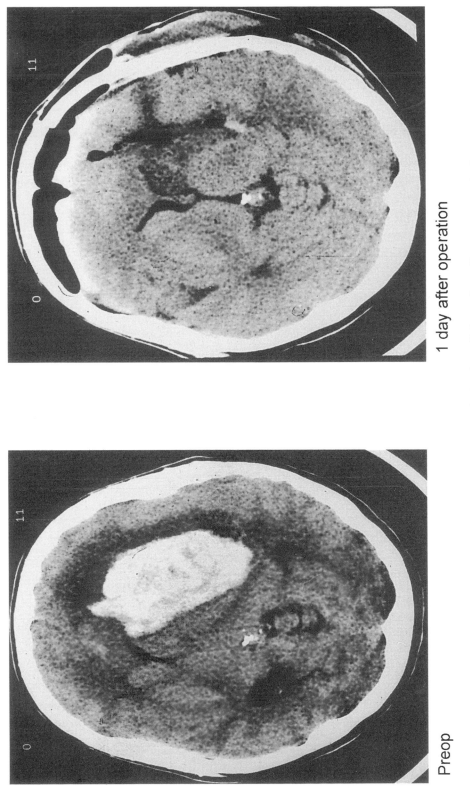

1 day after operation

Preop

Figure 14-10. Intercerebral hemorrhage surgery: 41-year-old patient with a hypertensive basal ganglia hemorrhage. (Preop = preoperative.)

Table 14-12. Summary of Randomized Controlled Surgical Trials for Spontaneous Supratentorial Intracranial Hemorrhage

| Study | Number of Patients | | Time Window | Inclusion Criteria | Outcome | |
	Surgical Group	Medical Group			Surgical Group	Medical Group
Juvela et al.[44]	26	26	<48 hrs	Unconscious, severe hemiparesis	M6 = 46%	M6 = 38%
Auer et al.[45]	50	50	<48 hrs	>10 ml	M6 = 30%	M6 = 70%
Batjer et al.[46]	8	13	<24 hrs	Putaminal, >3 cm	M6 = 50%	M6 = 85%
Morgenstern et al.[47]	17	17	<12 hrs	>9 ml	M1 = 6%, M6 = 17%	M1 = 24%, M6 = 24%
Zuccarello et al.[48]	9	11	<27 hrs	>10 ml, GOS >4	GOS >3:56%	GOS >3:36%

M1 = mortality after 1 month; M3 = mortality after 3 months; M6 = mortality after 6 months; GOS = Glasgow Outcome Scale.

however, and is not indicated for thalamic hemorrhages. If cerebral amyloid angiopathy is suspected to be the cause of hemorrhage, surgical treatment should be considered carefully, as severe postoperative hemorrhages have been observed. Signs of secondary brain stem compression by supratentorial hemorrhage, such as pupillary dilation or bilateral extensor limb posturing for more than several hours, are generally associated with poor outcome, regardless of whether medical or surgical therapy is undertaken. Table 14-13 summarizes recommendations regarding surgical or nonsurgical treatment in special subgroups of patients. New approaches, such as stereotactic or endoscopic aspiration of hematomas or thrombolytic therapy of intracerebral or intraventricular blood clots, offer promising treatment strategies[49–52]; however, except for stereotaxically guided endoscopic evacuation, these have not been validated in randomized clinical trials.[45]

In summary, early surgical treatment for acute ICH is difficult to achieve but feasible at specialized centers. The trend toward lower morbidity and mortality with surgical intervention in subgroups of patients with spontaneous supratentorial ICH warrants further investigation of early clot removal in large randomized clinical trials.

Table 14-13. Current Recommendations Regarding Surgical or Surgical Treatment in Special Subgroups of Patients

ICH Location	Clinical/CT Features	Treatment
Putamen	Alert, small ICH (<30 ml)	Nonsurgical
	Comatose, large ICH (>60 ml)	Nonsurgical
	Drowsy, intermediate ICH (30–60 ml)	Consider evacuation
Caudate	Alert or drowsy, with intraventricular hemorrhage and hydrocephalus	Consider ventriculostomy
Thalamus	Drowsy or lethargic, with blood in the third ventricle and hydrocephalus	Consider ventriculostomy
Lobar white matter	Drowsy or lethargic, with intermediate ICH (20–60 ml), progressive decline in level of consciousness	Consider evacuation
Pons, midbrain, medulla	—	Nonsurgical
Cerebellum	Noncomatose, with ICH >3 cm in diameter, and/or hydrocephalus, and/or effacement of quadrigeminal cistern	Evacuation recommended, preceded by ventriculostomy if patient is actively deteriorating

ICH = intracerebral hemorrhage; CT = computed tomography.
Source: Modified from K Minematsu, T Yamaguhi. Management of Intracerebral Hemorrhage. In Fisher M (ed), Stroke Therapy. Boston: Butterworth–Heinemann, 1995;351–372.

Infratentorial Hemorrhage

In contrast to supratentorial hematomas, the indication for surgery in cerebellar hematomas is undisputed. The prognosis worsens rapidly with a hematoma volume of 20 ml (mean diameter of 3 cm) or more. Only small hemispheric hemorrhages with no consciousness disturbances on CT should be treated conservatively; all other patients should be operated on immediately, because even patients with massive cerebellar hemorrhage can survive if they have only been comatose for a short time.[53,54]

No recommendation can be made for surgical evacuation of brain stem hematomas, because the tissue destruction caused by the initial bleeding precludes any benefit. Instances of successful surgical treatment of hematomas located in the vicinity of the fourth ventricle constitute neurosurgical rarities, with only anecdotal reports.

Treatment of Intraventricular Hemorrhage

Intraventricular hemorrhage (IVH) occurs in up to 40% of all patients with ICH and in up to 20% of all patients with SAH. There is strong evidence that IVH contributes to mortality after cerebral hemorrhage. Routine clinical management consists of EVD, which lowers the ICP immediately but should be continued until the ventricular clot has dissolved and CSF circulation has normalized. However, clotted blood often blocks the drain, which makes removal and insertion of a second catheter necessary. Prolonged drainage, however, increases the risk of infection with increased rates of ventriculitis after the first week of intraventricular catheter placement. The drainage itself prevents acute hydrocephalus, but does not affect resolution of the clot or incidence of communicating hydrocephalus. Therefore, intraventricular thrombolysis was proposed to be an effective measure to hasten the resolution of the intraventricular blood clot, reduce the duration of EVD, decrease the degree and incidence of communicating hydrocephalus, and thereby reduce the deaths associated with IVH. Clinical experience with this approach has grown since the 1990s. However, a wide variety of dosages and substances (urokinase or recombinant t-PA) have been used. No randomized controlled trial results are available to show the beneficial effect of this therapy. In our institution we perform intraventricular lysis in patients with a large amount of intraventricular blood after ICH with 4 mg recombinant t-PA every 12 hours over 2 days, and a multicenter trial is being planned. Before administration, vascular malformations are ruled out using either CT angiography or conventional angiography (Figure 14-11).

Subarachnoid Hemorrhage

Aneurysmal SAH accounts for 5–10% of all strokes and has a combined mortality and morbidity that exceeds 40%. Because the lesion is treatable and even curable at particular stages, management decisions are critical. They largely depend on individual CT findings. Because loss of functional independence is a common consequence of aneurysmal bleeding, despite surgical clipping of the aneurysm, aggressive medical management may complement efforts to improve outcome.

Intensive Care Unit Treatment

Intraparenchymatous bleeding with a tendency to expand may entail an emergency operative decompression to remove blood clots, stop the progression of bleeding, and reduce the risk of rebleeding by eliminating or clipping the vascular malformation. Early surgery, once believed to be associated with a high perioperative rate of complications, is now widely recommended for patients with Hunt and Hess grades I–IV. If immediate intervention is not necessary, the patient should be transferred to the ICU. The timing for angiography depends on the intended operative treatment. For detailed information about surgical management of aneurysmal SAH, see Chapter 18.

Basic Treatment

Intensive care should focus on (1) basic treatment, and (2) prevention, close monitoring, and treatment of complications.

For basic medical treatment of patients with acute SAH, the same principles apply as described for spontaneous ICH. Medical treatment of SAH concerning fluid and BP management radically changed during the 1990s. Although fluid restriction and aggressive BP reduction (induced hypotension)

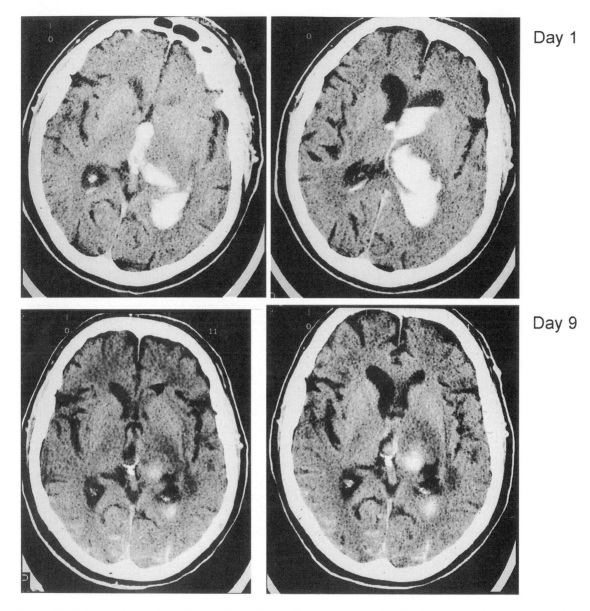

Day 1

Day 9

Figure 14-11. Intraventricular lysis: thalamic hemorrhage with intraventricular blood before and after lysis with recombinant tissue plasminogen activator.

were suggested in the past, now hypervolemic treatment is performed, and a comparatively high BP after clipping of the aneurysm is accepted.[55–57]

Treatment of Complications

Hydrocephalus

Symptomatic hydrocephalus occlusus or malresorptivus occurs in 15–20% of patients with SAH.[58] A char-

acteristic history consists of gradual obtundation after a lucid interval of a few hours. Insertion of an external ventricular catheter results in dramatic improvement within 1 or 2 days, but at the cost of a higher risk of rebleeding. Ventriculostomy is recommended even in patients with Hunt and Hess grades IV and V.[59]

Vasospasm

Up to 25% of patients with a ruptured aneurysm develop cerebral ischemia, mainly between 5 and

Table 14-14. Transcranial Doppler Ultrasound Signs Indicating Vasospasms

Ultrasound Measurements	Ultrasound Values
Intensity-weighted mean velocity	>3 kHz (120 cm/sec) = borderline
	>4 kHz (160 cm/sec) = significant
	>5 kHz (200 cm/sec) = critical
Maximum systolic velocity	>4 kHz (160 cm/sec) = relevant
	>7.5 kHz (300 cm/sec) = critical
MCA/ICA index	>3.0
Velocity increase during the first 6 days	>50%/die or >1 kHz (40 cm/sec)/die
Pulsatility of signals	Pulsatility index >1.0
	Resistance index >0.6

MCA = middle cerebral artery; ICA = internal carotid artery; die = diastole.
Source: Reprinted from permission from B Widder. Subarachnoidalblutungen: Intrakranielle Dopplerbefunde. In B Widder (ed), Doppler- und Duplexsonographie der hirnversorgenden Arterien. Berlin: Springer, 1999;444–447.

14 days after initial bleeding. It is the most prominent cause of death and disability after SAH. The time course of vasospasm is consistent with an immune-mediated response, and more recent observations suggest that immunologic processes, including activation of the complement system, may be involved.[60] The total amount of subarachnoid blood is a strong risk factor but its distribution does not predict the site of ischemia.

Monitoring for vasospasms includes close clinical observation and daily transcranial Doppler evaluation. Clinically, the level of consciousness gradually decreases in conjunction with focal neurologic signs. Transcranial Doppler sonographic signs indicating vasospasms are given in Table 14-14.

Measures to prevent ischemic stroke after aneurysmal SAH include (1) hypertensive hypervolemic treatment, and (2) the use of calcium-entry–blocking drugs, such as nimodipine.

Hypervolemic-Hypertensive Therapy. The first line of treatment is hypervolemic-hypertensive-hemodilution therapy (known as *triple-H therapy*) to increase CBF in the microcirculation (Tables 14-15 and 14-16). The first large patient series, reported by Kassel et al.,[61] showed that combined induced hypertension and volume expansion reversed neurologic deficits in the vast majority of patients. It is indicated when severe vasospasm is found by trans-

Table 14-15. Hypervolemic-Hypertensive Therapy

High-volume colloidal infusion (hetastarch 500–1,500 ml)
Ringer's solution (5,000–10,000 ml)
Hemoglobin solution if necessary
Sympathomimetics (norepinephrine 0.2–1.2 mg/hr or dopamine 10–30 mg/kg/min)

cranial Doppler ultrasound. Hypervolemia is induced by infusion of isotonic saline, hypertonic saline, or plasma expanders, aiming at a CVP of 8 mm Hg. If no clinical improvement is achieved, the additional use of vasopressors, such as norepinephrine, should be considered. Starting at 0.2 mg/kg, the continuous infusion is titrated until mean arterial BP has increased to 20–30 mm Hg above the baseline value, with systolic BP values up to 180 mm Hg.

Although the benefit of this therapy has not yet been proven by randomized studies, the rate of permanent ischemic deficits seems to be lower.[62] However, pulmonary and cerebral edema, cardiac dysregulation due to volume overload, myocardial infarction, and the risk of rebleeding seem to be more common under this treatment.

Nimodipine

Nimodipine significantly reduces delayed cerebral ischemia and improves outcome.[63,64] Working mechanisms of nimodipine comprise blockade of calcium channels of the vascular muscles and direct neuroprotection with increased tolerance to anoxia. In Europe, an initial intravenous formula is approved (for 1–2 hours, 1 mg/hour, followed by continuous infusion of 1–6 mg/hour), which may be substituted later by oral nimodipine (4–6 × 60 mg). Side effects include pulmonary right-to-left shunts and hypotension, which affects the coronary blood flow and the digestive tract muscles.

Table 14-16. Required Monitoring for Hypervolemic-Hypertensive Therapy

Laboratory tests, including osmolarity of urine and serum
Mean arterial BP (systolic BP → 160–180 mm Hg)
Central venous pressure (CVP → 10–12 mm Hg)
Fluid status and weight control (hematocrit → 33–38%)
Daily chest x-ray
If available: wedge pressure (Swan-Ganz catheter) (WP <20 mm Hg)

BP = blood pressure.

Promising new approaches for the treatment of vasospasm include endovascular techniques, such as balloon angioplasty, intra-arterial administration of papaverine, or a combination thereof.[65]

Rebleeding

Without coiling or surgical clipping, there is at least a 30% risk of rebleeding over the subsequent 4 weeks. The primary sign of rebleeding is a sudden decrease in the level of consciousness, often in combination with apnea. However, other causes may contribute to this as well (e.g., epilepsy, ischemia, or hydrocephalus). Therefore, a repeated CT scan is mandatory. In cases of rebleeding, emergency clipping of the aneurysm seems justified.

Surgical and Endovascular Treatments

Surgical and endovascular treatments are presented in detail in Chapters 18 and 19. In brief, the following techniques have been established:

Angioplasty and stenting: When neurologic manifestations of delayed cerebral ischemia due to vasospasm cannot be reversed by medical therapy, balloon catheters may be used to dilate the stenosed arteries. With this technique, the carotid artery, vertebral artery, proximal MCA, and entire basilar artery can be treated; however, this technique does not seem to be safe enough to go beyond the proximal portion of the anterior, middle, and posterior arteries. Early results with angioplasty for vasospasms with delayed ischemia are encouraging.[65] Stenting is an option for short, massive vasospasm.

Intra-arterial papaverine: The vasodilator papaverine may be administered in patients with severe vasospasm who cannot be treated with angioplasty.[65,66] Intra-arterial administration of doses of approximately 300 mg may be infused for 20 minutes to 1 hour. Angiographically, 50% of patients show noticeable changes in diameter, whereas clinical improvement is less impressive (approximately one in four patients). The vasodilatory effect of papaverine is significantly reduced when vasospasm has existed for several days, resulting in secondary histologic changes of the vessel wall.

Endovascular occlusion of the aneurysm: Saccular aneurysms can be occluded angiographi-cally by application of electrically detachable coils. Follow-up angiograms show persistent occlusion in approximately 90% of patients, and clinical results at up to 3 years were excellent.[67] Long-term follow-up studies must be completed before this technique can be claimed as an alternative for surgical clipping of aneurysms. However, patients with a high associated medical comorbidity, high surgical risk, and poor grade of SAH may be particularly suitable for this approach (Figures 14-12 and 14-13).

Sinus Venous Thrombosis

The thrombotic process of the cerebral venous system is almost the same as that for venous thrombosis in other parts of the body. There are numerous etiologic factors, including local infections, sepsis, and hypercoagulopathies of varying origin.[68] Diagnosis has been aided by magnetic resonance imaging and MRA. Reasons for patients' admission to the NCCU are either development of hemorrhagic infarction, seizures, or increased ICP. Clinically, the coincidence of headache, fluctuating course of focal neurologic deficits, and seizures are characteristic. Possible causes of sinus venous thrombosis are listed in Table 14-17.

In patients with impaired consciousness, focal or generalized seizures, or signs of septic thrombosis (fever, chemosis, and meningitis), further observation in an NCCU is mandatory.[69]

The basic regimen for all patients with aseptic thrombosis is intravenous administration of heparin with therapeutic partial thromboplastin time levels (50–120 seconds). Heparin is indicated even in patients with intracranial bleeding or hemorrhagic infarcts.[70] Long-term anticoagulation treatment with warfarin should be initiated in patients with coagulation disorders, and elevated ICP should be treated as described previously.

Because seizures occur frequently, prophylactic antiepileptic treatment should be considered. Further clinical deterioration with anticoagulant therapy is relatively uncommon. However, deterioration from an enlarging hematoma may require further aggressive therapy, including craniotomy to relieve ICP. An attempt to lyse the clotted sinus with thrombolytics has occasionally been undertaken. However, the value of this approach is difficult to estimate because patients may recover from coma with conservative management alone.

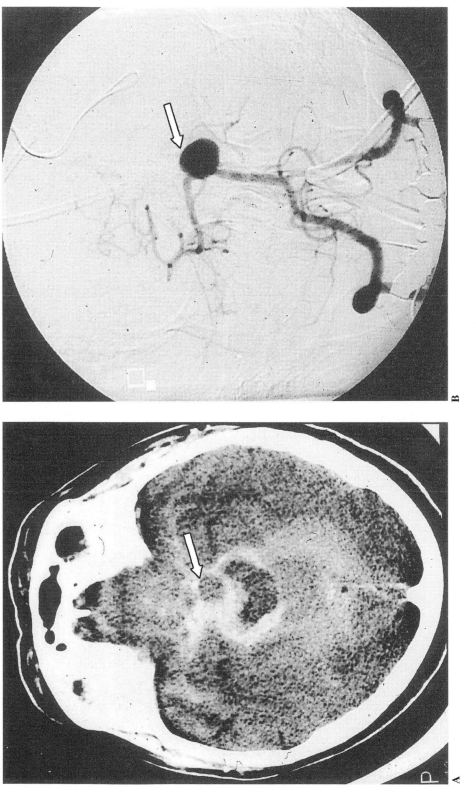

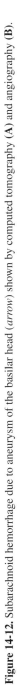

Figure 14-12. Subarachnoid hemorrhage due to aneurysm of the basilar head (*arrow*) shown by computed tomography (**A**) and angiography (**B**).

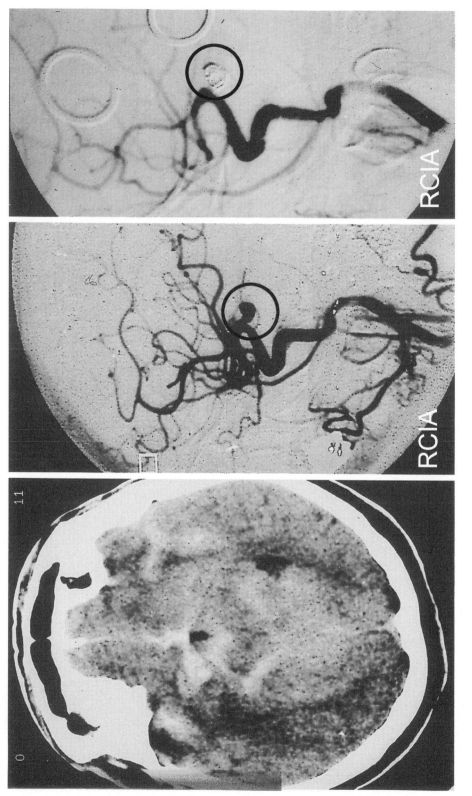

Figure 14-13. Subarachnoid hemorrhage (Hunt and Hess grade IV) in a 54-year-old woman with blood pronounced in the right sylvian fissure. Aneurysm of the right carotid artery before and after endovascular coiling (*circles*).

Table 14-17. Possible Causes of Sinus Venous Thrombosis

Coagulation disorders (among others)
    Protein C and S deficiency
    Homocystinemia
    Factor Leyden mutation
    Activated protein C resistance
    Infections of middle ear, mastoid, and paranasal sinus
Sepsis of any origin
Drugs
    Oral contraceptives
    Chemotherapeutics
        Asparaginase
        Methotrexate
        Tamoxifen
Trauma
Endocrine imbalance
    Pregnancy and postpartum state
Hematologic disorders
(Para)neoplasm
Autoimmune disorders

Mildly elevated ICP due to minor brain swelling should not be treated with antiedematous agents. In severe cases with risk of herniation, invasive ICP monitoring and lowering of ICP by infusion of 20% mannitol is recommended. In some cases of major edema, craniotomy may be considered.

References

1. Bounds JV, Wiebers DO, Whisnant JP, Okazaki H. Mechanisms and timing of deaths from cerebral infarction. Stroke 1981;19:1119–1124.
2. Malik AB. Mechanisms of neurogenic pulmonary edema. Circ Res 1985;57:1–18.
3. Samuels MA. Cardiopulmonary Aspects of Acute Neurologic Disease. In AH Ropper (ed), Neurological and Neurosurgical Intensive Care (3rd ed). New York: Raven, 1993;103–120.
4. Aidinis SJ, Lafferty J, Shapiro HM. Intracranial response to PEEP. Anesthesiology 1976;45:275–286.
5. Robertson GL, Aycinena P, Zerbe RL. Neurogenic disorders of osmoregulation. Am J Med 1982;72:339–353.
6. Brown RG. Disorders of water and sodium balance. Postgrad Med 1993;93:231–240.
7. Long CL, Schaffel N, Geiger JW, et al. Metabolic response to injury and illness: estimation of protein and energy needs from direct calorimetry and nitrogen balance. JPEN J Parenter Enteral Nutr 1979;3:442–456.
8. Ott L, Young B. Nutrition in the neurologically injured patient. Nutr Clin Prac 1991;6:223–229.
9. Zander JF, Bourke DB. Pain Relief and Sedation. In Hacke W (ed), Neuro Critical Care. Berlin: Springer, 1995;116–124.
10. Hacke W, Schwab S, De Georgia M. Intensive care of acute ischemic stroke. Cerebrovasc Dis 1994;4:385–392.
11. Schwab S, Aschoff A, Spranger M, et al. The value of intracranial pressure monitoring in acute hemispheric stroke. Neurology 1996;47:393–398.
12. Wolf A, Levi L, Marmorou A, et al. Effect of THAM on outcome in severe head injury: a randomized prospective clinical trial. J Neurosurg 1993;78:54–59.
13. Hacke W, Schwab S, Horn M, et al. "Malignant" middle cerebral artery infarction. Arch Neurol 1996;53:309–315.
14. Krieger DW, Demchuk AM, Kasner SE, et al. Early clinical and radiological predictors of fatal brain swelling in ischemic stroke. Stroke 1999;30:287–292.
15. Wijdiks EF, Diringer MN. Middle cerebral artery territory infarction and early brain swelling: progression and effect of age on outcome. Mayo Clin Proc 1989;73:829–836.
16. Tijssen CC, Schulte BP, Leyten AC. Prognostic significance of conjugate eye deviation in stroke patients. Stroke 1991;22:200–202.
17. Plum F, Posner JB. The Diagnosis of Stupor and Coma (3rd ed). Philadelphia: FA Davis, 1983.
18. Grotta J, Pasteur W, Khwaja G, et al. Elective intubation for neurological deterioration after stroke. Neurology 1995;45:640–644.
19. Hacke W, Kaste M, Fieschi C, et al. Intravenous thrombolysis with recombinant tissue plasminogen activator for acute hemispheric stroke. JAMA 1995;274:1017–1025.
20. von Kummer R, Meyding-Lamadé U, Forsting M, et al. Sensitivity and prognostic value of early computed tomography in middle cerebral artery trunk occlusion. AJNR Am J Neuroradiol 1994;15:9–15.
21. von Kummer R, Nolte PN, Schnittger H, et al. Detectability of cerebral hemisphere ischaemic infarcts by CT within 6 h of stroke. Neuroradiology 1996;38:31–33.
22. Moulin T, Cattin F, Crépin-Leblond T, et al. Early CT signs in acute middle cerebral artery infarction: predictive value for subsequent infarct locations and outcome. Neurology 1996;47:366–375.
23. Manelfe C, Larrue V, von Kummer R, et al. Association of hyperdense middle cerebral artery sign with clinical outcome in patients treated with tissue plasminogen activator. Stroke 1999;30:769–772.
24. Lutsep HL, Albers GW, DeCrespigny A, et al. Clinical utility of diffusion-weighted magnetic resonance imaging in the assessment of ischemic stroke. Neurology 1997;41:574–580.
25. Fisher M, Albers GW. Applications of diffusion-perfusion magnetic resonance imaging in acute ischemic stroke. Neurology 1999;52:1750–1756.
26. Jansen O, Schellinger P, Fiebach J, et al. Early recanalisation in acute ischaemic stroke saves tissue at risk defined by MRI. Lancet 1999;353:2036–2037.
27. Schwab S, Steiner T, Aschoff A, et al. Early hemicraniectomy in patients with complete middle cerebral artery infarction. Stroke 1998;29:1888–1893.

28. Marion D, Penrod L, Kelsey S, et al. Treatment of traumatic brain injury with moderate hypothermia. N Engl J Med 1997;336:540–546.

29. Schwab S, Schwarz S, Spranger M, et al. Efficacy and safety of moderate hypothermia in the therapy of patients with acute MCA stroke. Stroke 1998;29:2461–2466.

30. Levy EI, Firlik AD, Wisniewski S, et al. Factors affecting survival rates for acute vertebrobasilar artery occlusions treated with intra-arterial thrombolytic therapy: a meta-analytical approach. Neurosurgery 1999;45:539–548.

31. Hacke W, Zeumer H, Ferbert A, et al. Intra-arterial thrombolytic therapy improves outcome in patients with acute vertebrobasilar occlusive disease. Stroke 1988;19:1216–1222.

32. Rieke K, Krieger D, Adams HP, et al. Therapeutic strategies in space-occupying cerebellar infarction based on clinical, neuroradiological, and neurophysiological data. Cerebrovasc Dis 1993;3:45–55.

33. Heros RC. Surgical treatment of cerebellar infarction. Stroke 1992;23:937–938.

34. Chen HJ, Lee TC, Wei CP. Treatment of cerebellar infarction by decompressive suboccipital craniectomy. Stroke 1992;23:957–961.

35. Diringer MN. Intracerebral hemorrhage: pathophysiology and management. Crit Care Med 1993;21:1591–1603.

36. Wijman CA, Kase SK. What Should Become the Treatment of Cerebral Hemorrhage? In J Bogousslavsky (ed), Acute Stroke Treatment. London: Martin Dunitz, 1997;245–258.

37. Fredericksson K, Norrving B, Strömblad L. Emergency reversal of anticoagulation. Stroke 1992;23:972–977.

38. Wijdicks EF, Schievink WI, Brown RD, Mullany CJ. The dilemma of discontinuation of anticoagulation therapy for patients with intracranial hemorrhage and mechanical heart valves. Neurosurgery 1998;42:769–773.

39. Bertram M, Bonsanto M, Hacke W, Schwab S. Managing the therapeutic dilemma: patients with spontaneous intracerebral hemorrhage and urgent need for anticoagulation. J Neurol 2000;247:209–214.

40. Schwarz S, Häffner K, Aschoff A, Schwab S. Incidence and prognostic significance of fever following spontaneous supratentorial intracerebral hemorrhage. Neurology 2000;54:354–361.

41. Caplan LR. General Symptoms and Signs. In Kase CS, LR Kaplan (eds), Intracerebral Hemorrhage. Boston: Butterworth–Heinemann, 1994;31–43.

42. Brott T, Broderick J, Kothari R, et al. Early hemorrhage growth in patients with intracerebral hemorrhage. Stroke 1997;28:1–5.

43. McKissok W, Richardson A, Taylor J. Primary intracerebral hemorrhage: a controlled trial of surgical and conservative treatment in 180 unselected cases. Lancet 1961;2:221–226.

44. Juvela S, Heiskanen O, Poranen A, et al. The treatment of spontaneous intracerebral hemorrhage. A prospective randomized trial of surgical and conservative treatment. J Neurosurg 1990;72:152–155.

45. Auer LM, Deinsberger W, Niederkorn K, et al. Endoscopic surgery versus medical treatment for spontaneous intracerebral hematoma: a randomized study. J Neurosurg 1989;70:530–535.

46. Batjer HH, Reisch JS, Allen BC, et al. Failure of surgery to improve outcome in hypertensive putaminal hemorrhage: a prospective randomized controlled trial. Arch Neurol 1990;47:1103–1106.

47. Morgenstern MD, Frankowski RF, Shedden P, et al. Surgical treatment for intracerebral hemorrhage (STICH): a single-center, randomized clinical trial. Neurology 1998; 51:1359–1363.

48. Zuccarello M, Brott T, Derex L, et al. Early surgical treatment for supratentorial intracerebral hemorrhage: a randomized feasibility study. Stroke 1999;30:1833–1839.

49. Backlund E-O, Holst H. Controlled subtotal evacuation of intracerebral hematomas by stereotactic technique. Surg Neurol 1978;9:99–101.

50. Matsumoto K, Hondo H. CT-guided stereotaxic evacuation of hypertensive intracerebral hematomas. J Neurosurg 1984;61:440–448.

51. Niizuma H, Otzuki T, Juhkura H, et al. CT-guided stereotactic aspiration of intracerebral hematoma: result of hematolysis method using urokinase. Appl Neurophysiol 1985;48:427–430.

52. Schaller C, Rohde V, Meyer B, Hassler W. Stereotactic puncture and lysis of spontaneous intracerebral hemorrhage using recombinant tissue plasminogen activator. Neurosurgery 1995;36:328–335.

53. Minematsu K, Yamaguhi T. Management of Intracerebral Hemorrhage. In Fisher M (ed), Stroke Therapy. Boston: Butterworth–Heinemann, 1995;351–372.

54. Ott KH, Kase CS, Ojemann RG, Mohr JP. Cerebellar hemorrhage: diagnosis and treatment. A review of 56 cases. Arch Neurol 1974;31:160–167.

55. Hasan D, Vermeulen M, Wijdicks EF, et al. Effect of fluid intake and antihypertensive treatment on cerebral ischemia after subarachnoid hemorrhage. Stroke 1989;20: 1511–1515.

56. Wijdicks EF, Vermeulen M, ten Haaf JA, et al. Volume depletion and natriuresis in patients with a ruptured intracranial aneurysm. Ann Neurol 1985;18:211–216.

57. Wijdicks EF, Vermeulen M, Murray GD, et al. The effects of treating hypertension following aneurysmal subarachnoid hemorrhage. Clin Neurol Neurosurg 1990;92:111–117.

58. Heros RC. Acute hydrocephalus after subarachnoid hemorrhage. Stroke 1989;20:715–717.

59. Bailes JE, Spetzler RF, Hadley MN, Baldwin HZ. Management morbidity and mortality of poor-grade aneurysm patients. J Neurosurg 1990;72:559–566.

60. Ostergaard JR. Risk factor in intracranial saccular aneurysms. Aspects on the formation and rupture of aneurysms, and development of cerebral vasospasm. Acta Neurol Scand 1989;80:81–89.

61. Kassel NF, Peerless SJ, Durward QJ, et al. Treatment of ischemic deficits from vasospasm with intravascular volume expansion and induced arterial hypertension. Neurosurgery 1982;11:337–343.

62. Wijdicks EF. New Management Trends in Aneurysmal Subarachnoid Hemorrhage. In J Bogousslavsky (ed), Acute Stroke Treatment. London: Martin Dunitz, 1997;259–269.

63. Hongo K, Kobayashi S. Calcium antagonists for the treatment of vasospasm following subarachnoid hemorrhage. Neurol Res 1993;15:218–224.

64. Barker FG II, Ogilvy CS. Efficacy of prophylactic nimodipine for delayed ischemic deficit after subarachnoid hemorrhage: a meta-analysis. J Neurosurg 1996; 84:405–414.

65. Newell DW, Eskridge JM, Mayberg MR, et al. Angioplasty for the treatment of symptomatic vasospasm following subarachnoid hemorrhage. J Neurosurg 1989;71:654–660.

66. Kaku Y, Yonekawa Y, Tsukahara T, Kazkawa K. Supraselective intra-arterial infusion of papaverine for the treatment of cerebral vasospasm after subarachnoid hemorrhage. J Neurosurg 1992;77:842–847.

67. Casasco AE, Aymard A, Gobin JP, et al. Selective endovascular treatment of 71 intracranial aneurysms with platinum coil. J Neurosurg 1993;79:3–10.

68. Ameri A, Bousser MG. Cerebral venous thrombosis. Neurol Clin 1992;10:87–111.

69. Di Nubile MJ, Boom WH, Southwick FS. Septic cortical thrombophlebitis. J Infect Dis 1990;161:1216–1220.

70. Einhäupl KM, Villringer A, Meister W, et al. Heparin treatment of sinus venous thrombosis. Lancet 1991;333: 597–600.

Chapter 15
Thrombolytic Therapy

Gregory J. del Zoppo, Gerhard Hamann,
and Naoshia Hosomi

Based on phase II and phase III trial experience, which supports the potential safety and efficacy of acute intravenous and intra-arterial infusion of several plasminogen activators (PAs) in acute ischemic stroke, progress has been made toward the goal of injury reduction and improved recovery. Prospective clinical studies in ischemic stroke have tested acute administration of urokinase-type PA (u-PA), streptokinase (SK), recombinant tissue PA (rt-PA), recombinant prourokinase (rpro-UK), or the defibrinating agent ancrod. When given within 3 hours of symptom onset, rt-PA was associated with a significant increase in the number of patients with little or no disabling defect within 3 months[1] and 12 months[2] of treatment. On the basis of that experience, rt-PA has been licensed for intravenous delivery for ischemic stroke patients within 3 hours of symptom onset in the United States and several other countries.[1]

Efforts to evaluate the efficacy of thrombus lysis in acute ischemic stroke rest on the observation that 80–90% of focal cerebral ischemic events presenting within 6–24 hours of symptom onset are associated with atherothrombotic or embolic occlusive disease.[3] Nearly 50–70% of all strokes prospectively studied are associated with migratory arterial occlusions (e.g., cardiogenic embolism or local artery-to-artery embolism) or thrombus superimposed on the atherosclerotic lesion. Thrombi and emboli may originate from atheromas in large extracranial (carotid and vertebral) arteries or distal dependent intracranial vessels (e.g., proximal middle cerebral artery [MCA]). Additional causes of focal symptoms not generally associated with major vascular obstructions include small, deep infarcts of the lacunar type and intracerebral hemorrhage.

Prospective angiographic studies of patients presenting with symptoms of ischemic stroke confirmed the presence of occlusions within the territory of the ischemic signs (MCA) and an increase in arterial patency in time from symptom onset.[4–9] Recanalization can occur spontaneously in 4–18% of patients with documented proximal MCA lesions within 6 hours of symptom onset.[5–7] The "spectacular shrinking deficit" described by some investigators most probably represents downstream translocation of an embolus secondary to endogenous thrombus lysis.[10,11] A composite of five prospective angiography-based studies demonstrates a successive reduction in carotid territory occlusions from 6 hours to 7 days after the ictus.[3,7–9,12] In one report, in which initial angiograms were performed between 2 to 9 days after initial symptoms of embolic stroke, reperfusion of carotid territory occlusions were observed from 10 minutes to 8 days after the initial angiogram.[4] Whether angiography per se accelerates recanalization is not certain, but anecdotal experience suggests that mechanical disruption of the occlusion may facilitate recanalization. The potential for spontaneous recanalization is the rationale for proper control groups in prospective clinical trials, which have been used in several angiographic studies.[6,13,14]

The presence of arterial occlusion was determined in a number of phase I and II clinical safety and efficacy outcome trials, and a prospective controlled phase III study.[6] A number of prospective controlled phase III clinical outcome trials have been completed in which precise vascular diagnosis was not obtained. Experience with MCA territory stroke suggests that (1) the neurologic status at symptom onset has prognostic value (e.g., patients with mild or moderate deficits are more likely to fare better than those with severe deficits),[12,15] (2) mortality or the final neurologic status is generally a poor indicator of the anatomic location of the occlusion,[12,16] (3) clinical deficit and clinical outcome depend to some degree on occlusion location,[6] and (4) although neurologic deficits may reflect occlusion location, the clinical deficits do not invariably correlate.[17] Although most trials have used neurologic scoring instruments for baseline, post-treatment and delayed outcome, completed phase III trials have used disability outcome measures, including the Barthel Index and the Modified Rankin Scale (mRS). There is little published prospectively derived information to validate either disability outcome instrument in acute stroke trial management.[18] A report by Wityk et al. demonstrates the lesion-dependence of outcomes measured by one neurologic scoring instrument and the variation of outcome with time from onset.[19]

Technical Aspects

Direct intra-arterial delivery of PAs with cerebral angiography allows diagnosis and direct delivery of the agent via superselective catheters. Advances in catheter design and imaging techniques have resulted in the ability to demonstrate and reach small intracerebral branch arteries. Image digitization and road mapping are invaluable in aiding the neuroradiologist to guide less traumatic soft microcatheters with steerable guidewires to the site of occlusion.[20]

Intravenous delivery is technically easier to perform; however, thrombolytic agents are given in systemic doses. Intra-arterial infusions can be regional (intracarotid) or local (into or abutting the occlusion). Experience from peripheral vascular thrombolysis suggests that catheter placement into the thrombus results in more rapid and efficacious recanalization.[21]

Zeumer et al. described the use of balloon occlusion of the ipsilateral internal carotid artery (ICA) while delivering thrombolytic agent directly to increase local concentration to the thrombus.[22] Steerable microcatheter placement abutting the site of occlusion[20] or positioned into the clot[6,23] has been used most commonly. There are no clear data on whether catheter placement adjacent to, or into, the occlusion is the superior technique; however, perfusion past the thrombus enhances PA-assisted reperfusion. Studies have suggested that intra-arterial drug delivery with a high dose of contrast may result in extravasation and thus be misinterpreted as petechial hemorrhage.[24,25]

Zeumer et al. found that rt-PA and u-PA instilled locally lasted a median of 120 minutes for complete recanalization (which occurred in 56% of patients), whereas 97% of patients had partial or complete recanalization.[20] In comparison, using intravenous rt-PA, del Zoppo et al. noted a 1-hour recanalization incidence of 8% (extracranial ICA occlusion), 26% (MCA occlusion), and 38% (more distal MCA occlusion).[7] Among angiography-based studies, perfusion was achieved in 45–100% patients with direct intra-arterial delivery of u-PA, SK, or rt-PA, compared to approximately 30% of patients receiving intravenous rt-PA.

The benefits of highly selective angiography and local instillation of thrombolytic agents must be weighed against the time taken to arrange and perform the procedure, the availability of a highly skilled neuroradiologist who is able to perform the study, and the risks inherent in performing cerebral angiography. Arterial rupture with concomitant hemorrhage (1.5%)[26] and dissection can occur with intracerebral catheter manipulations.[26–28] Several studies have shown a higher incidence of neurologic deficit in patients with underlying cerebral disease, suggesting a significant potential complication rate in acute stroke, particularly if an embolism complicates the procedure.[27,29]

Contemporary studies using intra-arterial digital subtraction angiography have demonstrated a low but significant incidence of complications. These include local complications in the groin or brachial region, such as hematoma formation, arterial occlusion, or arterial dissection (0.5–7.3%), and systemic reactions to contrast (0.5–1.8%).[30–32] The incidence of transient neurologic deficits in predominantly elective and semielective series range from 0.45% to a mean of 3.1% in eight prospective studies reviewed by Hankey et al.[33] Persistent neurologic deficits occurred in 0.09% of radiographic studies performed by Grzyska et al.[34] and a mean of 1% in Hankey's review.[33] The use of digital subtraction angiography does not appear to decrease this incidence of complications.

A role for duplex and transcranial Doppler ultrasonography (TCD) has been suggested. TCD has been used to demonstrate and resolve reperfusion in intracranial arteries. Although not consistently applied, carotid duplex ultrasonography can be used to exclude complete ICA occlusions, which occur in approximately 25% of MCA-territory strokes treated within 8 hours and have been shown to be resistant to thrombolysis.[7]

Other diagnostic options that are available, particularly when intravenous thrombolysis is being considered, include magnetic resonance imaging combined with magnetic resonance angiography, TCD in association with CT or magnetic resonance imaging, or CT angiography. These modalities do not carry the risk of angiography but are less accurate. However, this tradeoff in accuracy may be considered worthwhile. Assessing reperfusion of the ischemic brain by TCD or single photon emission computed tomography (SPECT) has been performed. Baird et al.[35] used ^{99}mTc-hexamethylpropyleneamine oxime SPECT to monitor reperfusion after treatment of patients with intravenous SK. Ringelstein et al. monitored recanalization in patients who presented with documented carotid territory thrombosis with serial TCD after the use of fibrinolytic agents.[36]

Safety Considerations

The theoretical risk of extending hemorrhage by using PAs in stroke has limited the spread of this potential therapeutic approach outside specialized medical centers and universities.[37] It is essential that hemorrhagic transformation associated with the developing infarction be excluded by neuroimaging procedures (e.g., CT scan) before treatment with any fibrinolytic agent. Hemorrhage accompanies the action of PAs, which alter the vascular matrix and increase vascular permeability as well as to proteolytic cleavage and consumption of fibrin(ogen). An understanding that PAs may

extend or worsen a developing hemorrhage associated with the consequences of ischemia has been one result of the prospective study of fibrinolytic agents in the setting of focal cerebral ischemia.

Hemorrhagic transformation may be subcategorized as hemorrhagic infarction (HI) or parenchymal hematoma (PH).[38] *Hemorrhagic infarction* refers to petechial or confluent petechial hemorrhage confined to the region of ischemic injury, which may have few clinical consequences. PHs, on the other hand, are masses of blood that may encroach on surrounding structures, resulting in midline shift, and are often associated with clinical worsening. Experience in prospective open phase I trials of fibrinolytic agents in acute thrombotic stroke have confirmed improvement in neurologic outcome with HI.[13,14] More recent experimental data suggests that HI may result from loss of microvascular matrix integrity.[39,40] Although not proven, the pathophysiologic basis of HI and PH may be similar,[41] and only the extent of the bleeding may vary.[42–44]

Acute Myocardial Infarction

The mean incidence of intracerebral hemorrhage after fibrinolysis for acute myocardial infarction (MI) was calculated as 0.32% by Sloan and Price in a retrospective review of 46,000 patients.[45] Trials with different PAs have suggested different risks: for SK, 0.18%; anisolyl plasminogen SK activator complex, 0.32%; rt-PA, 0.47%; and pro-UK, 0.79% rate of symptomatic intracranial hemorrhage in acute MI. For rt-PA, the occurrence of intracerebral hemorrhage was dose-dependent: Patients receiving 150 mg rt-PA had a 1.3% incidence of symptomatic hemorrhage, whereas patients receiving 100 mg rt-PA had a risk of 0.4%.[46]

Significant predictors for high risk of symptomatic cerebral hemorrhage in MI were older age (older than 65 years), hypertension on admission, low body weight (less than 79 kg), and the use of single-chain rt-PA.[47,48] In the Global Utilization of Streptokinase and t-PA for Occluded Coronary Arteries trial, the more aggressive and recommended treatment branches ("accelerated" rt-PA dose with intravenous heparin, SK, and rt-PA with heparin) displayed a higher frequency of hemorrhagic stroke (0.72% and 0.94%, respectively) than other strategies (SK with subcutaneous heparin

[0.49%] or SK with intravenous heparin [0.54%]).[49] Despite the higher frequency of cerebral complications, however, the improvement in cardiac survival surpassed overall deterioration.

Certain pre-existing conditions may result in a higher risk for intracerebral hemorrhage and lead to exclusion from thrombolysis in acute MI.[50,51] Typically, arteriovenous malformations,[45] cerebral amyloid angiopathy,[52] previous head trauma,[46] and cerebrovascular accidents increase the risk for cerebral hemorrhagic complications.[46,53] The central nervous system pathology underlying symptomatic hemorrhage in MI patients treated with PAs is generally unknown, whereas the development of HI in stroke patients treated acutely involves the evolving ischemic lesion.

Acute Cerebral Ischemia: Hemorrhagic Transformation

Natural History of Ischemia-Related Hemorrhage

The transformation of an ischemic cerebral lesion into an HI is a common event, whereas gross intracerebral hemorrhage (PH) after an ischemic stroke is less frequent.[38] Pathologic findings indicate that 50–70% of all ischemic strokes develop some kind of hemorrhagic change (petechial to gross hemorrhage).[54–56] Clinical studies indicate a frequency of hemorrhagic transformation of approximately 40%.[57,58] The highest frequencies of hemorrhagic complications occur in cerebral embolic infarctions,[3,57] whereas the risk in thrombotic stroke may be low (1.9%).[3] Hemorrhagic transformation is most often seen within the area of infarction,[3,7] but has been reported to occur outside it in approximately 10% of patients with MCA-territory ischemic strokes treated with rt-PA.[7]

Experimental Models and Intracerebral Hemorrhage

In various animal models, possible relationships between fibrinolysis and the occurrence of hemorrhagic complications have been studied.[59] Slivka and Pulsinelli, using a rabbit model, suggested that cerebral hemorrhagic complications for late (24-hour) fibrinolysis surpassed those for early treatment (within 1 hour).[60] Increased intracerebral hemorrhage was not found in different experimental settings when rt-PA was used by Zivin et al.[61] and Overgaard et al.[62] Those data were confirmed by the absence of a correlation among dose, time of administration, recanalization, and the rate of hemorrhagic complications in a rabbit study using rt-PA.[63]

Using a primate model of focal cerebral ischemia, which probably is most comparable to the situation in humans, Hamann and del Zoppo demonstrated the appearance of microvascular hemorrhage in regions of decreased microvascular matrix.[39,40] Primate model experiments involving a glycoprotein IIb/IIIa inhibitor have clearly shown the role of normal platelet reactivity in preventing ischemia-dependent HI.[64] In a separate study, no dose relationship of rt-PA to the incidence or volume of hemorrhage was detected when the agent was applied within 3 hours of MCA occlusion.[65] Also, intra-arterial fibrinolysis with u-PA did not increase the incidence or severity of hemorrhage.[65,66] From limited experimental model studies in stroke, early fibrinolysis would appear to be safe, but late administration of a PA in focal ischemia is associated with an increase in hemorrhage frequency.[60]

Clinical Experience

Because of the hemorrhagic complications experienced in the early studies of thrombolysis in stroke,[67,68] ischemic stroke was considered a major contraindication for fibrinolysis.[69] Pilot (phase I and II) studies prospectively tested this concept.[70] The risk of symptomatic hemorrhage has been further refined in more recent phase III trials. The issue of whether a PA may contribute to the development of intracerebral hemorrhage appears to depend on the severity of the initial ischemic insult, the dose-rate of PA, and other factors.[7,71,72] The mode of delivery may also contribute to risk. With intra-arterial fibrinolysis, the incidence of hemorrhagic complications has been reported to vary between 9.3% and 32.5%, depending on which agent (u-PA or SK) and which arterial territory (carotid or vertebrobasilar) was under investigation. HI was seen in 4.7–22.5% of treated patients and PH in 4.7–16.7%.[73]

Table 15-1. Hemorrhagic Transformation: Carotid Territory Ischemia, Intra-Arterial Delivery (Angiography-Based)

| Study | Patients (N) | Hemorrhage | | | With Deterioration (%)[b] |
		HI	PH	%[a]	
del Zoppo et al.[5]	20	4	0	20	0
Mori et al.[15]	22	1	3	18	14
Theron et al.[86]	12	1	2	25	17
Zeumer et al.[20]	31	6	0	19	0
Overgaard et al.[62]	17	2	0	12	0
Lee et al.[88]	20	5	4	20	15
Sasaki et al.[89]	35	7	1	23	3
del Zoppo et al.[6]					
rpro-UK	26	11[c]	—	42	15
Placebo	14	1[c]	—	7	14

HI = hemorrhagic infarction; PH = parenchymatous hemorrhage; rpro-UK = recombinant prourokinase.
[a]Percent of total number of patients who demonstrated hemorrhagic transformation.
[b]Percent with hemorrhagic transformation and deterioration (most often PH).
[c]HI + PH.

The Prolyse in Acute Cerebral Thromboembolism (PROACT) trial was the first randomized, double-blind, multicenter trial comparing the safety, recanalization frequency, and clinical efficacy of direct intra-arterial infusion of rpro-UK with placebo in patients with symptomatic MCA occlusion of less than 6 hours duration (Table 15-1).[6] The phase II trial randomized 26 patients to intra-arterial infusion of 6 mg rpro-UK and 14 patients to placebo infusion. A high-dose heparin (100 IU/kg bolus, followed by 1,000 IU/hour infusion for 4 hours) administration to the first 16 patients (11 rpro-UK and 5 placebo) resulted in a high recanalization frequency of 82% in the rpro-UK arm (vs. 0% in the placebo group), but also produced a high incidence of intracranial hemorrhage (73% vs. 20% in the placebo group). Reduction of the heparin dosage to a bolus of 2,000 IU, followed by a 500 IU per hour infusion in 24 successive patients, resulted in a lower recanalization rate in the rpro-UK patients (40% vs. 22% in the placebo group) and reduced incidence of intracerebral hemorrhage (20% and 0%, respectively). Overall, 24-hour results in the high- and the low-dose heparin group yielded 58% and 14% recanalization ($P = .017$), and 42% and 7% intracranial hemorrhage ($P = .03$). This experience underscored the contribution of other antithrombotic agents to the risk of intracerebral hemorrhage with PAs.

In two placebo-controlled intravenous fibrinolysis trials,[13,14] hemorrhagic complications were seen in 52.6% and 54.9% of the treated and 41.7% and 57.5% of the control patients (Table 15-2). The slightly higher frequencies in the treated group were mainly caused by an increase in HI (from 33.3% and 46.8% to 41.7% and 47.1%, respectively), whereas the frequency of PH was similar. Among 12 intravenous delivery trials of u-PA, SK, or rt-PA, the incidence of symptomatic hemorrhage (predominantly PH) ranged from 1.0% to 19.8%. Among phase III placebo-controlled trials, the lowest incidence of symptomatic hemorrhage associated with rt-PA was observed in the trial sponsored by the National Institute of Neurological Disorders and Stroke (NINDS).[1]

The importance of the interval between the onset of stroke symptoms and treatment was emphasized by the results of del Zoppo et al.[7] Twenty-five percent of patients treated with rt-PA within 6 hours had hemorrhagic complications, whereas 53% of the patients treated between 6 and 8 hours developed these complications. In a retrospective analysis of the NINDS pilot trials, Levy et al. confirmed a time relationship and found that patients with PH received a higher rt-PA dose (0.97–0.17 mg/kg) than those without symptomatic hemorrhage (0.74–0.22 mg/kg, $P < .05$).[72] Known risk factors for cere-

Table 15-2. Hemorrhagic Transformation: Carotid Territory Ischemia, Intravenous Delivery (Angiography-Based)

Study	Agent	Patients (Total Patients Treated)	Hemorrhage			With Deterioration (%)[b]
			HI	PH	%[a]	
del Zoppo et al.[7]	rt-PA	93 (104)	21	11	31	11
Mori et al.[13]	rt-PA	19	8	2	53	11
	C	12	4	1	42	0
Von Kummer and Hacke[81]	rt-PA	22	9	3	10	14
Yamaguchi[14]	rt-PA	47 (51)	20	4	47	8
	C	46 (47)	17	5	47	11

HI = hemorrhagic infarction; PH = parenchymal hemorrhage; rt-PA = recombinant tissue plasminogen activator; C = control.
[a]Percent of total number of patients who demonstrated hemorrhagic transformation.
[b]Percent with hemorrhagic transformation and deterioration (most often PH).

bral hemorrhage are hypertension[71] and cerebral amyloid angiopathy,[52] whereas old age, large infarct, early ischemic signs, or the use of anticoagulants, such as heparin, are potential risk factors for hemorrhagic complications in individual acute stroke trials. In a separate study, hemorrhagic change was high in 34 patients with markedly reduced regional cerebral blood flow demonstrated by SPECT before treatment.[74]

Experience with rt-PA in the two European Cooperative Acute Stroke Study (ECASS) presentations suggests that the risk of symptomatic hemorrhage depends on the severity of the initial ischemic lesion (Table 15-3).[75] In ECASS-I, rt-PA at 1.1 mg/kg

Table 15-3. Clinical Outcome Studies: Intravenous Delivery

Study	Agent	Patients (N)	Δ (T-O) (hrs)	Outcome	Improvement (%)	Hemorrhage		
						HI	PH	%[a]
MAST-E[90,91]	SK	156	<6.0	EM	34[b]	63	33	21.0[b]
	C	154	—	—	18	57	4	3.0
ASK[92,93]	SK	165	<4.0	M	36[b]	33	23	13.2[b]
	C	163	—	—	21	23	5	3.1
MAST-I[94]	SK	313	<6.0	EM	25[b]	60	21	6.7[b]
	C	309	—	—	12	27	2	0.7
ECASS-I[75]	rt-PA	313	<6.0	D	36	72	62	19.8[b]
	C	307	—	—	29	93	30	6.5
NINDS (I)[1]	rt-PA	144	0.0–3.0	NO	47	—	13	5.6[b]
	C	147	—	—	39	—	3	0.0
NINDS (II)[2]	rt-PA	168	0.0–3.0	D/NO	48	—	21	7.1[b]
	C	165	—	—	39	—	8	2.1
ECASS-II[76]	rt-PA	409	0.0–6.0	NO	40	142	48	11.7[b]
	C	391	—	—	37	141	12	3.1

MAST-E = Multicentre Acute Stroke Trial-Europe; ASK = Australian Streptokinase Trial; MAST-I = Multicentre Acute Stroke Trial-Italy; ECASS = European Cooperative Acute Stroke Study; NINDS = National Institute of Neurological Disorders and Stroke rt-PA Stroke Trial; Δ (T-O) = interval from onset to treatment; HI = hemorrhagic infarction; PH = parenchymatous hemorrhage; SK = streptokinase; C = control; rt-PA = recombinant tissue plasminogen activator; EM = early mortality; M = mortality (3 or 6 months); D = best disability outcome (3 months); NO = neurologic outcome.
[a]Percent with hemorrhagic transformation (most often PH) and deterioration.
[b]Statistically significant.

given to patients within 6 hours of symptom onset produced a 19.8% frequency of symptomatic PH compared to placebo (6.5%). When the data were adjusted in post hoc analysis for the number of patients displaying "early signs of ischemia" on baseline CT scan, the efficacy outcomes became significant. Attention to excluding patients with "early signs of ischemia" in ECASS-II was associated with a lower baseline National Institutes of Health Stroke Scale (NIHSS) score and a lower frequency of PH (11.7%) compared to placebo (3.1%).[76] Among three prospective trials of SK, all of which were terminated because of safety concerns, injury severity was a major accompaniment of increased hemorrhage in the Multicentre Acute Stroke Trial-Europe. The baseline NIHSS scores and hemorrhagic risks among the rt-PA, rpro-UK, and SK trials offer support for the presence of discrete subpopulations of ischemic stroke patients who have significantly increased risk for hemorrhage when exposed to PAs. For future studies, new diagnostic methods, including cerebral blood flow measurement and assessment of the extent of initial injury, may help to identify high-risk patients.

Outcomes

Since Sussman and Fitch first described the use of fibrinolysin in carotid territory stroke in 1958,[68] more than 400 reports of the use of thrombolytic agents in acute stroke have appeared in the literature. The vast majority of those have been published since 1985. Trials fall into two broad categories: (1) symptom-based studies that measure clinical outcome only, and (2) angiography-based studies, which have been designed to assess recanalization or clinical outcome, or both.

Symptom-Based Trials

Symptom-based trials (see Table 15-3), which assess clinical outcome, have several advantages and disadvantages compared to angiography-based studies. Evaluation (neurologic examination and admission CT to exclude hemorrhage) and therapy can be commenced within 3 hours of symptom onset. Although these strict entry criteria are feasible, they also limit the number of ischemic stroke patients that can be successfully treated. Such early acquisition of stroke

patients also raises concerns about accuracy of diagnosis and clinical efficacy. However, the findings of symptom-based trials of rt-PA suggest that even treatment within 6 hours of symptom onset may be associated with benefit in select patients.

The ECASS-I trial, a placebo-controlled study, compared disability outcome and mortality at 90 days after intravenous infusion of rt-PA (1.1 mg/kg, maximum 100 mg) with placebo.[75] At 75 European centers, 620 patients were randomized within 6 hours of symptom onset. Prospectively applied rules sought to exclude patients with evidence of large regions of hemispheric injury ("early infarct signs") by neuroradiographic criteria. A post hoc re-evaluation of baseline CT scans in all patients by the Neuroradiology Core Committee defined a population with "early infarct signs" not apparent to investigators. A post hoc re-evaluation of clinical outcomes counted 109 patients who should have been excluded, of whom 60.6% should have been excluded by CT scan criteria, mostly because of the presence of major "early infarct signs." The "intention-to-treat" analysis demonstrated no apparent difference between the rt-PA and placebo groups with regard to median Barthel Index and mRS scores. The "target" analysis yielded an 11–12% absolute improvement in best outcome (mRS scores of 0 and 1) favoring the rt-PA–treated group. Median neurologic and disability outcomes at 30 days and 90 days were better in the rt-PA–treated "target" patients only. When the data were subsequently reanalyzed using the dichotomized outcome thresholds of the NINDS-sponsored trial, significant outcomes favoring the rt-PA group were noted, according to the NIHSS and mRS.[77] In ECASS-I, the "intention-to-treat" analysis demonstrated a significantly higher proportion of patients with intracerebral hemorrhage causing neurologic deterioration or death (PH) with rt-PA compared to placebo. No significant difference in cumulative mortality ("intention-to-treat") at 90 days (22.7% rt-PA group vs. 15.8% placebo group) was seen. A singular interpretation of the data from ECASS-I is that the lack of benefit in functional outcome and neurologic recovery was "driven" by a subgroup of patients with clinically significant cerebral injury at increased risk for hemorrhage or further deterioration after intravenous thrombolysis. An overall analysis suggests that when a subgroup of patients at high risk for poor outcome or hemorrhage (e.g., with "early infarct signs") would be excluded, 90-day disability outcome would be favorably affected.

To address the hypothesis that exclusion of patients with "early signs of ischemia" would lead to improved outcome, ECASS-II was initiated in 1996.[76] ECASS-II was a prospective, multicenter, randomized, double-blind, placebo-controlled trial of intravenous rt-PA at 0.9 mg/kg, with patients receiving treatment within 6 hours of symptom onset. By 90 days, 165 of 409 (40.3%) rt-PA patients and 143 of 391 (36.6%) placebo patients ($P = .277$) had mRS scores of 0 or 1. There were no significant differences in outcome, regardless of whether the patients were treated within 3 hours or 3–6 hours from symptom onset. Symptomatic intracerebral hemorrhage was significantly more frequent in the rt-PA group than the placebo group. Although the ECASS-I and ECASS-II outcomes were similar, the patients entered into ECASS-II were more mildly affected than either the ECASS or NINDS trials. When outcome data for ECASS-II was dichotomized to mRS scores of 0, 1, and 2, versus 3–6 in an unspecified retrospective analysis, benefit was associated with the rt-PA group. The ECASS experience has underscored the need to define subtle alterations on the initial CT scan consistent with ischemia that may place those patients at high risk for poor outcome.

After a series of pilot studies to assess the relative safety of rt-PA (alteplase) in acute ischemic stroke, a two-part, four-armed, placebo-controlled clinical outcome study of rt-PA with entry at ≤90 minutes or 91–180 minutes from symptom onset was completed by the NINDS (see Table 15-3).[1] In part I, 291 patients were randomized to rt-PA (0.9 mg/kg) or placebo within the two treatment time intervals. According to the NIHSS, no difference in neurologic status was observed between the rt-PA ($n = 144$) and placebo ($n = 147$) groups at 24 hours. In part II, 168 rt-PA recipients displayed a significant (11–13%) absolute improvement in Barthel Index, mRS, Glasgow Outcome Scale, and NIHSS scores, with minimal or no disability (deficit) at 3 months over 165 patients receiving placebo. No difference in mortality was observed, however, and the benefit was observed in patients with all stroke etiologies. In the combined experience of both parts of the NINDS study, the frequency of symptomatic hemorrhage was significantly greater among those patients treated with rt-PA (6.4%) than those who received placebo (0.6%) ($2P <.001$). In this study, a substantial increase in the number of patients displaying no or minimal disability was achieved among patients treated within 3 hours of symptom onset with rt-PA. Based on these findings, alteplase was approved with strict limitations by the U.S. Food and Drug Administration for clinical use in acute ischemic stroke in the United States. Taken together, the ECASS and NINDS studies indicate the enormous importance of patient selection to reduce the hemorrhagic risk that accompanies the use of PAs in stroke. The interval between symptom onset and treatment to achieve clinical improvement varies individually. Both studies suggest that CT scans and neurologic scores at study entry do not completely identify those at risk for hemorrhage, although proper attention to the presence and extent of ischemic injury on initial CT scan is likely to address hemorrhagic risk. Evidence of large (>33%) hemispheric regions of ischemic injury on entry CT scan are associated with poor outcome. It is not possible to separate benefit from hemorrhagic risk in a given patient based on simple clinical criteria. However, the three studies indicate that outcome improvement is feasible with a longer interval before treatment.

Angiography-Based Trials

Prospective angiography-based trials that have assessed the efficacy of intravenous rt-PA on recanalization or neurologic outcome have used a 60- to 90-minute infusion initiated within 6–8 hours of symptom onset (Table 15-4).

In an open, prospective, multicenter, dose-escalation trial, del Zoppo et al. demonstrated no relationship between the dose of rt-PA (duteplase) and recanalization frequency.[7] At 60 minutes postinfusion, the total recanalization incidence at doses 0.12–0.76 mIU/kg was 34.4%. That study demonstrated a marked difference in recanalization for different anatomic occlusions: 8.0% for ICA occlusion, 26.1% for MCA stem occlusion, and 38.1% for more distal MCA occlusions. This is consistent with the findings of other intravenous studies[78,79] and the experience of Ohtaki et al. using local intra-arterial infusion techniques.[80]

In a three-arm, placebo-controlled, double-blind trial comparing 20 mIU and 30 mIU of rt-PA (duteplase) with placebo, Mori et al. demonstrated

Table 15-4. Recanalization Outcome: Carotid Territory Ischemia, Intravenous Delivery (Angiography-Based)

Study	Agent	Patients	Δ (T-O) (hrs)	Recanalization	
				N	%[a]
del Zoppo et al.[7]	rt-PA	93 (104)[b]	<8	32	—
Mori et al.[13]	rt-PA	19	<6	9	47
	C	12	—	2	17
Von Kummer and Hacke[81]	rt-PA	22	<6	13	59
Yamaguchi[14]	rt-PA	47	<6	10	21
	C	46	—	2	4

Δ (T-O) = interval from onset to treatment; rt-PA = recombinant tissue plasminogen activator; C = control.
[a]Percent of total number of patients who demonstrated recanalization.
[b]Total number of patients treated.

increased recanalization and a significantly better clinical improvement at 30 days in patients receiving the higher dose of rt-PA than those treated with placebo or 20 mg rt-PA.[13] That was the first report suggesting that recanalization was associated with improved clinical outcome.

In a multicenter, placebo-controlled trial using 20 mIU rt-PA, Yamaguchi et al. reported successful reperfusion in 10 of 47 (21%) patients receiving rt-PA (duteplase) compared to 2 of 46 (4.4%) patients treated with placebo.[79] Evidence that rt-PA was associated with a significantly more favorable outcome at 30 days did not show a dose effect. The overall recanalization frequencies found in some angiography-based studies using intravenous thrombolysis have been 21–67% in the carotid territory and 40–80% in the vertebrobasilar circulation.

The value of acutely applied angiography has been seen in the assessment of collateral patency. Two studies demonstrated an association between the presence of robust collaterals at initial angiography and good clinical outcome in a study of the safety and recanalization of rt-PA (alteplase).[12,81]

Intra-arterial studies using regional infusion or local infusion techniques have shown efficacy in cerebral arterial recanalization (Tables 15-5 and 15-6).

Table 15-5. Recanalization Outcome: Carotid Territory Ischemia, Intra-Arterial Delivery (Angiography-Based)

Study	Agent	Patients (N)	Δ (T-O) (hrs)	Recanalization	
				N	%*
del Zoppo et al.[5]	SK/UK	20	1–24	18	90
Mori et al.[15]	UK	22	0.8–7.0	10	45
Theron et al.[86]	SK/UK	12	2–504	12	100
Zeumer et al.[20]	rt-PA/UK	31	<4	29	94
Overgaard et al.[62]	rt-PA	17	<6	12	71
Lee et al.[88]	UK	20	<24	9	45
Sasaki et al.[89]	rt-PA/UK	35	<8	16	46
Freitag et al.[95]	rt-PA/UK	22	<6	14	64
	PA + lys-plg	14	<6	12	86
Endo et al.[96]	rt-PA/UK	21	<6	8	38
del Zoppo et al.[6]	rpro-UK	26	<6	15	58
	Placebo	14	—	2	14

Δ (T-O) = interval from onset to treatment; SK = streptokinase; UK = urokinase; rt-PA = recombinant tissue plasminogen activator; PA = plasminogen activator; lys-plg = lys-plasminogen; rpro-UK = recombinant prourokinase.
*Percent of total number of patients with recanalization.

Table 15-6. Recanalization Outcome and Hemorrhagic Transformation: Vertebrobasilar Territory, Intra-Arterial Delivery (Angiography-Based)

Study	Agent	Patients (N)	Recanalization		Hemorrhage		
			N	%[a]	HI	PH	%[b]
Hacke et al.[84]	SK/UK	43	19	44	2	2	9
Zeumer et al.[23]	UK	7	7	100	1	0	14
Möbius et al.[97]	SK/UK	18	14	78	0	0	0
Matsumoto and Satoh[98]	UK	10	4	40	0	1	10
Zeumer et al.[20]	rt-PA/UK	28	28	100	2	0	0
Brandt et al.[99]	UK	44	23	52	3	3	7
Becker et al.[100]	UK	12	10	83	—	2	17
Wijdicks et al.[101]	UK	9	7	78	—	1	11
Cross et al.[102]	UK	20	13	65	—	3	15

HI = hemorrhagic infarction; PH = parenchymatous hemorrhagic; rt-PA = recombinant tissue plasminogen activator; SK = streptokinase; UK = urokinase.
[a]Percent of total number of patients who demonstrated recanalization.
[b]Percent of total number of patients who demonstrated hemorrhagic transformation.

Initial reports of single or small case studies[82,83] were followed by larger prospective trials using u-PA or SK, which demonstrated efficacy in the recanalization of occlusions within either the carotid and vertebrobasilar arterial systems.[5,15,23,84–86] A report by Zeumer et al. showed partial or complete recanalization in 29 of 31 (94%) patients in the carotid territory and in all 28 (100%) patients with vertebrobasilar occlusions.[20] Arterial recanalization has been reported in 46–100% of acutely treated patients with carotid territory focal ischemia.

Two randomized and prospectively conducted placebo or nonplacebo competing approach trials have examined direct intra-arterial infusion of the proenzyme of u-PA, prourokinase. The PROACT trial was designed to compare rpro-UK with placebo in a double-blind, prospective dose-rate–finding phase I/II format.[6] A significant increase in 2-hour recanalization was associated with 6 mg/kg rpro-UK over placebo when the mode of delivery was controlled. Both the frequency of recanalization and hemorrhagic transformation were directly dependent on heparin dose. When the heparin dose (required for preventing delivery catheter thrombosis or embolism) was decreased in view of an apparent increase in hemorrhage frequency, both recanalization efficacy and hemorrhage frequency decreased. A second randomized, controlled clinical efficacy trial (PROACT-2) of intra-arterial rpro-UK (9 mg/kg) and intravenous heparin com-

pared to intravenous heparin alone within 6 hours demonstrated superior recanalization in the group receiving direct microcatheter PA delivery over no intervention.[87] Symptomatic intracranial hemorrhage at 24 hours was higher in the rpro-UK group (10.2%) than the noninterventional group (1.9%). Clinical efficacy remains controversial. Based on the more subjective primary outcome dichotomization of mRS scores of 0, 1, and 2 (independent) versus 3–6 (dependent and demise), a marginally superior ($P = .043$) improvement was found with intra-arterial rpro-UK over no PA. However, when the dichotomization assessed normal neurologic outcome as mRS scores 0 and 1,[87] no significant difference in outcome was noted. That result raises a number of issues, including the formatting of prospective clinical trials in this arena. However, it is clear that the use of intra-arterial delivery techniques have entered the era of controlled trials.

Experience with fibrinolytic agents in vertebrobasilar occlusions has been limited. In a retrospective analysis, Hacke et al. suggested a survival benefit in patients undergoing recanalization after fibrinolysis.[82] More recent smaller series have resulted in recanalization rates of 40–100% (see Table 15-6). Although thrombolysis may well be effective in this context because the outcome of unsuccessful or conservative treatment may be poor, there are insufficient data to support this conclusion.

Defibrinating Agents

A different therapeutic strategy was used in the Stroke Treatment with Ancrod Trial. The defibrinating agent ancrod reduces fibrinogen concentration and enhances endogenous fibrinolysis by activating endothelial cells, but does not dissolve existing thrombi. Because of the acute aspect of this trial and the massive changes in coagulation and endogenous fibrinolysis, its inclusion in the group of ongoing acute intervention trials in thrombolysis can be justified.

Practical Recommendations

Clinical and experimental studies of PAs acutely applied have increased knowledge of the pathophysiology of ischemic stroke and attendant hemorrhage, and have offered several ischemic therapeutic avenues for stroke. But this approach is not generally recommended for each stroke patient or stroke center. At the time of this writing, only rt-PA (alteplase) at 0.9 mg/kg infusion (maximum 100 mg) is approved in the United States and several countries for use within 3 hours of symptom onset in select patients with ischemic stroke. Case reports and uncontrolled, single-center studies are not appropriate to solve the general questions of thrombolysis in stroke.

The recurrent issue of safety and the experimental character of each clinical use of PAs in ischemic stroke urges a careful clinical examination and follow-up evaluation to prove benefit for the patient. Of utmost importance is the resolution of which outcome measures can best describe benefit in the setting of ischemic stroke.

Conclusion

At the time of this writing, a number of questions remain unanswered. These offer opportunities for rational treatment of ischemic stroke.

1. Despite the acceptance of intravenous rt-PA (alteplase) for treatment within 3 hours of symptom onset, the optimal dose rate and agent to provide significant recanalization and clinical improvement by the intravenous route have not been developed.

2. Phase II and phase III studies of intra-arterial infusion require more careful attention to study design and outcome issues.

3. Despite experimental work that indicates the importance of the precise timing of intervention, there are few clinical data available to suggest how early (e.g., less than 180 minutes from symptom onset) intervention would produce a superior outcome compared to later entry time (e.g., 6 hours). The differences in study design and outcome measurement make comparison among studies difficult, and no direct comparison study has been undertaken.

4. Although aggregate information suggests that intra-arterial and intravenous infusion routes are equally safe (with similar incidences of hemorrhagic transformation), this issue remains unresolved.

5. Diagnostic efforts are required to define those patients at high risk for poor outcome with thrombolysis.

6. Specific differences in the vascular pathology associated with vertebrobasilar ischemia and carotid territory ischemia suggest that the use of ancillary antithrombotics (e.g., heparin) might be of some benefit in the former. The value of ancillary therapies has not been directly addressed in either setting.

7. The effect of reperfusion on the ischemic microvasculature is under active study experimentally, but no intervention to preserve microvascular integrity has been approached so far.

8. With growing experience, it is important to know something of the profile of successfully treated patients (e.g., which patients are at particularly high risk for hemorrhagic complications and which patients may be most likely to undergo recanalization). Patients with the most distal occlusions (in the carotid territory) may develop smaller infarcts and have a better clinical outcome.

These are some of the questions that arise from ongoing work in this field. The role of thrombolysis as a treatment strategy in stroke has highlighted the importance of early patient entry and concerns about symptomatic hemorrhage. Benefit of the acute intervention with one PA has been shown and suggests that restoration of blood flow early after arterial occlusion may lead to functional recovery. The validation of this hypothesis is fundamental to the rational conduct of trials that may promote recovery of neuronal function and improved neurologic outcome. Adherence to principles of appropriate clinical trial design and patient care insure that the outcomes measured in clinical trials are suitable for safe treatment of the ischemic stroke patient.

References

1. The National Institute of Neurological Disorders and Stroke rt-PA Stroke Study Group. Tissue plasminogen activator for acute ischemic stroke. N Engl J Med 1995;333:1581–1587.
2. Kwiatkowski TG, Libman RB, Frankel M, et al. Effects of tissue plasminogen activator for acute ischemic stroke at one year. National Institute of Neurological Disorders and Stroke Recombinant Tissue Plasminogen Activator Stroke Study Group. N Engl J Med 1999;340:1781–1787.
3. Solis OJ, Roberson GR, Taveras JM, et al. Cerebral angiography in acute cerebral infarction. Rev Interam Radiol 1977;2:19–25.
4. Dalal PM, Shah PM, Sheth SC, Deshpande CK. Cerebral embolism: angiographic observations on spontaneous clot lysis. Lancet 1965;1:61–64.
5. del Zoppo GJ, Ferbert A, Otis S, et al. Local intra-arterial fibrinolytic therapy in acute carotid territory stroke. A pilot study. Stroke 1988;19:307–313.
6. del Zoppo GJ, Higashida RT, Furlan AJ, et al. PROACT: a phase II randomized trial of recombinant pro-urokinase by direct arterial delivery in acute middle cerebral artery stroke. PROACT Investigators. Prolyse in Acute Cerebral Thromboembolism. Stroke 1998;29:4–11.
7. del Zoppo GJ, Poeck K, Pessin MS, et al. Recombinant tissue plasminogen activator in acute thrombotic and embolic stroke. Ann Neurol 1992;32:78–86.
8. Fieschi C, Argentino C, Lenzi GL, et al. Clinical and instrumental evaluation of patients with ischemic stroke within the first six hours. J Neurol Sci 1989;91:311–321.
9. Irino T, Taneda M, Minami T. Angiographic manifestations in postrecanalized cerebral infarction. Neurology 1977;27:471–475.
10. Minematsu K, Yamaguchi T, Omae T. "Spectacular shrinking deficit:" rapid recovery from a major hemispheric syndrome by migration of an embolus. Neurology 1992;42:157–162.
11. Mohr JP, Barnett HJ. Classification of Ischemic Strokes. In HJ Barnett, BM Stein, JP Mohr, et al (eds), Stroke: Pathophysiology, Diagnosis and Management. New York: Churchill Livingstone, 1986;281–291.
12. Yamaguchi T, Minematsu K, Choki J, Ikeda M. Clinical and neuroradiological analysis of thrombotic and embolic cerebral infarction. Jpn Circ J 1984;48:50–58.
13. Mori E, Yoneda Y, Tabuchi M, et al. Intravenous recombinant tissue plasminogen activator in acute carotid artery territory stroke. Neurology 1992;42:976–982.
14. Yamaguchi T, Hayakawa T, Kikuchi H. Intravenous tissue plasminogen activator ameliorates the outcome of hyperacute embolic stroke. Cerebrovasc Dis 1993;3:269–272.
15. Mori E, Tabuchi M, Yoshida T, Yamadori A. Intracarotid urokinase with thromboembolic occlusion of the middle cerebral artery. Stroke 1988;19:802–812.
16. Saito I, Segawa H, Shiokawa Y, et al. Middle cerebral artery occlusion: correlation of computed tomography and angiography with clinical outcome. Stroke 1987;18:863–868.
17. Adams RD, Victor M. Cerebrovascular Diseases. Principles of Neurology (3rd ed). New York: McGraw-Hill, 1988;569–640.
18. Lesaffre E, Sheys I, Fröhlich J, et al. On the Estimation of the Sample Size for the ECASS Study. In GJ del Zoppo, E Mori, W Hacke (eds), Thrombolytic Therapy in Acute Ischemic Stroke (2nd ed). Heidelberg, Germany: Springer, 1992;72–79.
19. Wityk RJ, Pessin MS, Kaplan RF, Caplan LR. Serial assessment of acute stroke using the NIH Stroke Scale. Stroke 1994;25:362–365.
20. Zeumer H, Freitag H-J, Zanella F, et al. Local intra-arterial fibrinolytic therapy in patients with stroke: urokinase versus recombinant tissue plasminogen activator (rt-PA). Neuroradiology 1993;35:159–162.
21. McNamara TO, Fischer JR. Thrombolysis of peripheral arterial and graft occlusions: improved results using high-dose urokinase. AJR Am J Roentgenol 1985;144:769–775.
22. Zeumer H, Hundgen R, Ferbert A, Ringelstein EB. Local intra-arterial fibrinolytic therapy in inaccessible internal carotid occlusion. Neuroradiology 1984;26:315–317.
23. Zeumer H, Freitag HJ, Grzyska U, Neunzig HP. Local intra-arterial fibrinolysis in acute vertebrobasilar occlusion. Technical developments and recent results. Neuroradiology 1989;31:336–340.
24. Komiyama M, Nishijima Y, Nishio A, Khosla VK. Extravasation of contrast medium from the lenticulostriate artery following local intracarotid fibrinolysis. Surg Neurol 1993;39:315–319.
25. Wildenhain SL, Jungreis CA, Barr J, et al. CT after intracranial intra-arterial thrombolysis for acute stroke. AJNR Am J Neuroradiol 1994;15:487–492.
26. Halbach VV, Higashida RT, Dowd CF, et al. Management of vascular perforations that occur during neurointerventional procedures. AJNR Am J Neuroradiol 1991;12:319–328.
27. Chapman AB, Rubinstein D, Hughes R, et al. Intracranial aneurysms in autosomal-dominant polycystic kidney disease. N Engl J Med 1992;327:916–920.
28. Higashida RT, Halback VV, Dowd CF, et al. Intravascular balloon dilation therapy for intracranial arterial vasospasm: patient selection, technique and clinical results. Neurosurg Rev 1992;15:89–95.
29. Hellmann DB, Roubenoft R, Healy RA, Wang H. Central nervous system angiography: safety and predictors of a positive result in 125 consecutive patients evaluated for possible vasculitis. J Rheumatol 1992;19:568–572.
30. Davies KN, Humphrey PR. Complications of cerebral angiography in patients with symptomatic carotid territory ischemia screened by carotid ultrasound. J Neurol Neurosurg Psychiatry 1993;56:967–972.
31. Hankey GJ, Warlow CP, Molyneux AJ. Complications of cerebral angiography for patients with mild carotid territory ischemia being considered for carotid endarterectomy. J Neurol Neurosurg Psychiatry 1990;53:542–548.
32. Waugh JR, Sacharias N. Arteriographic complications in the DSA era. Radiology 1992;182:243–246.
33. Hankey GJ, Warlow CP, Sellar RJ. Cerebral angiographic risk in mild cerebrovascular disease. Stroke 1990;21:209–222.

34. Grzyska V, Freitag J, Zeumer H. Selective cerebral intracranial DSA. Neuroradiology 1990;32:296–299.

35. Baird AE, Austin MC, McKay J, et al. Reperfusion after thrombolytic therapy in ischemic stroke. Stroke 1994; 25(abstract):256.

36. Ringelstein EB, Biniek R, Weiller C, et al. Type and extent of hemispheric brain infarctions and clinical outcome in early and delayed middle cerebral artery recanalization. Neurology 1992;42:289–298.

37. Wardlaw JM, Warlow CP. Thrombolysis in acute ischemic stroke: does it work? Stroke 1992;23:1826–1839.

38. Pessin MS. Hemorrhagic Transformation in the Natural History of Acute Embolic Stroke. In W Hacke, GJ del Zoppo, M Hirschberg (eds), Thrombolytic Therapy in Acute Ischemic Stroke. Heidelberg, Germany: Springer, 1991;67–74.

39. Hamann GF, Okada Y, del Zoppo GJ. Hemorrhagic transformation and microvascular integrity during focal cerebral ischemia/reperfusion. J Cereb Blood Flow Metab 1996;16:1373–1378.

40. Hamann GF, Okada Y, Fitridge R, del Zoppo GJ. Microvascular basal lamina antigens disappear during cerebral ischemia and reperfusion. Stroke 1995;26:2120–2126.

41. Savage M, Fischman D, Leon M, et al. Efficacy of coronary stents in the treatment of refractory restenosis following balloon angioplasty. J Am Coll Cardiol 1993; 32(abstract):33A.

42. Globus JH, Epstein JA. Massive cerebral hemorrhage: spontaneous and experimentally induced. J Neuropathol Exp Neurol 1953;12:107–133.

43. Globus JH, Epstein JA, Green MA, et al. Focal cerebral hemorrhage experimentally induced. J Neuropathol Exp Neurol 1949;8:653–670.

44. Molinari GF. Pathogenesis of Secondary Brain Hemorrhage after Ischemia: Lessons from Animal Models. . . And a Few From Man, Too! In GJ del Zoppo, E Mori, W Hacke (eds), Thrombolytic Therapy in Acute Ischemic Stroke (2nd ed). Heidelberg, Germany: Springer, 1993; 29–36.

45. Sloan MA, Price TR. Intracranial hemorrhage following thrombolytic therapy for acute myocardial infarction. Semin Neurol 1991;11:385–399.

46. Gore JM, Sloan M, Price TR, et al. Intracerebral hemorrhage, cerebral infarction, and subdural hematoma after acute myocardial infarction and thrombolytic therapy in the Thrombolysis in Myocardial Infarction Study. Thrombolysis in Myocardial Infarction, Phase II, pilot and clinical trial. Circulation 1991;83:448–459.

47. Simoons ML, de Jaegere P, van Domburg R, Boersma E. Intracranial hemorrhage after thrombolysis therapy. A perspective. Z Kardiol 1993;82(Suppl 2):153–156.

48. Simoons ML, Maggioni AP, Knatterud G, et al. Individual risk assessment for intracranial hemorrhage during thrombolytic therapy. Lancet 1993;342:1523–1528.

49. An international randomized trial comparing four thrombolytic strategies for acute myocardial infarction. The GUSTO Investigators. N Engl J Med 1993;329:673–682.

50. Califf RM, Fortin DF, Tenaglia AN, Sane DC. Clinical risks of thrombolytic therapy. Am J Cardiol 1992;69:12A–20A.

51. Fennerty AG, Levine MN, Hirsh J. Hemorrhagic complications of thrombolytic therapy in the treatment of myocardial infarction and venous thromboembolism. Chest 1989;95(Suppl):88S–97S.

52. Leblanc R, Haddad G, Robitaille Y. Cerebral hemorrhage from amyloid angiopathy and coronary thrombolysis. Neurosurgery 1992;31:586–590.

53. Kase CS, Pessin MS, Zivin JZ, et al. Intracranial hemorrhage following coronary thrombolysis with tissue plasminogen activator. Neurology 1990;40(Suppl 1):191.

54. Fisher CM, Adams RD. Observations on Brain Embolism with Special Reference to Hemorrhage Infarction. In AJ Furlan (ed), The Heart and Stroke. Exploring Mutual Cerebrovascular and Cardiovascular Issues. New York: Springer, 1987;17–36.

55. Fisher CM, Adams RD. Observations on brain embolism with special reference to the mechanism of hemorrhagic infarction. J Neuropathol Exp Neurol 1951;10:92–94.

56. Jörgensen L, Torvik A. Ischaemic cerebrovascular diseases in an autopsy series. 2. Prevalence, location, pathogenesis, and clinical course of cerebral infarcts. J Neurol Sci 1969;9:285–320.

57. Hornig CR, Dorndorf W, Agnoli AL. Hemorrhagic cerebral infarction: a prospective study. Stroke 1986;17:179–185.

58. Okada Y, Yamaguchi T, Minematsu K, et al. Hemorrhagic transformation in cerebral embolism. Stroke 1989;20: 598–603.

59. del Zoppo GJ, Okada Y, Hamann G, et al. Mechanisms of Fibrinolysis-Associated Hemorrhagic Transformation. In T Yamaguchi, K Minematsu, E Mori, et al (eds), Thrombolytic Therapy in Acute Ischemic Stroke (3rd ed). Tokyo: Springer-Verlag, 1995;254–268.

60. Slivka A, Pulsinelli WA. Hemorrhagic complications of thrombolytic therapy in experimental stroke. Neurology 1987;37(Suppl 1):82.

61. Zivin JA, Lyden PD, De Girolami U, et al. Tissue plasminogen activator. Reduction of neurologic damage after experimental embolic stroke. Arch Neurol 1988;45:387–391.

62. Overgaard K, Sereghy T, Pedersen H, Boysen G. Effect of delayed thrombolysis with rt-PA in a rat embolic stroke model. J Cereb Blood Flow Metab 1994;14:472–477.

63. Lyden PD, Zivin JA, Clark WA, et al. Tissue plasminogen activator-mediated thrombolysis of cerebral emboli and its effect on hemorrhagic infarction in rabbits. Neurology 1989;39:703–708.

64. Abumiya T, Fitridge R, Mazur C, et al. Integrin alpha(IIb)beta(3) inhibitor preserves microvascular patency in experimental acute focal cerebral ischemia. Stroke 2000;31:1402–1410.

65. del Zoppo GJ, Copeland BR, Anderchek K, et al. Hemorrhagic transformation following tissue plasminogen activator in experimental cerebral infarction. Stroke 1990;21: 596–601.

66. del Zoppo GJ, Copeland BR, Waltz TA, et al. The beneficial effect of intracarotid urokinase on acute stroke in a baboon model. Stroke 1986;17:638–643.

67. Meyer JS, Gilroy J, Barnhart MI, Johnson JF. Anticoagulants plus streptokinase therapy in progressive stroke. JAMA 1964;189:373.

68. Sussman BJ, Fitch TS. Thrombolysis with fibrinolysin in cerebral arterial occlusion. JAMA 1958;167:1705–1709.

69. Sharma GV, Cella G, Parisi AF, Sasahara AA. Drug therapy: thrombolytic therapy. N Engl J Med 1982;306:1268–1276.

70. del Zoppo GJ, Pessin MS, Mori E, Hacke W. Thrombolytic intervention in acute thrombotic and embolic stroke. Semin Neurol 1991;11:368–384.

71. Larrue V, von Kummer R, del Zoppo GJ, Bluhmki E. Hemorrhagic transformation in acute ischemic stroke. Potential contributing factors in the European Cooperative Acute Stroke Study. Stroke 1997;28:957–960.

72. Levy DE, Brott TG, Haley EC, Jr, et al. Factors related to intracranial hematoma formation in patients receiving tissue-type plasminogen activator for acute ischemic stroke. Stroke 1994;25:291–297.

73. Wildemann B, Hacke W. Thrombolytic Therapy of Basilar and Middle Cerebral Artery Occlusion. In M Tomita, A Mchedlishvili, W Rosenblum, et al (eds), Microcirculatory Stasis in the Brain. Amsterdam: Elsevier, 1993;517–524.

74. Ueda T, Hatakeyama T, Kumon Y, et al. Evaluation of risk of hemorrhagic transformation in local intra-arterial thrombolysis in acute ischemic stroke by initial SPECT. Stroke 1994;25:298–303.

75. Hacke W, Kaste M, Fieschi C, et al. Intravenous thrombolysis with recombinant tissue plasminogen activator for acute hemispheric stroke. The European Cooperative Acute Stroke Study. JAMA 1995;274:1017–1025.

76. Hacke W, Kaste M, Fieschi C, et al. Randomised double-blind placebo-controlled trial of thrombolytic therapy with intravenous alteplase in acute ischaemic stroke (ECASS II). Second European-Australasian Acute Stroke Study Investigators. Lancet 1998;352:1245–1251.

77. Hacke W, Bluhmki E, Steiner T, et al. Dichotomized efficacy end points and global end-point analysis applied to the ECASS intention-to-treat data set: post hoc analysis of ECASS I. Stroke 1998;29:2073–2075.

78. Mori E, Yoneda Y, Ohkawa S, et al. Double-blind placebo-controlled trial of intravenous recombinant tissue plasminogen activator (rt-PA) in acute carotid stroke. Neurology 1991;41(Suppl 1)(abstract):347.

79. Yamaguchi T. Intravenous Tissue Plasminogen Activator in Acute Thromboembolic Stroke: A Placebo-Controlled, Double-Blind Trial. In The Second International Symposium on Thrombolytic Therapy for Acute Ischemic Stroke Proceedings, 1992.

80. Ohtaki M, Shinya T, Yamamura A, et al. Local Fibrinolytic Therapy Using Superselective Catheterization for Patients with Acute Cerebral Embolism within 10 hours. In M Tomita, A Mchedlishvili, W Rosenblum, et al (eds), Microcirculatory Stasis in the Brain. Amsterdam: Elsevier, 1993;539–545.

81. von Kummer R, Hacke W. Safety and efficacy of intravenous tissue plasminogen activator and heparin in acute middle cerebral artery. Stroke 1992;23:646–652.

82. Atkin N, Nitzberg S, Dorsey J. Lysis of intracerebral thromboembolism with fibrinolysin. Report of a case. Angiology 1964;15:346–439.

83. Herndon RM, Meyer JS, Johnson JF, Landers J. Treatment of cerebrovascular thrombosis with fibrinolysin. Preliminary report. Am J Cardiol 1960;30:540–545.

84. Hacke W, Zeumer H, Ferbert A, et al. Intra-arterial thrombolytic therapy improves outcome in patients with acute vertebrobasilar occlusive disease. Stroke 1988;19:1216–1222.

85. Nenci GG, Gresele P, Taramelli M, et al. Thrombolytic therapy for thromboembolism of vertebrobasilar artery. Angiology 1983;34:561–571.

86. Theron J, Courtheoux P, Casasco A, et al. Local intra-arterial fibrinolysis in the carotid territory. AJNR Am J Neuroradiol 1989;10:753–765.

87. Furlan A, Higashida R, Wechsler L. Intra-arterial prourokinase for acute ischemic stroke. JAMA 1999;282:2003–2011.

88. Lee BI, Lee BC, Park SC, et al. Intracarotid thrombolytic therapy in acute ischemic stroke of carotid arterial territory. Yonsei Med J 1994;35:49–61.

89. Sasaki O, Takeuchi S, Koike T, et al. Fibrinolytic therapy for acute embolic stroke: intravenous, intracarotid, and intra-arterial local approaches. Neurosurgery 1995;36:246–252.

90. Hommel M, Boissel JP, Cornu C, et al and for the MAST Group. Termination of trial of streptokinase in severe acute ischemic stroke (Letter). 1995;345:578–579.

91. The Multicenter Acute Stroke Trial—Europe Study Group. Thrombolytic therapy with streptokinase in acute ischemic stroke. N Engl J Med 1996;335:145–150.

92. Donnan GA, Davis SM, Chambers BR, et al. Trials of streptokinase in severe acute ischaemic stroke. Lancet 1995;345:578–579.

93. Donnan GA, Davis SM, Chambers BR, et al and for the Australian Streptokinase (ASK) Trial Study Group. Streptokinase for acute ischemic stroke with relationship to time of administration. JAMA 1996;276:961–966.

94. Multicentre Acute Stroke Trial—Italy (MAST-I) Group. Randomized controlled trial of streptokinase, aspirin, and combination of both in treatment of acute ischaemic stroke. Lancet 1995;346:1509–1514.

95. Frietag H-J, Zeumer H, Knospe V. Acute Central Retinal Artery Occlusion and the Role of Thrombolysis. In GJ del Zoppo, E Mori, W Hacke (eds), Thrombolytic Therapy in Acute Ischemic Stroke II. Heidelberg, Germany: Springer-Verlag, 1993;103–105.

96. Endo S, Kuwayama N, Hirashima Y. Results of urgent thrombolysis in patients with major stroke and atherothrombotic occlusion of the cervical internal carotid artery. AJNR Am J Neuroradiol 1998;19:1169–1175.

97. Möbius E, Berg-Dammer E, Kuhne D, et al. Local Thrombolytic Therapy in Acute Basilar Artery Occlusion. In W Hacke, GL del Zoppo, M Hirschberg (eds), Thrombolytic Therapy in Acute Ischemic Stroke. Berlin: Springer-Verlag, 1991;213–215.

98. Matsumoto K, Satoh K. Topical Intra-arterial Urokinase Infusion for Acute Stroke. In W Hacke, GJ del Zoppo, M Hirschberg (eds), Thrombolytic Therapy in Acute Ischemic Stroke. Heidelberg, Germany: Springer-Verlag, 1991;207–212.

99. Brandt T, von Kummer R, Müller-Kuppers M, et al. Thrombolytic therapy of acute basilar artery occlusion: variables affecting recanalization and outcome. Stroke 1996;27:875–881.

100. Becker KJ, Monsein LH, Ulatowski J, et al. Intra-arterial thrombolysis in vertebrobasilar occlusion. AJNR Am J Neuroradiol 1996;17:255–262.

101. Wijdicks EFM, Nichols DA, Thielen KR, et al. Intra-arterial thrombolysis in acute basilar artery thromboembolism: the initial Mayo Clinic experience. Mayo Clin Proc 1997;72:1005–1013.

102. Cross DT, Moran CJ, Akins PT, et al. Relationship between clot location and outcome after basilar artery thrombolysis. AJNR Am J Neuroradiol 1997;18:1221–1228.

Chapter 16

Pharmacologic Neuroprotection for Stroke

Wolf-Rüdiger Schäbitz and Marc Fisher

Pathophysiologic Targets for Neuroprotection

Neuroprotective agents and strategies have been studied for years and appear to be effective in a variety of preclinical stroke models. However, none of the drugs have proven conclusively to be effective in humans. The difficulty of translation from animal to human studies relates to issues of drug dosage, time window, gender differences, and, in particular, the stroke target population.[1] Misunderstanding of these issues may have caused negative trial results, nonapproval of drugs, and a pessimistic view for neuroprotection of stroke in general. A closer look at some studies clearly demonstrates that there is evidence that subpopulations of patients can benefit from the neuroprotective approach. It is probably a matter of time before the first neuroprotectant is available for the treatment of acute stroke.

The occlusion of a cerebral vessel with subsequent energy failure in the supplied arterial territory initiates the cascade that leads to cerebral infarction (Figure 16-1). All of the downstream events, from cellular depolarization to cell death and apoptosis, do not affect the ischemic territory homogeneously. The ischemic core, with a reduction of cerebral blood flow (CBF) to less than 20% of normal values, develops ischemic injury within minutes, and cells are rapidly killed by lipolysis, proteolysis, disaggregation of microtubules as a consequence of the energy failure, and breakdown of ion homeostasis.[2] The brain tissue between the dead core and surrounding normal brain has been defined as the *tissue at risk* or the so-called penumbra, which can be salvaged by neuroprotection and

is the prime target of this therapy. Without treatment, the penumbra becomes involved in the ischemic cascade and progresses to infarction within hours. There is evidence that the penumbra also exists in human stroke, although the extent and temporal dynamics of this area are still unclear.[3]

Neuroprotective agents have been developed and tested for nearly all aspects of the ischemic cascade (Figure 16-2). As seen with some mechanisms, such as gene expression or the role of zinc after stroke, new agents may be developed and new chances to treat may occur. The discovery that Ca^{2+}-induced excitotoxicity occurs after ischemia is relatively old (identified in approximately 1980) and has been widely accepted as a key event after cerebral ischemia. The ischemia-induced energy failure causes membrane depolarization and release of excitatory amino acids, such as glutamate, into the extracellular space.[4,5] Glutamate receptors become activated, resulting in Ca^{2+} overload of neurons (Figure 16-3). This step can be efficiently blocked by Ca^{2+}, N-methyl-D-aspartate (NMDA), and alpha-amino-3-hydroxy-5-methyl-4-isoxazole propionic acid (AMPA) antagonists. Subsequently, water moves into the cell with Na^+ and Cl^- via monovalent ion channels causing so-called cytotoxic edema. The large amount of intracellular Ca^{2+} activates proteolytic enzymes that degrade cytoskeletal and extracellular matrix proteins. Ca^{2+} also activates phospholipase A_2 and cyclooxygenase, producing oxygen-free radicals, as well as nitric oxide (NO) and its free radical product, peroxynitrite, which is synthesized by the Ca^{2+}-dependent NO synthase (NOS). The free radical release promotes further

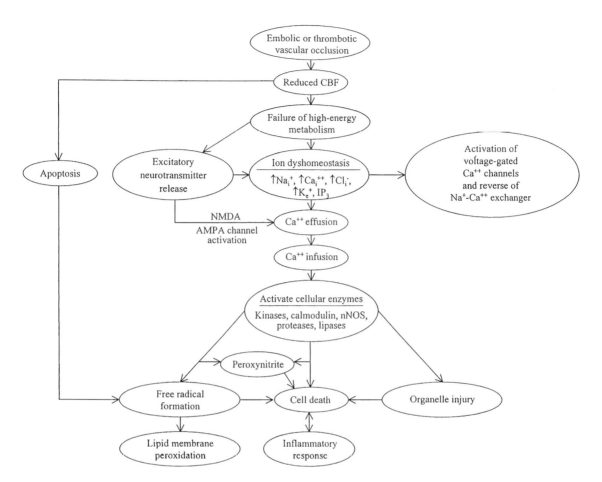

Figure 16-1. Ischemic cascade shows the major downstream events after vessel occlusion, from excitotoxicity to neuronal death. (CBF = cerebral blood flow; IP = inositol 1,4,5-triphosphate; NMDA = N-methyl-D-aspartate; AMPA = alpha-amino-3-hydroxy-5-methyl-4-isoxazole propionic acid; nNOS = neuronal nitric oxide synthase.)

membrane damage and subsequent damage to the mitochondrial function; it can efficiently be blocked by antioxidants and free radical scavengers.

Secondary to these events, expression of proinflammatory genes is induced by the synthesis of transcription factors and release of mediators of inflammation, such as platelet activating factor, tumor necrosis factor-α (TNF-α), and interleukin-1β (IL-1β).[6] Consequently, expression of the adhesion molecules intercellular adhesion molecule 1 (ICAM-1), P-selectins, and E-selectins occur on the endothelial surface.[7–9] After binding to adhesion molecules, neutrophils adhere to the endothelium, cause microvascular obstruction, cross the vascular wall, and enter the brain parenchyma, followed by macrophages and monocytes. Blocking of adhesion molecules can prevent these mechanisms. Furthermore, activated inflammatory cells and injured neu-

rons produce a number of toxic mediators that may worsen ischemia. For example, infiltrating neutrophils produce toxic amounts of NO through activation of inducible NOS (iNOS).[10] Pharmacologic blockade of iNOS inhibitors consequently reduces ischemic brain injury.[11] Ischemic neurons also express cyclooxygenase-2, an enzyme that mediates ischemic injury by producing superoxide and toxic prostanoids.[12] Inhibition of the enzyme by cyclooxygenase-2 blockers significantly reduces ischemic brain damage. Furthermore, injured neurons produce IL-1, which can be blocked by IL-1 inhibitors to reduce infarct size after ischemia.[13]

Another mechanism that contributes to ischemic injury is apoptosis. Triggered by a number of pathophysiologic events, including excitotoxicity, free oxygen radicals, an inflammatory reaction, and mitochondrial and DNA damage, apoptosis

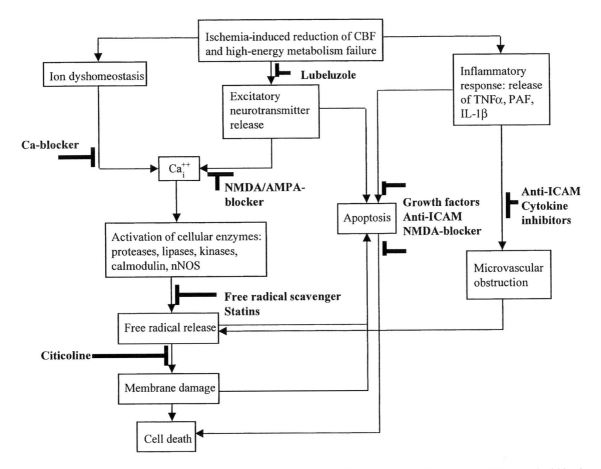

Figure 16-2. Blockage of key pathways in the ischemic cascade by available neuroprotective agents. (CBF = cerebral blood flow; NMDA = *N*-methyl-D-aspartate; AMPA = alpha-amino-3-hydroxy-5-methyl-4-isoxazole propionic acid; nNOS = neuronal nitric oxide synthase; TNFα = tumor necrosis factor α; PAF = platelet activating factor; IL 1β = interleukin-1β; ICAM = intercellular adhesion molecule.) (Reproduced with permission from Arch Int Med 2000;160:3196–3206.)

occurs after milder ischemic injury, particularly within the penumbra.[14] Apoptosis is mediated by a cascade of gene expression, including the caspases, a family of aspartate-specific cysteine proteases, as well as genes that suppress (e.g., Bcl-2) or augment (e.g., Bax) cell death.[15,16] Caspase activity can be blocked by caspase inhibitors, reducing infarct size and apoptosis as well as improving outcome.[17,18] Other candidates that may counteract apoptosis after focal cerebral ischemia via Bcl-2/Bax–dependent mechanisms are growth factors (GFs), such as brain-derived neurotrophic GF.[19]

Recovery and reorganization occurs weeks after focal lesions and may have a major impact on outcome after stroke.[20,21] The underlying mechanisms include neuronal sprouting and synaptogenesis, which are part of the spontaneous recovery process, particularly after smaller focal lesions. Enhancement of recovery followed by an improvement of behavioral outcome can be pharmacologically achieved with drugs, such as GFs and nootropic agents.[22,23]

Acute Treatment

Ca²⁺ Antagonists

Ca²⁺-channel antagonists were among the first drugs to be evaluated for neuroprotection after stroke. They reduce the Ca²⁺ influx into the cell via voltage-sensitive calcium channels and therefore should have antiexcitotoxic effects. Ca²⁺ antagonists have been shown in several experimental studies to be neuroprotective after focal cerebral ischemia.[24] The best investigated drug is the dihydropyridine compound, nimodipine, that typically

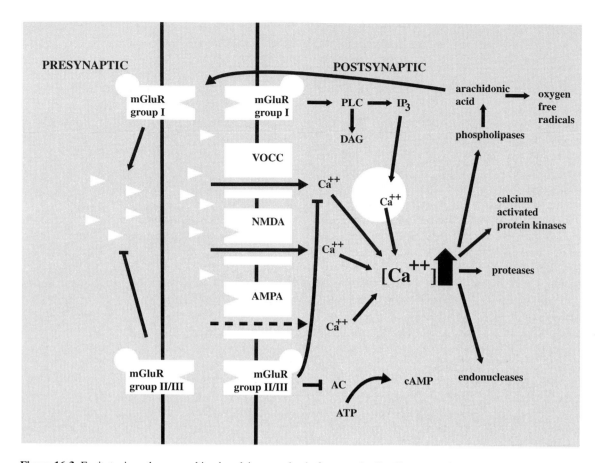

Figure 16-3. Excitotoxic pathway resulting in calcium overload of neuronal cells. Glutamate triggers calcium influx into the cell, activating endonucleases, proteases, calcium-activated protein kinase, and phospholipases. (mGluR = metabotropic glutamate receptor; PLC = phospholipase C; IP_3 = inositol 1,4,5-triphosphate; DAG = diacylglycerol; VOCC = voltage-operated calcium channel; NMDA = Nmethyl-D-aspartate; AMPA = alpha-amino-3-hydroxy-5-methyl-4-isoxazole propionic acid; AC = adenylcyclase; ATP = adenosine triphosphate; cAMP = cyclic adenosine monophosphate.) (Reproduced with permission from Arch Int Med 2000;160:3196–3206.)

blocks the L-type Ca^{2+} channel. Nimodipine was tested in at least 10 randomized, placebo-controlled stroke trials. Beside positive results with reduction of mortality and improved neurologic outcome at 6 months after stroke in an early trial,[25] all other trials were negative. Adverse effects of intravenous (i.v.) nimodipine include hypotension that was directly correlated to an increase in mortality.[26] A meta-analysis of nine trials including 3,719 patients showed a benefit for oral nimodipine (30 mg over 6 hours) in the subgroup treated within 12 hours of stroke onset.[27] Therefore, oral nimodipine was again studied within 6 hours of symptom onset in the Very Early Nimodipine Use in Stroke trial. The study was negative and probably

precludes further considerations of voltage-regulated Ca^{2+}-channel antagonists for the treatment of acute stroke. Nevertheless, nimodipine is the standard treatment for prevention of ischemic neurologic deficits after subarachnoid hemorrhage.[28]

N-*Methyl-D-Aspartate Antagonists*

NMDA antagonists reduce the calcium influx into neurons through postsynaptic agonist-operated calcium channels. They were the first drugs that remarkably reduced infarct size (40–70%) after experimental focal cerebral ischemia, primarily in the penumbra.[29,30] This effect can be achieved with competitive and noncompetitive NMDA antagonists. Competitive NMDA antagonists, such as phosphonates or CGS19755 (selfotel), block the glutamate recognition site of the receptor. Noncompetitive NMDA antagonists, including phencyclidine, ketamine, MK801, dextrorphan, or CNS-1102, block the NMDA-associated ion channel in a use-dependent manner. Negative modulation of receptor activity can be achieved by Zn^{2+}. Mg^{2+} blocks the channel in a voltage-dependent manner and has been shown to reduce infarct size after focal cerebral ischemia. Apart from the main recognition site for glutamate, the receptor also contains a glycine site, where inhibition reduces NMDA receptor activity. Antagonists of the glycine site of the receptor, such as GV150526 and ACEA1021, also reduce infarct size after experimental focal cerebral ischemia.[31,32] Although preclinical studies demonstrated potent infarct-reducing effects in a variety of species, clinical trials using NMDA antagonists (selfotel, eliprodil, CNS-1102, and dextrorphan) were negative or discontinued due to adverse effects.[33–36] Side effects likely occurred before a neuroprotective plasma level of the drugs could be achieved. Side effects occurred in a dose-dependent manner and included neuropsychiatric symptoms (agitation, confusion, hallucination, catatonia, ataxia, dysarthria) and hypertension. These side effects are known to be phencyclidine-related and should not occur when targeting another subunit of the NMDA receptor. Indeed, antagonists of the glycine site of the NMDA receptor (GV150526, ACEA1021) were generally better tolerated without neuropsychiatric adverse effects.[37,38] A phase III trial of GV150526 was negative. Another compound that acts on the NMDA receptor and is being studied in a multicenter clinical trial is Mg^{2+}. A pilot study showed the drug was well tolerated and associated with a trend toward fewer early deaths in the Mg^{2+}-treated group.[39]

A randomized, double-blind, placebo-controlled, multicenter, collaborative trial designed to test the efficacy of magnesium sulfate given within 12 hours after stroke onset is proceeding.

Alpha-Amino-3-Hydroxy-5-Methyl-4-Isoxazole Propionic Acid Antagonists

AMPA receptor antagonists prevent Na^+ influx into the cell by blockading the AMPA/kainate receptor, preventing cell depolarization and the subsequent Ca^{2+} overload of the cell. AMPA receptor antagonists, such as 2,3-dihydroxy-6-nitro-7-sulfamoyl-benzo(f)quinoxaline (NBQX) and ZK200775, have potent neuroprotective capacities when given after experimental focal cerebral ischemia[40]; however, adverse effects include nephrotoxicity (NBQX) and sedation (ZK200775).

Lubeluzole

Lubeluzole, a benzothiazole compound, is an Na^+-blocker that prevents presynaptic glutamate release and reduces postsynaptic excitotoxicity. Lubeluzole also prevents glutamate-mediated increases in NO production by inhibiting the NOS activity. Experimental studies demonstrated neuroprotective effects after focal cerebral ischemia.[41,42] Two large clinical, multicenter, placebo-controlled trials, one conducted in Northern America and one conducted in Europe/Australia, have been completed.[43,44] Beside occasional and transient electrocardiographic QT prolongations, lubeluzole was well tolerated at the concentrations given in both trials (7.5 mg every 1 hour i.v., followed by 10 mg/day for 5 days i.v.). However, there was no significant effect on the primary endpoint (mortality), although the American trial showed a significant 7% increase in patients with little or no disability at 3 months after stroke. A meta-analysis including 1,375 patients suggested a positive effect on mild to moderate stroke, but no effect on severe stroke.[45] Therefore, a third trial has been completed, designed to detect approximately 7% of a functional benefit in the treated group. The results were negative, and lubeluzole should not be considered for further development for stroke therapy.

Free Radical Scavengers

Tirilazad mesylate, a 21-aminosteroid, acts as a free radical scavenger and has antioxidant effects. Tirilazad reduces infarct size after transient ischemia but not after permanent focal cerebral ischemia.[46] Tirilazad has been tested in several clinical trials with inconclusive results. Although well tolerated at a dose of 6 mg per kg per day,[47] the study was terminated for lack of efficacy.[48] A parallel study showed that mortality at 3 months was reduced in patients treated with tirilazad when compared to placebo (19% vs. 33%).[49] Although not significant (111 patients), the results of one phase III high-dose study showed a trend of reduced mortality and improved outcome in the tirilazad-treated group.[50]

NO and peroxynitrite release can be inhibited by neuronal (n) or inducible (i) NOS blockers. The selective nNOS blocker 7-nitroindazole and 1-(2-trifluoromethylphenyl) imidazole significantly reduce infarct size after focal and global cerebral ischemia.[51,52] Blockage of iNOS can be achieved relatively selectively by aminoguanidines. Aminoguanidines have been reported to be potent neuroprotectants after focal cerebral ischemia.[53] Aminoguanidines seem to be protective when the treatment is delayed for 24 hours, making them promising for future human use.[54]

Another promising antioxidant is the seleno-organic compound ebselen. Ebselen acts through a glutathione peroxidase–like action. It inhibits the peroxidation of membrane phospholipids and the lipoxygenase in the arachidonate cascade. Ebselen also blocks the production of superoxide anions by activated leukocytes, inhibits iNOS, and protects against peroxynitrite. Ebselen has been shown to be neuroprotective after transient and permanent experimental focal cerebral ischemia.[55,56] A clinical pilot study showed that oral ebselen (300 mg/day) was well tolerated and significantly improves functional outcome when given within 24 hours of stroke.[57] When given within 12 hours (150 mg/day) after ischemia, there was a trend toward reduced infarct volume and better outcome in ebselen-treated patients. A significant reduction in infarct volume and outcome occurred only in the 6-hour subgroup.[58]

Antibodies to Intercellular Adhesion Molecules

Monoclonal antibodies against the ICAM-1 receptor on the vascular endothelium prevent leukocyte activation and plugging. ICAM-1 antibodies have been shown to reduce infarct size and improve outcome after transient but not permanent experimental focal cerebral ischemia.[59] Consequently, results of a randomized, placebo-controlled trial (625 patients) using the anti-ICAM antibody enlimomab were negative. The treatment group received i.v. 160 mg the first day and 40 mg the next 4 days (time window = 6 hours), and experienced worse outcome and increased mortality due to higher rates of fever, infection, and pneumonia.[60] The adverse effects were thought to be due to a complement reaction triggered by enlimomab.

Inhibition of Cytokines

The best-studied cytokines that have key roles after ischemia and can pharmacologically be inhibited are IL-1 and TNF-α. IL-1 mediates excitotoxicity through NMDA receptor activation and activates surface adhesion molecules.[61] Consequently, overexpression of endogenous IL-1 receptor antagonists or treatment with the IL-1 antagonist (ZnPP) reduces infarct and edema size during temporary focal ischemia.[62,63] Another cytokine, TNF-α may also exacerbate ischemic and, in particular, reperfusion injury.[64] Inhibiting TNF-α improves CBF and reduces infarct size after focal cerebral ischemia.[64,65] Other cytokines involved in the reperfusion damage after ischemia are ILs 1 and 6, platelet activating factor, and transforming GF-β. As indicated by a few studies, inhibition of these cytokines may have neuroprotective effects after cerebral ischemia.[66–69] Further experimental studies evaluating dosage and timing of cytokine antagonists in different models of focal ischemia and in different species should be completed before future clinical development becomes promising.

Statins

Some trials of 3-hydroxy-3-methylglutaryl coenzyme A reductase inhibitors (statins) have demonstrated a significant reduction of ischemic stroke in patients with history of coronary artery disease.[70,71] Because this reduction was independent of the serum cholesterol level, statins are thought to have neuroprotective capacities aside from their anti-atherosclerotic effects. Prophylactic statin therapy has been shown to improve CBF through upregulation of endothelial NOS and to reduce infarct size (30%).[72] Statins also inhibit the cytokine-mediated (IL-1β, TNF-α) upregulation of iNOS and production of NO in rat astrocytes and macrophages.[73] Furthermore, statins may reduce lipoprotein oxidation and attenuate free radical injury.[74,75] Despite these encouraging results, more studies are needed to define the time window for administration, dosage, and mechanisms of action before statins should be considered as neuroprotective stroke therapy.

Recovery Treatment

Growth Factors

GFs are endogenously occurring polypeptides that have not only neuroprotective but also regenerative and proliferative capacities, and may therefore be unique candidates for stroke therapy. Several GFs have been shown to be neuroprotective after experimental ischemia in vivo and in vitro. The best-studied GFs after focal cerebral ischemia are basic fibroblast GF (bFGF), brain-derived neurotrophic GF, insulin-like GF, and osteogenic protein-1. All of these GFs have robust neuroprotective effects after experimental stroke and reduce infarct size 35–50%.[76–79] Potential mechanisms of action after stroke include attenuation of excitotoxicity, improvement of CBF, and reduction of apoptosis.[78,80,81] The regenerative and proliferative capacities of GFs after focal ischemic lesions have been convincingly shown for bFGF and osteogenic protein-1. Both compounds achieved a significant improvement of behavioral outcome without changes in infarct size when given 24 hours after ischemia.[82,83] GF treatment improved synaptogenesis and dendritic sprouting. In a clinical, placebo-controlled, multicenter trial for the treatment of acute stroke, bFGF was well tolerated.[84] A subsequent phase III study has been stopped, and the results were negative.[85]

Citicoline

Citicoline (cytidine 5'-diphosphate choline), a naturally occurring endogenous compound that serves as an intermediary in the synthesis of the membrane phosphatidylcholine, is thought to have membrane-stabilizing functions and to reduce free fatty acid formation during stroke. Citicoline reduces the size of infarction and improves neurologic outcome in experimental models of focal cerebral ischemia.[86,87] In clinical studies, treatment with citicoline improved cognitive and behavioral function in patients with memory deficits.[88,89] After human stroke, treatment with citicoline improved the neurologic outcome and reduced the ischemic lesion volume, as demonstrated by diffusion-weighted magnetic resonance imaging.[90,91] The drug was well tolerated without any known side effects. Therefore, citicoline has been tested in a dose-response study at 0.5 g, 1.0 g, and 2.0 g, beginning within 24 hours after stroke. The outcome, based on the Barthel Index, was significantly better only for patients in the group receiving 0.5 g.[92] A randomized, double-blind, placebo-controlled, phase III study of the 0.5 g dose of citicoline was negative, however, although post hoc analysis indicated that medium and severe stroke patients benefited from the treatment.[93] A follow-up study based on the National Institutes of Health Stroke Scale and magnetic resonance imaging–derived lesion volume 12 weeks after stroke was also negative, although citicoline significantly reduced infarct volume and improved neurologic outcome in patients with baseline diffusion-weighted lesions of 1–120 cm^3.[91,92]

Nootropics

Piracetam is a γ-aminobutyric acid derivative and a nootropic agent with neuroprotective capacities mediated through restoration of cell membrane fluidity and maintenance of membrane-bound cell functions. Experimental studies demonstrated a neuroprotective and regenerative effect of piracetam after focal lesions.[94] However, a randomized, placebo-controlled i.v. trial including 927 patients was negative for mortality and outcome at 12 weeks poststroke. Only a subgroup of patients treated within 7 hours showed a trend toward better neurologic outcome.[95] Another randomized, placebo-controlled, multicenter trial with a 7-hour time window has been launched.

Clomethiazole, a γ-aminobutyric acid agonist, showed neither severe adverse nor beneficial effects after acute stroke in a large multicenter trial, although subgroup analysis indicated that patients with large infarctions may have benefited from the treatment.[96] Therefore, the Clomethiazole Acute Stroke Study was started, including patients within

12 hours after onset of symptoms with large cerebral infarctions, intracerebral hemorrhages, and patients who received recombinant tissue plasminogen activator (rt-PA). The portion of the CLASS study for ischemia was recently reported to be negative.

Amphetamines increase the release at the noradrenergic terminals of norepinephrine, dopamine, and serotonin, and could be future candidates for recovery studies after stroke. D-amphetamine has been demonstrated to improve behavioral outcome and memory function up to 60 days after focal cerebral ischemia. This was correlated with enhanced neocortical sprouting and synaptogenesis in the D-amphetamine–treated group.[97]

Combination Treatment

The exploration of the effectiveness of combination therapies for stroke seems rational because cerebral ischemia triggers a multitude of pathophysiologic and biochemical events that affect the evolution of focal ischemia differently. Impeding different steps in this cascade with different therapeutic agents may not only synergistically enhance the neuroprotective effect, but may also allow for use of lower doses of each drug and consecutively reduce side effects. This approach has been demonstrated to be promising in several experimental studies and may serve as a future strategy for stroke therapy in humans. For example, combining low doses of citicoline and MK-801 or bFGF significantly reduces infarct size after focal cerebral ischemia, whereas the single compounds were not effective.[98,99] Strategies include not only the combination of different neuroprotective agents but also the combination of thrombolysis and neuroprotection. Adding free radical scavengers (tirilazad), AMPA antagonists (NBQX), NMDA antagonists (MK-801), or citicoline to rt-PA treatment extends the time window for administration and enhances the effect of thrombolysis after stroke.[100–103] Combining agents for acute (e.g., rt-PA, NMDA antagonists, free radical scavengers) and recovery treatment (e.g., GFs, nootropics) may be the future of stroke therapy. However, the combination of lubeluzole and rt-PA for the treatment of human stroke achieved no benefit compared to rt-PA alone, which is not surprising because no lubeluzole study has shown any neuroprotective effect after human stroke. To achieve synergistic effects, combination studies should combine compounds that have convincingly been shown to be neuroprotective as a single treatment in clinical and preclinical studies.

References

1. Stroke Therapy Academic Industry Roundtable. Recommendations for standards regarding preclinical neuroprotective and restorative drug development. Stroke 1999;30:2752–2758.
2. Hossmann KA. Viability thresholds and the penumbra of focal ischemia. Ann Neurol 1994;36:557–565.
3. Read SJ, Hirano T, Abbott DF, et al. Identifying hypoxic tissue after acute ischemic stroke using PET and 18F-fluoromisonidazole. Neurology 1998;51:1617–1621.
4. Siesjo BK. Pathophysiology and treatment of focal cerebral ischemia. Part II. Mechanisms of damage and treatment. J Neurosurg 1992;77:337–354.
5. Kristian T, Siesjo BK. Calcium in ischemic cell death. Stroke 1998;29:705–718.
6. Rothwell NJ, Hopkins SJ. Cytokines and the nervous system II: actions and mechanisms of action. Trends Neurosci 1995;18:130–136.
7. Lindsberg PJ, Hallenbeck JM, Feuerstein G. Platelet-activating factor in stroke and brain injury. Ann Neurol 1991;30:117–129.
8. Haring HP, Berg EL, Tsurushita N, et al. E-selectin appears in nonischemic tissue during experimental focal cerebral ischemia. Stroke 1996;27:1386–1391.
9. Zhang R, Chopp M, Zhang Z, et al. The expression of P- and E-selectins in three models of middle cerebral artery occlusion. Brain Res 1998;785:207–214.
10. Forster C, Clark HB, Ross ME, Iadecola C. Inducible nitric oxide synthase expression in human cerebral infarcts. Acta Neuropathol (Berl) 1999;97:215–220.
11. Iadecola C, Zhang F, Casey R, et al. Delayed reduction of ischemic brain injury and neurological deficits in mice lacking the inducible nitric oxide synthase gene. J Neurosci 1997;17:9157–9164.
12. Nogawa S, Zhang F, Ross ME, Iadecola C. Cyclo-oxygenase-2 gene expression in neurons contributes to ischemic brain damage. J Neurosci 1997;17:2746–2755.
13. Loddick SA, Rothwell NJ. Neuroprotective effects of human recombinant interleukin-1 receptor antagonist in focal cerebral ischaemia in the rat. J Cereb Blood Flow Metab 1996;16:932–940.
14. Li Y, Chopp M, Jiang N, et al. Temporal profile of in situ DNA fragmentation after transient middle cerebral artery occlusion in the rat. J Cereb Blood Flow Metab 1995;15:389–397.
15. Thornberry NA, Lazebnik Y. Caspases: enemies within. Science 1998;281:1312–1326.
16. Adams JM, Cory S. The Bcl-2 protein family: arbiters of cell survival. Science 1998;281:1322–1366.
17. Fink K, Zhu J, Namura S, et al. Prolonged therapeutic window for ischemic brain damage caused by delayed

caspase activation. J Cereb Blood Flow Metab 1998;18: 1071–1076.

18. Endres M, Namura S, Shimizu-Sasamata M, et al. Attenuation of delayed neuronal death after mild focal ischemia in mice by inhibition of the caspase family. J Cereb Blood Flow Metab 1998;18:238–247.

19. Schäbitz WR, Sommer C, Zoder W, et al. Intravenous brain-derived neurotrophic factor reduces infarct size and counterregulates Bax and Bcl-2 expression after temporary focal cerebral ischemia. Stroke 2000;31:2212–2217.

20. Nudo RJ, Milliken GW. Reorganization of movement representations in primary motor cortex following focal ischemic infarcts in adult squirrel monkeys. J Neurophysiol 1996;75:2144–2149.

21. Nudo RJ, Wise BM, SiFuentes F, Milliken GW. Neural substrates for the effects of rehabilitative training on motor recovery after ischemic infarct. Science 1996;272: 1791–1794.

22. Kawamata T, Alexis NE, Dietrich WD, Finklestein SP. Intracisternal basic fibroblast growth factor (bFGF) enhances behavioral recovery following focal cerebral infarction in the rat. J Cereb Blood Flow Metab 1996;16:542–547.

23. Stroemer RP, Kent TA, Hulsebosch CE. Enhanced neocortical neural sprouting, synaptogenesis, and behavioral recovery with D-amphetamine therapy after neocortical infarction in rats. Stroke 1998;29:2381–2393.

24. Grotta JC. Clinical aspects of the use of calcium antagonists in cerebrovascular disease. Clin Neuropharmacol 1991;14:373–390.

25. Gelmers HJ, Gorter K, de Weerdt CJ, Wiezer HJ. A controlled trial of nimodipine in acute ischemic stroke. N Engl J Med 1988;318:203–207.

26. Wahlgren N, MacMahon PG, Dekeyes J, et al. Intravenous Nimodipine West European Stroke Trial (INWEST) of nimodipine in the treatment of acute ischemic stroke. Cerebrovasc Res 1994;4:204–210.

27. Mohr J, Dragozzo JM, Harrison MJG, et al. Metaanalysis of oral nimodipine trials in acute ischemic stroke. Cerebrovasc Res 1994;4:194–203.

28. Feigin VL, Rinkel GJ, Algra A, et al. Calcium antagonists for aneurysmal subarachnoid haemorrhage. Cochrane Database Syst Rev 2000;2:CD000277.

29. Park CK, Nehls DG, Graham DI, et al. The glutamate antagonist MK-801 reduces focal ischemic brain damage in the rat. Ann Neurol 1988;24:543–551.

30. Choi DW. Methods for antagonizing glutamate neurotoxicity. Cerebrovasc Brain Metab Rev 1990;2:105–147.

31. Tatlisumak T, Takano K, Meiler MR, Fisher M. A glycine site antagonist, ZD9379, reduces number of spreading depressions and infarct size in rats with permanent middle cerebral artery occlusion. Stroke 1998;29:190–195.

32. Takano K, Tatlisumak T, Formato JE, et al. Glycine site antagonist attenuates infarct size in experimental focal ischemia. Postmortem and diffusion mapping studies. Stroke 1997;28:1255–1262.

33. Lees KR. Cerestat and other NMDA antagonists in ischemic stroke. Neurology 1997;49:66–69.

34. Davis SM, Lees KR, Albers GW, et al. Selfotel in acute ischemic stroke: possible neurotoxic effects of an NMDA antagonist. Stroke 2000;31:347–354.

35. Albers GW, Atkinson RP, Kelley RE, Rosenbaum DM. Safety, tolerability, and pharmacokinetics of the N-methyl-D-aspartate antagonist dextrorphan in patients with acute stroke. Dextrorphan Study Group. Stroke 1995; 26:254–258.

36. Fisher M, for CNS1102 Investigators. Cerestat (CNS 1102), a noncompetitive NMDA antagonist, in ischemic stroke patients: dose escalating safety study. Cerebrovasc Dis 1994;4:245–254.

37. Albers GW, Clark WM, Atkinson RP, et al. Dose escalation study of the NMDA glycine-site antagonist ACEA 1021 in acute ischemic stroke. Stroke 1997;28:233–239.

38. Lees KR, Lavelle JF, Hobbinger SF. GAIN European Study Group. Safety and tolerability of GV150526 in acute stroke. Cerebrovasc Dis 1998;8:20–29.

39. Muir KW, Lees KR. A randomized, double-blind, placebo-controlled pilot trial of intravenous magnesium in acute stroke. Stroke 1995;26:1183–1186.

40. Turski L, Huth A, Sheardown M, et al. ZK200775: a phosphonate quinoxalinedione AMPA antagonist for neuroprotection in stroke and trauma. Proc Natl Acad Sci U S A 1998;95:10960–10965.

41. Aronowski J, Strong R, Grotta JC. Treatment of experimental focal ischemia in rats with lubeluzole. Neuropharmacology 1996;35:689–693.

42. Culmsee C, Junker V, Wolz P, et al. Lubeluzole protects hippocampal neurons from excitotoxicity in vitro and reduces brain damage caused by ischemia. Eur J Pharmacol 1998;342:193–201.

43. Grotta J. Lubeluzole treatment of acute ischemic stroke. The US and Canadian Lubeluzole Ischemic Stroke Study Group. Stroke 1997;28:2338–2346.

44. Diener HC. Multinational randomised controlled trial of lubeluzole in acute ischaemic stroke. European and Australian Lubeluzole Ischaemic Stroke Study Group. Cerebrovasc Dis 1998;8:172–181.

45. Hantson L, Wessel T. Therapeutic effects of lubeluzole in ischemic stroke (abstract). Stroke 1998;29:287.

46. Xue D, Slivka A, Buchan AM. Tirilazad reduces cortical infarction after transient but not permanent focal cerebral ischemia in rats. Stroke 1992;23:894–899.

47. Safety study of tirilazad mesylate in patients with acute ischemic stroke (STIPAS). Stroke 1994;25:418–423.

48. Peters GR, Hwang LW, Musch B, Brosse DM, Dragozzo JM. Safety and efficacy of 6mg/kg/d tirilazad mesylate in patients with acute ischemic stroke. Stroke 1996;27:195–245.

49. A randomized trial of tirilazad mesylate in patients with acute ischemic stroke (RANTTAS). The RANTTAS investigators. Stroke 1996;27:1453–1458.

50. Saver JL, Johnston KC, Homer D, et al. Infarct volume as a surrogate or auxiliary outcome measure in ischemic stroke clinical trials. The RANTTAS Investigators. Stroke 1999;30:293–298.

51. Escott KJ, Beech JS, Haga KK, et al. Cerebroprotective effect of the nitric oxide synthase inhibitors, 1-(2-trifluoromethylphenyl) imidazole and 7-nitro indazole, after transient focal cerebral ischemia in the rat. J Cereb Blood Flow Metab 1998;18:281–287.

52. Nanri K, Montecot C, Springhetti V, et al. The selective inhibitor of neuronal nitric oxide synthase, 7-nitroindazole,

reduces the delayed neuronal damage due to forebrain ischemia in rats. Stroke 1998;29:1248–1253.

53. Cockroft KM, Meistrell M III, Zimmerman GA, et al. Cerebroprotective effects of aminoguanidine in a rodent model of stroke. Stroke 1996;27:1393–1398.

54. Iadecola C, Zhang F, Xu X. Inhibition of inducible nitric oxide synthase ameliorates cerebral ischemic damage. Am J Physiol 1995;268:286–292.

55. Dawson DA, Masayasu H, Graham DI, Macrae IM. The neuroprotective efficacy of ebselen (a glutathione peroxidase mimic) on brain damage induced by transient focal cerebral ischaemia in the rat. Neurosci Lett 1995;185:65–69.

56. Takasago T, Peters EE, Graham DI, et al. Neuroprotective efficacy of ebselen, an antioxidant with anti-inflammatory actions, in a rodent model of permanent middle cerebral artery occlusion. Br J Pharmacol 1997;122:1251–1256.

57. Yamaguchi T, Sano K, Takakura K, et al. Ebselen in acute ischemic stroke: a placebo-controlled, double-blind clinical trial. Ebselen Study Group. Stroke 1998;29:12–17.

58. Ogawa A, Yoshimoto T, Kikuchi H, et al. Ebselen in acute middle cerebral artery occlusion: a placebo-controlled, double-blind clinical trial. Cerebrovasc Dis 1999;9:112–118.

59. Zhang RL, Chopp M, Jiang N, et al. Anti-intercellular adhesion molecule-1 antibody reduces ischemic cell damage after transient but not permanent middle cerebral artery occlusion in the Wistar rat. Stroke 1995;26:1438–1442.

60. The enlimomab acute stroke trial final results. Enlimomab Acute Stroke Trial Study Group (abstract). Neurology 1997;48:A270.

61. Jean WC, Spellman SR, Nussbaum ES, Low WC. Reperfusion injury after focal cerebral ischemia: the role of inflammation and the therapeutic horizon. Neurosurgery 1998;43:1382–1396.

62. Betz AL, Yang GY, Davidson BL. Attenuation of stroke size in rats using an adenoviral vector to induce overexpression of interleukin-1 receptor antagonist in brain. J Cereb Blood Flow Metab 1995;15:547–551.

63. Kadoya C, Domino EF, Yang GY, et al. Preischemic but not postischemic zinc protoporphyrin treatment reduces infarct size and edema accumulation after temporary focal cerebral ischemia in rats. Stroke 1995;26:1035–1038.

64. Barone FC, Arvin B, White RF, et al. Tumor necrosis factor-alpha. A mediator of focal ischemic brain injury. Stroke 1997;28:1233–1244.

65. Dawson DA, Martin D, Hallenbeck JM. Inhibition of tumor necrosis factor-alpha reduces focal cerebral ischemic injury in the spontaneously hypertensive rat. Neurosci Lett 1996;218:41–44.

66. Panetta T, Marcheselli VL, Braquet P, Bazan NG. Arachidonic acid metabolism and cerebral blood flow in the normal, ischemic, and reperfused gerbil brain. Inhibition of ischemia-reperfusion–induced cerebral injury by a platelet-activating factor antagonist (BN 52021). Ann N Y Acad Sci 1989;559:340–351.

67. Matsumoto T, Ikeda K, Mukaida N, et al. Prevention of cerebral edema and infarct by an antibody to interleukin-8. Lab Invest 1997;77:119–125.

68. Prehn JH, Backhauss C, Krieglstein J. Transforming growth factor-beta 1 prevents glutamate neurotoxicity in rat neocortical cultures and protects mouse neocortex

from ischemic injury in vivo. J Cereb Blood Flow Metab 1993;13:521–525.

69. Gross CE, Bednar MM, Howard DB, Sporn MB. Transforming growth factor-beta 1 reduces infarct size after experimental cerebral ischemia in a rabbit model. Stroke 1993;24:558–562.

70. Sacks FM, Pfeffer MA, Moye LA, et al. The effect of pravastatin on coronary events after myocardial infarction in patients with average cholesterol levels. Cholesterol and Recurrent Events Trial investigators. N Engl J Med 1996;335:1001–1009.

71. Stalenhoef AF. Scandinavian simvastatin study (4S). Lancet 1994;344:1766–1767.

72. Endres M, Laufs U, Huang Z, et al. Stroke protection by 3-hydroxy-3-methylglutaryl (HMG)-CoA reductase inhibitors mediated by endothelial nitric oxide synthase. Proc Natl Acad Sci U S A 1998;95:8880–8885.

73. Pahan K, Sheikh FG, Namboodiri AM, Singh I. Lovastatin and phenylacetate inhibit the induction of nitric oxide synthase and cytokines in rat primary astrocytes, microglia, and macrophages. J Clin Invest 1997;100:2671–2679.

74. Hussein O, Schlezinger S, Rosenblat M, et al. Reduced susceptibility of low-density lipoprotein (LDL) to lipid peroxidation after fluvastatin therapy is associated with the hypocholesterolemic effect of the drug and its binding to the LDL. Atherosclerosis 1997;128:11–18.

75. Chen L, Haught WH, Yang B, et al. Preservation of endogenous antioxidant activity and inhibition of lipid peroxidation as common mechanisms of antiatherosclerotic effects of vitamin E, lovastatin, and amlodipine. J Am Coll Cardiol 1997;30:569–575.

76. Fisher M, Meadows ME, Do T, et al. Delayed treatment with intravenous basic fibroblast growth factor reduces infarct size following permanent focal cerebral ischemia in rats. J Cereb Blood Flow Metab 1995;15:953–959.

77. Loddick SA, Liu XJ, Lu ZX, et al. Displacement of insulin-like growth factors from their binding proteins as a potential treatment for stroke. Proc Natl Acad Sci U S A 1998;95:1894–1898.

78. Schäbitz WR, Schwab S, Spranger M, Hacke W. Intraventricular brain-derived neurotrophic factor reduces infarct size after focal cerebral ischemia in rats. J Cereb Blood Flow Metab 1997;17:500–506.

79. Lin SZ, Hoffer BJ, Kaplan P, Wang Y. Osteogenic protein-1 protects against cerebral infarction induced by MCA ligation in rats. Stroke 1999;30:126–133.

80. Freese A, Finklestein SP, DiFiglia M. Basic fibroblast growth factor protects striatal neurons in vitro from NMDA-receptor mediated excitotoxicity. Brain Res 1992;575:351–355.

81. Tanaka R, Miyasaka Y, Yada K, et al. Basic fibroblast growth factor increases regional cerebral blood flow and reduces infarct size after experimental ischemia in a rat model. Stroke 1995;26:2154–2158.

82. Kawamata T, Ren J, Chan TC, et al. Intracisternal osteogenic protein-1 enhances functional recovery following focal stroke. Neuroreport 1998;9:1441–1445.

83. Kawamata T, Dietrich WD, Schallert T, et al. Intracisternal basic fibroblast growth factor enhances functional recovery and up-regulates the expression of a molecular

marker of neuronal sprouting following focal cerebral infarction. Proc Natl Acad Sci U S A 1997;94:8179–8184.

84. Clinical safety of intravenous bFGF in acute stroke. The FIBLAST Safety Study Group. Stroke 1998;29:287–293.

85. Clark WM, Shim JO, Kasner SE, Victor S. Trafermin in acute ischemic stroke: results of a phase II/III randomized efficacy study. Neurology 2000;54:A88.

86. Schabitz WR, Weber J, Takano K, et al. The effects of prolonged treatment with citicoline in temporary experimental focal ischemia. J Neurol Sci 1996;138:21–25.

87. Aronowski J, Strong R, Grotta JC. Citicoline for treatment of experimental focal ischemia: histologic and behavioral outcome. Neurol Res 1996;18:570–574.

88. Spiers PA, Myers D, Hochanadel GS, et al. Citicoline improves verbal memory in aging. Arch Neurol 1996;53: 441–448.

89. Alvarez XA, Laredo M, Corzo D, et al. Citicoline improves memory performance in elderly subjects. Methods Find Exp Clin Pharmacol 1997;19:201–210.

90. Tazaki Y, Sakai F, Otomo E, et al. Treatment of acute cerebral infarction with a choline precursor in a multicenter double-blind placebo-controlled study. Stroke 1988;19:211–216.

91. Warach SJ, LuAnn AS. ECCO 2000 study of citicoline for treatment of acute ischemic stroke: effects on infarct volumes measured by MRI. 25th International Stroke Conference, February 10–12, 2000.

92. Clark WM, Warach SJ, Pettigrew LC, et al. A randomized dose-response trial of citicoline in acute ischemic stroke patients. Citicoline Stroke Study Group. Neurology 1997;49:671–678.

93. Clark WM, Williams BJ, Selzer KA, et al. A randomized efficacy trial of citicoline in patients with acute ischemic stroke. Stroke 1999;30:2592–2597.

94. Coq JO, Xerri C. Acute reorganization of the forepaw representation in the rat SI cortex after focal cortical injury:

neuroprotective effects of piracetam treatment. Eur J Neurosci 1999;11:2597–2608.

95. De Deyn PP, Reuck JD, Deberdt W, et al. Treatment of acute ischemic stroke with piracetam. Members of the Piracetam in Acute Stroke Study (PASS) Group. Stroke 1997;28:2347–2352.

96. Wahlgren NG, Ranasinha KW, Rosolacci T, et al. Clomethiazole Acute Stroke Study (CLASS): results of a randomized, controlled trial of clomethiazole versus placebo in 1,360 acute stroke patients. Stroke 1999;30:21–28.

97. Stroemer RP, Kent TA, Hulsebosch CE. Enhanced neocortical neural sprouting, synaptogenesis, and behavioral recovery with D-amphetamine therapy after neocortical infarction in rats. Stroke 1999;29:2381–2393.

98. Önal MZ, Li F, Tatlisumak T, et al. Synergistic effects of citicoline and MK-801 in temporary experimental focal ischemia in rats. Stroke 1997;28:1060–1065.

99. Schäbitz WR, Li F, Irie K, et al. Synergistic effects of a combination of low-dose bFGF and citicoline after temporary experimental focal ischemia. Stroke 1999;30: 427–432.

100. Meden P, Overgaard K, Sereghy T, Boysen G. Enhancing the efficacy of thrombolysis by AMPA receptor blockage with NBQX in a rat embolic stroke model. J Neurol Sci 1993;119:209–216.

101. Meden P, Overgaard K, Pedersen H, Boysen G. Effect of early treatment with tirilazad combined with delayed thrombolytic therapy in rat embolic stroke. Cerebrovasc Dis 1996;6:141–148.

102. Zivin JA, Mazzarella V. Tissue plasminogen activator plus glutamate antagonists improves outcome after embolic stroke. Arch Neurol 1991;48:1235–1240.

103. Anderson M, Meden P, Overgaard K, Boysen G. Effects of citicoline combined therapy in a rat embolic stroke model. Stroke 1999;30:1464–1471.

Chapter 17
Management of Intracerebral Hemorrhage

Kazuo Minematsu and Takenori Yamaguchi

Incidence and Pathogenesis

Intracerebral hemorrhage (ICH), or brain hemorrhage, is defined as bleeding within the brain parenchyma. It accounts for approximately 10–15% of all strokes in the United States and European countries[1–3] and approximately 20–30% of strokes in Japan and other Asian countries.[4–6] ICH is usually classified according to the anatomic sites of hemorrhage as putaminal, thalamic, caudate, subcortical (or lobar), cerebellar and pontine (brain stem) hemorrhage (Figure 17-1).

Potential mechanisms producing ICH are listed in Table 17-1. Nontraumatic ICH in adults most commonly results from hypertensive arteriopathies in the brain. Epidemiologic studies have indicated that 70–80% of ICH patients have hypertension, especially uncontrolled hypertension.[2,7] Because hypertensive arteriopathies develop predominantly in the basal perforating arteries, most hypertensive ICHs occur in the putamen, thalamus, pons, and dentate nucleus of the cerebellum. In contrast, approximately 55% of lobar hemorrhages are nonhypertensive in nature and may be caused by cerebral amyloid angiopathy (CAA) or vascular malformations.[8,9] Brain tumors, anticoagulants, thrombolytic agents, and sympathomimetic drugs, including amphetamines, are other potential pathogenic factors associated with ICH.

Clinical Syndromes

The majority of clinical studies, except for some series in the United States, demonstrated that the most common location of ICH is the putamen, accounting for between 25% and 46% of all ICHs.[3,10–14] The typical syndrome of putaminal hemorrhage (see Figure 17-1A), which has been recognized as representative for that of ICH, consists of the abrupt onset of flaccid hemiplegia, a complete hemisensory deficit, homonymous hemianopsia, paralysis of conjugate gaze to the side opposite the lesion, mild to moderate impairment of consciousness with or without headache and vomiting, and in some cases, neuropsychological disorders. In thalamic hemorrhage (22–42% of ICH, see Figure 17-1B), similar syndromes may occur, but a sensory deficit usually predominates over the other manifestations. Oculomotor signs, such as forced downward gaze, convergence paralysis, and unreactive miotic pupils, suggest the diagnosis of thalamic hemorrhage. The sudden onset of severe headache may be the sole manifestation of caudate hemorrhage, which is usually accompanied by ventricular hemorrhage (see Figure 17-1C).

Neurologic manifestations are more variable in lobar hemorrhage (9–32% of ICH, see Figure 17-1D) than in deep hemorrhage and depend on the location and size of the hematoma. Relatively small hemorrhages may present with only a simple cortical syndrome, such as homonymous hemianopsia, monoparesis, or aphasia. Headache is common, but disturbance of consciousness is milder than deep hemorrhage with a similar hematoma size.

Dysequilibrium, ataxia, vertigo, nausea, and vomiting are characteristic symptoms and signs in cerebellar hemorrhage (4–10% of ICH, see Figure 17-1E). Neurologic signs indicative of brain stem

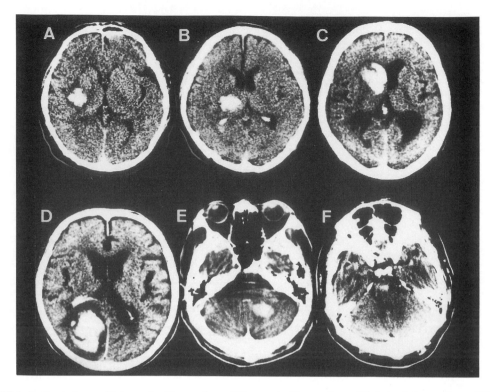

Figure 17-1. Anatomic types of intracerebral hemorrhage: **(A)** putaminal hemorrhage, **(B)** thalamic hemorrhage, **(C)** caudate hemorrhage, **(D)** subcortical (or lobar) hemorrhage, **(E)** cerebellar hemorrhage, **(F)** pontine (or brain stem) hemorrhage.

dysfunction, such as facial palsy of the peripheral type, nystagmus, miosis, decreased corneal reflex, and abducens palsy, may be detected in a large hematoma. Pontine hemorrhage (5–9% of ICH, see Figure 17-1F) is characterized by the rapid development of coma, quadriplegia, conjugate gaze devia-tion opposite to the lesion or ocular bobbing, and abnormal respiration. Small pontine hemorrhages occur more frequently than previously thought and produce milder syndromes, such as "pure motor hemiparesis" and "ataxic hemiparesis."

Diagnosis

Studies have suggested that ICH may present with milder clinical symptoms and signs than previously considered, which cannot reliably be distinguished from manifestations of brain infarction.[15–17] Drury et al.[18] estimated that 24% of ICHs were misdiagnosed as brain infarction before the era of computed tomography (CT) scan. The clinical diagnosis of ICH, therefore, should be made by CT or magnetic resonance imaging (MRI). Hematomas can easily and reliably be demonstrated by CT scans if the examination is done early after the onset of stroke. Because the hematoma becomes hypodense and sometimes leaves no trace with a late CT examination,[19] it may be misdiagnosed as an infarct.

Table 17-1. Mechanisms Producing Intracerebral Hemorrhage

Traumatic

Nontraumatic

  Hypertensive (due to hypertensive arteriopathy)

  Nonhypertensive

    Cerebral amyloid angiopathy

    Vascular malformations

    Other arteriopathies: moyamoya disease, dural sinus thrombosis, arterial dissection

    Brain tumors, metastatic and primary

    Blood dyscrasias: leukemia, clotting factor deficiencies, platelet abnormality

    Medications: anticoagulant or thrombolytic therapy, drug abuse (amphetamines and other sympathomimetic drugs)

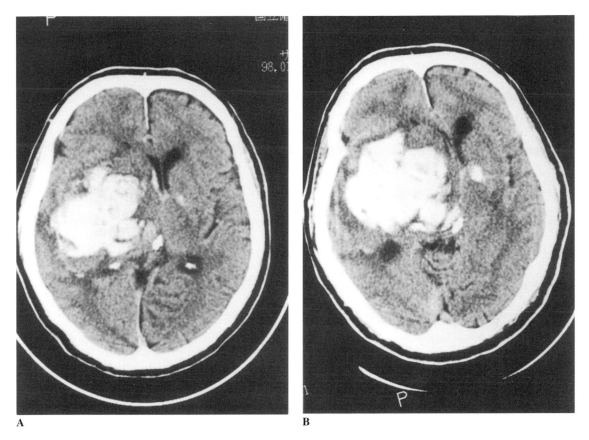

Figure 17-2. Early hematoma enlargement. A 76-year-old man with hypertension developed disturbance of consciousness and left hemiparesis. **(A)** A computed tomography (CT) scan 2 hours after stroke onset demonstrated right putaminal hemorrhage. **(B)** One hour later, when the patient became comatose, the second CT examination revealed that the hematoma expanded with compression of ventricular systems and midline structures.

The conventional MRI methods, such as T1- and T2-weighted images, are not superior to CT scan in the acute phase of ICH. Strong susceptibility-weighted MRI, such as echoplanar gradient-echo image, can detect a fresh hematoma within hours of hemorrhage onset as regions of marked signal loss due to susceptibility effects.[20] MRI is useful to diagnose hemorrhage later after onset because it is sensitive to hemosiderin deposition, the final metabolite of hemoglobin.[21]

Early Hematoma Enlargement

An increase in a volume of hematoma (hematoma enlargement or hematoma growth) can occur several hours after stroke onset. It is frequently associated with neurologic deterioration (Figure 17-2).[13,22–24] In a study by Kazui et al.[24] on 204 patients with

ICH, early expansion of hematoma was not uncommon: 35% in patients examined with the initial CT scan <3 hours, 16% at 3–6 hours, 15% at 6–12 hours, and 6% at 12–24 hours. Clinical deterioration was more frequently observed in patients with hematoma enlargement than in those with unchanged hematoma size (66% vs. 14%, respectively; odds ratio, 11.7). In a prospective study of patients with ICH within 3 hours of hemorrhage onset, hematoma growth occurred in 26% between the baseline and 1-hour CT scans and additionally in 12% between the 1- and 20-hour scans.[13]

In the other study by Kazui et al.[25] using multivariate analysis in 186 ICH patients, a patient examined >6 hours after ictus who had a hematoma volume <25 cm^3 was unlikely to experience further hematoma growth. History of brain infarction, liver disease, and high blood glucose (>141 mg/dl) or high glycosylated hemoglobin A_{1C}

Table 17-2. Thirty-Day Mortality from Intracerebral Hemorrhage

Author (Reference)	Country	Period	Number of Patients	Mortality (%)
Foulkes et al.[2]	United States	1983–86	237	30
Tuhrim et al.[28]	United States	1980–81	94	34
Broderick et al.[26]	United States	1980–84	?	48
Broderick et al.[29]	United States	1988	188	44
Brott et al.[13,a]	United States	1989–94	103	37
Silver et al.[30]	Canada	1975–80	106	56
Garde et al.[31]	Sweden	1977–79	100	28
Daverat et al.[10]	France	?	166	31
Schuetz et al.[27]	Germany	1978–81	148	49
		1982–85	167	42
		1986–89	173	31
Kutsuzawa[32]	Japan	1982–86	335	13
Hashimoto et al.[33]	Japan	1978–85	194	13
Terayama et al.[12]	Japan	1984–88	1,701	23
Fujii et al.[14,b]	Japan	1987–95	627	17[c]

[a]Patients admitted within 3 hours after stroke onset.
[b]Patients admitted within 24 hours after stroke onset.
[c]Three-month mortality.

(>5.1%) with high systolic blood pressure (BP) (>200 mm Hg) were factors independently predisposing to hematoma enlargement. In a study by Fujii et al.,[14] who examined 627 patients with ICH admitted within 24 hours, independent predictors of hematoma enlargement were a short time interval between onset and admission, habitual alcohol consumption, consciousness disturbance, an irregularly shaped hematoma shown on initial CT scan, and low levels of fibrinogen.

Outcome

Before the 1970s, ICH was considered to be associated with an extremely high mortality. The clinical severity of ICH has become consistently milder since the CT era began.[18] In a population-based study in Rochester, Minnesota, the 30-day mortality rate from ICH decreased dramatically from 90% between 1945 and 1974 to less than 50% in between 1980 and 1984.[26] Similar reductions in mortality were also reported in Japan.[5] An increased detection rate of milder ICH with CT and MRI, a decrease in the prevalence of hypertension, and improved antinypertensive therapy are likely to have reduced the severity of ICH.[5,8,27] The early mortality rate within 30 days in ICH patients, however, varied from 13% to 56% among some studies (Table 17-2),[2,10,12–14,26–33] a fact that is probably a reflection of differences in study design, race, or country, and the medical backgrounds of subjects in the studies.

Death from ICH occurs most frequently within the first several days. Early death within the first week accounted for 53–82% of 30-day mortality and usually results from transtentorial or tonsillar herniation secondary to the hematoma itself and brain edema.[27,30] Early mortality and morbidity can be predicted by the volume of the hematoma on CT and initial neurologic severity (level of consciousness).[10,28,29,34]

Increased understanding of the etiologies and sites of ICH has been particularly emphasized in the United States.[9,35,36] In a study by Brott et al.,[35] 50% or more of the cases were not related to chronic hypertension, and these ICHs occurred most frequently in the subcortex (47%). The relative frequency of nonhypertensive ICH varies from 25% to 50%, depending on the site of ICH.

Medical Therapy

General Management

Each patient with ICH should be managed according to the location, size, and potential mechanism of hematoma, and the patient's age, BP, and underlying illness and complications. Many patients with ICH are best managed in an intensive care unit or stroke unit.

Emergency Procedures

Appropriate maintenance of the airway, breathing, BP, and heart rate must be achieved before establishing the diagnosis of ICH. Patients with a deeply depressed level of consciousness or abnormal breathing, such as ataxic respiration, need endotracheal intubation to avoid asphyxia and systemic hypoxia. Prophylactic intubation is recommended in patients with frequent vomiting or dysphagia to avoid potential aspiration and asphyxia. Supplemental oxygen may be given to maintain arterial oxygen saturation above 90–95%. A venous route must be secured for parenteral supply of water, electrolytes, and nutrition, and for delivering pharmacologic agents.

Hydration and Nutrition

Patients are often unable to complain about thirst or to take sufficient amounts of water and food because of consciousness disturbance, nausea and vomiting, or dysphagia. For such patients, 1,600–2,200 ml per day of water should be given intravenously or through a gastric tube. The volume of water may be increased if the patient has experienced excessive loss of water, such as with hyperthermia, hyperhidrosis, diarrhea, and vomiting. If the patient has already developed dehydration, it should be gradually corrected over several days. Overhydration should be avoided, because it worsens brain edema and may cause heart failure. Hyponatremia is likely to accelerate the development of brain edema. To maintain an appropriate electrolyte balance, patients should be given 50–70 mEq of sodium and 40–50 mEq of potassium daily. At least 75–100 g of carbohydrate should be given daily to prevent metabolic acidosis.

Management of Hypertension

Acute ICH is frequently accompanied by significant increases in systemic BP, which is usually an acceleration of pre-existing hypertension by stress, a response to acute increases in intracranial pressure (ICP) by the hematoma or brain edema (Cushing's phenomenon), or both. Terayama et al.[12] analyzed 1,701 patients with ICH and reported that increases in mean BP and volume of hematoma on admission were related to increased mortality in putaminal and thalamic hemorrhage, but not in subcortical, cerebellar, and pontine hemorrhage. In a study by Fogelholm et al.,[37] the most important predictor of the 28-day survival in patients with supratentorial ICH was the level of consciousness on admission, followed by day 1 mean BP.

The best strategy to manage elevated BP during the first few days after stroke onset remains controversial. Hypertension may prolong the period of active bleeding and augment brain edema. Some authors recommend using antihypertensive agents to prevent hematoma expansion and reduce brain edema.[38]

A rapid drop in BP may, however, induce ischemia in regions around and, in some instances, distant from the hematoma, because cerebral autoregulation may be impaired in these regions within days and weeks after ICH. Brain tissues surrounding an acute hematoma have profound and extensive ischemia,[39] and a significant decrease in BP may produce tissue ischemia.[40–42]

Antihypertensive agents should not be used in patients with an acute ICH unless systolic BP is persistently higher than 180–200 mm Hg, an increase in hematoma volume or active bleeding is present, or the patient has an illness, such as congestive heart failure, requiring antihypertensive therapy. If the BP is to be reduced, it should be done cautiously, but not aggressively, with a short-acting hypotensive agent and intra-arterial BP monitoring. Antihypertensive agents with cerebral vasodilating activity, such as sodium nitroprusside, may induce further increases in ICP and, therefore, should be avoided. The authors prefer to use trimethaphan, a ganglion blocker, for controlling BP in acute ICH because it is short-acting and does not elevate ICP. Labetalol, a beta-adrenergic blocker, is an agent to be recommended in this situation.

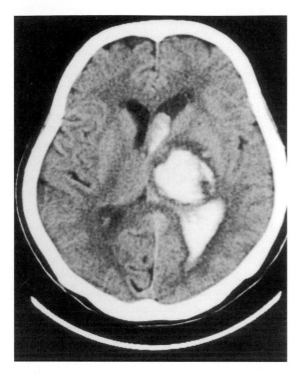

Figure 17-3. Brain edema on computed tomography scan in a 65-year-old woman with left thalamic hemorrhage. On day 2, the hematoma was surrounded by edema. Ventricular extension of the hemorrhage was also evident.

Calcium-channel blockers, such as nicardipine, may be effective when used carefully.

Medical Management of Nonhypertensive Intracerebral Hemorrhage

The treatment must be specified according to the underlying illness or condition in patients with nonhypertensive ICH.

Hemostatic Agents

If the patient has a coagulopathy, it must be reversed as soon as possible. Fresh frozen plasma and vitamin K should be used for patients on warfarin therapy. Effects of heparin can be neutralized by an intravenous infusion of protamine. Protamine and epsilon-aminocaproic acid may be recommended for ICH patients on thrombolytic agents. Patients with a deficiency of a specific coagulation factor, such as hemophilia, must receive their deficient fac-

tor or fresh plasma. These measures help to prevent a further increase in hematoma volume, recurrence of ICH, and other systemic complications.

Platelet Transfusion

Patients with platelet disorders, such as leukemia or aplastic anemia, should receive a platelet transfusion. Patients on aspirin or other antiplatelet agents should stop taking the agents but do not need platelet transfusion.

Withdrawal from a Particular Agent

Some studies suggest that ICH in young patients is often attributed to the abuse of illicit and prescription drugs, including methamphetamine, phenylpropanolamine, cocaine, phencyclidine, pentazocine-pyribenzamine (Talwin-pyribenzamine), or methylphenidate. If such a drug can be identified, the patient should be withdrawn from the agent.

Treatment for Brain Edema and Intracranial Hypertension

Brain edema begins to develop in the brain tissues surrounding the hematoma within the first several hours after ICH (Figure 17-3). A hematoma combined with brain edema causes compression of the surrounding brain structures and elevation of ICP and may cause transtentorial or tonsillar herniation, the most serious consequence after ICH. The majority of acute deaths within the first days after stroke onset result from these processes. Extensive brain edema with increased ICP may cause secondary brain damage. To minimize these hazards, treatment of brain edema should be initiated immediately after admission.

Corticosteroids

Corticosteroids are widely used for reducing brain edema in patients with brain tumors, abscesses, and so forth. However, they are contraindicated to acute ICH patients because clinical trials failed to prove beneficial effects with corticosteroids on ICH.[43] The use of corticosteroids often results in complications, such as infection and deterioration of diabetes mellitus.

Hyperosmolar Agents

Hyperosmolar agents, such as mannitol and glycerol, are potential agents for reducing brain edema. A 20% solution of mannitol given intravenously (5 to 15 ml/kg body weight in 10 to 30 ml/minute) often induces rapid but transient decrease in raised ICP. The agent causes systemic hypervolemia, followed by remarkable diuresis. Attention should be paid to avoiding acute cardiac failure, dehydration, and electrolyte imbalance. Rebound increase in ICP may occur hours after the administration of the agent.

A 10% solution of glycerol in saline (200 ml in 2 hours two to four times daily) acts more slowly and mildly than mannitol. Sasaki et al.[44] demonstrated that intravenous infusion of 200 ml of 10% glycerol over 30 minutes significantly increased cerebral blood flow in the affected hemisphere of patients with acute ICH. Hemodilution and a reduction in raised ICP after glycerol administration were probably attributable to the clinical effects. A randomized clinical trial, however, failed to demonstrate benefits from the agent in patients with ICH as judged by 6-month outcome.[45] Further investigations are needed to establish benefits and limitations of hyperosmolar agents in acute ICH.

Other Therapies

Hyperventilation or barbiturate administration reduces ICP through diffuse vasoconstriction of the brain. A tris-hydroxy-methyl-aminomethane buffer can be infused through a central venous catheter to control elevated ICP. This approach requires frequent ICP measurement and blood gas analyses. These strategies are not popular but may be useful for ICH patients with severe brain edema if they are scheduled to undergo surgical intervention or are carefully managed in an intensive care unit or operating room.

Management of Complications

Infection

ICH is often complicated by respiratory and urinary tract infection. Body postures should be changed at appropriate intervals to prevent pneumonia and bedsores. An indwelling catheter into the bladder is needed in patients with a decreased level of con-sciousness, and the bladder must be irrigated at regular intervals. When infections are suspected, antibiotic therapy is recommended, preferably after a determination of pathogenic microorganisms.

Gastrointestinal Bleeding

Gastrointestinal bleeding is another important complication in acute ICH patients, particularly with massive hematoma and ventricular hemorrhage. In a previous study with endoscopic examination, more than one-half of acute ICH patients had erosion, petechial bleeding, or ulceration of the stomach. Use of histamine H_2-channel blockers has dramatically reduced the incidence and severity of this complication.

Syndrome of Inappropriate Secretion of Antidiuretic Hormone

Clinicians should watch for the syndrome of inappropriate secretion of antidiuretic hormone, which is not rare in patients with acute ICH. The syndrome is characterized by an excess of sodium excretion into urine associated with low plasma concentration. Although hyponatremia may exacerbate brain edema, correction should be made gradually by restricting the water intake (500–700 ml daily) or loading salt (9–12 g daily), and if necessary, with furosemide administration. Rapid normalization of the plasma sodium concentration may induce serious complications, such as central pontine myelinolysis.

Convulsions

Some investigators recommend the routine use of anticonvulsants for ICH patients. Convulsive seizures after acute ICH, however, are not frequently encountered except for subcortical (or lobar) hemorrhages and massive hematomas with ventricular extension. If a convulsion occurs, 5–20 mg of diazepam or 15–20 mg/kg of phenytoin should be given intravenously. Evidence of respiratory suppression or hypotension caused by the infusion should be carefully monitored.

Surgical Therapy

It is a reasonable concept that brain damage due to ICH may be minimized by removal of the hematoma

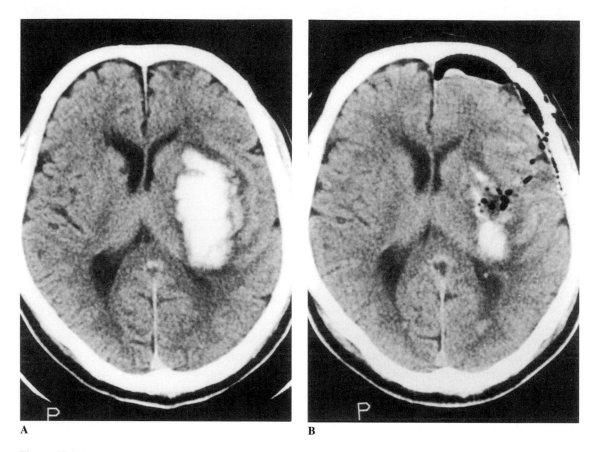

A   B

Figure 17-4. Surgical evacuation of massive putaminal hemorrhage in a 54-year-old man. **(A)** In the presurgical computed tomography (CT) scan taken 5 hours after stroke onset, the estimated volume of hematoma was 40 ml, with compression of the ventricular system and midline structures. The patient was semicomatose. **(B)** In the CT scan taken on the day after surgical evacuation, the mass effects by the hematoma were dramatically decreased. On day 60, the patient was transferred to a rehabilitation hospital with moderate disability.

(Figure 17-4). Evacuation of hematoma followed by craniotomy has been evaluated for many years. Needle aspiration of hematomas by a CT-guided stereotaxic technique has been investigated. This method is less invasive and therefore more promising than open hematoma evacuation. Although hematoma evacuations are performed frequently around the world (e.g., >7,000/year in the United States),[46] definite indications for these surgical therapies remain unestablished.

Evacuation of Hematoma

Earlier experiences demonstrated that surgical evacuation can be successful. In the first controlled trial by McKissock et al.,[47] no benefit from surgical evacuation was demonstrated in regard either to mortality or morbidity. Similar results were also reported in prospective randomized studies in a small number of patients with supratentorial ICH.[48,49] A meta-analysis of three randomized controlled trials of open craniotomy and one trial of endoscopic evacuation for supratentorial ICH indicated a nonsignificant increase in odds of death and dependency at 6 months for patients treated surgically.[50]

Some single-center and multicenter, randomized pilot trials of early hematoma removal in ICH patients were conducted (n = 34 or 20).[51,52] The studies demonstrated the trend toward better outcome with hematoma evacuation. An ongoing, large-scale, multicenter, randomized study is testing the effects of early surgical evacuation of ICH on mortality and morbidity at 6 months.[53]

Putaminal Hemorrhage

Kanaya[34] reported the result of a retrospective cooperative study in which data of 3,638 patients with putaminal hemorrhage treated surgically and 3,372 treated medically were compared. Patients were subdivided into several groups according to their presurgical consciousness level (neurologic grading), CT findings (CT classification), and hematoma volume. After comparing the mortality and morbidity in each subgroup, surgical treatment was recommended if the hematoma was larger than 30 ml in extent and the level of consciousness was somnolent to semicomatose (Table 17-3). This guideline for surgical therapy was introduced in the English literature.[54]

The results of this study have been criticized, however, mainly because of the lack of prospective randomized comparisons. In nonrandomized comparative studies performed in Japan, surgical evacuation of putaminal hemorrhage did not give better results than medical management.[55,56] In patients with mild to moderate severity, overall outcome was significantly better in the medical treatment group than in the surgical treatment group. Mortality in patients with severe neurologic deficits was better, but functional outcome was worse in the surgical treatment group.[56]

Cerebellar Hemorrhage

Cerebellar hemorrhage is often a surgical emergency. McKissok et al.[57] demonstrated that evacuation of cerebellar hematoma resulted in excellent outcome, and ventricular drainage alone was rather dangerous in these patients. Large cerebellar hematomas often cause lethal conditions due to brain stem compression and upward herniation. The surgery should be performed immediately after the diagnosis and the surgical indication is established, because the outcome is clearly related to the preoperative level of consciousness and to the timing of the surgery. The consensus is that patients should be promptly examined with CT when cerebellar hemorrhage is suspected, and a hematoma larger than 3 cm in diameter should be

Table 17-3. Recommendation of Surgical Evacuation or Aspiration

Site of Hematoma	Conditions	Indication
Putamen	Alert, hematoma ≤30 ml	–
	Hematoma volume >30 ml	±
	Deep coma	–
Thalamus		–
Subcortex	Young, progressive deficits	±
	Advanced age	–
Pons		–
Cerebellum	Hematoma >3 cm diameter	+

+ = surgical therapy recommended; ± = questionable; – = not recommended.

evacuated (see Table 17-3). Patients with a smaller hematoma without progressive neurologic deterioration and signs of brain stem compression can be treated medically but should be carefully observed to detect unpredictable deterioration during the first week. Even patients in deep coma may recover almost fully without significant deficits if the brain stem compression is promptly relieved by surgery.

Other Types of Intracerebral Hemorrhages

Patients with subcortical (or lobar) hemorrhage can be treated medically. Surgical evacuation may be recommended if the patient is young and has progressive neurologic deterioration (Figure 17-5).[58] Surgical interventions for CAA-related ICH have the potential of triggering recurrent hemorrhage, although this concept has been challenged by some clinical studies.[59] Surgical evacuation is not recommended for patients with thalamic and pontine hemorrhage.

Stereotaxic Aspiration

Needle aspiration of a hematoma was proposed as early as the 1930s. Backlund and von Holst[60] reported their successful experiences of subtotal evacuation of hematoma by a CT-guided stereotaxic technique. Its primary objective is decompression and reduction of increased ICP. The technique is easier to perform and less invasive than the conventional evacuation method and, therefore, may be more promising. The technique has been greatly

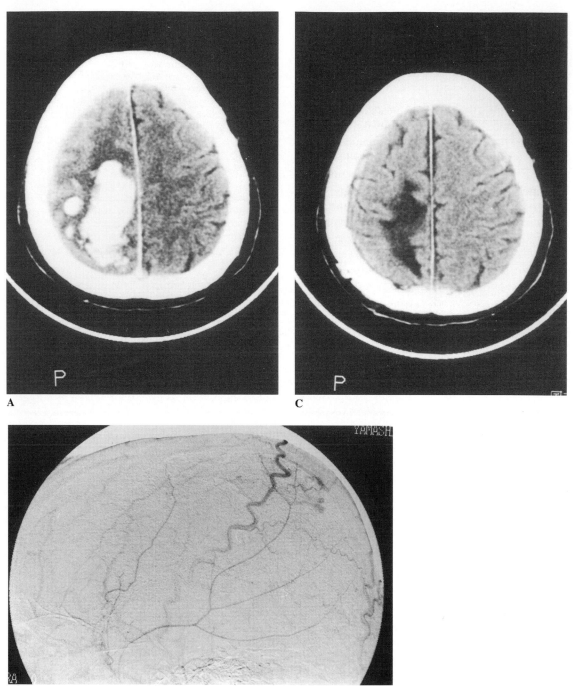

Figure 17-5. A subcortical hemorrhage in a 60-year-old man without hypertension. **(A)** On the day of stroke onset, a computed tomography (CT) scan demonstrated a right parietal hemorrhage. The patient had progressive neurologic deterioration with hematoma enlargement. **(B)** An emergency cerebral angiographic examination revealed a dural arteriovenous fistula (dural AVF) in the parietal cortex, fed by the right superficial temporal and occipital arteries and drained to the superior sagittal sinus. The hematoma was evacuated and the dural AVF was removed. **(C)** A CT scan after surgery. On day 58, the patient was transferred to a rehabilitation hospital with moderate disability.

improved by combining it with fibrinolytic agents,[61] modifications of needles, increased number of tracks, and endoscopic approaches.[62–65] An increase in the incidence of rebleeding after the aspiration, however, has been suggested.

In a collaborative study in Japan,[34] overall mortality rate in 811 ICH patients treated with stereotaxic aspiration was not significantly different from that in 2,561 patients treated with conventional evacuation. However, lower mortality with aspiration was observed in patients with no or mild disturbance in consciousness (aspiration 3% vs. evacuation 11%, P <.001), or in patients with hematoma of 11–50 ml in volume. Functional outcome was also better in the aspiration group if the patient's preoperative consciousness was normal or stuporous. Although the study was not performed in a randomized fashion, the data suggest the superiority of the aspiration technique over the conventional evacuation approach as a surgical therapy for patients with mild to moderate ICH.

Other Surgical Therapies

Acute hydrocephalus may develop in some ICH patients, particularly those with ventricular hemorrhage or ventricular compression by hematoma. In such patients, emergency ventricular drainage may be required.

Prevention of Recurrence

Earlier studies suggested that hypertensive ICH rarely rebleeds. Some clinical studies, however, indicated that rebleeding after the first ICH is not uncommon.[66,67] In a previous study by Hashimoto et al.[33] in 169 survivors with hypertensive ICH, recurrent hemorrhage was found to be not so rare, with a recurrence rate of 2.9% per year. BP remained uncontrolled in the majority of patients who experienced recurrent ICH.

Chronic hypertension should be treated in survivors with ICH. Irie et al.[68] reported that ICH patients with lower poststroke BP had less frequent recurrent strokes. The type of recurrent stroke in ICH patients receiving antihypertensive agents was usually ischemic. This observation was supported by a study by Arakawa et al.[69]

Subcortical (lobar) hemorrhage due to CAA often recurs over a period of months or years and may develop at multiple sites. Head trauma and prior neurosurgical procedures may precede the onset of CAA-related ICH.

References

1. Sivenius J, Heinonen OP, Pyorala J, et al. The incidence of stroke in the Kupio area of east Finland. Stroke 1985;16: 188–192.
2. Foulkes MA, Wolf PA, Price TR, et al. The Stroke Data Bank: design, methods, and baseline characteristics. Stroke 1988;19:547–554.
3. Massaro AR, Sacco RL, Mohr JP, et al. Clinical discriminators of lobar and deep hemorrhages: the Stroke Data Bank. Neurology 1991;41:1881–1885.
4. Suzuki K, Kutsuzawa T, Takita K, et al. Clinico-epidemiologic study of stroke in Akita, Japan. Stroke 1987;18: 402–406.
5. Ueda K, Hasuo Y, Kiyohara Y, et al. Intracerebral hemorrhage in a Japanese community, Hisayama: incidence, changing pattern during long-term follow-up, and related factors. Stroke 1988;19:48–52.
6. Kay R, Woo J, Kreel L, et al. Stroke subtypes among Chinese living in Hong Kong: the Shatin Stroke Registry. Neurology 1992;42:985–987.
7. Omae T, Ueda K. Hypertension and cerebrovascular disease: the Japanese experience. J Hypertens 1988;6:343–349.
8. Tanaka Y, Furuse M, Iwasa H, et al. Lobar intracerebral hemorrhage: etiology and a long-term follow-up study of 32 patients. Stroke 1986;17:51–57.
9. Kase CS. Intracerebral hemorrhage: nonhypertensive causes. Stroke 1986;17:590–595.
10. Daverat P, Castel JP, Dartigues JF, Orgogozo JM. Death and functional outcome after spontaneous intracerebral hemorrhage. A prospective study of 166 cases using multivariate analysis. Stroke 1991;22:1–6.
11. Yamaguchi T, Miyashita T, Minematsu K, et al. Incidence of thalamic infarction and hemorrhage, and their distribution in the thalamus (in Japanese with English abstract). Jpn J Stroke 1987;9:513–518.
12. Terayama Y, Tanahashi N, Fukuuchi Y, Gotoh F. Prognostic value of admission blood pressure in patients with intracerebral hemorrhage. Keio Cooperative Stroke Study. Stroke 1997;28:1185–1188.
13. Brott T, Broderick J, Kothari R, et al. Early hemorrhage growth in patients with intracerebral hemorrhage. Stroke 1997;28:1–5.
14. Fujii Y, Takeuchi S, Sasaki O, et al. Multivariate analysis of predictors of hematoma enlargement in spontaneous intracerebral hemorrhage. Stroke 1998;29:1160–1166.
15. Tapia JF, Kase CS, Sawyer RH, Mohr JP. Hypertensive putaminal hemorrhage presenting as pure motor hemiparesis. Stroke 1983;14:505–506.
16. Mori E, Tabuchi M, Yamadori A. Lacunar syndrome due to intracerebral hemorrhage. Stroke 1985;16:454–459.

17. Arboix A, Marti-Vilalta JL. Lacunar syndromes not due to lacunar infarcts. Cerebrovasc Dis 1992;2:287–292.

18. Drury I, Whisnant JP, Garraway WM. Primary intracerebral hemorrhage: impact of CT on incidence. Neurology 1984;34:653–657.

19. Sung CY, Chu NS. Late CT manifestations in spontaneous putaminal haemorrhage. Neuroradiology 1992;34:200–204.

20. Patel MR, Edelman RR, Warach S. Detection of hyperacute primary intraparenchymal hemorrhage by magnetic resonance imaging. Stroke 1996;27:2321–2324.

21. Gomori JM, Grossman RI, Goldberg HI, et al. Intracranial hematomas: imaging by high-field MR. Radiology 1985; 157:87–93.

22. Broderick JP, Brott TG, Tomsick T, et al. Ultra-early evaluation of intracerebral hemorrhage. J Neurosurg 1990;72: 195–199.

23. Fujii Y, Tanaka R, Takeuchi S, et al. Hematoma enlargement in spontaneous intracerebral hemorrhage. J Neurosurg 1994;80:51–57.

24. Kazui S, Naritomi H, Yamamoto H, et al. Enlargement of spontaneous intracerebral hemorrhage. Incidence and time course. Stroke 1996;27:1783–1787.

25. Kazui S, Minematsu K, Yamamoto H, et al. Predisposing factors to enlargement of spontaneous intracerebral hemorrhage. Stroke 1997;28:2370–2375.

26. Broderick JP, Phillips SJ, Whisnant JP, et al. Incidence rates of stroke in the eighties: the end of the decline in stroke? Stroke 1989;20:577–582.

27. Schuetz H, Dommer T, Boedeke R-H, et al. Changing pattern of brain hemorrhage during 12 years of computed axial tomography. Stroke 1992;23:653–656.

28. Tuhrim S, Dambrosia JM, Price TR, et al. Prediction of intracerebral hemorrhage survival. Ann Neurol 1988;24: 258–263.

29. Broderick JP, Brott T, Tomsick T, et al. Intracerebral hemorrhage more than twice as common as subarachnoid hemorrhage. J Neurosurg 1993;78:188–191.

30. Silver FL, Norris JW, Lewis AJ, Hachinski VC. Early mortality following stroke: a prospective review. Stroke 1984;15:492–496.

31. Garde A, Bohmer G, Selden B, Neiman J. 100 cases of spontaneous intracerebral hematoma. Diagnosis, treatment and prognosis. Eur Neurol 1983;22:161–172.

32. Kutsuzawa T. Recent trend in stroke: clinicoepidemiological analysis (in Japanese with English abstract). Jpn J Stroke 1987;9:473–480.

33. Hashimoto Y, Moriyasu H, Miyashita T, et al. Recurrence of hypertensive intracerebral hemorrhage (in Japanese with English abstract). Jpn J Stroke 1992;14:172–178.

34. Kanaya H. All Japan co-operative study on the treatment of hypertensive intracerebral hemorrhage (in Japanese). Jpn J Stroke 1990;12:509–524.

35. Brott T, Thalinger K, Hertzberg V. Hypertension as a risk factor for spontaneous intracerebral hemorrhage. Stroke 1986;17:1078–1083.

36. Caplan L. Intracerebral hemorrhage revisited. Neurology 1988;38:624–627.

37. Fogelholm R, Avikainen S, Murros K. Prognostic value and determinants of first-day mean arterial pressure in spontaneous supratentorial intracerebral hemorrhage. Stroke 1997;28:1396–1400.

38. Abdulrauf SI, Furlan AJ, Awad I. Primary intracerebral hemorrhage and subarachnoid hemorrhage. J Stroke Cerebrovasc Dis 1999;8:146–150.

39. Mendelow AD. Mechanisms of ischemic brain damage with intracerebral hemorrhage. Stroke 1993;24(Suppl I): I115–I117.

40. Strandgaard S, Olesen J, Skinhoj JE, Lassen NA. Autoregulation of brain circulation in severe hypertension. BMJ 1973;1:507–510.

41. Kawakami H, Kutsuzawa T, Uemura K, et al. Regional cerebral blood flow in patients with intracerebral hemorrhage. Stroke 1974;5:207–212.

42. Kaneko T, Sawada T, Niimi T, et al. Lower limit of blood pressure in treatment of acute hypertensive intracranial hemorrhage (AHCH). J Cereb Blood Flow Metabol 1983; 3(Suppl 1):S51–S52.

43. Poungvarin N, Bhoopat W, Viriyavejakul A, et al. Effects of dexamethasone in primary supratentorial intracerebral hemorrhage. N Engl J Med 1987;316:1229–1233.

44. Sasaki T, Matsuzaki T, Nakagawara J, et al. Improvement of CBF by glycerol administration in hypertensive intracerebral hemorrhage. Brain Nerve (Tokyo) 1983;35:505–510.

45. Yu YL, Kumana CR, Lauder IJ, et al. Treatment of acute cerebral hemorrhage with intravenous glycerol. A double-blind, placebo-controlled, randomized trial. Stroke 1992; 23:967–971.

46. Fayad PB, Awad IA. Surgery for intracerebral hemorrhage. Neurology 1998;51(Suppl 3):S69–S73.

47. McKissock W, Richardson A, Taylor J. Primary intracerebral hemorrhage. A controlled trial of surgical and conservative treatment in 180 unselected cases. Lancet 1961;2:221–226.

48. Juvela S, Heiskanen O, Poranen A, et al. The treatment of spontaneous intracerebral hemorrhage. A prospective randomized trial of surgical and conservative treatment. J Neurosurg 1989;70:755–758.

49. Batrjer HH, Reisch JS, Allen BC, et al. Failure of surgery to improve outcome in hypertensive putaminal hemorrhage. A prospective randomized trial. Arch Neurol 1990; 47:1103–1106.

50. Hankey GJ, Hon C. Surgery for primary intracerebral hemorrhage: is it safe and effective? A systematic review of case series and randomized trials. Stroke 1997;28: 2126–2132.

51. Morgenstern LB, Frankowski RF, Shedden P, et al. Surgical treatment for intracerebral hemorrhage (STICH): a single-center, randomized clinical trial. Neurology 1998;51:1359–1363.

52. Zuccarello M, Brott T, Derex L, et al. Early surgical treatment for supratentorial intracerebral hemorrhage: a randomized feasibility study. Stroke 1999;30:1833–1839.

53. Major ongoing trials: Surgical Trial in Intracerebral Hemorrhage (STICH). Stroke 1999;30:490.

54. Kaufman HH. Treatment of deep spontaneous intracerebral hemorrhage. Stroke 1993;24(Suppl I):I101–I106.

55. Waga S, Miyazaki M, Okada M, et al. Hypertensive putaminal hemorrhage: analysis of 182 patients. Surg Neurol 1986;26:159–166.

56. Gotoh F. Comparison of conservative treatment and surgical treatment for hypertensive putaminal hemorrhage in 819 cases. Keio Cooperative Stroke Study (in Japanese with English abstract). Jpn J Stroke 1990;12:493–500.

57. McKissock W, Richardson A, Walsh L. Spontaneous cerebellar haemorrhage. A study of 34 consecutive cases treated surgically. Brain 1960;83:1–9.

58. Maiuri F, Corriero G, Passarelli F, et al. CT indications for surgery and evaluation of prognosis in patients with spontaneous intracerebral haematomas. Br J Neurosurg 1990; 12:509–515.

59. Izumihara A, Ishihara T, Iwamoto N, et al. Postoperative outcome of 37 patients with lobar intracerebral hemorrhage related to cerebral amyloid angiopathy. Stroke 1999;30:29–33.

60. Backlund EO, von Holst H. Controlled subtotal evacuation of intracerebral hematomas by stereotactic technique. Surg Neurol 1978;9:99–101.

61. Wagner KR, Xi G, Hua Y, et al. Ultra-early clot aspiration after lysis with tissue plasminogen activator in a porcine model of intracerebral hemorrhage: edema reduction and blood-brain barrier protection. J Neurosurg 1999;90: 491–498.

62. Matsumoto K, Hondo H. CT-guided stereotaxic evacuation of hypertensive intracerebral hematomas. J Neurosurg 1984;61:440–448.

63. Kandel EI, Peresedov V. Stereotaxic evacuation of spontaneous intracerebral hematomas. J Neurosurg 1985;62: 206–213.

64. Niizuma H, Suzuki J. Stereotaxic aspiration of putaminal hemorrhage using a double track aspiration technique. Neurosurgery 1988;22:432–436.

65. Niizuma H, Shimizu Y, Yonemitsu T, et al. Results of stereotactic aspiration in 175 cases of putaminal hemorrhage. Neurosurgery 1989;24:814–819.

66. Gonzalez-Duarte A, Cantu C, Ruiz-Sandoval JL, Barinagarrementeria F. Recurrent primary cerebral hemorrhage: frequency, mechanisms, and prognosis. Stroke 1998;29: 1802–1805.

67. Hill MD, Silver FL, Austin PC, Tu JV. Rate of stroke recurrence in patients with primary intracerebral hemorrhage. Stroke 2000;31:123–127.

68. Irie K, Yamaguchi T, Minematsu K, Omae T. The J-curve phenomenon in stroke recurrence. Stroke 1993; 24:1844–1849.

69. Arakawa S, Saku Y, Ibayashi S, et al. Blood pressure control and recurrence of hypertensive brain hemorrhage. Stroke 1998;29:1806–1809.

Chapter 18
Subarachnoid Hemorrhage

John P. Weaver

Subarachnoid hemorrhage (SAH) from the rupture of an intracranial aneurysm can be a devastating neurologic disorder. Morbidity, mortality, and financial costs associated with the disease remain high despite advances in diagnostic imaging, medical management, and surgical intervention in the disease. This chapter reviews patient intensive care management and treatments of saccular aneurysms, without in-depth discussion of other types of aneurysms or surgical techniques.

Epidemiology

Demographics and Incidence

Intracranial hemorrhage secondary to the rupture of saccular aneurysms accounts for 6–10% of all strokes and 22–25% of cerebrovascular deaths and is not rare in the general population. The incidence of incidental aneurysms reported in autopsy studies ranges from 0.2% to 18.0%, with multiple aneurysms noted in 15–20%.[1–4] Modern imaging technology by magnetic resonance angiography (MRA) has demonstrated a prevalence of 7% overall; 10.5% and 6.8% in subgroups with and without family history, respectively. With regard to family history, women have a greater incidence of aneurysm than men (12.3% vs. 7.9%).[5] SAH occurs most frequently in the fifth and sixth decades of life, but can occur from adolescence to elderly age. SAH is also more common in females.

Mortality and morbidity rates after SAH have improved but remain significant, despite modern medical management and improvements in surgical techniques. Therefore, costs associated with SAH are high because of intensive medical and surgical intervention, rehabilitation, nursing care, and lost productivity. The International Cooperative Aneurysm Study showed that only 58% of patients who had an aneurysmal SAH returned to their premorbid state. Morbidity and mortality depended largely on the patient's age, the severity of the initial hemorrhage, rebleeding, cerebral vasospasm, and surgical complications.[6] An epidemiologic study of SAH in Finland reported an incidence of 33 out of 100,000 per year among men and 25 out of 100,000 per year among women; the fatality rate was 35% among men and 33% among women within 2 days of the ictus and 48% and 46%, respectively, at 1 month.[7] Finland, the United States, and Japan had the highest incidence of SAH among industrialized nations reviewed, whereas New Zealand had the lowest incidence. In a prospective study of 325 patients presenting with aneurysmal SAH in Sweden during a 1-year period, 56% made a good neurologic recovery, 23% experienced some morbidity, and 21% were dead at follow-up between 3 and 6 months. A subgroup of patients in the study had good Hunt and Hess grades (I–III), aneurysms in favorable supratentorial locations, and were operated on within 72 hours of SAH. In this subgroup, 81% made a good recovery, and unfavorable outcome was ascribed to delayed ischemia.[8] If the medical and surgical course of SAH is uncomplicated, patients can have an excellent outcome.[9,10]

Cognitive Outcome

Patients who survive SAH may have persistent cognitive problems with memory, the most common significant impairment.[11] There is a significant correlation between findings on computed tomography (CT) with deficits related to the affected arterial distribution. Damage to the anterior communicating artery (ACoA) perforating branches frequently cause severe amnestic deficits, memory problems, and personality changes.[12] The severity of SAH as demonstrated by CT correlates with poor performance on testing of memory, concentration, divided attention, and perseveration, especially with dominant brain injury. Nondominant injuries may cause poor visuoconstructional abilities; mesial frontal injury affects memory. Acute hydrocephalus, intraventricular hemorrhage, and frontal hematomas are also associated with cognitive deficits and exacerbate executive dysfunction more than SAH alone.[13]

Economic Impact

National Hospital Survey data served as the basis for analyzing the public health perspective of aneurysmal SAH in the United States. A tremendous lifetime cost for annual cases of patients hospitalized with aneurysmal SAH was documented.[14] This cost included direct costs of hospitalization and surgery, disability, and lost income from morbidity and mortality (stratified by age). The estimated lifetime costs for patients hospitalized with unruptured aneurysms was approximately one-third the overall cost for patients with SAH ($522,500,000 vs. $1,755,600,000). The comparison with unruptured aneurysms was based on an incidence of 5% in the general population and a rupture rate of 2% per year.

The cost-effectiveness of screening for unruptured aneurysms by high-resolution magnetic resonance imaging (MRI) is highly related to aneurysm rupture rate. If the rate is as low as 0.005, as published by the International Study of Unruptured Intracranial Aneurysms study, then screening asymptomatic populations to avoid the cost and medical risks of unruptured aneurysms may not be cost-effective.[15] However, the screening cost of MRA has been favorably compared to the 2.9% annual cost of screening mammography or the cumulative cost of treating one patient with aneurysm rupture.[16,17]

Pathogenesis

Saccular or berry aneurysms are distinguished from other types of intracerebral aneurysms, such as traumatic, dissecting, mycotic, and tumor-related aneurysms. Saccular aneurysms are characterized by a vascular wall lacking the normal muscular media and elastic lamina layers. Normal intracerebral vessels have a prominent muscular media layer, although the external elastic lamina is only found in extracranial vessels.[18]

Common sites for aneurysm formation are at the junction of the anterior cerebral artery (ACA) and ACoA, the junction of the posterior communicating artery (PCoA) and internal carotid artery (ICA), the middle cerebral artery (MCA) bifurcation, and the top of the basilar artery. Some 12–31% of patients have multiple aneurysms, which occurr more frequently when there is a familial incidence of aneurysms.[19] Multiple aneurysms may be located at identical sites bilaterally. The most common location of these mirror aneurysms is the MCA bifurcation.[20] Other sites, in order of lessening frequency, are PCoA, ICA, and ACA aneurysms. Rupture is usually demonstrated from the largest or most irregularly shaped aneurysm. Figure 18-1A demonstrates a case in which a woman in her 60s had an SAH resulting from the rupture of a large basilar apex aneurysm. A total of nine aneurysms were noted on her angiogram, including bilateral MCA and PCoA aneurysms. Figures 18-1B and 18-1C demonstrate multiple ICA and MCA aneurysms in the left and right carotid circulations, respectively.

Although larger aneurysms have a greater risk of rupture, most aneurysms that rupture are found to be small (<10 mm in diameter). Difference in histology between small and large aneurysm, including hyalinization and smooth muscle formation found primarily in small aneurysms, may affect the rupture risk.[21]

Aneurysms are also associated with arteriovenous malformations (AVMs), presumably due to chronically increased blood flow, and are usually located on afferent arteries supplying the AVM.[22,23]

Pathogenesis of Saccular Aneurysms

The pathogenesis of saccular aneurysms and the cause of subsequent rupture is uncertain. There is continued controversy over whether aneurysms are

Figure 18-1. (A) A woman in her 60s experienced subarachnoid hemorrhage from rupture of a large basilar apex aneurysm. **(B)** An anteroposterior view of the left common carotid injection (*arrows*).

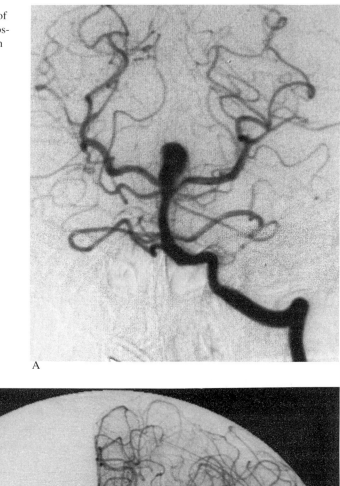

A

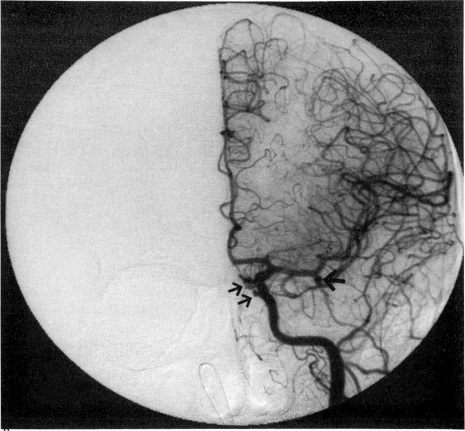

B

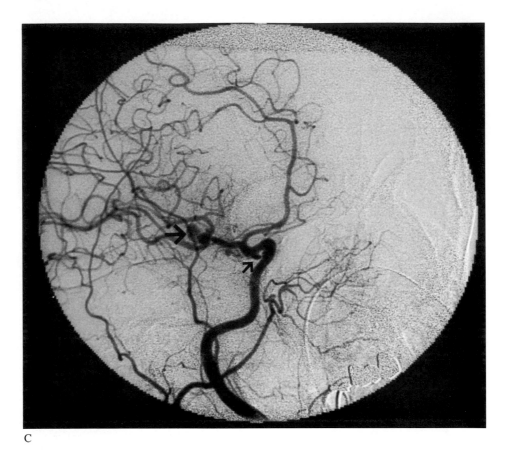

C

Figure 18-1. (*Continued*) (**C**) An oblique view of the right common carotid injection demonstrates multiple aneurysms (*arrow*) in a patient with bilateral middle cerebral artery and posterior communicating artery aneurysms.

congenital or acquired and to what extent environmental factors are involved. The congenital or medial defect hypothesis states that there is an arterial wall weakness due to maldevelopment. This hypothesis is supported by the frequency of multiple aneurysms, familial occurrence of aneurysms, and the association of aneurysms with AVMs and other systemic inherited disease.[24] Development of de novo aneurysms, which can occur in familial aneurysms, suggests a genetic factor influencing the development of new aneurysms rather than degenerative atherosclerotic mechanisms.[25] Alternatively, the degenerative theory suggests an acquired defect in the vessel wall and is supported by the increased frequency of aneurysms with age, hypertension, smoking, lean body mass, and atherosclerosis. Hypertension and connective tissue disorders reduce vessel wall tensile strength and may be contributory rather than causal to aneurysm formation.[26] Furthermore, pathologic specimens reveal intimal changes, inflammatory response, calcification, and thrombosis within aneurysms. Combinations of maldevelopment and degeneration co-exist; however, no theory of saccular aneurysm formation and rupture has been uniformly accepted.[27,28]

Family History

There is a significant correlation and association with family history of aneurysmal SAH, multiple aneurysms, and rupture risk. Among patients with a family history of SAH, family members who are first- or second-degree blood relations have incidence rates higher than the incidence rate in the general population. The incidence of aneurysms in first-degree blood relations is only 4% for relatives of patients with sporadic SAH, with the risk highest for siblings. Diagnostic screening for other relatives is not necessary.[29,30]

Associated Systemic Disease

A large health survey in Finland evaluating risk factors for SAH demonstrated that smoking and hypertension were positively associated and body mass index inversely associated with the risk of SAH. The study found no associations between SAH and serum cholesterol, hematocrit, known coronary artery disease, or diabetes.[27] Both the Framingham and International Cooperative studies have also demonstrated associations with hypertension.[4,6] Systemic diseases, such as polycystic kidney, Marfan's syndrome, Ehlers-Danlos syndrome, pseudoxanthoma elasticum, fibromuscular dysplasia, sickle-cell disease, and coarctation of the aorta, are associated with an increased incidence of intracerebral aneurysms.[31–36] Broderick et al. reported that young and middle-aged blacks have significantly higher risks for SAH and intracerebral hemorrhage than whites.[37] Blacks had 2.1 times the risk of SAH than whites and 2.3 times the risk of intracerebral hemorrhage younger than the age of 75 years.

Clinical Presentation

Signs and Symptoms

The signs and symptoms of intracranial aneurysms result from their expansion or rupture. Aneurysmal expansion can lead to localized headache, facial pain, pupillary dilation from compression of the pupilloconstrictor fibers of the oculomotor nerve, paresis from brain stem compression, and visual field defects due to compression of the optic nerve or chiasm. Warning signs preceding major hemorrhage are present in 20% or more of patients and are usually headache attributed to minor leak or sentinel hemorrhage, but ischemic symptoms have also been suggested. Sixty-two percent of warning signs occur within 1 month and 92% within 3 months before a major hemorrhage. These signs include headache, dizziness, visual or oculomotor disturbances, nausea and vomiting, transitory sensory or motor deficit, or both, and loss of consciousness.[38] Activities such as lifting, defecation, or sexual intercourse can cause elevated blood pressure (BP) and may predispose the patient to SAH. However, many ruptures occur during sleep or other nonspecific activity. Increased risk of SAH may also be associated with emotional lability and smoking. There is increased risk of SAH during

Table 18-1. Hunt and Hess Classification of Patients with Intracranial Aneurysms According to Surgical Risk

Category*	Criteria
Grade I	Asymptomatic, or minimal headache and slight nuchal rigidity
Grade II	Moderate to severe headache, nuchal rigidity, no neurologic deficit other than cranial nerve palsy
Grade III	Drowsiness, confusion, or mild focal deficit
Grade IV	Stupor, moderate to severe hemiparesis, possibly early decerebrate rigidity, and vegetative disturbances
Grade V	Deep coma, decerebrate rigidity, moribund appearance

*Serious systemic diseases, such as hypertension, diabetes, severe arteriosclerosis, chronic obstructive pulmonary disease, and severe vasospasm, result in placement of the patient in the next less favorable category.
Source: Adapted from WE Hunt, RM Hess. Surgical risk as related to time of intervention in the repair of intracranial aneurysms. J Neurosurg 1968;28:14–20.

pregnancy that may be associated with hypertension or albuminuria, or both, from which there is at least three times the risk of AVM hemorrhage, which usually occurs during the second trimester.[39]

Aneurysm rupture typically produces sudden severe headache, nuchal rigidity, back pain, nausea, vomiting, photophobia, and lethargy. At the time of rupture, 45% of patients lose consciousness, reflecting an acute rise in intracranial pressure (ICP) that may transiently equal or exceed mean arterial pressure. The elevation of ICP may result in an abducens nerve palsy, and funduscopy may demonstrate subhyaloid retinal hemorrhages and papilledema. Other symptoms, such as paresis, paresthesias, aphasia, visual hallucinations, vertigo, and ataxia, may also develop. Twenty-six percent of patients experience seizures after SAH, with the majority occurring shortly after bleeding. The occurrence of seizures has no relationship to the location of the aneurysm or the patient's prognosis and may reflect the acute rise in ICP.[40]

Clinical Grading and Prognosis

The clinical grading scale developed by Hunt and Hess is based on the presence or absence of neurologic deficits and significant associated diseases (Table 18-1).[41] The classifications of the clinical status correlate with surgical risk and prognosis. Treatment protocols are based on clinical grade to reduce the morbidity of rebleeding in good-grade patients and operation in poor-grade patients. The grading scale has proved to be a valuable guide in treatment, operative timing, and prognosis. Patients who are grade I or II at presentation have a relatively good prognosis, whereas grade IV or V patients have a poorer prognosis, and grade III patients are intermediate. The Glasgow Coma Scale is a clinical classification of brain injury that is reproducible, widely used, and a useful scoring tool when used in conjunction with the Hunt and Hess scale.

Diagnostic Evaluation

Computed Tomography

Noncontrast CT is the radiographic investigation of choice to identify, localize, and quantify the hemorrhage if SAH is suspected. The estimates of CT scan sensitivity for SAH vary with the series, but an initial scan may be negative in as many as 35% of patients with only a sentinel hemorrhage.[42] The distribution of SAH on a noncontrast CT study can occasionally suggest aneurysm location. Intraparenchymal hemorrhage occurs from PCoA and MCA aneurysm rupture more commonly than with other aneurysm locations. Interhemispheric and intraventricular extension of hemorrhage is characteristic of ACoA and some distal ACA aneurysms. The CT scan can also demonstrate abnormal ventricular size.

CT scans with intravenous contrast infusion and computer reformatted images can produce an angiographic image. Such a CT angiographic (CTA) image can demonstrate aneurysms larger than approximately 4 mm and can be useful if emergent operation is required and digital subtraction angiography (DSA) cannot be performed. Compared to DSA, CTA sensitivity and specificity for the detection of aneurysms has been reported to be 84–97% and 100%, respectively.[43,44] CTA may in many cases provide an accurate enough depiction of anatomic detail of the aneurysm and the surrounding vascular anatomy to proceed with surgery. It has the additional benefit of producing three-dimensional reconstructed images, which may assist surgical planning. However, most neurosurgeons rely on anatomic detail of DSA performed before surgery.

Lumbar Puncture

Lumbar puncture is indicated if the CT scan is nondiagnostic or is unavailable, the patient's neurologic examination is nonfocal, and the clinical history and presentation are convincing of SAH. Cerebrospinal fluid (CSF) will be xanthochromic in a centrifuged specimen if examined at least 2 hours after the initial hemorrhage. A traumatic puncture can yield bloody CSF and make the determination of SAH difficult, although the red blood cell count usually decreases in serial CSF samples, and xanthochromia is not usually apparent in spun specimens. Elevated opening pressure may reflect intracranial hypertension, fluid protein may be elevated, and glucose may be slightly depressed.

Magnetic Resonance Imaging and Angiography

Brain MRI and MRA are becoming more important in the evaluation of aneurysms because anatomic resolution has improved. Incidental aneurysms to approximately 4 mm are not uncommonly diagnosed (Figures 18-2A and 18-3A).[45] Because of the sensitivity to blood products, MRI may also be helpful in cases of multiple aneurysms in which the source of the hemorrhage is uncertain. MRA can provide a relatively high-quality diagnostic study, but it lacks the resolution of angiography, especially in the evaluation of the aneurysm neck and perforating arteries (see Figures 18-2B, 18-2C, and 18-3B).[45]

The resolution of MRA and MRI is good enough that these have become important and reliable examinations for screening first-degree relatives of patients with SAH for aneurysms or prospective follow-up of untreated or interventionally treated aneurysms.[46]

Cerebral Angiography

Cerebral angiography provides aneurysm localization with an image of the inner lumen. Angiography is used to determine the presence of multiple aneurysms, define the vascular anatomy and collateral circulation, and assess the degree of vasospasm. It is also the best way to evaluate the patient for AVMs or unusual vascular tumors that can also present with SAH.

A complete four-vessel angiogram is essential due to the frequency of multiple aneurysms and should be performed soon after admission if early surgery is contemplated. In approximately 15% of initial four-vessel angiograms, no aneurysm is identified.[47,48] A high index of suspicion for an occult aneurysm is based on CT finding when there is a dense focal clot or significant hemorrhage into the anterior interhemispheric fissure or sylvian fissure. If angiography does not reveal an aneurysm, it should be repeated in 2–3 weeks, as thrombus within the aneurysm or vasospasm that could interfere with angiographic visualization is usually resolved (Figure 18-4).[49,50] Insufficient examination of the posterior circulation may also explain why an aneurysm is not visualized. Only after subsequent negative angiography can other diagnoses be considered, such as trauma,

intracranial artery dissections, dural AVMs, mycotic aneurysms, trauma, bleeding disorders, substance abuse, or a cervical origin of hemorrhage. The patient without a detectable aneurysm has a good prognosis when the CT scan of a so-called "benign" SAH does not have a dense clot and shows a perimesencephalic pattern of hemorrhage.[47,48]

General Medical Management

The complications of SAH are fatal in 25% of cases, so the goal of medical management is to avoid these complications and provide the best situation for brain recovery from the neurologic insult. General medical

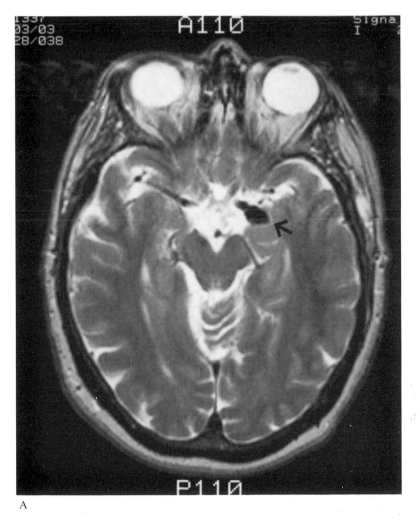

A

Figure 18-2. (A) An incidental left posterior communicating artery aneurysm is demonstrated by a second echo T2-weighted magnetic resonance image (*arrow*).

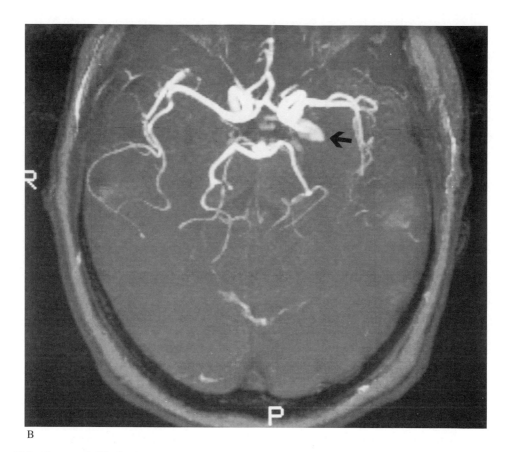

B

Figure 18-2. (*Continued*) **(B)** The three-dimensional magnetic resonance angiography image provides a clear image of the circle of Willis and also depicts the posterior communicating artery aneurysm (*arrow*). (A = anterior; P = posterior; R = right.) **(C)** A selective left internal carotid injection in subsequent conventional angiography shows the posterior communicating artery aneurysm and more details of the vascular anatomy. (Reprinted with permission from JP Weaver, M Fisher. Subarachnoid hemorrhage: an update of pathogenesis, diagnosis, and management. J Neurol Sci 1994;125:119–131.)

management to avoid aneurysm re-rupture includes quiet bed rest with subdued lighting to avoid patient stimulation and agitation. The head of the bed should be elevated to 30 degrees to facilitate intracranial venous drainage and provide good pulmonary toilet to avoid atelectasis and pneumonia. Bed rest requires prophylaxis against thrombophlebitis with pneumatic boots. All patients should receive stool softeners. Nausea and vomiting can be controlled with antiemetics other than phenothiazine derivatives. Pain control is best accomplished with analgesics, such as codeine or meperidine, so as not to mask changes in mental status. If necessary, sedation can be induced with diazepam or low doses of phenobarbital (30–60 mg q8h), which can also serve as an anticonvulsant.

The use of steroid therapy remains controversial; however, dexamethasone is often adminis-

tered, especially to poorer-grade patients with brain edema and intracranial hypertension. It may act as a brain protectant against further ischemic insult and as a blood-brain barrier stabilizer. Prophylactic antacids or H_2-blockers are administered with dexamethasone because its use further increases the risk of gastritis or gastrointestinal bleeding already present due to the stress of SAH.

Seizure Prophylaxis

Secondary epilepsy commonly complicates SAH and has a postoperative incidence of 4.5–27.5%.[51] Increased risk is associated with a history of seizures preoperatively, aneurysms in the MCA distribution, intraoperative temporary clipping, temporal lobe

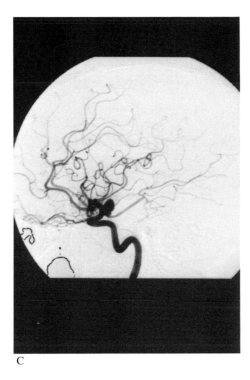
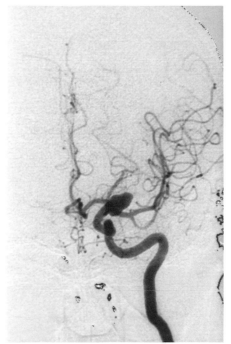

C

retraction, wrapping technique to treat the aneurysm, cortical lesions, and postoperative vasospasm, because ischemia can increase seizure risk.[52,53] Seizures can occur postoperatively even without SAH after surgery for unruptured intracranial aneurysms.

Although there is some controversy, most patients should receive anticonvulsant prophylaxis despite presentation in good neurologic condition.[54] Preoperative seizures can provoke aneurysm rupture and postoperatively complicate treatment of intracranial hypertension. Phenytoin is the preferred anticonvulsant because it is available as an intravenous preparation, which can be used in patients who have a depressed level of consciousness.

Intracranial Pressure Management

Elevated ICP is treated with hyperosmolar and diuretic therapy, with careful measurement of fluid balance, frequent evaluation of serum electrolytes and osmolarity, and central venous catheter monitoring. In poor-grade patients, an ICP-monitoring device is inserted so that intracranial hypertension can be measured. If possible, a ventriculostomy is the preferred method so that CSF drainage can be used as treatment.

Cardiac Complications

Electrocardiographic monitoring is important during the first few hours after SAH because hypothalamic dysfunction leads to cardiac dysrhythmias, due to excessive sympathetic stimulation in 20% of cases. This can cause subendocardial ischemia, focal areas of myocardial necrosis, and, subsequently, electrocardiographic changes, deterioration of cardiac indices, and pulmonary edema.[55] Increased levels of circulating catecholamines influence the alpha-receptors of the myocardium and can result in prolonged myofibril contraction, eventually causing myofibrillar degeneration and necrosis. Another theory suggests that coronary artery spasm is the mechanism for the myocytolysis; therefore, cautious use of nitrates or calcium channel blockers may be indicated in suspected cases.

Systolic BP greater than 180 mm Hg or a diastolic BP greater than 95 mm Hg should be treated, but agents that can depress consciousness, such as alpha-methyldopa, should be avoided. Hypertension can instead be managed with beta-blocking agents, which also reduce ventricular tachycardia and the risks of cardiac arrhythmias. The goal of treatment is not a normal BP; a systolic pressure between 120 mm Hg and 160 mm Hg and a diastolic pressure below 90 mm Hg is adequate. When cardiac arrhythmias occur, they respond well to sympathetic blocking agents, which may also have a subendocardial protective effect; however, there is no evidence that prophylactic administration of a beta-blocking agent alters the outcome in these patients.[56]

Syndrome of Inappropriate Antidiuretic Hormone

Another manifestation of hypothalamic dysfunction is the syndrome of inappropriate antidiuretic hormone with resultant hyponatremia. After SAH, there may be a salt-wasting diuresis due to an increase in circulating atrial natriuretic peptide levels. Accordingly, fluid input and output must be followed closely, along with serum electrolytes and osmolarity.[57]

Surgical Management

Surgical Timing and Patient Selection

The appropriate timing for surgical intervention remains controversial despite substantial investigation.[58] The findings of the International Cooperative Study on the Timing of Aneurysm Surgery are the most widely regarded by neurosurgeons.[9] There were no overall differences in outcome in patients operated on early (0–3 days post-SAH) or late (11–14 days post-SAH). Surgical mortality was higher with early surgery due to brain swelling, disturbed autoregulation, premature aneurysm rupture, hemorrhage, and the presence of tenacious clot surrounding the aneurysm and vessels.[59] Despite these difficulties, early clip ligation pre-

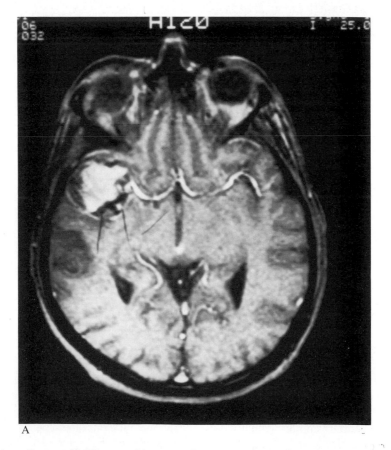

A

Figure 18-3. (A) A gradient-recalled flow-sensitive magnetic resonance image demonstrates a giant right middle cerebral artery aneurysm. Other images in the series suggested significant intraluminal thrombus within the aneurysm. **(B)** The three-dimensional magnetic resonance image reveals a large abnormality oriented toward the middle cerebral artery bifurcation consistent with a thrombosed aneurysm. (Reprinted with permission from JP Weaver, M Fisher. Subarachnoid hemorrhage: an update of pathogenesis, diagnosis, and management. J Neurol Sci 1994;125:119–131.)

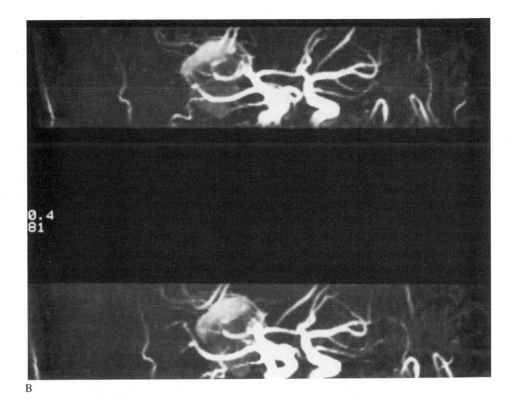

B

vents rebleeding and affords the opportunity to aggressively treat patients with hypertensive therapy should vasospasm subsequently occur. Patients who were alert preoperatively did well with early surgery, whereas those who were lethargic did better with delayed surgery. Surgery was most hazardous between days 7 and 10 due to the combined risks of rebleeding and vasospasm. Delaying surgery for 14 days was accompanied by a risk of rebleeding in 12% of patients and a focal ischemic deficit in 30%.

Current practice is for the patient with a grade I–III presentation to undergo microsurgical clip ligation within 48 hours of hemorrhage. Surgery for grade IV–V patients may be done early if ICP is normal or easily controlled, or may be delayed for 10–14 days. Advocates of early operative intervention for patients of a lower grade who are radiographically free of vasospasm point out that surgery reduces the risk of rebleeding and vasospasm.[60,61] Medical treatment only is offered for patients with elevated intracranial hypertension (ICP), poor brain stem function, or destruction of vital brain areas on CT.

Emergent surgical intervention is used in patients with an intracerebral clot causing significant mass effect. In these cases, the patient's neurologic status cannot tolerate further delay to surgical decompression, and angiography is sometimes bypassed.[62] Contrast CT or CTA can rapidly localize the aneurysm in many of these cases.[63] The surgical approach and evacuation of the hematoma is performed with careful consideration of the possible source of hemorrhage. Complete cerebral angiography must be performed postoperatively to evaluate the surgical result and identify other unruptured aneurysms.

General Principles

Modern neuroanesthetic techniques, use of the operating microscope, spinal CSF drainage, and temporary vessel occlusion are part of routine surgical management for clip occlusion of the aneurysm neck.[64,65] Mild systemic intraoperative hypotension is part of traditional neuroanesthetic practice to allow easier aneurysm neck dissection and reduce the risk of intraoperative rupture. There are significant additions to both the surgical and neuroanesthetic technique to allow for safer microdissection and brain protection from ischemia. Temporary occlusion of parent vessels with normal BP or induced hypertension is an alternative to hypotension during aneurysm dissection and clipping.[65] Methods to improve collateral circulation and protect potentially ischemic brain during temporary clip occlusion include hypertension, hypothermia, and medications that may have cytoprotective qualities.[66–69] Dilantin, decadron, mannitol, barbiturates, or barbiturate-acting drugs, such as etomidate and some neuroanesthetics, act as cytoprotective agents by stabilizing cellular membrane, improving cerebral blood flow (CBF) and rheology, or reducing oxygen consumption and metabolism ($CMRO_2$).[70]

Novel methods of intraoperative monitoring of brain metabolism can be performed by microelectrode recording on-line during aneurysm surgery. By monitoring brain tissue oxygen, CO_2, pH, and temperature, anesthetics, BP, and rheology can be adjusted to treat cortical ischemia, which may be secondary to brain swelling, temporary occlusion, hypotension, retraction, or hydrocephalus.[71–73]

Postoperative continuous cisternal CSF drainage is used to remove clot or bloody CSF and, by so doing, remove spasmogenic red blood cell degradation products. Although the intent is to reduce the incidence of vasospasm, higher incidence of vasospasm and hydrocephalus have been reported.[74]

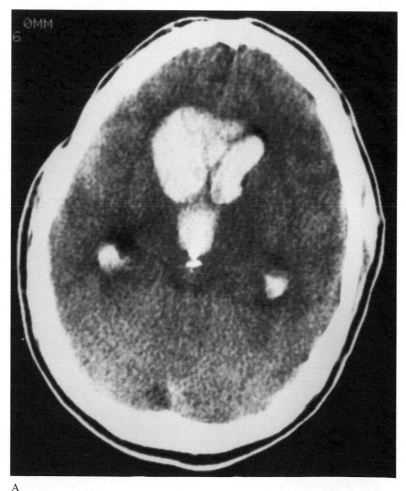

A

Figure 18-4. (A) A 39-year-old man enjoyed a good outcome from the previous rupture and surgical treatment of an anterior communicating artery aneurysm 9 years previous to his current presentation. This time he presents in coma, and computed tomography demonstrates ventriculomegaly and a large intraventricular hemorrhage consistent with rupture of an anterior cerebral artery aneurysm. **(B)** Angiograms performed acutely and again in 10 days after this rupture were normal. A follow-up study at 6 weeks showed a distal A2 aneurysm (*arrow*).

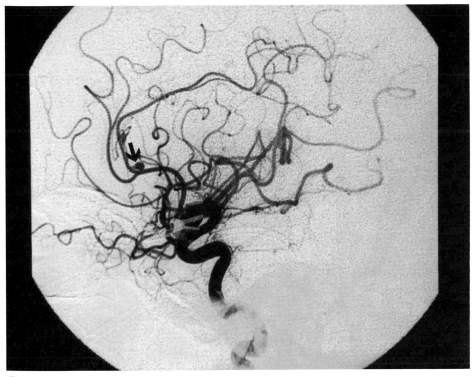

B

Giant and Complicated Aneurysms

More challanging aneurysms that dictate the use of specialized techniques include carotid cavernous and ophthalmic artery aneurysms, vertebral-basilar circulation aneurysms, and giant aneurysms (>25 mm).[75] Aneurysms with sessile or nonpedunculated bases may require external reinforcement or reconstruction of the parent vessel. Moreover, some giant aneurysms can be isolated from the intracerebral circulation by extracranial-intracranial microvascular bypass techniques. These can include superficial temporal artery to MCA bypass with subsequent trapping of a giant MCA aneurysm, saphenous vein graft from cervical to the intracranial ICA, or MCA with subsequent trapping of a giant paraclinoidal or ophthalmic artery aneurysm.[76–78] Common carotid ligation may continue to be an effective way to reduce intra-aneurysmal pressure, induce thrombosis, and reduce the occurrence of subsequent hemorrhage in certain aneurysms.[79] Various endovascular techniques are more common adjuncts to the surgical treatment of some giant aneurysms.[80,81]

Flexible and rigid endoscopes are used to demonstrate anatomic details of parts of the aneurysm and associated vessels not directly visualized through the microscope. Residual neck or inadvertent occlusion of distal vessels may be identified and the clip position readjusted.[82] Intraoperative angiography is another useful adjunct that may enhance the safety and efficacy of surgery.

Microvascular Doppler ultrasonography may also be used to assess patency of distal vessels. Aneurysm clip adjustment may be necessary to completely treat partially clipped aneurysms or restore patency of vessels with origin at the aneurysm neck.

Multiple and Unruptured Aneurysms

Multiple aneurysms are relatively common, especially in women. Their presence may be related to smoking history and sickle cell anemia and possibly chronic hypertension and AVMs.[5] Thoughtful treatment of multiple aneurysms includes issues of size, location, patient age and neurologic condition, anatomic relation to the ruptured aneurysm, the rupture rate based on location, and surgical timing.[83] The best surgical situation is when all aneurysms can be approached through a unilateral craniotomy in a single operation. In this case, one approach is to clip the deepest aneurysm first and work more superficially so that the clips do not obscure vision and cannot be caught under retractor blades. An alternative to this approach is to clip the ruptured or more difficult aneurysm first and treat the others secondarily.

Unruptured aneurysms are disclosed not only by angiography after SAH, but—perhaps with increasing frequency—as incidental findings by high-resolution CT or MRI. Other than their association with a ruptured aneurysm, unruptured aneurysms are discovered due to symptoms from mass effect (cranial nerve or brain stem compression), embolic stroke, and seizure.[84]

The natural history of unruptured intracranial aneurysms is better understood with the results of the International Study of Unruptured Intracranial Aneurysms. This study accrued 2,621 patients at 53 participating centers in the United States, Canada, and Europe, and included retrospective and prospective components. The risks of rupture and surgical intervention were evaluated to better understand the natural history of unruptured aneurysms and define optimal management. The study showed that the risk of aneurysm rupture for an aneurysm <10 mm in diameter without another associated ruptured aneurysm was <0.05% per year. With an associated ruptured aneurysm, the rupture rate was 0.5% per year. The rupture rate for giant (≥25 mm in diameter) aneurysms was 6%. Surgery-related morbidity and mortality was 17.5% without another aneurysm and 13.6% with an associated ruptured aneurysm. Hypertension, patient age, and aneurysmal location showed no significant correlation to annual growth rate or rupture rate.[15]

Controversy remains regarding the appropriate treatment of unruptured intracranial aneurysms. Some aggressive surgeons advocate surgical treatment of all aneurysms, regardless of size, if it is technically feasible and the patient's age and medical condition are not surgical contraindications. The cost of treating an unruptured aneurysm is low, and the outcome is better than ruptured aneurysms, at least for aneurysms >10 mm without an associated ruptured aneurysm.[85–91]

Thrombolytic Therapy

Fibrinolytic therapy to enhance the clearance of subarachnoid blood may reduce the amount of spasmogenic red blood cell degradation products, which probably contribute to the occurrence and severity of vasospasm. Recombinant tissue plasminogen activator can be applied in the cisternal spaces at surgery as well as postoperatively via a cisternal catheter. Results of clinical investigation using intracisternal application of recombinant tissue plasminogen activator are encouraging. The subarachnoid clot rapidly disappears by CT, and the treatment seems effective in reducing the incidence and severity of delayed vasospasm.[92–95]

Postoperative Management

Postoperative intensive care unit management is not dissimilar from preoperative management. It includes bed rest, head elevation, sequential compression boots, intravenous H_2-antagonists, anticonvulsant prophylaxis, corticosteroid, and supplemental oxygen to maintain partial pressure of oxygen in arterial gas at 100–120 mm Hg. Complete blood cell counts, electrolytes, blood urea nitrogen, creatinine, and glucose are repeated regularly. The patient usually returns from surgery volume-depleted, and this is reversed with crystalloids and colloids to a central venous pressure of 8–10 mm Hg. More aggressive hemodilution and hypertensive therapy to treat symptomatic vasospasm dictate the continuing use of pulmonary artery pressure monitoring.[96] The control of protracted elevated ICP may require continuing use of pressure-monitoring systems. The patient is usually discharged from the intensive care unit when the risk of vasospasm has passed, the aneurysm has been surgically obliterated, and other urgent medical problems have been successfully treated.

Follow-up care also includes angiography to assess the position of the clip, confirm the successful occlusion of the aneurysm, and identify unclipped aneurysms not seen on preoperative studies. Although aneurysm clipping has been shown to be an effective long-term treatment, even small residual portions of the aneurysm neck or sac can dilate to become a larger aneurysm or rupture.[97,98]

Cerebral Blood Flow and Metabolism

SAH causes disturbances in CBF, $CMRO_2$, cerebral autoregulation, CO_2 reactivity, neurotransmitter levels, and cerebral blood velocity.[99,100] Measurements of CBF are accomplished using [133]xenon, xenon CT, single-photon emission CT (SPECT), or positron emission tomography.[101,102] CBF measurement can also be used preoperatively to evaluate adequacy of collateral circulation in patients considered for temporary or permanent ICA occlusion and postoperatively to predict the risk of vasospasm and distinguish deficits caused by vasospasm and altered cerebral reactivity.[81]

In patients with a good-grade SAH, CBF usually remains within the normal range preoperatively and immediately postoperatively, with a significant increase during the 2 weeks after surgery. Autoregulation and CO_2 reactivity are significantly disturbed in these patients, even after early operation.[103] Patients with worse grades show no significant increase in CBF.[104] CBF measurement can be sensitive in the early detection of vasospasm and is useful in establishing a diagnosis in patients who deteriorate or do not improve after SAH.[105–107] $CMRO_2$ is reduced after SAH and is negatively correlated to the thickness of blood measured on CT, ventricular bleeding, and hematoma.[100]

Neurologic Complications

Hydrocephalus, rebleeding from aneurysmal rerupture, and cerebral vasospasm with ischemia are the three major neurologic complications after SAH. Clinical deterioration after SAH is a diagnosis of exclusion requiring investigation to detect hypotension, hypoxia, fever, electrolyte abnormalities, or expanding intracranial lesions.

Hydrocephalus

Hydrocephalus may develop acutely within the first 24 hours after bleeding due to blood within the basal cisterns or ventricular system causing obstruction of CSF outflow or increased resistance to CSF absorption. Ventricular drainage is indicated because it can dramatically and rapidly improve neurologic condition in some cases. There is some controversy, however, because spontaneous improvement in level of consciousness can occur within 24 hours without ventricular drainage.[108] The risk of rebleeding from an untreated aneurysm is associated with the potential abrupt decrease in ICP that may occur with CSF drainage. Presumably, this decrease in transmural pressure could increase the risk of rehemorrhage. The ICP should be carefully monitored and gradually reduced to a more normal pressure (12–15 mm Hg).

Hydrocephalus developing subacutely over a few days or weeks after SAH is manifest clinically by the loss of vertical gaze, impaired memory and intellectual function, abulia, urinary incontinence, disorders of gait, and progressive lethargy. Diuresis may be a therapeutic treatment for some patients and can be attempted before CSF diversion, but a ventriculoperitoneal or ventriculoatrial shunt is commonly indicated. There is an association of shunt-dependent hydrocephalus on the admission Hunt and Hess grade, Fisher CT grade, incidence of repeat SAH, aneurysm location at the ACoA, and intraventricular hemorrhage.[109–112]

Rebleeding

Aneurysm rebleeding, which is postulated to be due to breakdown of the perianeurysmal clot, is a serious and frequent neurologic complication with a mortality of approximately 50%.[113] The peak incidence of rebleeding occurs during the first day after SAH, and there may be a secondary peak at 1 week. The risk is as high as 20% in the first 2 weeks and 50% within 6 months if the aneurysm is not treated.[6,84] The results of the Cooperative Aneurysm Study showed that women had a recurrent hemorrhage rate 2.2 times that of men, hypertention (systolic BP >169 mm Hg) was more prominent in women, and clinical grade of women was worse than men at presentation.[114] The clinical presentation of rehemorrhage includes increasing headache, nausea, vomiting, depressed level of consciousness, and the appearance of new neurologic deficits.

Clot formation and tissue damage stimulate fibrinolytic activity in the CSF, resulting in potential risk of rebleeding. This provides the rationale for the use of antifibrinolytic agents to retard clot lysis by inhibiting the formation of proteolytic enzymes and reducing the concentration of fibrin degradation products in the CSF.

Antifibrinolytic treatment has no beneficial effect on outcome assessed at 3 months with the Glasgow Outcome Scale, but significantly reduces the occurrence of rebleeding. The occurrence of ischemic and other complications is the same with or without treatment.[115] The antifibrinolytic agents epsilon-aminocaproic acid and tranexamic acid both reduce the risk of rebleeding but are associated with an increased risk of deep venous thrombosis, pulmonary embolism, ischemic cardiac disease, and delayed cerebral ischemia. Their use to prevent secondary hemorrhage is controversial and is generally reserved for patients in whom surgery is delayed. Antifibrinolytic therapy is not administered to patients at high risk of vasospasm and should be immediately discontinued when clinical or angiographic evidence of vasospasm develops. Delayed fibrinolysis of clot-surrounding arteries at the base of the brain may account for the increased incidence of vasospasm and stroke. Attempts to otherwise prevent rebleeding by drug-induced hypotension and bed rest have not been successful.[108,116–119]

Vasospasm

Clinical Presentation and Diagnosis

Delayed cerebral ischemia associated with cerebral vasospasm is a major cause of morbidity and mortality in patients after SAH. Contraction of the arterial smooth muscle and morphologic changes in the vessel wall and along its endothelial surface occur in response to injury.[120] The location and amount of blood in the subarachnoid space is predictive of the degree and distribution of delayed cerebral ischemic events. Thus, vasospasm occurs more frequently in patients with a poor clinical grade or with thick focal blood clots or a diffuse layer of blood in the subarachnoid space. The pathogenesis of cerebral vasospasm is a complicated, partially understood multifactorial process. In theory, the pathogenesis of vasospasm is related to by-products of local erythrocyte breakdown that may be spasmogenic. Potential spasm inducers

include oxyhemoglobin, angiotensin, histamine, serotonin, prostaglandin, nitric oxide metabolites, and catecholamines.[112] Vasospasm may occur because of structural changes in the arterial wall rather than muscle contraction. The mechanism of arterial wall changes may be an inflammatory response, depressed metabolism of the vessel wall, or damage from prolonged active arterial wall contraction. Other theories include impairment of normal vasodilatation, the mechanical effects of arterial compression by clot, and development of a proliferative vasculopathy. There are secondary disturbances of cerebral autoregulation noted at the microcirculatory level as well. Pathologic specimens of affected vessels demonstrate intimal proliferation and medial necrosis.[58]

Unlike rebleeding, the clinical presentation of vasospasm is not sudden; rather, it develops over hours to days. Symptoms related to cerebral ischemia may be first noted on the third day after hemorrhage, peak between days 4–12, and may persist as long as 3 weeks after SAH.[112,113] Vessel narrowing is depicted angiographically in 70% of patients. Many patients are asymptomatic, however, despite various degrees of arterial narrowing on angiography; arterial narrowing is symptomatic in only 36% of patients. Neurologic deficits are certainly related to arterial stenosis, but the correlation between angiographic or transcranial Doppler (TCD) ultrasound criteria and clinical ischemia is not direct or always predictable.[121] The difference probably reflects the adequacy of collateral circulation in individual patients as well as the degree of spasm. Neurologic impairment during vasospasm may also be associated with older age, intracerebral hemorrhage, poor neurologic condition at admission, surgical complications, and lack of immediate improvement with hypervolemic therapy.[122] However, vasospasm detected early in the clinical course by angiography or TCD is prognostic, with a one-and-a-half to threefold increase in mortality during the 2 weeks after SAH.[114]

Diagnostic Testing

Transcranial Doppler. Although confirmation of neurologic deterioration from ischemia due to cerebral vasospasm was previously only possible by angiography, TCD techniques are also used to follow its course.[123,124] TCD is a noninvasive study used to assess the degree and extent of cerebral arterial stenosis. Patient treatment can be modified to prevent or minimize clinical neurologic deterioration from ischemia.

TCD uses pulsed rather than continuous Doppler to record signal velocities at preselected depths or distances from the probe. It penetrates the thin temporal bone by using a 2-mHz frequency, which is lower than that used for studies of other peripheral and extracranial vessels (3–10 mHz), enabling measurement of most of the circle of Willis. The transorbital route is used for the ophthalmic and internal carotid arteries, whereas the transoccipital/foramen magnum view is used to visualize the vertebral and basilar arteries.

Vasospasm creates resistance to CBF, which is a function of the degree of vessel stenosis and the length of stenosis. Blood flow velocity (BFV) increases at a rate proportional to the reduction in cross-sectional area or the square of the vessel radius. It is typically increased five to six times normal with symptomatic vasospasm.[125] When resistance to CBF is reduced to a critical level by vasospasm, regional CBF is reduced, and the brain in that vascular distribution becomes ischemic.

A preoperative TCD study often does not demonstrate the presence of vasospasm acutely after SAH. However, the study can be performed to gain experience with the individual patient's vasculature and determine acoustic imaging windows without postoperative artifacts (bandages, soft-tissue swelling, hematoma). It may be useful in managing circulating blood volume and BP (Figure 18-5A).[45] The MCA is the best vessel to study serially as it has the most limited collateral circulation in the circle of Willis, and there is good correlation of BFV to ischemic symptoms and to angiographic measurement of vessel narrowing when proximal vessels are involved. Mean MCA BFV is normally 30–80 cm per second and increases >120 cm per second for symptomatic vasospasm and >200 cm per second in severe vasospasm. Angiography shows details of the vascular involvement and severity of vasospasm (Color Plate 9; Figure 18-5B).[45] Other vessels do not have as reliable a correlation as the MCA; however, they provide useful measurements when observed serially and bilaterally. Serial TCD studies are important because an elevated BFV within 24 hours of surgery or rapid elevation in the early postoperative period can identify patients at increased risk of severe vasospasm and subsequent ischemic deficit.[126] These patients might benefit from early prophylactic therapy.

Brain Single-Photon Emission Computed Tomography. Brain SPECT imaging is a noninvasive study that provides a semiquantitative measure of cerebral perfusion by tomographic imaging. Regional hypoperfusion demonstrated by SPECT correlates with the presence and severity of delayed neurologic deficits due to vasospasm.[127–130] Regional hypoperfusion can be seen before abnormalities appear on CT and may even precede symptoms; thus, it can be used to establish the ischemic etiology of a neurologic change as well as the efficacy of treatment (Figure 18-6).

Treatment

Hyperdynamic Therapy. Although there is no proven treatment for cerebral vasospasm, the current mainstay of therapy is hyperdynamic, hypervolemic-hypertensive-hemodilution or "triple-H" therapy. The goals of this hyperdynamic therapy are to augment cerebral perfusion pressure by raising systolic BP, cardiac output, and intravascular volume, and to minimize cerebral ischemia from delayed vasospasm after SAH and early aneurysm clipping.[131] In theory, ischemic tissues lose normal autoregulatory mechanisms, and CBF becomes passively responsive to changes in systolic BP. Expansion of the intravascular volume and subsequent hemodilution leads to improvement in cerebral microcirculation due to decreased viscosity. Serial CBF examinations reveal sustained CBF elevations and improvement of neurologic status that correlates to CBF values.

In practice, this treatment is reserved primarily for the postoperative period due to the risks of aneurysmal re-rupture before surgery.[132] Hematocrit is reduced to 30 ± 3% by plasma volume expansion, although venesection is sometimes used. The central venous pressure is elevated to 8–12 mm Hg, pulmonary capillary wedge pressure elevated to 15–18 mm Hg, and systolic BP maintained at 130–150 mm Hg in patients with unclipped aneurysms and 150–180 mm Hg in patients with clipped aneurysms. Inotropic drugs are used to keep systolic BPs 20–40 mm Hg above pretreatment levels or high enough to effectively ameliorate the neuro-

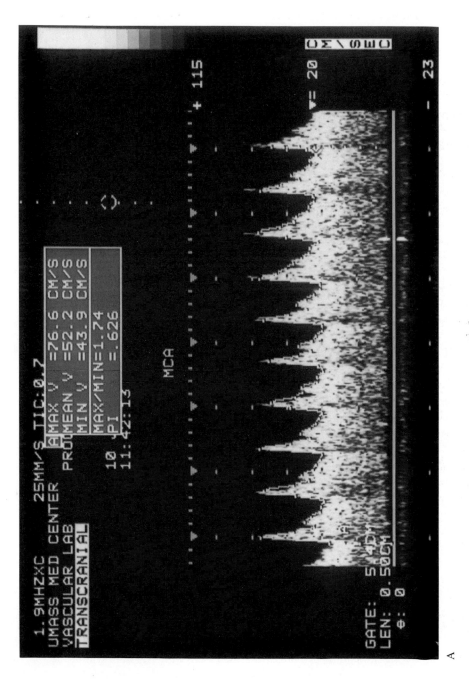

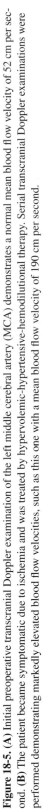

A

Figure 18-5. (A) Initial preoperative transcranial Doppler examination of the left middle cerebral artery (MCA) demonstrates a normal mean blood flow velocity of 52 cm per second. **(B)** The patient became symptomatic due to ischemia and was treated by hypervolemic-hypertensive-hemodilutional therapy. Serial transcranial Doppler examinations were performed demonstrating markedly elevated blood flow velocities, such as this one with a mean blood flow velocity of 190 cm per second.

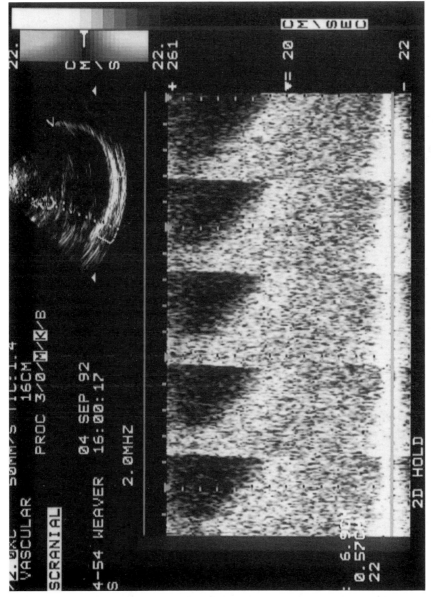

B

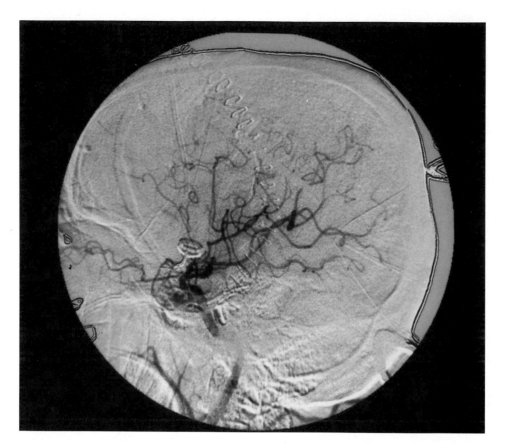

Figure 18-6. A good-grade patient after rupture of an anterior communicating artery aneurysm was well after early surgery until day 6 after the subarachnoid hemorrhage, at which time he became lethargic and developed a hemiparesis. This lateral projection of a right common carotid injection at mid-arterial phase demonstrated poor filling of the distal middle cerebral artery and opercular loops diffusely.

logic deficit caused by the vasospasm. Therapy is continued for at least 48–72 hours before it is gradually withdrawn under close observation for recurrent vasospasm based on changes in the neurologic examination and TCD studies. The aggressiveness of treatment may be tempered in the case of a large territory infarction already present on CT to avoid aggravated cerebral edema or hemorrhagic infarction.[133] Other risks of hyperdynamic therapy include myocardial infarction, congestive heart failure, dysrhythmias, rebleeding, hyponatremia, and hemothorax.

Calcium Antagonists. Although calcium channel blockers are widely used in current clinical practice to reduce the risk or severity of delayed cerebral ischemia, their mechanism of action and

clinical usefulness is controversial.[134] They probably do not reverse vasospasm, but they may reduce the incidence of symptoms due to vasospasm and delayed ischemic deficits in patients with SAH by various mechanisms, including cytoprotection by inhibition of calcium entry into mitochondria and subsequent preservation of oxidative metabolism despite ongoing ischemia, cell membrane stabilization, leptomeningeal vasodilation with improved collateral circulation, and microrheologic effects that improve erythrocyte deformability, reduce sludging, and exert an antiplatelet aggregating effect.[97,119,135,136]

Nimodipine is used in the United States, where it is administered as a 60-mg oral preparation every 4 hours for a 21-day course beginning at the onset of SAH. Intravenous preparations of nimodipine or nicardipine, another calcium channel blocker, are not available in the United States (except for investigational studies), but are available in Europe. The long-term efficacy of nimodipine therapy has been demonstrated by a significant decrease in morbidity and mortality due to delayed ischemic deterioration.[137,138] Results of a randomized controlled trial of intravenous nicardipine administered as a 14-day infusion demonstrated a reduced incidence of symptomatic vasospasm, fewer patients subsequently required aggressive triple-H therapy for symptomatic vasospasm, and antihypertensive agents were used less frequently.[139]

Investigational Therapies. Because the etiology and mechanism of vasospasm is unclear and multifactorial, there are several avenues of investigation to further elucidate the factors acting on the cerebral vasculature and affecting treatment. Among the factors that can cause delayed secondary injury after SAH are arachidonic acid metabolites, such as thromboxane A_2, which is a potent vasoconstrictor and platelet-aggregating agent released by platelets. Experimental therapies, such as thromboxane A_2, synthetase inhibitor, and leukotriene C4 antagonists, are intended to reduce the concentration or action of these potentially damaging metabolites.[138,140,141] Antagonists of the calmodulin and protein kinase C systems may inhibit vessel contraction.[142] Free radical scavengers and antiperoxidants, including 21-aminosteroids, are used to reduce oxygen free radical formation and lipid peroxidation, which induce vasoconstriction and morphologic damage to cerebral arteries.[143] Vasoconstrictor peptide endothelin-1 immunoreactivity is elevated after SAH and may have a role in vasospasm pathogenesis.

Interventional Neuroradiologic Techniques

Treatment of Inoperable or Incompletely Operated Aneurysms

Endovascular techniques may be applied to selectively exclude an aneurysm from cerebral circulation in cases in which surgical clipping is associated with a high risk because of size or site, presence of a wide or calcified neck, poor neurologic condition, or other medical contraindication.[145] Endovascular treatment may also be appropriate therapy for elderly patients. Microballoon and coil technologies with the Guglielmi detachable coil (GDC) (Boston Scientific/Target Therapeutics, Fremont, CA) method have proved to be useful adjuncts to surgery in high-risk patients. These endovascular therapies are used either for occlusion of the parent artery or preservation of the parent artery by selective occlusion of the aneurysm.[146] Endosaccular GDC treatment of giant and large aneurysms can be accomplished with procedure-related morbidity and mortality rates comparable to surgery and apparent long-term efficacy.[147] The most complete occlusion depends on the aneurysm geometry, with those aneurysms having a narrower neck relative to the dome. A dome to neck ratio of less than 2 to 1 yields a lower occlusion rate.[148]

The frequency and severity of vasospasm may be reduced by the endovascular treatment of ruptured aneurysms, suggesting that surgical factors may predispose the patient to increased risk and severity of vasospasm.[149] Aneurysm domes with a neck perpendicular to the parent artery blood flow direction, such as the basilar apex or ICA bifurcation, may be less well treated. Long-term follow-up has demonstrated that the coils can compact within the aneurysm, leaving an untreated aneurysm neck. Results of the U.S. Food and Drug Administration multicenter clinical trial showed, however, that 90% coil packing in 75% of patients was possible in basilar tip aneurysms.[150] The treatment offers a lower morbidity and mortality than the natural history of the disease and is a promising treatment for selected patients.

Flexible intravascular stents have been demonstrated to isolate an aneurysm from its parent blood supply or provide a scaffold to support intraaneurysmal GDC.[151] Some complex aneurysms may be treated by the combination of both surgical and endovascular techniques.[152–156]

Endovascular Balloon Occlusion

Intravascular detachable balloon embolization techniques have been demonstrated to be a useful therapeutic option in treating complex and surgically difficult aneurysms.[157,158] Balloons are especially useful for parent vessel occlusion in cases of fusiform aneurysms, vertebral artery dissections, paraclinoidal and intracavernous aneurysms, carotid-cavernous fistula, or trapping aneurysms with ectatic or broad-based necks.[146,158–160] Before definitive parent artery occlusion, test occlusion is performed as presurgical evaluation, with the neurologic examination and various other neurodiagnostic studies used to determine the potential neurologic risk, including electroencephalography, SPECT, and xenon CBF measurement. If test occlusion is not tolerated, antecedent extracranial-intracranial bypass to a vessel distal to the aneurysm can be performed.

Primary occlusion of an aneurysm with preservation of the parent artery is also possible, but it is associated with a significant rate of stroke, incomplete aneurysm obliteration, and embolic complications.[159,161] Its use has been largely abandoned due to risks (e.g., incomplete aneurysm sac filling and migrating into the parent artery lumen or through the aneurysm dome, and increased intraluminal pressure during balloon filling).[146,162]

Endovascular Detachable Coils

Occlusion of an aneurysm by placing detachable platinum coils into the aneurysm sac is a promising therapy. A major advancement in coil technology occurred with the development of the GDCs, which allow controlled placement and release in the aneurysm lumen. A low, positive direct electric current transmitted through the guidewire detaches the coil from the stainless steel microcatheter by electrolysis and promotes intra-aneurysmal electrothrombosis by the attraction of local blood components.[162] It is an investigational device used at designated centers, and early experience has supported its use as an alternative to surgical therapy in high-risk cases, including posterior circulation aneurysms.[163–165] Mortality and morbidity rates have been relatively low and generally comparable to surgery; in one review, mortality and morbidity were 11.3 and 4.2, respectively.[166] Complications include embolism due to the guiding catheter, puncture of the aneurysm sac by the coil or guidewire, coil migration, parent artery occlusion, and vasospasm induced by the guidewire. Aneurysm thrombosis is not always complete immediately after endovascular treatment, and the coils may compact or shift slightly within the lumen of the aneurysm. Although complete thrombosis may

be demonstrated in subsequent angiography, some studies demonstrate that the treatment may be safer than surgery, but it is not certain in many cases, and further follow-up is needed to determine long-term efficacy.[167–169]

Treatment for Cerebral Vasospasm

Angioplasty

Transluminal balloon angioplasty has been used successfully to recover patients with ischemic deficit from vasospasm of proximal or larger arteries. It is most useful for proximal arterial narrowing rather than distal vessel or diffuse vasospasm. Mechanical dilation of narrowed arteries is indicated when the patient is refractory to medical and pharmacologic treatment for neurologic deterioration, there is no CT or MRI evidence of significant cerebral infarction, and there is angiographic evidence of vasospasm.[170] It improves function in approximately 70% of patients treated and is most effective if used within 12 hours after the neurologic deficit occurs and the vascular territory treated correlates well with the observed neurologic deficit. Neurologic improvement can be dramatic and immediately observed after vessel dilation, and recurrent vasospasm in the treated vessel is rare. However, delayed treatment as a "salvage" procedure may produce little neurologic benefit or improved outcome. The treatment is usually reserved for patients who have already been treated surgically; however, reversal of the neurologic deficit in a poor-grade patient could allow earlier definitive surgical intervention and potentially more aggressive hemodynamic treatment.[171] Potential complications of angioplasty include rupture of an unclipped aneurysm, displacement of aneurysm clips, vessel rupture, or occlusion.

Intra-Arterial Papaverine Infusion

Another promising treatment for cerebral vasospasm is selective or super-selective infusion of intra-arterial papaverine into a spastic vessel. It has been shown by Kassell and others to safely and effectively change the angiographic and clinical course in preliminary studies.[172,173] Early experience demonstrates improvement in approximately

50% of patients treated, but also suggests that the changes in vessel caliber are sometimes transient, and the patient may require repeat treatment or alternative therapy.

Conclusion

Aneurysmal SAH remains a neurologic disease that causes death, disability, and consumes considerable medical resources in its treatment. Microsurgical clip ligation remains the best treatment for most aneurysms with endovascular treatment providing excellent alternatives and adjunctive treatment for posterior circulation, partially treated, and complicated aneurysms. Advances in endovascular treatments have provided treatment of previously inoperable or high-risk surgical aneurysms. Further technological improvements make the techniques even more applicable to aneurysms with complicated shapes and wide necks. Unruptured incidental aneurysms are more frequently discovered by MRI examination. The natural history and treatment recommendations are now also better understood.

References

1. Housepian EM, Pool JL. A systematic analysis of intracranial aneurysms from the autopsy file of the Presbyterian Hospital 1914 to 1956. J Neuropath Exp Neurol 1958;17:409–423.
2. McCormick WF, Nofziger JD. Saccular intracranial aneurysms: an autopsy study. J Neurosurg 1965;22:155–159.
3. McCormick WF, Acosta-Rua GJ. The size of intracranial saccular aneurysms: an autopsy study. J Neurosurg 1970; 33:422–427.
4. Sacco RL, Wolf PA, Bharucha NE, et al. Subarachnoid and intracerebral hemorrhage: natural history, prognosis, and precursive factors in the Framingham study. Neurology 1984;34:847–854.
5. Kojima M, Nagasawa S, Lee YE, et al. Asymptomatic familial cerebral aneurysms. Neurosurgery 1998;43:776–781.
6. Kassell NF, Torner JC, Haley C, et al. The International Cooperative Study on the Timing of Aneurysm Surgery. Part 1. Overall management results. J Neurosurg 1990;73:18–36.
7. Sarti CJ, Tuomilehto V, Salomaa J, et al. Epidemiology of subarachnoid hemorrhage in Finland from 1983 to 1985. Stroke 1991;22:848–853.
8. Saveland H, Hillman J, Brandt L, et al. Overall outcome in aneurysmal subarachnoid hemorrhage. A prospective study from neurosurgical units in Sweden during a 1-year period. J Neurosurg 1992;76:729–734.
9. Kassell NF, Torner JC, Jane JA, et al. The International Cooperative Study on the Timing of Aneurysm Surgery. Part 2. Surgical results. J Neurosurg 1990;73:37–47.
10. McKenna P, Willison JR, Phil B, et al. Cognitive outcome and quality of life one year after subarachnoid haemorrhage. Neurosurgery 1989;24:361–367.
11. Vilkki J, Holst P, Öhman J. Cognitive deficits related to computed tomographic findings after surgery for a ruptured intracranial aneurysm. Neurosurgery 1989;25:166–172.
12. Gade A. Amnesia after operations on aneurysms of the anterior communicating artery. Surg Neurol 1982;18:46–49.
13. Hutter BO, Kreitschmann-Andermahr I, Gilsbach JM. Cognitive deficits in the acute stage after subarachnoid hemorrhage. Neurosurgery 1998;43:1054–1065.
14. Wiebers DO, Torner JC, Meissner I. Impact of unruptured intracranial aneurysms on public health in the United States. Stroke 1992;23:1416–1419.
15. Unruptured intracranial aneurysms: risk of rupture and risks of surgical intervention. The International Study of Unruptured Intracranial Aneurysms Investigators. N Engl J Med 1998;339:1725–1733.
16. Yoshimoto T, Wakai S. Cost-effectiveness analysis of screening for asymptomatic, unruptured intracranial aneurysms. A mathematical model. Stroke 1999;30:1621–1627.
17. Brown BM, Soldevilla F. MR angiography and surgery for unruptured familial intracranial aneurysms in persons with a family history of cerebral aneurysms. AJR Am J Roentgenol 1999;173:133–138.
18. Stehbens WE. Ultrastructure of aneurysms. Arch Neurol 1975;32:798–807.
19. Wilkins RH. Subarachnoid hemorrhage and saccular intracranial aneurysm—an update. Surg Neurol 1981;15:92–101.
20. McKissock W, Richardson A, Walsh L, Owen E. Multiple intracranial aneurysms. Lancet 1964;1:623–626.
21. Kataoka K, Taneda M, Asai T, Yamada Y. Difference in nature of ruptured and unruptured cerebral aneurysms. Lancet 2000;355:203.
22. Deruty R, Mottolese C, Soustiel JF, Pelissou-Guyotat I. Association of cerebral arteriovenous malformation and cerebral aneurysm. Diagnosis and management. Acta Neurochir 1990;107:133–139.
23. Cunha e Sa MJ, Stein BM, Solomon RA, McCormick PC. The treatment of associated intracranial aneurysms and arteriovenous malformations. J Neurosurg 1992;77:853–859.
24. Forbus WD. On origin of miliary aneurysms of superficial cerebral arteries. Bull Johns Hopkins Hosp 1930;47: 239–284.
25. Lebland R. De novo formation of familial cerebral aneurysm: case report. Neurosurgery 1999;44:871–876.
26. Stehbens WE. Etiology of intracranial berry aneurysms. J Neurosurg 1989;70:823–831.
27. Knekt P, Reunanen A, Aho K, et al. Risk factors for subarachnoid hemorrhage in a longitudinal population study. J Clin Epidemiol 1991;44:933–939.
28. Sekhar LN, Heros RC. Origin, growth, and rupture of saccular aneurysms: a review. Neurosurgery 1981;8:248–260.
29. Nakagawa T, Hashi K, Kurokawa T, Yamamura A. Family history of subarachnoid hemorrhage and the incidence of asymptomatic unruptured cerebral aneurysms. J Neurosurg 1999;91:391–395.

30. Risks and benefits of screening for intracranial aneurysms in first-degree relatives of patients with sporadic subarachnoid hemorrhage. The Magnetic Resonance Angiography in Relatives of Patients with Subarachnoid Hemorrhage Study Group. N Engl J Med 1999;28:1344–1350.

31. Raaymakers TW. Aneurysms in relatives of patients with subarachnoid hemorrhage: frequency and risk factors. MARS Study Group. Magnetic Resonance Angiography in Relatives of patients with Subarachnoid hemorrhage. Neurology 1999;53:982–988.

32. Anson JA, Koshy M, Ferguson L, Crowell RM. Subarachnoid hemorrhage in sickle cell disease. J Neurosurg 1991;75:552–558.

33. Batjer HH, Adamson TE, Bowman GW. Sickle cell disease and aneurysmal subarachnoid hemorrhage. Surg Neurol 1991;36:145–149.

34. Oyesiku NM, Barrow DL, Eckman JR, et al. Intracranial aneurysm in sickle cell anemia: clinical features and pathogenesis. J Neurosurg 1991;75:356–363.

35. Chapman AB, Rubinstein D, Hughes R, et al. Intracranial aneurysms in autosomal dominant polycystic kidney disease. N Engl J Med 1992;327:916–920.

36. Lozano AM, Leblanc R. Cerebral aneurysms and polycystic kidney disease: a critical review. Can J Neurol Sci 1992;19:222–227.

37. Broderick JP, Brott T, Tomsick T, et al. The risk of subarachnoid and intracerebral hemorrhages in blacks as compared with whites. N Engl J Med 1992;326:733–736.

38. Bassi P, Bandera R, Loiero M, et al. Warning signs in subarachnoid hemorrhage: a cooperative study. Acta Neurol Scand 1991;84:277–281.

39. Dias MS, Sekhar LN. Intracranial hemorrhage from aneurysms and arteriovenous malformations during pregnancy and the puerperium. Neurosurgery 1990;27:855–866.

40. Hart RG, Byer JA, Slaughter JR, et al. Occurrence and implications of seizures in subarachnoid hemorrhage due to ruptured intracranial aneurysms. Neurosurgery 1981;8:417–421.

41. Hunt WE, Hess RM. Surgical risk as related to time of intervention in the repair of intracranial aneurysms. J Neurosurg 1968;28:14–20.

42. LeBlanc R. The minor leak preceding subarachnoid hemorrhage. J Neurosurg 1987;66:35–39.

43. Anderson GB, Steinke DE, Petruk KC, et al. Computed tomographic angiography versus digital subtraction angiography for the diagnosis and early treatment of ruptured intracranial aneurysms. Neurosurgery 1999;45:1315–1320.

44. Lai PH, Yang CF, Pan HB, et al. Detection and assessment of circle of Willis aneurysms in acute subarachnoid hemorrhage with three-dimensional computed tomographic angiography: correlation with digital subtraction angiography findings. J Formos Med Assoc 1999;98:672–677.

45. Weaver J, Fisher M. Subarachnoid hemorrhage: an update of pathogenesis, diagnosis, and management. J Neurol Sci 1994;125:119–131.

46. Kahara VJ, Seppanen SK, Ryymin PS, et al. MR angiography with three-dimensional time-of-flight and targeted maximum-intensity-projection reconstructions in the follow-up of intracranial aneurysms embolized with Guglielmi detachable coils. AJNR Am J Neuroradiol 1999;20:1470–1475.

47. Kawamura S, Yasui N. Clinical and long-term follow-up study in patients with spontaneous subarachnoid haemorrhage of unknown aetiology. Acta Neurochir (Wien) 1990;106:110–114.

48. Rinkel GJ, van Gijn J, Wijdicks EF. Subarachnoid hemorrhage without detectable aneurysm. Stroke 1993;24:1403–1409.

49. West HH, Mani RI, Eisenberg RL, et al. Normal cerebral arteriography in patients with spontaneous subarachnoid hemorrhage. Neurology 1972;27:592–594.

50. Kassell NF, Torner JC. The International Cooperative Study on Timing of Aneurysm Surgery: an update. Stroke 1984;15:566–570.

51. Keränen T, Tapaninaho A, Hernesniemi J, Vapalahti M. Late epilepsy after aneurysm operation. J Neurosurg 1985;17:897–900.

52. Ukkola V, Heikkinen ER. Epilepsy after operative treatment of ruptured cerebral aneurysms. Acta Neurochir (Wien) 1990;106:115–118.

53. Rabinowicz AL, Ginsburg DL, DeGiorgio CM, et al. Unruptured intracranial aneurysms: seizures and antiepileptic drug treatment following surgery. J Neurosurg 1991;75:371–373.

54. Auer LM, Brandt L, Ebeling U, et al. Nimodipine and early aneurysm operation in good condition SAH patients. Acta Neurochir (Wien) 1986;82:7–13.

55. Weintraub BM, McHenry LC Jr. Cardiac abnormalities in subarachnoid hemorrhage: a resume. Stroke 1974;5:384–392.

56. Marion DW, Segal R, Thompson ME. Subarachnoid hemorrhage and the heart. Neurosurgery 1986;18:101–106.

57. Norris JW. Effects of cerebrovascular lesions of the heart. Neurol Clin 1983;1:87–101.

58. Chyatte D, Sundt TM. Cerebral vasospasm after subarachnoid hemorrhage. Mayo Clin Proc 1984;59:498–505.

59. Auer LM. Unfavorable outcome following early surgical repair of ruptured cerebral aneurysms—a critical review of 238 patients. Surg Neurol 1991;35:152–158.

60. Suzuki J, Yoshimoto T, Onuma T. Early operations for ruptured intracranial aneurysms—study of 31 cases operated on within the first four days after ruptured aneurysm. Neurol Med Chir (Tokyo) 1978;18:82–89.

61. Whisnant JP, Phillips LH, Sundt TM. Aneurysmal subarachnoid hemorrhage. Mayo Clin Proc 1982;57:471–475.

62. Batjer HH, Samson DS. Emergent aneurysm surgery without cerebral angiography for the comatose patient. Neurosurgery 1991;28:283–287.

63. Le Roux PD, Dailey AT, Newell DW, et al. Emergent aneurysm clipping without angiography in the moribund patient with intracerebral hemorrhage: the use of infusion computed tomography scans. Neurosurgery 1993;33:189–197.

64. Drake CG. Management of cerebral aneurysm. Stroke 1981;12:273–283.

65. Farrar JK, Gamache FW, Ferguson GG, et al. Effects of profound hypotension on cerebral blood flow during surgery for intracranial aneurysms. J Neurosurg 1981;55:857–864.

66. Charbel FT, Ausman JI, Diaz FG, et al. Temporary clipping in aneurysm surgery: technique and results. Surg Neurol 1991;36:145–149.

67. Muizelaar JP. The use of electroencephalography and brain protection during operation for basilar aneurysms. Neurosurgery 1989;25:899–903.

68. Rosenwasser RH, Jimenez DF, Wending WW, Carlsson C. Routine use of etomidate and temporary vessel occlusion during aneurysm surgery. Neurol Res 1991;13:224–228.

69. Meyer FB, Muzzi DA. Cerebral protection during aneurysm surgery with isoflurane anesthesia. J Neurosurg 1992;76:541–543.

70. Ravussin P, de Tribolet N. Total intravenous anesthesia with propofol for burst suppression in cerebral aneurysm surgery: preliminary report of 42 patients. Neurosurgery 1993;32:236–240.

71. Hutchinson PJ, Al-Rawi PG, O'Connell MT, et al. Biochemical changes related to hypoxia during cerebral aneurysm surgery: combined microdialysis and tissue oxygen monitoring. Case report. Neurosurgery 2000;46:201–205.

72. Stendel R, Pietila T, Al Hassan AA, et al. Intraoperative microvascular Doppler ultrasonography in cerebral aneurysm surgery. J Neurol Neurosurg Psychiatry 2000;68:29–35.

73. Doppenberg EM, Watson JC, Broaddus WC, et al. Intraoperative monitoring of substrate delivery during aneurysm and hematoma surgery: initial experience in 16 patients. J Neurosurg 1997;87:809–816.

74. Kasuya H, Shimizu T, Kagawa M. The effect of continuous drainage of cerebrospinal fluid in patients with subarachnoid hemorrhage: a retrospective analysis of 108 patients. Neurosurgery 1991;28:56–59.

75. Pritz MB. Evaluation and treatment of aneurysms of the vertebral artery: different strategies for different lesions. Neurosurgery 1991;29:247–256.

76. Wakui K, Kobayashi S, Takemae T, et al. Giant thrombosed vertebral artery aneurysm managed with extracranial-intracranial bypass surgery and aneurysmectomy. Case report. J Neurosurg 1992;77:624–627.

77. Fitzpatrick BC, Spetzler RF, Ballard JL, Zimmerman RS. Cervical-to-petrous internal carotid artery bypass procedure. Technical note. J Neurosurg 1993;79:138–141.

78. Greene KA, Anson JA, Spetzler RF. Giant serpentine middle cerebral artery aneurysm treated by extracranial-intracranial bypass. Case report. J Neurosurg 1993;78:974–978.

79. Miller JD, Jawad K, Jannett B. Safety of carotid ligation and its role in the management of intracranial aneurysms. J Neurol Neurosurg Psychiatry 1977;40:64–72.

80. Linskey ME, Sekhar LN, Horton JA, et al. Aneurysms of the intracavernous carotid artery: a multidisciplinary approach to treatment. J Neurosurg 1991;75:525–534.

81. Taki W, Nishi S, Yamashita K, et al. Selection and combination of various endovascular techniques in the treatment of giant aneurysms. J Neurosurg 1992;77:37–42.

82. Taniguchi M, Takimoto H, Yoshimine T, et al. Application of a rigid endoscope to the microsurgical management of 54 cerebral aneurysms: results in 48 patients. J Neurosurg 1999;91:231–237.

83. Inagawa T. Multiple intracranial aneurysms in elderly patients. Acta Neurochir (Wien) 1990;106:119–126.

84. Ojemann RG. Management of the unruptured intracranial aneurysm. N Engl J Med 1981;304:725–726.

85. Samson DS, Hodosh RM, Clark WK. Surgical management of unruptured asymptomatic aneurysms. J Neurosurg 1977;46:731–734.

86. Wiebers DO, Whisnant JP, O'Fallon WM. The natural history of unruptured intracranial aneurysms. N Engl J Med 1981;304:696–698.

87. David CA, Vishteh AG, Spetzler RF, et al. Late angiographic follow-up review of surgically treated aneurysms. J Neurosurg 1999;91:396–401.

88. Winn HR, Almaani WS, Berga SL. The long-term outcome in patients with multiple aneurysms. J Neurosurg 1983;59:642–651.

89. Wirth FP, Laws ER, Piepgras D Jr, Scott RM. Surgical treatment of incidental intracranial aneurysm. Neurosurgery 1983;12:507–511.

90. Juvela S. Natural history of unruptured intracranial aneurysms: a long-term follow-up study. J Neurosurg 1993;79:174–182.

91. Raps EC, Rogers JD, Galetta SL, et al. The clinical spectrum of unruptured intracranial aneurysms. Arch Neurol 1993;50:265–268.

92. Findlay JM, Weir BKA, Kassell NF, et al. Intracisternal recombinant tissue plasminogen activator after aneurysmal subarachnoid hemorrhage. J Neurosurg 1991;75:181–188.

93. Ohman J, Servo A, Heiskanen O. Effect of intrathecal fibrinolytic therapy on clot lysis and vasospasm in patients with aneurysmal subarachnoid hemorrhage. J Neurosurg 1991;75:197–201.

94. Zabramski JM, Spetzler RF, Lee KS, et al. Phase I trial of tissue plasminogen activator for the prevention of vasospasm in patients with aneurysmal subarachnoid hemorrhage. J Neurosurg 1991;75:189–196.

95. Mizoi K, Yoshimoto T, Takahashi A, et al. Prospective study on the prevention of cerebral vasospasm by intrathecal fibrinolytic therapy with tissue-type plasminogen activator. J Neurosurg 1993;78:430–437.

96. Levy M, Giannotta SL. Cardiac performance indices during hypervolemic therapy for cerebral vasospasm. J Neurosurg 1991;75:27–31.

97. Drake CG, Vanderlinden RG. The late consequences of incomplete surgical treatment of cerebral aneurysm. J Neurosurg 1967;27:226–238.

98. Lin T, Fox AJ, Drake CG. Regrowth of aneurysm sacs from residual neck following aneurysm clipping. J Neurosurg 1989;70:556–560.

99. Archer DP, Shaw DA, LeBlanc RL, Tranmer BI. Haemodynamic considerations in the management of patients with subarachnoid haemorrhage. Can J Anaesth 1991;38:454–470.

100. Jakobsen M, Skjodt T, Enevoldsen E. Cerebral blood flow and metabolism following subarachnoid haemorrhage: effect of subarachnoid blood. Acta Neurol Scand 1991;83:226–233.

101. Powers WJ, Grubb RL Jr, Baker RP, et al. Regional cerebral blood flow and metabolism in reversible ischemia due

to vasospasm. Determination by positron emission tomography. J Neurosurg 1985;62:539–546.

102. Hino A, Mizukawa N, Tenjin H, et al. Postoperative hemodynamic and metabolic changes in patients with subarachnoid hemorrhage. Stroke 1989;20:1504–1510.

103. Dernbach PD, Little JR, Jones SC, Ebrahim ZY. Altered cerebral autoregulation and CO_2 reactivity after aneurysmal subarachnoid hemorrhage. Neurosurgery 1988;22:822–826.

104. Mountz JM, McGillicuddy JE, Wilson MW, et al. Pre- and post-operative cerebral blood flow changes in subarachnoid haemorrhage. Acta Neurochir (Wien) 1991;109:30–33.

105. Muizelaar JP. Cerebral Blood Flow Measurements in the Diagnosis and Treatment of Aneurysmal "Vasospasm." In RH Wilkins (ed), Cerebral Vasospasm. New York: Raven, 1988;63–72.

106. Yonas H, Sekhar L, Johnson DW, Gur D. Determination of irreversible ischemia by xenon-enhanced computed tomographic monitoring of cerebral blood flow in patients with symptomatic vasospasm. Neurosurgery 1989;24:368–372.

107. Fukui MB, Johnson DW, Yonas H, et al. L. Xe/CT cerebral blood flow evaluation of delayed symptomatic cerebral ischemia after subarachnoid hemorrhage. AJNR Am J Neuroradiol 1992;13:265–270.

108. Hasan D, Vermeulen M, Wijdicks EF, et al. Management problems in acute hydrocephalus after subarachnoid hemorrhage. Stroke 1989;20:747–753.

109. Gruber A, Reinprecht A, Bavinszski G, et al. Chronic shunt-dependent hydrocephalus after early surgical and early endovascular treatment of ruptured intracranial aneurysms. Neurosurgery 1999;44:503–509.

110. Kosteljanetz M. CSF dynamics in patients with subarachnoid and/or intraventricular hemorrhage. J Neurosurg 1984;60:940–946.

111. Prats AR, Barrow DL. Preoperative management of the aneurysmal subarachnoid hemorrhage patient—part I. Contemp Neurosurg 1987;9:1–6.

112. Kistler JP, Heros RC. Subarachnoid Hemorrhage Due to a Ruptured Saccular Aneurysm. In AH Ropper, SF Kennedy (eds), Neurological and Neurosurgical Intensive Care. Rockville, MD: Aspen, 1988;219–232.

113. Biller J, Godersky JC, Adams HP. Management of aneurysmal subarachnoid hemorrhage. Stroke 1988;19:1300–1305.

114. Torner JC, Kassell NF, Wallace RB, Adams HP Jr. Preoperative prognostic factors for rebleeding and survival in aneurysm patients receiving antifibrinolytic therapy: report of the Cooperative Aneurysm Study. Neurosurgery 1981;9:506–513.

115. Roos Y. Antifibrinolytic treatment in subarachnoid hemorrhage: a randomized placebo-controlled trial. STAR Study Group. Neurology 2000;54:77–82.

116. Nibbelink DW. Cooperative Aneurysm Study: Antihypertensive and Antifibrinolytic Therapy Following Subarachnoid Hemorrhage from Ruptured Intracranial Aneurysm. In JP Whisnant, BA Sandok (eds), Cerebral Vascular Diseases. New York: Grune & Stratton, 1975;155.

117. Nibbelink DW, Torner JC, Henderson WG. Intracranial aneurysms and subarachnoid hemorrhage: report on a randomized treatment study. IV-A. Regulated bedrest. Stroke 1975;8:202–218.

118. Kassell NF, Torner JC, Adams HP. Antifibrinolytic therapy in the acute period following aneurysmal subarachnoid hemorrhage: preliminary observations from the Cooperative Aneurysm Study. J Neurosurg 1984;61:225–230.

119. Solomon RA, Fink ME. Current strategies for the management of aneurysmal subarachnoid hemorrhage. Arch Neurol 1987;44:769–774.

120. Wilkins RH. Cerebral vasospasm. Contemp Neurosurg 1988;10:18.

121. Vermeulen M, Lindsay KW, Murray GD, et al. Antifibrinolytic treatment in subarachnoid hemorrhage. N Engl J Med 1984;311:432–437.

122. Shimoda M, Oda S, Tsugane R, Sato O. Prognostic factors in delayed ischemic deficit with vasospasm in-patients undergoing early aneurysm surgery. Br J Neurosurg 1997;11:210–215.

123. Sekhar LN, Wechsler LR, Yonas H, et al. Value of transcranial Doppler examination in the diagnosis of cerebral vasospasm after subarachnoid hemorrhage. Neurosurgery 1988;22:813–821.

124. Newell DW, Winn HR. Transcranial Doppler in cerebral vasospasm. Neurosurg Clin N Am 1990;1:319–328.

125. Klingelhöfer J, Sander D, Holzgraefe M, et al. Cerebral vasospasm evaluated by transcranial Doppler ultrasonography at different intracranial pressures. J Neurosurg 1991;75:752–758.

126. Grosset DG, Straiton J, McDonald I, et al. Use of transcranial Doppler sonography to predict development of a delayed ischemic deficit after subarachnoid hemorrhage. J Neurosurg 1993;78:183–187.

127. Soucy JP, McNamara D, Mohr G, et al. Evaluation of vasospasm secondary to subarachnoid hemorrhage with technetium-99m-hexamethyl-propyleneamine oxime (HM-PAO) tomoscintigraphy. J Nucl Med 1990;31:972–977.

128. Davis S, Andrews J, Lichtenstein M, et al. A single-photon emission computed tomography study of hypoperfusion after subarachnoid hemorrhage. Stroke 1990;21:252–259.

129. Lewis DH, Eskridge JM, Newell DW, et al. Brain SPECT and the effect of cerebral angioplasty in delayed ischemia due to vasospasm. J Nucl Med 1992;33:1789–1796.

130. Tranquart F, Ades PE, Groussin P, et al. Postoperative assessment of cerebral blood flow in subarachnoid haemorrhage by means of 99mTc-HMPAO tomography. Eur J Nucl Med 1993;20:53–58.

131. Origitano TC, Wascher TM, Reichman OH, Anderson DE. Sustained increased cerebral blood flow with prophylactic hypertensive hypervolemic hemodilution ("Triple-H" therapy) after subarachnoid hemorrhage. Neurosurgery 1990;27:729–740.

132. Heros RC, Zervas NT, Varsos V. Cerebral vasospasm after subarachnoid hemorrhage: an update. Ann Neurol 1983;14:599–608.

133. Shimoda M, Oda S, Tsugane R, Sato O. Intracranial complications of hypervolemic therapy in patients with a delayed ischemic deficit attributed to vasospasm. J Neurosurg 1993;78:423–429.

134. Adams HP. Calcium antagonists in the management of patients with aneurysmal subarachnoid hemorrhage: a review. Angiology 1990;41:1010–1016.

135. Peters T. Calcium in physiological and pathological cell function. Eur Neurol 1986;25:27–44.

136. Siesjo BK. Calcium and ischemic brain damage. Eur Neurol 1986;25:45–56.

137. Ohman J, Heiskanen O. Effect of nimodipine on the outcome of patients after aneurysmal subarachnoid hemorrhage and surgery. J Neurosurg 1988;69:683–686.

138. Kobayashi HH, Ide Y, Handa H, et al. Effect of leukotriene antagonist on experimental delayed cerebral vasospasm. Neurosurgery 1992;31:550–556.

139. Haley EC Jr, Kassell NF, Torner JC. A randomized controlled trial of high-dose intravenous nicardipine in aneurysmal subarachnoid hemorrhage. J Neurosurg 1993;78: 537–547.

140. Juvela S. Cerebral infarction and release of platelet thromboxane after subarachnoid hemorrhage. Neurosurgery 1990;27:929–935.

141. Tokiyoshi K, Ohnishi T, Nii Y. Efficacy and toxicity of thromboxane synthetase inhibitor for cerebral vasospasm after subarachnoid hemorrhage. Surg Neurol 1991;36: 112–118.

142. Nishizawa S, Peterson JW, Shimoyama I, Uemura K. Relation between protein kinase C and calmodulin systems in cerebrovascular contraction: investigation of the pathogenesis of vasospasm after subarachnoid hemorrhage. Neurosurgery 1992;31:711–716.

143. Takahashi S, Kassell HF, Toshima M, et al. Effect of U88999E on experimental cerebral vasospasm in rabbits. Neurosurgery 1993;32:281–288.

144. Suzuki R, Masaoka H, Hirata Y, et al. The role of endothelin-1 in the origin of cerebral vasospasm in patients with aneurysmal subarachnoid hemorrhage. J Neurosurg 1992;77:96–100.

145. Hodes JE, Aymard A, Gobin YP, et al. Endovascular occlusion of intracranial vessels for curative treatment of unclippable aneurysms: report of 16 cases. J Neurosurg 1991;75:694–701.

146. Nichols DA, Meyer FB, Piepgras DG. Endovascular treatment of intracranial aneurysms. Mayo Clin Proc 1994;69:272–285.

147. Lot G, Houdart E, Cophignon J, et al. Management of intracranial aneurysms by surgical and endovascular treatment—modalities and results from a series of 395 cases. Neurologia Med Chir (Tokyo) 1998;38(Suppl):21–25.

148. Debrun GM, Aletich VA, Kehrli P, et al. Aneurysm geometry: an important criterion in selecting patients for Guglielmi detachable coiling. Neurol Med Chir (Tokyo) 1998;38(Suppl):1–20.

149. Yalamanchili K, Rosenwasser RH, Thomas JE, et al. Frequency of cerebral vasospasm in patients treated with endovascular occlusion of intracranial aneurysms. AJNR Am J Neuroradiol 1998;19:553–558.

150. Eskridge JM, Song JK. Endovascular embolization of 150 basilar tip aneurysms with Guglielmi detachable coils: results of the Food and Drug Administration multicenter clinical trial. J Neurosurg 1998;89:81–86.

151. Lanzino G, Wakhloo AK, Fessler RD, et al. Efficacy and current limitations of intravascular stent for intracranial internal carotid, vertebral and basilar artery aneurysms. J Neurosurg 1999;91:538–546.

152. Martin NA. The combination of endovascular and surgical techniques for the treatment of intracranial aneurysms. Neurosurg Clin N Am 1998;9:897.

153. LeRoux PD, Winn HR. Surgical approaches to basilar bifurcation aneurysms. Neurosurg Clin N Am 1998;9:835–849.

154. Lempert TE, Malek AM, Halbach VV, et al. Endovascular treatment of ruptured posterior circulation cerebral aneurysms. Clinical and angiographic outcomes. Stroke 2000;31:100–110.

155. Cockroft KM, Marks MP, Steinberg GK. Planned direct dual-modality treatment of complex broad-necked intracranial aneurysms: four technical case reports. Neurosurgery 2000;46:226–230.

156. Hacein-Bey L, Connolly ES Jr, Mayer SA, et al. Complex intracranial aneurysms: combined operative and endovascular approaches. Neurosurgery 1998;43:1304–1312.

157. Higashida RT, Halbach VV, Cahan LD, et al. Detachable balloon embolization therapy of posterior circulation intracranial aneurysms. J Neurosurg 1989;71:512–519.

158. Higashida RT, Halbach VV, Dowd CF, et al. Intracranial aneurysms: interventional neurovascular treatment with detachable balloons. Results in 215 cases. Radiology 1991;178:663–670.

159. Fox AJ, Viñuela F, Pelz D, et al. Use of detachable balloons for proximal artery occlusion in the treatment of unclippable cerebral aneurysms. J Neurosurg 1987;66:40–46.

160. Halbach VV, Higashida RT, Dowd CF, et al. Endovascular treatment of vertebral artery dissections and pseudoaneurysms. J Neurosurg 1993;79:183–191.

161. Forsting M, Resch KM, von Kummer R, Sartor K. Balloon occlusion of a giant lower basilar aneurysm: death due to thrombosis of the aneurysm. AJNR Am J Neuroradiol 1991;12:1063–1066.

162. Lane B, Marks MP. Coil embolization of an acutely ruptured saccular aneurysm. AJNR Am J Neuroradiol 1991;12:1067–1069.

163. Guglielmi G, Viñuela F, Sepetka I, Macellari V. Electrothrombosis of saccular aneurysms via endovascular approach. Part 1: Electrochemical basis, technique, and experimental results. J Neurosurg 1991;75:1–7.

164. Guglielmi G, Viñuela F, Dion J, et al. Electrothrombosis of saccular aneurysms via endovascular approach. Part 2: Preliminary clinical experience. J Neurosurg 1991;75:8–14.

165. Dowd CF, Halbach VV, Higashida RT, et al. Endovascular coil embolization of unusual posterior inferior cerebellar artery aneurysms. Neurosurgery 1990;27:954–961.

166. Casasco AE, Aymard A, Gobin P, et al. Selective endovascular treatment of 71 intracranial aneurysms with platinum coils. J Neurosurg 1993;79:3–10.

167. Brilstra EH, Rinkel GH, van der Graaf Y, et al. Treatment of intracranial aneurysms by embolization with coils: a systematic review. Stroke 1999;30:470–476.

168. Guglielmi G, Viñuela F, Duckwiler G, et al. Endovascular treatment of posterior circulation aneurysms by electrothrombosis using electrically detachable coils. J Neurosurg 1992;77:515–524.

169. Knuckey NW, Haas R, Jenkins R, Epstein MH. Thrombosis of difficult intracranial aneurysms by the endovascular placement of platinum-Dacron microcoils. J Neurosurg 1992;77:43–50.

170. Higashida RT, Halbach VV, Cahan LD, et al. Transluminal angioplasty for treatment of intracranial arterial vasospasm. J Neurosurg 1989;71:648–653.

171. Dion JE, Duckwiler GR, Viñuela F, et al. Pre-operative micro-angioplasty of refractory vasospasm secondary to subarachnoid hemorrhage. Neuroradiology 1990;32: 232–236.

172. Kaku Y, Yonekawa Y, Tsukahara T, Kazekawa K. Superselective intra-arterial infusion of papaverine for the treatment of cerebral vasospasm after subarachnoid hemorrhage. J Neurosurg 1992;77:842–847.

173. Kassell NF, Helm G, Simmons N, et al. Treatment of cerebral vasospasm with intra-arterial papaverine. J Neurosurg 1992;77:848–852.

Chapter 19

Endovascular Therapy of Cerebral Aneurysms and Arteriovenous Malformations

Peter A. Rasmussen, Alex Abou-Chebl, and Anthony J. Furlan

Intracranial Arteriovenous Malformations

Arteriovenous malformations (AVMs) of the brain are the third most common cause of intracranial hemorrhage. In young adults, AVMs are one of the most common causes of parenchymal hemorrhage.[1] Until 1970, surgical therapy for AVMs was frequently complicated and often unsuccessful. As with the therapy of intracranial aneurysms, the development of modern microvascular neurosurgical techniques has allowed for the successful management of most patients. However, large lesions with deep vascular supply have remained a formidable surgical challenge. With the aid of endovascular therapy, patients with previously untreatable AVMs may have a treatment option other than observation. Unlike endovascular therapy of aneurysms, however, endovascular therapy of AVMs is usually adjunctive to definitive surgical excision, rather than a separate therapeutic option.

Epidemiology

The frequency of AVMs is 0.5% in autopsy series.[2] The annual incidence of AVMs is one-seventh to one-tenth that of aneurysms and ranges from 0.15% to 3.0%. There is a slight male preponderance, with a reported male to female ratio ranging from 1:1 to 2:1.[3] Most AVMs become symptomatic

by age 40 years; the peak age of hemorrhage is between 15 and 20 years of age.[2,3]

AVMs can occur throughout the brain and have three morphologic components: (1) the feeding artery or arteries, (2) the draining vein(s), and (3) the dysplastic nidus or abnormal connection between arteries and veins without an intervening capillary bed.[4] AVMs are commonly classified using the Spetzler-Martin classification schema (Table 19-1), which is based on three radiologic characteristics: (1) the size of the AVM, (2) the location and, therefore, the eloquence of the surrounding brain, and (3) the pattern of venous drainage, either deep or superficial.[5] On initial presentation, 30% of AVMs are <3 cm in diameter, 60% are between 3 cm and 6 cm, and the remainder are >6 cm in size.[6] In approximately 15–20% of AVMs, an associated intracranial aneurysm is found.[6]

Clinical Presentation

The initial presenting symptom for AVMs is a hemorrhage in 42–53% of patients, a seizure in 33–46% of patients, a headache in 14–34% of patients, and a progressive neurologic deficit in 21–23% of patients.[2] Large AVMs (those larger than 7 cm^3) are more likely to present with a seizure (72%) than with a hemorrhage (28%), whereas smaller AVMs (those smaller than 7 cm^3)

329

Table 19-1. The Spetzler-Martin Scale for Evaluating Risk of Neurologic Deterioration after Surgery for Arteriovenous Malformation Resection

Characteristic	Points Assigned
Size of lesion	
Small (<3 cm)	1
Medium (3–6 cm)	2
Large (>6 cm)	3
Location	
Non-eloquent site	0
Eloquent site	1
Sensorimotor, language, visual cortex, Hypothalamus, thalamus, brain stem, Cerebellar nuclei, or regions directly adjacent to these structures	
Direction of venous drainage	
Superficial	0
Deep (any vein)	1

are more likely to present with a hemorrhage (75%) than a seizure (25%). In cases in which the initial presentation is a hemorrhage, larger AVMs tend to have a higher risk of rebleeding.[2,3]

Hemorrhage is the most devastating complication of AVMs and may be secondary to rupture of the AVM itself, an associated aneurysm, or both. By age 40 years, 40% of all patients with AVMs will have experienced a hemorrhage.[3] The hemorrhage may be intraparenchymal or subarachnoid in location. Unlike aneurysmal subarachnoid hemorrhage (SAH), intraparenchymal hemorrhage secondary to an AVM is rarely associated with early rebleeding or vasospasm and delayed ischemic deficit.[7] The annual risk of hemorrhage is 3–4%, or 30–40% per decade, with a higher risk associated with smaller AVMs.[2,3,6,8]

The annual mortality risk for AVMs is 0.9–1.0%; however, the risk decreases after 15 years from the last hemorrhage.[2] With each episode of hemorrhage, there is a 20% risk of a major neurologic deficit and a 10% risk of mortality.[2,3,6,8] The risk of a neurologic deficit is decreased if the hemorrhage has a subarachnoid component.[2]

The location of the AVM correlates with the risk of epilepsy. The risk of seizures is highest in those patients with AVMs located in the frontal lobes (75%), lowest in patients with AVMs in the occipital lobes (0%), and intermediate in those with AVMs located in the parietal (57%) and temporal lobes (29%).[9] In one study of 545 patients, 44% of initial seizures were nonfocal.[3] Progressive neurologic deficits are thought to arise from a "steal phenomenon" that diverts blood away from viable brain tissue or from venous stasis and venous hypertension, both leading to chronic ischemia.[2]

Diagnosis

As with aneurysmal SAH, the mainstay for the correct diagnosis of an AVM, ruptured or unruptured, is a contrast-enhanced cranial computed tomography (CT) scan. CT scans readily detect hemorrhage and are also sensitive to calcification, which is frequently associated with AVMs.[2,6,7] On a noncontrast-enhanced CT scan, areas of acute hemorrhage or calcification appear as hyperdense regions with or without surrounding hypodensity representing edema. In cases without acute hemorrhage or calcification, the lesion may appear as isodense; however, with contrast enhancement, the AVM enhances intensely, typically in a "serpentine" pattern as the abnormal and dilated vessels fill with contrast material.[6] Cranial magnetic resonance imaging (MRI) is more sensitive for detecting AVMs than CT.[7] On MRI, hemorrhages have varying signal intensities, depending on the age of the hematoma and the oxidation state of the hemoglobin within the lesion. Vessels within the AVM appear as hypointense "flow voids" in a pattern not typical of the normal vascular anatomy of the affected region of the brain.[6] In addition, MRI allows for the accurate localization of associated normal and abnormal brain tissue, which is crucial for the adequate determination of eloquence, as defined in the Spetzler-Martin scale.[5] Conventional four-vessel cerebral angiography is the gold standard for evaluating AVMs preoperatively and before embolization. It is important to emphasize that magnetic resonance angiography is not an adequate substitute for conventional angiography.[6] Functional studies, such as xenon CT, single-photon CT, or positron emission tomography, have also been used to help predict the risk of AVM hemorrhage, infarction, or normal perfusion pressure breakthrough.[6,10]

Therapy

Therapeutic options for AVMs include observation, embolization, stereotactic radiosurgery, microsurgery, or combinations of these.[11] Given the poor natural history of AVMs, most patients should be considered for some form of therapeutic intervention. Spetzler-Martin grade I–III AVMs are amenable to microsurgical excision with 0.0–4.2% reported morbidity in many series.[12] Surgery in this patient group results in a cure and should be considered the treatment of choice.[11–13] Lesions that warrant endovascular therapy either alone or in combination with microsurgery or stereotactic radiosurgery are large high-risk lesions with deep venous drainage or those located in an eloquent location (i.e., Spetzler-Martin grades IV and V).[11,14–19] Microsurgery alone is associated with a long-term morbidity of 21.9% and 16.7% in grade IV and V AVMs, respectively.[12] The multidisciplinary management goal of AVM therapy is the complete removal or obliteration of the AVM. Partial therapy does not decrease the risk of rehemorrhage, although it may offer a palliative effect for headaches, seizures, and progressive neurologic deficits.[6,11,20]

Results Overview

Complete cure or obliteration of an AVM with endovascular therapy alone is feasible in only 5–20% of cases, most of which are small lesions that are also readily excised surgically.[6,20,21]

Embolization before microsurgery, however, is usually effective in decreasing surgical bleeding. Embolization makes distinguishing boundaries between AVM and normal brain easier, decreases operative time, and increases the chance of complete excision in high-grade lesions.[11,14–18] In one series of AVMs located in eloquent areas, combined endovascular embolization followed by microsurgery resulted in a 5% rate of new major deficits, compared to a rate of 31% in the surgery only group.[22] In another comparison of surgery alone or in combination with preoperative embolization, there was no difference in complication rates between the two groups despite the fact that the embolized group consisted of larger and higher Spetzler-Martin grade lesions.[23]

Optimal results are obtained when surgery is performed within 2–14 days of embolization. This decreases the risk of developing new leptomeningeal or deep collaterals as well as AVM recanalization.[11,20] Early and frequent recanalization has been observed with virtually all of the embolic materials used except the cyanoacrylates.[20] Except for cases treated with cyanoacrylate glue, endovascular therapy should be followed by early microsurgery.[6,11,20] In patients with large AVMs, staged embolization decreases the potential for perfusion pressure breakthrough and hemorrhage.[18,20] The combined approach of endovascular embolization and radiosurgery is controversial and has not been adequately studied.[20,24–26]

Complications of endovascular therapy include thromboembolic stroke, intracranial hemorrhage, pulmonary embolism, and microcatheter retention.[6,11,20] Endovascular complications occur in 3–25% of cases; however, serious neurologic complications or death occur in only 3–8% of cases.[11,15,27] Complications can be reduced by careful attention to technique, staged embolization of large AVMs, careful use of cyanoacrylates, and rapid withdrawal of the microcatheter after injection.[6,11,20]

Treatment Strategies

The development of the field of interventional neuroradiology or endovascular neurosurgery has been driven by improvements in the technology of catheter and device design and fabrication. As advances have entered the clinical arena, the scope and complexity of vascular lesions that may be addressed by endovascular techniques has broadened. Paralleling the explosion of advances in this field have been equally compelling improvements in stereotactic gamma knife radiosurgery for treatment of AVMs. Consequently, a multi-modal approach to the treatment of complex AVMs that includes surgery, radiosurgery, and endovascular embolization has evolved, allowing for the treatment of even high-risk lesions.

The goal of treatment for any AVM is the durable and complete angiographic elimination of the lesion. Historically, the only treatment available for AVMs has been microsurgical excision. If the AVM nidus can be completely removed, there is no chance that the AVM can recur, and the patient is cured. However, large AVMs or those located deep in the cerebral or cerebellar mantle have unacceptably high rates of neurologic morbidity associated with surgical extirpation. Some curative embolizations with liquid cyanoacrylates have been reported, but only 10% of AVMs treated this way are angiographically occluded and these have an average diameter of only 2.3 cm.[21]

Selecting the appropriate therapeutic strategy, observational or active, is dependent on both clinical and radiographic factors. Patients with Spetzler-

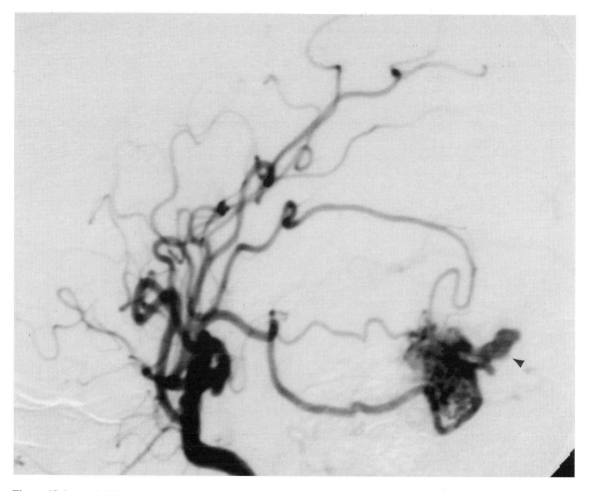

Figure 19-1. Arterial phase lateral left carotid artery angiogram reveals a Spetzler-Martin grade III posterior temporal arteriovenous malformation with three feeding arterial pedicles. The arrowhead identifies an associated nidal aneurysm, an angiographic finding known to increase the risk of hemorrhage.

Martin grade I and II AVMs can be treated with an acceptably low rate of neurologic morbidity (see Table 19-1).[5] Based on the clinical situation and the imaging findings, a subset of patients with grade III AVMs may also benefit from active treatment. Those patients with grade IV and V lesions generally have such a high rate of neurologic deterioration after treatment that observational management is favorable. However, if these patients have repeated hemorrhages, debilitating seizures, or cognitive impairments secondary to ischemia or "steal," multimodality curative therapy may be beneficial.

Full radiographic evaluation includes MRI and catheter angiography with selective injections of feeding pedicles and high-speed filming rates (≥4 frames/second). These studies provide information about the location of the lesion with respect to "eloquent" brain, the operative corridor needed to access the lesion surgically, and the technical feasibility of preoperative (surgical or radiosurgical) reductive or ablative embolization. A careful high-resolution angiographic study reveals the number and type of arterial pedicles, their relationship to the blood supply of surrounding normal brain tissue, the size of the nidus, the presence of associated fistulae and aneurysms (both intra-nidal and remote), and the type of venous drainage (superficial or deep). Radiographic features that have been associated with greater risk of hemorrhage are deep venous drainage (especially if a venous stenosis is present), periventricular location, and intranidal aneurysms (Figures 19-1 and 19-2).[28]

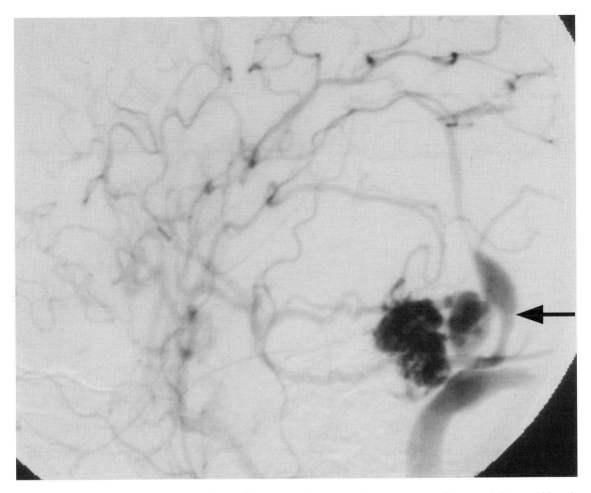

Figure 19-2. Late arterial phase lateral left carotid artery angiogram showing the pattern of venous drainage. Although superficial, the associated outflow venous stenosis (*arrow*) and retrograde venous drainage are risk factors for arteriovenous malformation hemorrhage.

Superselective angiographic studies disclose the exact nature of the arterial supply. Any number of arteries may feed the nidus, arterial feeders may terminate directly in the nidus, or they may send feeders or twigs to the nidus while the main trunk continues to supply normal brain distal to the branch point. These latter vessels are known as *en passage* (or vessel in passage) feeders. AVMs with *en passage* supply carry a higher risk of post-treatment neurologic deficit with both surgical and endovascular treatment because of the risk of injury to the parent vessel and subsequent infarction. Frequently, superselective angiography of AVMs with multiple feeders demonstrates that each feeder supplies only one portion or compartment of the AVM (Figure 19-3). This is of critical importance during endovascular embolization, as occlusion of one compartment of a large AVM may reduce the overall size sufficiently to improve the likelihood that radiosurgery may successfully obliterate the lesion.

Large supratentorial AVMs frequently are wedge- or pyramid-shaped, with their bases at the cortical surface and their apices extending down to the lateral ventricle. Superficially located AVMs usually have arterial supply from only one or a few cortical arteries; however, large AVMs or those found exclusively in a deep location frequently are supplied by the choroidal and lenticulostriate systems. This deep supply may increase the risk of surgical morbidity and certainly leads to a more technically demanding operation with an increased

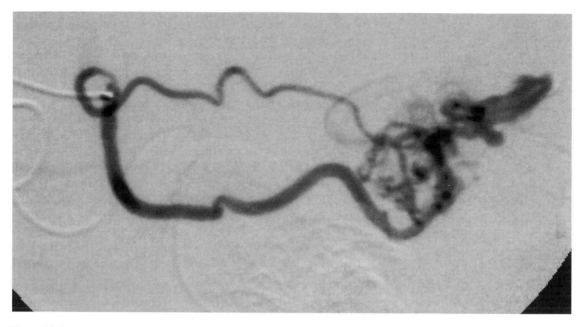

Figure 19-3. Superselective microcatheter injection angiogram demonstrating the supply of the arteriovenous malformation (AVM) from two of the three feeding pedicles. Note that the entire nidus does not opacify with this injection, suggesting compartmentalization of the nidus. On the outflow side of the AVM, there is an irregular nidal aneurysm pointing posteriorly.

risk of significant blood loss. Deep vessels are ideal targets for embolization because occlusion of these vessels prevents bleeding from a source that would otherwise be among the last to be seen surgically. Therefore, strategies using endovascular embolization target the reduction in both the rate of blood flow and the size of the AVM (i.e., to "downgrade" it). This should decrease operative morbidity or reduce the AVM size so that the probability of successful treatment with radiosurgery is higher.

Technique of Embolization

The success of endovascular therapy of AVMs depends on the equipment and embolic agents used, the quality of the angiographic equipment, and the experience and clinical judgment of the endovascular surgeon.

Embolization is performed in a neuroradiologic suite or operating room equipped with bi-planar fluoroscopy. Ideally, the patient is awake, facilitating neurologic assessment during the procedure. A transfemoral route is usually used, and a 6–8 Fr guiding catheter is positioned in the internal carotid or vertebral artery, depending on the vascular sup-

ply of the AVM. A microcatheter is used to superselectively catheterize the feeding arterial pedicles.

Microcatheters

Small size is a requisite for access to these potentially diminutive arteries. Catheters capable of reaching the distal cerebral arteries range in size from 2.3 Fr to 3.0 Fr. Two general types are available: an over-the-wire system and a flow-directed system. Both types have a hydrophilic coating that improves their performance and facilitates advancing them up a vessel. Over-the-wire catheters require accessing vessels with a steerable microguidewire, then advancing the catheter over the wire until the desired location is reached. Because AVMs usually have high-flow feeding pedicles, the preferential blood flow to these vessels may be used to the operator's advantage by using a catheter that has an extremely floppy, low mass, bulb-shaped tip. Such flow-directed catheters move like a sail in the wind and are drawn to the nidus by the flow of blood. Flow-directed techniques work best for accessing the nidus during the early stages of embolization when there is still a high-flow state through the AVM and its feeders. As the embolization proceeds and the shunt decreases, the ease with which these catheters "sail" to the nidus diminishes.

Guidewires

Like microcatheters, microguidewires also need to be small (0.010–0.014 in.) and flexible. Generally, a balance must be struck between the stiffness of the wire (which supports forward pushing of the catheter) and the softness of the tip to reduce the risk of vessel perforation. Usually manufactured from stainless steel or nitinol, the wire provides torqueability to steer the wire into the desired vessels while navigating several bends through tortuous vessel loops. Movements of guidewire-supported microcatheters are flow-independent and, consequently, these systems are best suited for accessing small feeders arising from a main vessel trunk.

Embolic Agents

Before delivering embolic material to an AVM, the interventionist should assess the risk of causing a permanent neurologic deficit. Angiography through the microcatheter after it has obtained its final position reveals whether there is any normal brain being irrigated distal to the tip of the microcatheter. If there is any question as to whether functional brain is embolized, a provocative neurologic challenge can be performed by injecting amobarbital through the microcatheter. Careful examination of the patient's neurologic function subserved by the brain in question is then performed. If there are no deficits, embolization is not likely to lead to a significant neurologic deficit.

Embolic agents can be categorized into two main groups: liquids and particles. The cyanoacrylates ("glue") are the prototypical liquid embolic agents and are the only agents that can lead to a permanent endovascular cure. The most widely used cyanoacrylate, N-butyl cyanoacrylate (NBCA) (Trufill, Cordis Corp., Miami, FL), exists as a liquid that polymerizes immediately on contact with an ionic solution containing free hydrogen ions. Because of its low viscosity, it can be injected through the smallest microcatheters, a limitation in delivering the larger particulates.

The technique of glue embolization requires a thorough knowledge of the polymerization characteristics of the agent, the rate of blood flow through the nidus, the degree of pedicle occlusion by the microcatheter, and the rate of material delivery through any given microcatheter. Endovascular cure demands that the entire AVM nidus be occluded, including the components nearest to the venous side, or the nidus may recruit a new arterial supply. Because NBCA polymerizes so rapidly, an agent must be added that retards its polymerization rate. The oily contrast medium lipiodol is used for this purpose and has the added advantage of opacifying the otherwise radio-transparent NBCA, allowing for visualization under fluoroscopy. By varying the ratios of the components, an experienced physician can mix a cocktail that penetrates the entire nidus before polymerizing without reaching the draining vein(s). Should the draining vein(s) be occluded, the blood pressure head within the nidus may rise to high levels that cannot be supported by the fragile walls of the dysplastic AVM vessels, resulting in rupture and hemorrhage. In addition, care must be taken to avoid gluing the microcatheter to the nidus, usually an irreversible situation.

Despite their complexities and potentially serious complications, cyanoacrylates' adhesive properties have made them useful in reducing the size of selected AVMs before stereotaxic radiosurgery. Other nonpermanent embolic agents (i.e., particulates) cannot fulfill this role, as the AVM nidus recannulates within a few weeks after their delivery. In contrast, particulates are somewhat safer and easier to use and are particularly helpful as an adjunct to open surgical therapy.

Particulates are manufactured from a variety of materials and come in a range of sizes. The smallest are polyvinyl alcohol (PVA) particles, which are engineered in sizes ranging from 50 to 1,500 µm and injected as a suspension in radiographic contrast media. The exact size used depends on the rate of flow through the nidus and the presence of intranidal shunts and fistulae. If too much PVA traverses the nidus without lodging in it, an inflammatory pulmonary reaction can develop with transient pulmonary failure. To minimize this complication, intranidal shunts can be partially occluded by mixing the PVA with fibrillary collagen or by using Berenstein liquid coils (Boston Scientific/Target Therapeutics, Fremont, CA). These are fine injectable platinum threads that promote thrombus formation. When delivered to small feeding pedicles, they lead to thrombosis and occlusion of the vessel (Figure 19-4). If the fistulae or

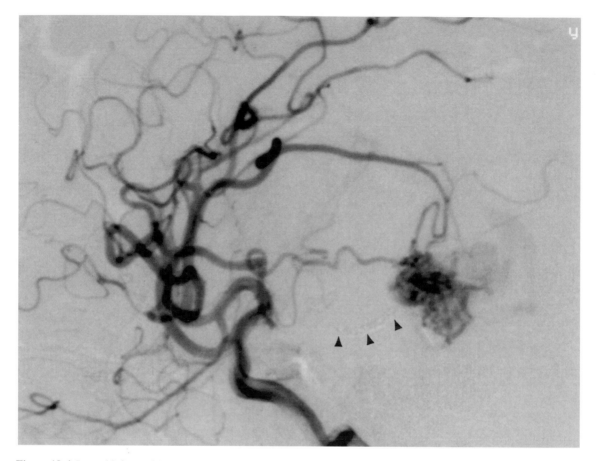

Figure 19-4. Lateral left carotid angiogram after occlusion of the inferior pedicle with Berenstein liquid coils (*arrowheads*). Limited treatment was authorized, and this pedicle was occluded to obtain a deconstructive treatment of the nidal aneurysm that no longer fills angiographically.

feeding vessels are large in diameter (3–5 mm), platinum coils that assume the configuration of vortices or tornadoes can be pushed through the microcatheter. These coils are usually coated with fibered threads that readily promote thrombosis and occlusion.

None of these materials, however, constitute the ideal embolic agent. The search for better devices and materials continues. The future holds the promise of new liquids and adhesives that use controlled delivery systems and possess more favorable polymerization characteristics. Additional cyanoacrylates are under clinical investigation that polymerize more slowly and are more viscous, allowing for deeper penetration into the nidus with a decreased risk of gluing the catheter in place. A novel polymer, Onyx (Microtherapeutics, Inc., San Clemente, CA), is dissolved in di-methyl sulfoxide and solidifies as the di-methyl sulfoxide diffuses. This agent lacks the adhesive quality of cyanoacrylates, making it safer to use, and its rate of polymerization is partly dependent on blood flow, hardening faster as flow increases. Another polymer is being developed that has an inherent magnetic moment. It is injectable and its flow and distribution is controlled by external, stereotactically placed, high-strength magnetic fields. Hopefully, the liquid agent that has the correct polymerization rate, flow characteristics, delivery system, and adhesive qualities can be found, rendering most of these lesions curable by endovascular methods.

Intracranial Aneurysms

The treatment of intracranial aneurysms has advanced significantly since the first direct surgical clipping of an aneurysm by Dandy in 1937.[29] With the development of microsurgical techniques and other technical advances, craniotomy with clipping remains the most widely accepted method of treating patients with intracranial aneurysms. As technologic breakthroughs were made in interventional neuroradiology in the 1970s, it was inevitable that these techniques would be applied to the treatment of intracranial aneurysms. Initial trials used balloons to occlude the parent vessel.[30,31] Endovascular techniques were further refined to involve packing and occlusion of the aneurysm itself with detachable balloons.[32] Both of these approaches were fraught with difficulties and complications, including aneurysm rupture and balloon deflation.[33,34]

The most recent advance in endovascular therapy has been the development of the Guglielmi detachable coil (GDC) (Boston Scientific/Target Therapeutics, Fremont, CA).[35,36] The coils are made of soft platinum and are deployed within an aneurysm by a microcatheter. Although controversial initially, multiple trials and reports have confirmed the efficacy and safety of this technique in carefully selected patients. In 1995, the FDA approved the use of GDCs in patients with high-risk of surgical morbidity. Since 1990, more than 15,000 patients have been treated by this method.[37]

Epidemiology of Subarachnoid Hemorrhage

SAH is one of the most dramatic and serious cerebrovascular disorders. The most common causes of SAH, in order of decreasing frequency, are trauma, rupture of intracranial aneurysms, AVMs, and benign nonaneurysmal peri-mesencephalic hemorrhage. Intracranial aneurysms are relatively common and have a prevalence of 0.3–8.0% in the general population.[38–40] Aneurysmal rupture and SAH occur in approximately 25,000 individuals annually in the United States, and 18,000 of these hemorrhages result in death or severe disability.[1] These figures represent an incidence of SAH of 10 per 100,000 individuals and account for approximately 5% of all strokes. The anatomic distributions of ruptured aneurysms in the large International Cooperative Study on the Timing of Aneurysm Surgery are summarized in Table 19-2.

Approximately 80% of intracranial aneurysms are congenital or saccular in nature and are formed

Table 19-2. Distribution of Aneurysms Among the 3,521 Patients of the International Cooperative Study on the Timing of Aneurysm Surgery

Vessel	Percent of Patients
Anterior cerebral	39.0
Internal carotid	29.8
Middle cerebral	22.3
Vertebrobasilar	7.6
Other	2.0

Source: Adapted from NF Kassell, JC Torner, JA Jane, et al. International Cooperative Study on the Timing of Aneurysm Surgery. 1. Overall management results. J Neurosurg 1990;73:18–36.

from defects of the arterial wall at arterial bifurcations.[1] Nearly 20% of individuals have multiple saccular aneurysms. Other types of aneurysms include fusiform or atherosclerotic aneurysms, mycotic or infectious aneurysms, and traumatic aneurysms usually arising from antecedent arterial dissections.

Clinical Presentation

The classic presentation of SAH is the sudden ("thunderclap") onset of severe headache accompanied by loss of consciousness, nausea, and vomiting. If the patient survives this initial event (approximately 25% of patients die before hospital admission), nuchal rigidity, focal neurologic deficits, seizures or fever, and depressed level of consciousness may develop.[1] In 20–50% of cases, patients do not have a dramatic presentation; rather, they have "sentinel" bleeds.[41] Sentinel bleeds or headaches are of sudden but lesser severity and are not associated with neurologic deficits other than mild signs of meningeal irritation.

Not all aneurysms present with SAH. Larger aneurysms usually present with symptoms of mass effect: headache, cranial neuropathies, especially oculomotor and abducens nerve palsies, and hydrocephalus. If the aneurysm is arising in the cavernous segment of the internal carotid artery, the patient may present with cavernous sinus syndrome.

Time to presentation and severity of neurologic deficit after SAH are predictive of potential therapeutic success and overall outcome.[42,43] Patients who present with a high Hunt and Hess grade (i.e., depressed level of consciousness, hemiparesis, and vegetative signs) have the worst prognosis, with a two-fold risk of death compared to patients in good neurologic condition (see Table 18-1 in Chapter 18). Patients treated for unruptured aneurysms have a better prognosis than patients with ruptured aneurysms. Aneurysms rupture at a rate of 0.05–2.30% per year depending on the size and location of the aneurysm.[44,45] Most aneurysms are >5 mm in size when they rupture.

Diagnosis

SAH should be considered in all patients who present with a sudden, severe headache, especially if there are other neurologic signs. Radiologic diagnosis is made with a CT scan, which has a reported sensitivity of 92% and a specificity of nearly 100%.[46] When there is strong clinical suspicion of SAH but a negative CT scan, a lumbar puncture should be performed. It may be difficult to differentiate true SAH from a "traumatic tap" because xanthochromia of the supernatant may take up to 12 hours to appear after the onset of SAH.[41] Cerebral angiography remains the gold standard for determining the etiology of SAH and is also the basis for making a therapeutic plan after SAH. Four-vessel cerebral angiography should be performed urgently in all patients with a Hunt and Hess grade III. Particular attention should be paid to the location of the aneurysm(s), its size, shape, presence and size of a neck, and the relationship of the aneurysm to the parent vessel and its adjacent branches. Cerebral angiography may be negative in approximately 15% of patients with SAH.[47,48] In such instances, angiography should be repeated 1–4 weeks later to definitively exclude a structural source of the SAH.[49] Aneurysms are classified as small if they are 8 mm in diameter at their largest point, large if between 9 mm and 25 mm in diameter, and giant if larger than 25 mm in diameter.

Therapy

The natural history of untreated cerebral aneurysms is dismal. Within the first 3 months after SAH there is an 81% mortality rate, 44% of which is due to rebleeding.[50] During the first week, the risk of rebleeding is 6–9%; at 30 days, the risk of rebleeding increases to more than 20%. The mortality rate with rebleeding approaches 70%.[42,50] Therapy for intracranial aneurysms remains controversial. Controversy exists over the merits of endovascular therapy versus surgical therapy, as well as over the timing of aneurysm surgery. In addition, the indications for therapy of unruptured aneurysms are controversial.

Endovascular therapy with GDCs is approved by the FDA only for high-risk patients with ruptured aneurysms. The general indications for endovascular aneurysm therapy are[51]

1. Technical difficulties with surgical approach secondary to anatomic factors
2. Aneurysms with high surgical risk (itself controversial)
3. Incomplete surgical clipping
4. Underlying severe medical illness(es) predisposing to high mortality from general anesthesia

The primary issues regarding the timing of aneurysm surgery are the technical aspects and the higher risks associated with early surgery. These risks are due partly to the presence of brain swelling and large amounts of subarachnoid blood that obscure the surgical field. Surgery is often delayed in patients in poor medical and neurologic condition (i.e., those with a Hunt and Hess grade III). However, delaying surgery increases the likelihood of rebleeding. The International Cooperative Study on the Timing of Aneurysm Surgery was conducted to address the timing of aneurysm surgery.[52] Investigators found that the overall results in patients treated with clipping in the first few days after SAH were equivalent to those treated after 10 days (although therapy at 7–10 days was high-risk due to vasospasm). Patients who were alert on presentation and underwent surgery within 3 days had the best outcomes. Generally, the accepted practice is to clip ruptured aneurysms as soon as practical after initial presentation, especially in patients with Hunt and Hess grade III.

Results of Endovascular Therapy

When comparing the results of endovascular therapy with surgical clipping, it should be remembered that most of the available data are from series of patients who were poor surgical candidates, many of whom had a poor neurologic grade (Hunt and Hess grades IV and V). The first 403 patients treated in the United States were reported by Vinuela and colleagues.[53] In this group, 53.6% of patients were Hunt and Hess grades III–V and were excluded from surgery. All of the patients were treated within 15 days of the initial ictus; 36.5% were treated within 48 hours. The treated aneurysms were located primarily in the posterior circulation (57%), and the size distribution was small (60.8%), large (34.7%), and giant (4.5%). The success rate, defined as complete occlusion of the aneurysm, was 70.8% in small aneurysms with a small neck but only 31.2% in small aneurysms with a wide neck. Of large aneurysms, 35% were successfully completely occluded, as were 50% of giant aneurysms. Twenty-three patients (5.7% overall) were classified as treatment failures due to inability to achieve even partial occlusion as a result of technical factors. Of the treatment failures, one-half were patients with small, wide-necked aneurysms. Patients with better clinical grades before therapy had better outcomes. For Hunt and Hess grade I patients, 93% were improved or unchanged, compared to 54% of patients with Hunt and Hess grade V. Overall, 84.9% of patients improved or remained the same clinically on discharge, 8.9% deteriorated after embolization, and 6.2% died within 1 week of embolization. Early rebleeding rates were decreased. Morbidity and mortality attributed to the endovascular procedure were 8.9% and 6.2%, respectively. Technical complications included aneurysm perforation (2.7%), parent artery occlusion (3.0%), and distal embolization (2.5%). Aneurysmal perforation occurred almost exclusively in patients with small aneurysms (9 of 11 cases). Although there was no follow-up beyond 36 months, nine aneurysms (2.2%) rebled, all of which were incompletely occluded aneurysms.

Other smaller series also reported complete occlusion rates of approximately 80%.[37] As clinical experience has increased, morbidity and mortality figures and technical success rates have improved, approaching the results achieved with surgery.[37,51,54–58] Factors that increase the chance of complete angiographic occlusion include a small neck (= 4 mm), a small aneurysm, indirect inflow

of the blood stream into the aneurysm, and technical experience of the interventionalist.[57,59,60] The differences between success rates in the anterior and posterior circulation are minor, but some reports have suggested improved success in posterior circulation aneurysms.[53,56,60,61] Immediate technical results are the best predictors of the likelihood of persistent occlusion.[57,60] Complications of therapy, including macro- and microembolization with resultant ischemia, parent artery occlusion, and aneurysm perforation, occur in 2.8–28.0% of patients.[37,53,54,56,61]

Direct comparisons with surgical series are problematic because patients treated early in the GDC experience with endovascular techniques were deemed not to be surgical candidates. Poor clinical condition or the high risk and complexity of the surgical approach were the major reasons for exclusion from surgery.[37,56] Although the risk of early rebleeding is decreased with successful endovascular therapy, there are few available data on long-term results and hemorrhage recurrence in patients treated endovascularly. Results of follow-up angiography performed up to 72 months after embolization have shown that 61–86% of aneurysms do not demonstrate any change in the degree of aneurysm occlusion.[55,59,60] As the length of follow-up increases, so does the risk of recanalization and rebleeding. The risk of rebleeding has been reported to be as low as 0.0–3.2% in small aneurysms but as high as 4% for large aneurysms and 33% for giant aneurysms.[55,60,62]

Asymptomatic and unruptured symptomatic aneurysms have also been treated by endovascular embolization with GDCs. Results are better than for acutely ruptured aneurysms because of the better clinical condition of the patients. In a series of 120 aneurysms reported by Murayama et al.,[63] 91% of incidental aneurysms were successfully treated (complete or near-complete occlusion) with a morbidity of 4.3%. All of the complications occurred in the first 50 patients, indicating that technical proficiency increases with experience. In another series of consecutive unruptured MCA aneurysms, only 2 (6%) of 34 aneurysms were successfully treated with GDCs.[64] Unfavorable anatomy—primarily a dome to neck ratio of less than 2 and the presence of an arterial branch at the aneurysm base—prompted primary clipping in two-thirds of these patients and resulted in failure of attempted embolization in the remaining one-third. Coil embolization has also been used to successfully treat cranial neuropathies and other clinical deficits associated with the mass effect of aneurysms.[65,66] As with ruptured aneurysms, long-term follow-up is lacking, and the durability of endovascular occlusions remains unknown.

Treatment Strategies

In contrast to the strategic planning needed for successful treatment of AVMs, therapeutic options for managing aneurysms are less complex. An extensive assessment of the relative benefits and risks of surgery versus endovascular therapy for the treatment of aneurysms is beyond the scope of this chapter. Both treatment modalities aim to achieve complete angiographic resolution of the aneurysm. Although complete occlusion is desirable, a 90% occlusion of an aneurysm at the basilar apex by endovascular methods in a debilitated 80-year-old person may be a more satisfying treatment than a 100% occlusion via craniotomy.

Treatment Techniques

Successful obliteration of intracranial aneurysms requires developing a stable or permanent thrombosis of the aneurysmal sac. Two general principles can be used to achieve this state: a constructive embolization or a deconstructive embolization. A constructive treatment technique is designed to re-create the parent vessel's normal lumen that gave rise to the aneurysm, preserving the patient's normal vessel anatomy and hemodynamics (e.g., surgical clipping). A deconstructive treatment is a planned sacrifice of the parent vessel and subsequent antegrade thrombosis of the aneurysm, as thrombus propagates beyond the point of occlusion. Success of this treatment without infarction depends on the patient's native collateral circulation.

Endovascular Tools

Constructive Treatment. The most familiar endovascular device for the treatment of intracranial aneurysms is the GDC. Now available in several different forms, the GDC technology and its delivery technique have evolved and can be successfully applied to aneurysms previously considered impossible to treat from the luminal side. Occlusion (thrombosis) of the aneurysm or isolation of the aneurysmal dome from the systemic circulation is accomplished by delivering the GDCs into the sac of the aneurysm through a microcatheter. Similar to the treatment of AVMs, the microcatheter is advanced through a previously positioned guiding catheter in the cervical internal carotid or vertebral artery. Once the microcatheter is in proper position, the coils are pushed into the aneurysm. After the full length of the coil has been deployed, potential impingement on the parent vessel lumen by the coil mass or individual loops is assessed with angiography. If there is compromise of the parent vessel, the coil can be withdrawn and then repositioned, or, alternatively, a different size coil can be used. Once satisfactory position is obtained, a low-amplitude electrical current dissolves a solder joint between the coil and the delivery wire by electrolysis. Contrary to previous thinking, electrothrombosis plays only a minor role in aneurysm occlusion.

Filling of the aneurysmal sac begins by creating a "basket" with the first coil and then filling the basket with progressively smaller and shorter coils. Dense packing is attempted because the resistance to future aneurysmal rupture is related to the thrombus created within the interstices of the coil mass. The more metal (thrombus nidus) that can be placed in a given volume, the more likely a stable thrombus can develop.

The main barrier to the successful application of this technique to all aneurysms is the width of the aneurysm's neck (or "face," if viewed from the vessel's lumen). Most endovascular surgeons have been reluctant to treat aneurysms with a dome to neck ratio of less than 2.[67] Wide-necked or broad-faced aneurysms are rarely completely obliterated with coils because of the risk of coil migration into the parent vessel. However, clinical experience, technical progress, and human resourcefulness have yielded several devices and techniques that have expanded application of GDC technology to these lesions. The most widely used and accepted technique for treating broad-faced aneurysms is the balloon remodeling method.[68] This technique requires the use of a soft distensible balloon that conforms to the shape of the parent vessel. The usual sequence is to position the noninflated balloon adjacent to the aneurysm's face and then position the

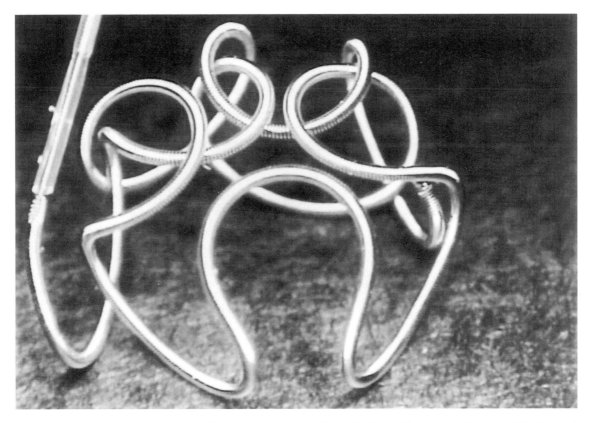

Figure 19-5. Guglielmi detachable three-dimensional coil (Boston Scientific/Target Therapeutics, Fremont, CA) deployed ex vivo. This coil is designed to be the first coil deployed to create the "basket" into which all subsequent coils will be placed and confined.

microcatheter into the aneurysm. Immediately before deploying a coil, the balloon is inflated. The distensible, silastic balloon assumes the normal shape of the parent vessel. The GDC is then positioned in the aneurysm with the balloon confining the coil's deployment only to the aneurysmal sac. Once the full length of the coil has been delivered, the balloon is deflated and angiography is performed to assess the stability of the coil in relationship to the parent vessel. If there has been no shift of the coil's position with balloon deflation, the coil is detached, and the sequence is repeated until the entire sac has been densely packed with coils.

An alternative method known as the *two-catheter technique* involves two microcatheters positioned inside the aneurysm.[69] GDCs are deployed through both catheters before detaching either with the hope that the coils orient themselves perpendicular to each other. Experience has shown that multiple coils, especially when positioned at right angles to

each other, tend to have a stabilizing effect, thus minimizing subsequent shift and migration as additional coils are introduced. After the deployment of the initial two coils, angiography is performed to assess stability and possible prolapse or migration into the parent vessel. Only after the coils' positions are deemed satisfactory are they detached and additional coils placed seriatim.

The coil-stabilizing concept has been incorporated into the fundamental design and native configuration of the three-dimensional GDC (Boston Scientific/ Target Therapeutics, Fremont, CA) (Figure 19-5). A variant of the original circular coil design, the three-dimensional coil is shaped on a mandrel so that it assumes a spheric cage-like configuration when deployed with coil segments at angles to each other. The first coil deployed is a three-dimensional coil that forms the initial "basket" and, due to its shape, is able to take purchase of any portion of the aneurysm wall that may be contributing to the neck. Another

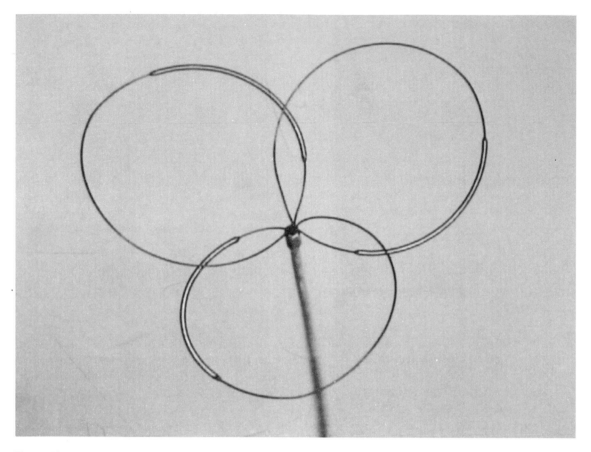

Figure 19-6. The Tri-Span Guglielmi detachable coil (GDC; Boston Scientific/Target Therapeutics, Fremont, CA). The "petals" are designed to be applied against the walls of a wide-necked aneurysm and support additional standard GDCs deployed through the interstices of the petals.

next-generation product is the Tri-Span coil (Boston Scientific/Target Therapeutics, Fremont, CA) (Figure 19-6). Use of this device requires the two-catheter technique. The Tri-Span coil is deployed first and assumes a flower petal configuration designed to mechanically create a small neck out of a wide-necked aneurysm. Once this device is positioned, standard GDCs are deployed to stabilize the "petals" against the aneurysm walls. After the sac has been filled, the petal is detached by electrolysis. All of these strategies have been used to expand the application of GDC technology to the therapy of wide-necked aneurysms.

Deconstructive Treatment. Although preserving the parent vessel that gives rise to an intracranial aneurysm is always preferred, sacrificing the parent vessel is the best means to treat some aneu-

rysms because of their location and available pattern of collateral circulation. Generally, aneurysms that arise in the cavernous segment of the internal carotid artery or from the distal branches of the cerebellar arteries are most favorably treated by vessel sacrifice due to the technical difficulties in approaching these locations surgically or the associated high surgical morbidity. Ideally, aneurysms in the cavernous carotid should be treated by a constructive technique; however, they almost always have a wide neck or arise from, or incorporate, the anterior loop of the carotid artery as it emerges from the cavernous sinus. Attempts to treat cavernous aneurysms with GDCs, including newer techniques, have frequently ended with coils prolapsed into the carotid artery or inadvertent carotid occlusion. Planned carotid sacrifice (Hunterian occlusion) preceded by a functional test measuring the robustness of the collateral circulation (test balloon occlusion) may provide the best long-term protection with a minimum of procedural morbidity in these patients.

If a patient has passed the test balloon occlusion, two different devices may be used to occlude the carotid artery. (Details, technique, controversies, and pitfalls of the test balloon occlusion are beyond the scope of this chapter.) Optimally, the aneurysm would be trapped between two occlusive devices, one proximal and one distal to the neck of the aneurysm, preventing any retrograde circulation to the aneurysm. In practice, aneurysms of the cavernous carotid have such broad necks that placing a device distal to the neck imperils the origin of the ophthalmic artery and risks ischemic insults to the retina. Usually, occlusion of the carotid artery proximal to the neck results in thrombus propagating up to the point of the next branch artery, the ophthalmic.

The most rapid method of occluding the carotid and the one associated with the fewest periprocedural ischemic complications involves detachable silicone balloons (Boston Scientific/Target Therapeutics, Fremont, CA).[70] The balloons are friction-mounted to and delivered on a microcatheter to the desired site of occlusion. They are rapidly inflated with an iso-osmolar concentration of contrast and then detached by simple mechanical traction. Two or three detachable silicone balloons are usually deployed serially to guard against the unlikely but observed possibility of balloon deflation and migration. Alternatively, the vessel may be blocked with large fiber-coated coils that rapidly promote thrombus formation and subsequent occlusion. This technique has been successfully used both with and without flow arrest in the parent vessel before coil delivery.[71,72] Position of the balloons then may be documented and followed with plain-skull radiography. With both techniques, patients are treated with coumadin for 6 months to allow for stabilization of the thrombus and to minimize the risk of embolization from the distal end of the thrombus.

References

1. Chicoine MR, Dacey RG. Clinical Aspects of Subarachnoid Hemorrhage. In KMA Weilch, LR Caplan, B Weir, BK Siesjo (eds), Primer on Cerebrovascular Diseases. San Diego: Academic, 1997;425–432.

2. Wilkins RH. Natural history of intracranial vascular malformations. Neurosurgery 1985;16:421–430.

3. Perret G, Nishioka H. Report on the cooperative study of intracranial aneurysms and subarachnoid hemorrhage. VI. Arteriovenous malformations: an analysis of 545 cases of cranio-cerebral arteriovenous malformations and fistulae reported to the cooperative study. J Neurosurg 1966;25:467–490.

4. McCormick WF. Pathology of Vascular Malformations of the Brain. In CB Wilson, BM Stein (eds), Intracranial Vascular Malformations. Baltimore: Williams & Wilkins, 1984;44–63.

5. Spetzler RF, Martin NP. A proposed grading system for arteriovenous malformations. J Neurosurg 1980;65:476–483.

6. Misra M, Aletich V, Charbel FT, et al. Multidisciplinary Approach to Arteriovenous Malformations. In AH Kaye, PM Black (eds), Operative Neurosurgery. London: Churchill Livingstone, 2000;1138–1151.

7. Lewis AI, Sathi S, Tew JM Jr. Intracranial Vascular Malformations. In RG Grossman, CM Loftus (eds), Principles of Neurosurgery. Philadelphia: Lippincott–Raven, 1999.

8. Ondra SI, Troupp H, George ED, Schwab K. The natural history of symptomatic arteriovenous malformations of the brain: a 24-year follow-up assessment. J Neurosurg 1990;73:387–391.

9. Waltimo O. The relationship of size, density, and localization of intracranial arteriovenous malformations to the type of initial symptom. J Neurol Sci 1973;19:13–19.

10. Batjer HH, Devous MD. The use of acetazolamide-enhanced regional cerebral blood flow measurements to predict risks to arteriovenous malformation patients. Neurosurgery 1992;33:312–316.

11. Rosenblatt SS, Lewis AI, Tew JM Jr. Combined interventional and surgical treatment of arteriovenous malformations. Neuroimaging Clin N Am 1998;8:469–482.

12. Hamilton MG, Spetzler RF. The prospective application of a grading system for arteriovenous malformations. Neurosurgery 1994;26:570–578.

13. Heros RC, Krosue K, Diebold PM. Surgical excision of cerebral arteriovenous malformations: late results. Neurosurgery 1990;26:570–578.

14. DeMeritt JS, Pile-Spellman J, Mast H, et al. Outcome analysis of preoperative embolization with N-butyl cyanoacrylate in cerebral arteriovenous malformations. AJNR Am J Neuroradiol 1995;16:1801–1807.

15. Fox AJ, Pelz DM, Lee DH. Arteriovenous malformations of the brain: recent results of endovascular therapy. Radiology 1990;177:51–57.

16. Grzyska U, Westphal M, Zanella F, et al. A joint protocol for the neurosurgical and neuroradiologic treatment of cerebral arteriovenous malformations: indications, technique, and results in 76 cases. Surg Neurol 1993;40:476–484.

17. Lawton MT, Hamilton MG, Spetzler RF. Multimodality treatment of deep arteriovenous malformations: thalamus, basal ganglia, and brain stem. Neurosurgery 1995;37:29–35.

18. Vinuela F, Dion JE, Duckwiler GR, et al. Combined endovascular embolization and surgery in the management of cerebral arteriovenous malformations: experience with 101 cases. J Neurosurg 1991;75:856–864.

19. Sasaki T, Kurita H, Saito I, et al. Arteriovenous malformations in the basal ganglia and thalamus: management and results in 101 cases. J Neurosurg 1998;88:285–292.

20. Deveikis JP. Endovascular therapy of intracranial arteriovenous malformations of the brain. Neuroimaging Clin N Am 1998;8:401–424.

21. Wikholm G. Occlusion of cerebral arteriovenous malformations with N-butyl cyano-acrylate is permanent. AJNR Am J Neuroradiol 1995;16:479–482.

22. Pasqualin A, Scienza R, Cioffi F, et al. Treatment of cerebral arteriovenous malformations with a combination of preoperative embolization and surgery. Neurosurgery 1991;29:358–368.

23. Jafar JJ, Rezai AR. Acute surgical management of intracranial arteriovenous malformations. Neurosurgery 1994; 34:8–13.

24. Dawson III RW, Tarr RW, Hecht ST, et al. Treatment of arteriovenous malformations of the brain with combined embolization and sterotactic radiosurgery. Results after 1 and 2 years. AJNR Am J Neuroradiol 1990;11:857–864.

25. Mathis JA, Barr JD, Horton JA, et al. The efficacy of particulate embolization combined with stereotactic radiosurgery for treatment of large arteriovenous malformations of the brain. AJNR Am J Neuroradiol 1995;16:299–306.

26. Flickinger JC, Kondziolka D, Pollock BE, Lunsford LD. Radiosurgical management of intracranial vascular malformations. Neuroimaging Clin N Am 1998;8:483–492.

27. Deruty R, Pelissou-Guyotat I, Amat D, et al. Complications after multidisciplinary treatment of cerebral arteriovenous malformations. Acta Neurochir (Wien) 1996;138: 119–131.

28. Marks MP, Lane B, Steinberg GK, Chang PJ. Hemorrhage in intracerebral arteriovenous malformations: angiographic determinants. Radiology 1990;176:807–813.

29. Dandy WE. Intracranial aneurysms of the internal carotid artery: cured by operation. Ann Surg 1938;107:654–659.

30. Serbinenko FA. Balloon catheterization and occlusion of major cerebral vessels. J Neurosurg 1974;41:125–145.

31. Debrun GM, Fox AJ, Drake CG, et al. Giant unclippable aneurysms: treatment with detachable balloons. AJNR Am J Neuroradiol 1981;2:167–173.

32. Higashida RT, Halbach VV, Barnwell SF. Treatment of intracranial aneurysms with preservation of the parent vessel: results of percutaneous balloon embolization with 84 patients. AJNR Am J Neuroradiol 1990;11:633–640.

33. Higashida RT, Halbach VV, Dormandy B, et al. Endovascular treatment of intracranial aneurysms with a new silicone microballoon device: technical considerations and indications for therapy. Radiology 1990;174:687–691.

34. Higashida RT, Halbach VV, Dowd CF, et al. Intracranial aneurysms: interventional neurovascular treatment with detachable balloons—results in 215 cases. Radiology 1991;178:663–670.

35. Guglielmi G, Vinuela F, Dion JE. Electrothrombosis of saccular aneurysms via endovascular approach. II. Preliminary clinical experience. J Neurosurg 2000;75:8–14.

36. Guglielmi G, Vinuela F, Sepetka I. Electrothrombosis of saccular aneurysms via endovascular approach. I. Electrochemical basis, technique, and experimental results. J Neurosurg 1991;75:1–7.

37. Bryan RN, Rigamonti D, Mathis JM. The treatment of acutely ruptured aneurysms: endovascular therapy versus surgery. AJNR Am J Neuroradiol 1997;18:1826–1830.

38. Jellinger K. Pathology and Etiology of Intracranial Aneurysms. In HW Pia, C Langmaid, J Zieski (eds), Cerebral Aneurysms. Advances in Diagnosis and Therapy. New York: Springer, 1979;5–19.

39. Kassell NF, Torner JC. Epidemiology of intracranial aneurysms. Int Anesthesiol Clin 1982;20:13–17.

40. Weir B. Epidemiology. In B Weir (ed), Aneurysms Affecting the Nervous System. Baltimore: Williams & Wilkins, 1987;357–360.

41. Edlow JA, Caplan LR. Avoiding pitfalls in the diagnosis of subarachnoid hemorrhage. N Engl J Med 2000;342:29–36.

42. Kassell NF, Torner JC, Jane JA, et al. The International Cooperative Study on the Timing of Aneurysm Surgery. Part 2: Surgical results. J Neurosurg 1990;73:37–47.

43. Hunt WE, Hess RM. Surgical risk as related to time of intervention in the repair of intracranial aneurysms. J Neurosurg 1968;28:14–20.

44. Asari S, Ohmoto T. Natural history and risk factors of unruptured cerebral aneurysms. Clin Neurol Neurosurg 1993;95:205–214.

45. Unruptured intracranial aneurysms: risk of rupture and risks of surgical intervention. The International Study of Unruptured Intracranial Aneurysms Investigators. N Engl J Med 1998;339:1725–1733.

46. Vespa PM, Gobin YP. Endovascular treatment and neurointensive care of ruptured intracranial aneurysms. Crit Care Clin 1999;15:667–684.

47. Rinkel GJE, van Gijn J, Wijdicks FM. Subarachnoid hemorrhage without detectable aneurysm: a review of the causes. Stroke 1993;24:1403–1409.

48. Rinkel GJE, Wijdicks FM, Hasan D, et al. Outcome in patients with subarachnoid haemorrhage and negative angiography according to pattern of haemorrhage on computed tomography. Lancet 1991;38:964–968.

49. Bradac GB, Bergui M, Ferrio MF, et al. False-negative angiograms in subarachnoid haemorrhage due to intracranial aneurysms. Neuroradiology 1997;39:772–776.

50. Graf CJ. Prognosis for patients with nonsurgically treated aneurysms. Analysis of the Cooperative Study of Intracranial Aneurysms and Subarachnoid Hemorrhage. J Neurosurg 1971;35:438–443.

51. Pruvo JP, Leclerc X, Ares GS, et al. Endovascular treatment of ruptured intracranial aneurysms. J Neurol 1999; 246:244–249.

52. Kassell NF, Torner JC, Jane JA, et al. International Cooperative Study on the Timing of Aneurysm Surgery. 1. Overall management results. J Neurosurg 1990;73:18–36.

53. Vinuela F, Duckwiler G, Mawad M. Guglielmi detachable coil embolization of acute intracranial aneurysm: perioperative anatomical and clinical outcome in 403 patients. J Neurosurg 1997;86:475–482.

54. Eskridge JM, Song JK. Endovascular embolization of 150 basilar tip aneurysms with Guglielmi detachable coils: results of the Food and Drug Administration multicenter clinical trial. J Neurosurg 1998;89:81–86.

55. Bavinzski G, Killer M, Gruber A, et al. Treatment of basilar artery bifurcation aneurysms by using Guglielmi

detachable coils: a 6-year experience. J Neurosurg 1999; 90:843–852.

56. Lempert TE, Malek AM, Halbach VV, et al. Endovascular treatment of ruptured posterior circulation cerebral aneurysms: clinical and angiographic outcomes. Stroke 2000; 31:100–110.

57. Turjman F, Massoud TF, Sayre J, Vinuela F. Predictors of aneurysmal occlusion in the period immediately after endovascular treatment with detachable coils: a multivariate analysis. AJNR Am J Neuroradiol 1998;19:1645–1651.

58. Bavinzski G, Killer M, Ferraz-Leite H, et al. Endovascular therapy of idiopathic cavernous aneurysms over 11 years. AJNR Am J Neuroradiol 1998;19:559–565.

59. Zubillaga AF, Guglielmi G, Vinuela F, Duckwiler G. Endovascular occlusion of intracranial aneurysms with electrically detachable coils: correlation of aneurysm neck size and treatment results. AJNR Am J Neuroradiol 1994; 15:815–820.

60. Hope JK, Byrne JV, Molyneux AJ. Factors influencing successful angiographic occlusion of aneurysms treated by coil embolization. AJNR Am J Neuroradiol 1999;20: 391–399.

61. Kremer C, Groden C, Hansen HC, et al. Outcome after endovascular treatment of Hunt and Hess grade IV or V aneurysms: comparison of anterior versus posterior circulation. Stroke 1999;30:2617–2622.

62. Malisch TW, Guglielmi G, Vinuela F, et al. Intracranial aneurysms treated with the Guglielmi detachable coil: midterm clinical results in a consecutive series of 100 patients. J Neurosurg 1997;87:176–183.

63. Murayama Y, Vinuela F, Duckwiler GR, et al. Embolization of incidental cerebral aneurysms by using the Gugliclmi detachable coil system. J Neurosurg 1999;90: 207–214.

64. Regli L, Uske A, de Tribolet N. Endovascular coil placement compared with surgical clipping for the treatment of unruptured middle cerebral artery aneurysms: a consecutive series. J Neurosurg 1999;90:1025–1030.

65. Birchall D, Khangure MS, McAuliffe W. Resolution of third nerve paresis after endovascular management of aneurysms of the posterior communicating artery. AJNR Am J Neuroradiol 1999;20:411–413.

66. Molyneux AJ. Management of unruptured intracranial aneurysms: endovascular treatment. 25th International Stroke Conference. New Orleans, 2000.

67. Debrun GM, Aletich VA, Kehrli P, et al. Selection of cerebral aneurysms for treatment using Guglielmi detachable coils: the preliminary University of Illinois at Chicago experience. Neurosurgery 1998;43:1281–1297.

68. Moret J, Cognard C, Weill A, et al. The "remodeling technique" in the treatment of wide-neck intracranial aneurysms. Intervent Neuroradiol 1997;3:21–35.

69. Baxter BW, Rosso D, Lownie SP. Double microcatheter technique for detachable coil treatment of large, wide-necked intracranial aneurysms. AJNR Am J Neuroradiol 1998;19:1176–1178.

70. Vazquez-Anon V, Aymard A, Gobin YP, et al. Balloon occlusion of the internal carotid artery in 40 cases of giant intracavernous aneurysm: technical aspects, cerebral monitoring, and results. Neuroradiology 1992;34:245–251.

71. Graves VB, Perl II J, Strother CM, et al. Endovascular occlusion of the carotid or vertebral artery with temporary proximal flow arrest and microcoils: clinical results. AJNR Am J Neuroradiol 1997;18:1201–1206.

72. Barr JD, Lemley TJ. Endovascular arterial occlusion accomplished using microcoils deployed with and without proximal flow arrest: results in 19 patients. AJNR Am J Neuroradiol 1999;20:1452–1456.

Chapter 20
Therapy for Unusual Causes of Stroke

Ursula E. Anwer

Cessation of blood flow to the brain can lead to irreversible damage and stroke. The most common underlying pathologies for stroke are atherosclerotic large and small blood vessel disease and cardiac emboli. Unusual causes of stroke are mostly identified in young stroke patients but are also recognized in the elderly. Relatively unusual causes of stroke are due to vascular, embolic, or hematologic abnormalities.

Vasculopathies can be congenital, as seen in vascular malformations, homocystinuria, Marfan's syndrome, pseudoxanthoma elasticum, cerebral autosomal dominant arteriopathy with subcortical infarcts and leukoencephalopathy (CADASIL); however, most vasculopathies are acquired. For example, they may be inflammatory, drug-related, or due to other causes (Table 20-1).

Emboli (Table 20-2) usually originate in the heart, either from cardiac valves or from akinetic segments of the ventricle or atrium. The origin of emboli expands significantly, including the venous system, if there is intracardiac shunting, as in atrioseptal defects or a patent foramen ovale (PFO). It has been increasingly recognized that emboli can originate in proximal arteries, including the aortic arch, and travel distally to occlude smaller intracranial blood vessels.

Hematologic causes (Table 20-3) of stroke can be categorized into hyperviscosity syndromes, cellular disorders, immune-mediated prothrombic states, and increasingly diagnosable problems in the coagulation-thrombolysis cascade.

Only knowledge of the factors leading to stroke helps prevent and treat this condition. Because unusual causes of stroke are seen rather infrequently, most of them are treated empirically or according to the experiences published in small patient series or case reports.

Migrainous Stroke

Migraine is a common disorder. It is experienced by 4–29% of the population.[1,2] The American Migraine Study reported that 17.6% of females and 6% of males in the United States experience severe migraine.[3] Migraine has been frequently implicated as a risk factor for stroke. In older publications, however, "other causes" of infarction have often not been exhaustively ruled out (e.g., excluding the presence of antiphospholipid antibodies [APLs] or a PFO). Migrainous cerebral infarction has been defined by the International Headache Society as one or more migrainous aura symptoms not fully reversible within 7 days or associated with neuroimaging confirmation of ischemic infarction, or both, associated with the following:

1. Patient has previously fulfilled criteria for migraine with neurologic aura.
2. The present attack is typical of previous attacks but the neurologic deficits are not completely reversible within 7 days or neuroimaging demonstrates ischemic infarction in the relevant area, or both.
3. Other causes of infarction are ruled out by appropriate investigations.[4]

Not all publications adhere to this definition, which implies that migrainous stroke can only occur

Table 20-1. Vasculopathies as Unusual Causes of Stroke

Infectious vasculitis
Noninfectious vasculitis
   Polyarteritis nodosa
   Churg-Strauss syndrome
   Giant cell arteritis
   Granulomatous angiitis
   Hypersensitivity angiitis
   Drug-induced
   Associated with systemic disease
Thromboangiitis obliterans
Vasospasm
Dissection
Fibromuscular hyperplasia
Moyamoya
Amyloid angiopathy
Migraine
Postirradiation angiopathy
Sneddon's syndrome
Homocystinuria
Marfan's syndrome

Table 20-2. Embolic Sources for Unusual Strokes

Cardiac
  Valvular
    Infectious endocarditis
    Marantic endocarditis
    Libman-Sacks endocarditis
    Prosthetic valves
    Rheumatic heart disease
    Mitral annulus calcification
    Mitral valve prolapse
  Hypokinesis
    Ischemic cardiomyopathy
    Nonischemic cardiomyopathy
    Sick sinus syndrome
  Intracardiac tumors
Vessel to vessel
  Aortic arch
  Extracranial vertebral arteries
  Extracranial carotid arteries
  Vascular malformations
  Dissection
  Aneurysm
Intracardiac shunt
  Atrial septal defect
  Patent foramen ovale

Table 20-3. Hematologic Causes for Stroke

Hyperviscosity
  Dysproteinemias
  Myeloproliferative disorders
  Polycythemia vera
  Thrombocythemia
Cellular disorders
  Sickle-cell disease
  Paroxysmal nocturnal hemoglobinuria
  Platelet hyperaggregability
Immune-mediated prothrombolytic states
  Thrombotic thrombocytopenic purpura
  Antiphospholipid antibody syndrome
Coagulopathies
  Antithrombin III deficiency
  Protein S, C deficiency
  Plasminogen deficiency
  Decreased factor VIII
  Decreased factor XII
  Disseminated intravascular coagulation
  Activated protein C resistance

in patients having migraine with aura (classic migraine). Welch and Levine reviewed this complex issue of migraine and stroke[5] and proposed a different classification of migraine-related stroke (Table 20-4). The general use of this classification would probably help to not only define the risk of stroke in this population but also help to develop proper therapies.

Additional Risk Factors

In spite of the high frequency of migraine, especially in young women, migrainous stroke is a relatively rare occurrence. Only 64 cases were reported

Table 20-4. Classification of Migraine-Related Stroke

Category	Features
I	Coexisting stroke and migraine
II	Stroke with clinical features of migraine
IIa	Established (symptomatic migraine)
IIb	New onset (migraine mimic)
III	Migraine-induced stroke
IIIa	Without risk factors
IIIb	With risk factors
IV	Uncertain

before 1983.[6] Rothrock et al. compared the clinical data of 310 patients with migraine to 30 patients with acute migrainous infarction and found migraine with aura to be significantly more common in the migrainous stroke group.[7] They also concluded that a prior history of a migrainous stroke was a high-risk factor for a recurrent stroke. They did not find a meaningful difference between migrainous stroke patients as compared to controls in terms of mitral valve prolapse, hypertension, active smoking, or estrogen use. Migraine seemed to be a risk factor predominantly in young women, and the risk for stroke was found to double in migraine with aura patients.[8] This doubled risk for migraine with aura was also found in a study of 77 female stroke patients by Tzourio et al.[9] In this study, the risk for stroke increased substantially in migrainous women smokers (odds ratio, 10.2) and those using oral contraceptives (odds ratio, 13.9). Smoking and migraine were more likely to be associated with stroke in the 212 patients studied by Iglesias et al.[10] Bogousslavsky et al. studied 22 patients with classic migraine who had a stroke during a migraine attack and concluded that migraine stroke accounts for 10.4% of strokes in patients younger than the age of 45 years.[11] By using migraineurs and nonmigraineurs who had experienced a remote cerebral infarction, they further noted that migraine stroke was not associated with a higher prevalence of mitral valve prolapse, arterial dissection, or oral contraceptive use, although these are independent risk factors for stroke.

Some publications indicate that traditional risk factors for stroke may also be risk factors for migraine with aura. The prevalence of a PFO in migraine with aura patients was found to be similar to that in young stroke patients, which was twice as often as in a control group or in migraine without aura patients.[12,13] Does this imply that microemboli cause the aura and potentially a stroke? Or is there a genetic abnormality causing dysfunctional platelets, as seen in migraine as well as endocardial abnormalities leading to the PFO?[12]

Migraine is a common initial complaint in patients with CADASIL.[14,15] CADASIL is a nonatherosclerotic vasculopathy with deposition of granular material into the smooth muscle cells of the small blood vessel media, leading to ischemic changes and eventually vascular dementia. Its inheritance is autosomal dominant linked to the Notch 3 gene on chromosome 19.[16]

Migraine may also be the presenting symptom in patients with mitochondrial encephalopathy, lactic acidosis, and stroke-like episodes.[17,18] This raises the question of whether the common denominator for migraine and stroke is an impaired energy supply.

Treatment

If migraine with aura is a significant risk factor for migrainous stroke or if it enhances other potential stroke risk factors, then therapy should focus on the pathophysiology of this entity. However, no distinct pathophysiologic mechanism has been discovered. Reduced blood flow is probably the reason for the migraine aura, which either originates in the nervous system, demonstrated as spreading depression, or could be due to a vascular disorder.[19] One should also be aware that low flow due to a structural lesion can mimic migraine with aura as described in five patients who initially were misdiagnosed as having migraine stroke and later were found to have marantic endocarditis (one), atherosclerotic disease (one), and carotid dissection (three).[20] Olesen et al. reported two cases of internal carotid dissection causing hypoperfusion and cases of atherosclerosis presenting as migraine with aura as well as typical migraine with aura resulting in infarction.[21] They proposed an interrelationship between migraine and stroke, suggesting that primary cerebral ischemia can both trigger migraine aura and stroke.

If hypoperfusion can cause both migraine with aura and stroke, then the therapy of migrainous stroke should be the prevention of hypoperfusion, which implies exclusion of structural lesions, especially vascular pathology, embolic sources, and immunologic etiologies (e.g., APLs). Anticoagulation stopped migraine with aura in one of Olesen et al.'s cases who was known to have atherosclerotic changes.[21]

The therapy of true migrainous infarction should be to prevent migraine with aura. Because the cause of a migraine attack and, specifically, an aura remain unknown, clinicians probably have to rely on the drugs used to prevent migraine. Migrainous strokes have been reported while on prophylaxis, however, especially in patients on propranolol.[22–26] Propranolol is one of the few medications approved by the U.S. Food and Drug Administration for migraine prophylaxis, which could at least in part explain the relatively high frequency of stroke occurrence associated with its use. One can argue for and against using propranolol. Welch proposes that beta blockers may work at the level of the descending orbitofrontal brain stem pathway or directly on the noradrenergic system to prevent migraine.[27] On the other hand, beta blockers have been shown to decrease cerebral blood flow, increase cerebral vascular resistance, and decrease cerebral oxygen consumption and glucose metabolism, which could predispose to stroke.[28,29] Migrainous stroke has also been reported in patients on other prophylactic agents: a combination of verapamil, amitriptyline, and prednisone[30]; cyproheptadine[23]; amitriptyline[23]; and after using ergotamine.[6,23]

Various therapies have been tried for acute strokes associated with migraine, but these are only anecdotal case reports. Bernsen et al.[31] treated a basilar migraine patient with bilateral cerebellar infarcts who also developed hydrocephalus with flunarizine, corticosteroids, carbasalate-calcium, and acetazolamide. Rothrock[23] showed reopening of a stenosed carotid artery (presumably arteriospasm) after intra-arterial injection of tolazoline hydrochloride and followed the therapy with dextran, dextramethasone, and heparin intravenously along with oral verapamil.

In summary, migrainous stroke should be treated initially by excluding all known risk factors for stroke and subsequently by avoidance, especially in patients who have already had one ischemic event. It is unknown whether one prophylactic agent (e.g., a calcium channel blocker) would be more effective than a beta blocker. Because migrainous stroke is rare, it is difficult to conduct meaningful clinical trials.

Stroke Associated with Antiphospholipid Antibodies

Numerous studies have indicated that there is an association between APLs and cerebral ischemic events.[32–38] Approximately 4% of the population has APLs on appropriate testing, but most are asymptomatic.[39] Patients with the primary antiphospholipid syndrome have antiphospholipids and various symptoms, including venous and arterial thrombosis, thrombocytopenia, recurrent fetal loss, and livedo reticularis.[40–42] The secondary antiphospholipid syndrome is equivalent to the primary but occurs in the context of an autoimmune disease, most often systemic lupus erythematosus (SLE).

APLs are a family of antibodies mostly directed against negatively charged or neutral phospholipids, or both. The lupus anticoagulant interferes with in vitro phospholipid-dependent coagulation tests, especially the activated partial thromboplastin time. The other antiphospholipids are usually identified using enzyme-linked immunosorbent assays. Cardiolipin is usually used as the antigen and serves as a target for the other negatively charged APLs as well, because most of them bind to it with similar avidity.[43,44] However, there are a significant number of other phospholipids that could be missed if only cardiolipin is used as antigen.[45–47]

Pathophysiology and Stroke Risk

Treatment of APL-associated stroke preferably should be based on the mechanism of action of these antiphospholipids. Many mechanisms have been proposed.[48,49] There may be different mechanisms or a combination of mechanisms at work for the different APLs, which may characterize the different syndromes. Ginsburg et al. showed that an anticardiolipin titer above the ninety-fifth percentile is an important risk factor for deep venous thrombosis and pulmonary emboli, but not stroke.[50] Only 3% of 667 SLE patients were found to have arterial occlusion, mostly in the form of cerebral ischemic events. In contrast, 30% had livedo reticularis, 20% thrombocytopenia, 17% recurrent fetal loss, and 11% venous thrombosis.[42] Some of the APLs may even cross-react with phosphodiester linkages in nucleic acids.[51–53] The effect on the coagulation system could be due to binding to endothelial cells, actively promoting thrombosis, or by inhibiting the role of endothelial cells in anticoagulation. Prostaglandin I_2 is a vasodilator and has a platelet-stabilizing function. There may also be an interaction with platelets, because patients often have thrombocytopenia[54] as well as a reduced number of erythrocytes, causing anemia. APLs may interact with protein C activation and function,[55–57] which can impair fibrinolysis. Some antiphospholipids require cofactors to bind to their specific site. Prothrombin[58,59] and beta-glycoprotein-I, also known as *apolipoprotein H* (*apoH*),[59,60] were discovered to improve binding of phospholipids to their targets. Gharavi[61] suggests that apoH may bind to phospholipid molecules in such a way that their phosphodiester portions are better exposed for the APL to bind. He suggests that APL could interfere with apoH's function (e.g., inhibiting the intrinsic pathway of coagulation[62,63] and, thereby, adenosine 5'-diphosphate–mediated platelet aggregation), resulting ultimately in thrombosis and platelet aggregation.

Because the heart is embryologically part of the vascular system, it is frequently involved with APL. Libman-Sacks–type changes have been identified in patients with APL.[64,65] In the presence of valvular vegetations, it can be difficult to decide whether a cerebroischemic event is thrombotic or embolic in origin.

APL was found to be an independent risk factor in stroke patients.[66,67] In a prospective study of patients with lupus anticoagulant or cardiolipin antibodies, or both, two independent risk factors for thrombotic events were identified: a previous thrombosis and immunoglobulin G anticardiolipin titer above 40 units.[68] There are conflicting reports about stroke recurrence rates in antiphospholipid-positive patients. The risk was not increased in the Antiphospholipid Antibodies in Stroke Study cohort followed prospectively, but the cohort was too small.[66] In other studies, the prospective average recurrence rate for a stroke in the context of APL was estimated to be 13–14% per year.[33,66] The association between anticardiolipin antibodies and stroke appears to be relatively specific because it was not found in patients with other central nervous system disease.[67] The prevalence of these antibodies increases with age[69,70] and seems to be associated with other stroke risk factors (e.g., congestive heart failure and atrial fibrillation). In this population, the antibodies may be "innocent bystanders" but could of course have caused the stroke. Tanne et al. caution against overdiagnosis and speculate that anticardiolipin antibodies, such as immunoglobulin G, may be markers of cardiovascular disease.[70]

Therapy

It is unclear whether any therapy is required for primary stroke prevention in healthy people with an elevated APL titer. Only long-term follow-up study can indicate whether they eventually become symptomatic. Another subset of patients who may not need active therapy are those with APL in association with certain medications (e.g., procainamide), neoplasia, and acquired immunodeficiency syndrome. There are probably different subpopulations of APL antibodies with different risks for stroke. Every patient who presents with a stroke should be rigorously evaluated for risk factors other than the antiphospholipids and treated accordingly.

As described previously, the mechanism of action of various APLs is largely speculative and may differ from antibody to antibody, yet it is largely similar for certain syndromes. Therefore, no clear avenue of therapy has evolved. Therapy is either directed toward the coagulation disturbances or determined by the autoimmune character of these antibodies.[49,71] No large case series has been published comparing primary and secondary APL syndromes. Review of therapies used in the past is further complicated by the fact that a single agent has rarely been used. Levine and Welch[72] found six cases of cerebrovascular ischemia in patients with APL who were on antiplatelet therapy. One case was asymptomatic after 3 months of follow-up, two cases after 4–6 months, and two "responded well" with an unspecific follow-up time. Three of their four cases were treated with a combination of therapies, two with aspirin and dipyridamole and one with aspirin, dipyridamole, and prednisone. The latter case persisted with transient ischemic attacks (TIAs). One of the aspirin-dipyridamole cases did well 6 months later, but the other developed thrombosis; this patient was treated with warfarin and did well 2 months later. Brey et al.[73] report two patients with recurrent strokes on aspirin who were then converted to warfarin. One of them had a recurrence on warfarin and dipyridamole and then received prednisone as well. At 1–3 years follow-up, 9 of 10 patients in the series of Montalbán et al. had no recurrence while on 1,000 mg aspirin per day.[74] Seventy percent of patients in a study by Nencini et al. received antiplatelet agents, 20% received antiplatelets and steroids, and 10% received anticoagulation.[75] During a mean follow-up time of 35 months, 40% of these patients had a stroke or systemic thrombotic event. At least three of nine patients must have had the recurrence on antiplatelet agents. Aspirin withdrawal may have precipitated a stroke in two postpartum women with the APL syndrome.[76]

Warfarin alone did not prevent TIAs in a patient with the lupus anticoagulant, but the addition of aspirin abolished them.[64] Warfarin controlled amaurosis fugax in two of six patients with anticardiolipin antibodies; warfarin plus aspirin failed in two patients; one patient was controlled with aspirin alone.[77]

Resove and Brewer[78] studied 70 patients with APL syndrome; 51 (73%) had primary APL syndrome. In 14 of these (20%) it was associated with SLE and in five (7%) with chronic idiopathic thrombocytopenic purpura. The authors stated that the site of the first event, in terms of arterial or venous thrombosis, tended to predict the site of subsequent events. Review of the rate of recurrence within groups (no treatment; aspirin; low-, intermediate- and high-warfarin) detected a better prophylaxis in the intermediate-dose warfarin (international normalized ration [INR], 2.0–2.9) and high-dose warfarin groups (INR ≥3.0).

The boundaries between primary APL syndrome and lupus-like illnesses are not distinct.[32] Because of the autoimmune issue, patients have been treated with immunosuppressants. The response to steroids is inconsistent. An early review[72] showed that seven of nine patients treated with steroids experienced further TIAs or strokes. Patients with adequate anticoagulation (prolonged prothrombin time of more than 1.3 times control) did better than those on corticosteroids or antiplatelet agents.[79] Steroids were rarely used alone; when successfully given, patients usually also received warfarin[80,81] or cytotoxic agents. Methyl-prednisolone and cyclophosphamide were the therapeutic agents used for repetitive flare-ups in four SLE cases with moderately to severely high APL titers.[82] In most cases, immunosuppressive therapy was not used for primary APL patients.

It is still unclear whether plasma exchange can reduce the risk of ischemia over time. Derksen et al.[83] studied anticardiolipin antibodies and lupus anticoagulants in four patients with SLE after one plasma exchange and found the anticardiolipin titer to be back at the pretreatment level in 7 days, whereas the lupus anticoagulant titer stayed below pretreatment level. Plasma exchange might be the therapy of choice for acutely ill patients with encephalopathy or seizures or those rapidly deteriorating with high antiphospholipid levels[84,85] who then may need to go onto immunosuppression and anticoagulation.

Immunoglobulin infusions have been successfully used in autoimmune diseases.[86] Their use in the APL syndromes had mostly been reported in the obstetrics literature for treatment of fetal loss[87,88] and thrombocytopenia.[89]

Considerable time and studies of larger series of patients with the same APL syndromes are needed to establish clear guidelines for therapy. The presence of APLs alone should not be treated because of its occurrence in the normal population, nor is treatment necessary, except for medication withdrawal if an increased APL level is due to medication. It might be worthwhile to try patients with mild symptoms on antiplatelet agents. Patients with recurrent strokes on an antiplatelet drug need anticoagulation with a moderate to high INR.[77] Patients with severe disease, such as multiple strokes, encephalopathy, thrombosis, or fetal loss, might benefit from plasma exchange during the acute phase; however, in terms of long-term therapy, such patients might need both immunosuppression and anticoagulation.

Patent Foramen Ovale

A PFO facilitates flow from the right atrium into the left atrium and thus allows venous emboli to reach the arterial circulation, especially the brain, causing stroke. The foramen ovale is delineated inferiorly by the septum primum and superiorly by the septum secundum. After birth, with cessation of the fetal circulation, the foramen closes like a valve and later in life closes permanently with fibrous adhesions. An intra-atrial shunt is formed whenever there is a higher pressure in the right as compared to the left atrium (e.g., during pulmonary hypertension, Valsalva maneuvers, and mechanical ventilation with positive end-expiratory pressure). According to autopsy studies, the foramen ovale stays patent in approximately 27% of the population.[90] One prospective study found a similar prevalence, identifying a PFO by transesophageal echocardiography in 25.6% of residents 45 years or older.[91] Lechat showed a significantly higher prevalence of PFO in patients having a cryptogenic stroke who were younger than 55 years old compared to controls (54% vs. 10%),[92] as did Webster in patients younger than 40 years of age (50% vs. 15%).[93] Ranoux et al.[94] observed a PFO in 40% of the 68 stroke patients they studied who were younger than 55 years old; Itoh et al.[95] observed a PFO in 77% of their younger than 55-year-old patients. Di Tullio[96] and deBelder[97] expanded these studies to all age groups and again demonstrated a significantly higher prevalence of PFO in patients experiencing cryptogenic stroke.

Since the advent of transesophageal echocardiography, PFO became more easily identifiable, and it has also become apparent that there is a frequent association between atrial septal aneurysms (ASAs) and stroke, with most of these patients also having a PFO.[98–102] There might be an increased risk for stroke in patients who have both a PFO and an ASA.[103] The risk probably also increases with the size of the PFO. The frequency of medium to large PFOs was found to be higher in patients with cryptogenic stroke compared to patients with a determined cause.[104,105]

In spite of the clinical evidence, it is difficult to prove that a stroke was actually caused by a paradoxical embolus via a PFO. A venous embolus lodged in a PFO has only rarely been demonstrated to have caused a stroke.[106,107] Most cases of PFO associated with stroke are presumptive. Meister[108] proposed certain clinical criteria for the diagnosis of paradoxical emboli during life, the documentation of the second criteria being the most challenging:

1. An arterial embolus, cerebral or systemic, with no evidence of left-sided circulatory origin
2. The presence of a venous thrombosis or pulmonary embolism, or both
3. An intracardiac defect that permits right-to-left shunt
4. An elevation of right heart pressure, either constant or transitory

Therapy

Because there also seems to be a higher stroke recurrence rate[109] in patients with PFO, especially in a high-risk subgroup (interatrial communication, posterior cerebral artery stroke, coexisting cause of stroke, and history of migraine),[110] an appropriate preventive therapy is required. A number of different options are available to stroke patients as prophylaxis against recurrent paradoxical emboli. In general, there are five options: (1) no therapy, (2) antiplatelet therapy, (3) anticoagulation, (4) surgical closure, or (5) transcatheter clo-

sure. If a thrombus is detected in the foramen ovale, prompt surgery might be life-saving.[111–113] Thrombolysis of a transit thrombus was achieved by Müller and Axthelm[114] and attempted by Siebenlist and Gattenlöhner.[106] Patients with embolic stroke, a PFO, and proved peripheral vein thrombosis should probably be treated with anticoagulation until the peripheral thrombus disappears.[92] Bogousslavsky et al.[110] treated all patients who were not referred to surgery but ended up on antiplatelet therapy with anticoagulation for 3 months. Documentation of the peripheral thrombosis itself is a challenging task. It may escape clinical detection in more than 50% of cases.[115] Peripheral thrombosis should also be expected in patients who have risk factors (e.g., patients who are immobilized, very obese, or known to be in a hypercoagulable state). These underlying risk factors should be eliminated or treated if possible. Thrombosis can be transient and should be looked for as soon as possible in patients with embolic events.

There is no consensus on how to treat patients with stroke associated with PFO because there have not been any randomized clinical trials. According to Chambers, the reasoning for existing treatment is "intuitive."[116] deBelder[97] does not treat patients unless there is a second cerebral ischemic event or definitive evidence of venous thrombosis. If this occurs, he then recommends anticoagulation. Aspirin may be an appropriate therapy for symptomatic patients with known PFO but no source of paradoxical emboli,[117] especially because the natural history for recurrence is unknown. This was also reflected in a retrospective review of 15 PFO patients treated with aspirin, warfarin, or surgery.[101] Jeanrenaud and Kappenberger[118] treat with antiplatelet drugs after the first stroke. Patients with proven deep vein thrombosis receive anticoagulation (2–3 times INR for longer than 3 months) and consideration of surgical closure for recurrence. Another option to prevent recurrence, especially in patients with persistent peripheral thrombosis while on anticoagulation, is the placement of an umbrella filter into the inferior vena cava[119] or its ligation.[120]

Since 1989, there have been investigational procedures to close intracardiac defects with nonsurgical transcatheter closure. Bridges[121] described successful closure of ventricular septal defects with an umbrella-like device. A similar approach was used for 35 patients with arterial thrombosis, predominantly cerebrovascular, using the Bard clamshell septal umbrella in a prospective trial.[122] Most patients had been on anticoagulants before the procedure but were kept on low-dose aspirin, except for three patients (two with morbid obesity and immobilization and one with amaurosis fugax and residual right-to-left atrial shunt). Eighty-two percent of the patients had complete closure; the rest had minimal leaks. In follow-up, patients have done well, but there was a 30% incidence of fractures of one or more arms of the umbrella, which prompted redesign of the device and another prospective study.

Nendaz et al.[123] took a theoretical approach to determine which therapy would be best to prevent secondary stroke caused by a PFO. They evaluated four treatment options (no therapy, antiplatelet therapy, anticoagulation, and surgery) with a Markov-based decision analysis in a hypothetical cohort of 55 patients using different presumed risks for stroke recurrence. The overall risk is probably 0–4% per year.[103,110] If the presumed recurrence risk was under 0.8% per year, no therapy would be preferred. In higher-risk patients, surgery is probably the best treatment and, to a lesser extent, anticoagulation: Both were determined better than no or antiplatelet therapy to prolong life and quality-adjusted life-years.

Devuyst et al.[124] recommend surgical closure of a PFO if the patient has no other demonstrated cause for stroke and at least two of the following four criteria: recurrent cerebrovascular events or multiple ischemic lesions on a brain magnetic resonance imaging (MRI), a PFO with an ASA, a massive right-to-left shunt through the PFO, or Valsalva strain preceding the stroke onset. If only one of these four criteria is present, they suggest 300 mg aspirin per day.

In summary, so far without prospective clinical trials, it is unclear how to treat patients with presumptive paradoxical emboli. In selected low-risk patients, antiplatelet therapy might be justified; however, most cases probably need anticoagulation or surgical closure of the PFO.

Carotid and Vertebral Artery Dissection

Signs and symptoms of internal carotid and vertebral artery dissection are cerebro- and occuloischemic in nature. Frequently, they are heralded or accompanied by local symptoms (e.g., ipsilateral headache, facial pain, Horner's syndrome, and lower cranial nerve dysfunction).[125–128] The local manifestations of vertebral artery dissection are neck pain and unilateral posterior headache.[128–130] The most frequently seen ischemic effects in vertebral artery dissection are the lateral medullary syndrome and lower brain stem ischemia.[129–131]

Dissection was originally thought to be exclusively caused by trauma; however, in the 1950s, it was increasingly recognized to also occur on a spontaneous basis,[132–134] especially in younger patients. Minor trauma cannot always be excluded, because ischemic symptoms after trauma can occur hours to days after the event. Dissections have been reported after rapid head turning,[135] swimming,[136] exercise,[137] and even coughing.[131] It is conceivable that microtrauma to the extradural vertebral or carotid arteries is the first step to dissection, because dissection frequently occurs where these arteries are most vulnerable to torsion or extension forces (e.g., compression of the internal carotid artery [ICA] against the transverse processes of the upper cervical vertebrae during head turning).

Vascular pathology predisposes to dissection as well. There is an increased incidence with fibromuscular dysplasia,[130,138–142] cystic medial necrosis,[128,143,144] Marfan's syndrome,[128,145,146] and Ehlers-Danlos syndrome.[145] Whether hypertension predisposes arteries to injury and subsequently dissection is unclear. Some authors find hypertension to be a risk factor,[126,127,129,147] whereas others do not.[128]

As the ICA and vertebral artery enter the skull and perforate the dura, the character of their wall structure changes. The thickness of the media and adventitia decreases, and there is loss of elastic fibers in the media and external elastic lamina,[148,149] which predisposes the intracranial arteries to subadventitial dissection and, subsequently, subarachnoid hemorrhage (SAH).[147,150] The development of SAH is an important factor in the management of dissection. It is mostly seen in intracranial vertebral artery dissection, possibly because the intracranial ICA has bony protection.

Angiography used to be the "gold standard" for diagnosis. The combination of MRI visualizing morphologic details and MRA visualizing the intravascular blood flow are commonly used as diagnostic tools when available.[151] They may not be sensitive enough to be used alone, especially in vertebral artery dissection.[152,153] Three-dimensional time-of-flight MRA and MRI were shown to have a high sensitivity and specificity and may be the reliable tool for diagnosis.[154] It is conceivable that transcranial Doppler may play a more important role in the diagnostic work-up by indicating whether a stroke is embolic from the dissection site or due to proximal vascular compromise, and in monitoring for evidence of recanalization of the dissected vessel.[155,156]

The therapeutic approach to dissection is subject to debate. There are no clear guidelines for optimal therapy. No controlled studies are available. Management spans the gamut from no therapy to complex surgery. In general, internal carotid dissection has a favorable outcome in 80–90% of cases,[127,128,157] as does vertebral artery dissection.[129,140,151,158] Patients who recall trauma should avoid known precipitating activity. A soft collar might be advisable for 1–3 months to limit neck movements.[131] Anecdotally, patients have done well after a dissection without any therapy.[127,152,158,159] In a series of 68 patients, Ast et al.[126] did not treat patients with massive stroke or those who only had minor local symptoms. Those with massive stroke had a poor outcome. Patients with stroke had similar outcome whether treated with anticoagulation or antiplatelet medications.

In general, anticoagulation is recommended and used for external carotid artery/ICA dissection[125,128] as well as external vertebral artery dissection.[152,154,160] Anticoagulation probably should be continued for 1–6 months and stopped when recanalization is established. Easton and Hart recommend antiplatelet therapy for those patients who cannot tolerate anticoagulation.[128]

The therapy of intracranial dissection requires a more cautious approach because of the association with SAH, especially in the posterior circulation. Some authors recommend lumbar puncture before anticoagulation, then anticoagulation for 3–6 months,[160] stopping as soon as the artery is recanalized or at 6 months. Recanalization can be shown by Doppler ultrasonography and confirmed by arteriography. Anticoagulation is recommended for patients with evidence of distal embolism, minor stroke, and recurrent TIAs.

Surgical therapy should be reserved for patients who continue to have cerebral ischemic attacks despite adequate anticoagulation, or those who are unable to tolerate anticoagulation (e.g., with SAH). There are no series of patients with one particular intervention. According to Pozzati et al.,[158] the only effective and safe management of an arterial dissection with SAH is the sacrifice of the parent artery. Vertebral artery ligation was performed in 13 cases of vertebral dissection with SAH[147] and a case of fibrovascular dysplasia with a left vertebral dissecting aneurysm.[161] Intramural hematoma removal with interposition of a venous graft, distal thrombectomy, dilation, and surgical occlusion of the distal extracranial carotid artery sometimes combined with superficial temporal-middle cerebral artery anastomosis were reviewed previously.[128] A Dacron sleeve was used successfully to close an ICA-dissecting aneurysm.[162] More recent types of intervention include intra-arterial balloon placements by interventional radiologists, as described in two case reports.[154,163] This is less invasive than surgery, but long-term outcome is unknown.

In summary, the therapy of carotid and vertebral artery dissection ranges from none to surgical intervention. Anticoagulation or possibly antiplatelet agents are advised to avoid distal embolization and for recurrent TIAs. Surgery is only recommended if anticoagulation fails or is contraindicated.

Cerebral Venous Thrombosis

The signs and symptoms of cerebral venous thrombosis (CVT) are nonspecific, often making an early diagnosis difficult. Ameri and Bousser[164] have probably the largest series of CVT patients and found headache to be the presenting symptom in 75% of their 110 patients; papilledema in 49%; motor or sensory deficits in 34%; seizures in 37%; and drowsiness, mental status changes, or coma in 33%; with the remaining patients presenting in various other ways. Symptoms depend on the site and extent of the thrombosis. Rapid increase in tissue impedance and an acute rise in intracranial pressure (ICP), as shown in experimental superior sinus thrombosis in rats, might be responsible for the headache, mimicry of pseudotumor cerebri, and eventually the mental status changes.[165] Involvement of the cortical veins seems to be a prerequisite for the development of focal signs and symptoms and for irreversible tissue damage.[165–168] The natural

Table 20-5. Causes of Cerebral Venous Thrombosis

Low flow
    Venous obstruction
    Congestive heart failure
    Dehydration
Septic thrombosis
    Local infection
    Systemic infection
Hypercoagulable state
    Coagulopathy
    Malignancy
    Infection
    Pregnancy
Trauma
Neurosurgical procedures
Connective tissue disorders

course of CVT is unpredictable. Some patients may have only transient symptoms, whereas patients with deep venous thrombosis seem to have a much poorer prognosis,[169] with a reported mortality rate of 37%,[170] possibly because the vein of Galen is a single vein with poor collaterals draining the thalami, basal ganglia, and midbrain.

Risk Factors for Cerebral Venous Thrombosis

Local or systemic infection used to be the main predisposing pathology for CVT. Since the era of antibiotics began, it has been recognized that the etiology of CVT can also be due to low-flow venous stasis, a hypercoagulable state, or changes in the vessel wall (Table 20-5). Low-flow can be due to local obstruction or systemic problems (e.g., dehydration or congestive heart failure). Septic thrombosis of the lateral sinus seems to be a major complication of middle ear or mastoid infections and can follow acute or chronic otitis media. Facial infections and sphenoid sinusitis can involve the cavernous sinus and cause local thrombosis. Hypercoagulable states are recognized in a variety of medical conditions, including coagulopathies, malignancies, and infections. A subclinical hypercoagulable state may need another predisposing factor (e.g., pregnancy or surgery) to precipitate thrombosis.[171] There is an increased risk of developing CVT during or after pregnancy; the inci-

dence is approximately 1 in 2,500 pregnancies.[172] It was found to occur 13 times more often during the puerperium than during pregnancy itself and seems to have a better prognosis than that of other causes.[173] Injury of a sinus or vessel wall can induce thrombosis as well.

Therapy of Cerebral Venous Thrombosis

Therapy of CVT depends on the underlying pathology. Systemic infections have to be treated aggressively with intravenous antibiotics. In addition, local infections should be approached surgically for appropriate drainage or resection (e.g., mastoidectomy in lateral sinus thrombosis).[174] Patients with seizures have to be started on anticonvulsants. The endpoint of the anticonvulsant therapy is less clear. Bousser[166] treats for 2 years and then tapers the anticonvulsants in those patients who have been seizure-free and have a normal computed tomography scan and electroencephalogram.

Most patients become symptomatic because of increased ICP. Reversal of the thrombotic process and recanalization of the thrombotic vessel or vessels is the primary objective and should normalize the ICP. Because management of the thrombosis itself is somewhat controversial and may not be immediately effective, other modalities have to be administered to avoid blindness and—in severe cases—herniation. Ameri and Bousser[164] reviewed the literature and reported diverse approaches, such as steroids, mannitol, acetazolamide, daily lumbar punctures, ventricular/cerebrospinal fluid drainage, lumbar/peritoneal shunting, barbiturate coma, and craniectomy. Most of their patients only required antiedema agents, such as acetazolamide, and repeated lumbar punctures. Only 3 of their 110 patients needed shunting.

In spite of the fact that the management of the thrombosis itself is still somewhat controversial, there is a growing tendency to use anticoagulation with three goals in mind: (1) to stop progression of the thrombus, (2) to salvage venous collaterals, and (3) to possibly facilitate lysis. Patients who have hemorrhagic venous infarcts theoretically have a higher risk of hemorrhage. These patients should be monitored closely. They account for 10–30% of CVT patients.[166,167] The use of anticoagulation is based on case reports but mainly on a study by Einhäupl et al.,[175] who report their experience with 102 aseptic venous sinus thrombosis patients. Twenty of these patients were randomized in a placebo-controlled blinded study of heparin versus placebo. The heparinized patients were noted to do better after 3 days of therapy. After 3 months, eight of the heparin-treated patients had completely recovered, with the remaining two having slight neurologic deficits. In the control group, one patient had complete recovery, six patients had neurologic deficits, and three patients died. Of all heparinized patients, 43 had intracranial hemorrhage before treatment. Twenty-seven of these patients were treated with heparin and had significantly better outcomes than the 13 untreated patients. The conclusion is that heparin may be an effective therapy for CVT. Heparinization apparently does not promote intracranial hemorrhage, and this should therefore not be a contraindication for heparin use in CVT. Ameri and Bousser comment that 82 of their patients were treated with heparin, and it apparently did not cause death or worsening symptoms.[164]

Isensee et al.[176] studied the clot evolution by serial MRIs in 23 consecutive CVT patients who were treated with heparin for 4 weeks and then with oral anticoagulants for 6 months. They speculate that early heparin treatment might accelerate thrombus dissolution. Heparin reversed the pathologic impedance increase in two animals with experimental sinus thrombosis, again supporting its beneficial effect.[165]

Krayenbühl studied a case series of 67 patients and recommends antibiotics and anticoagulation.[177] He states that he did not see an intracranial hemorrhage in 7 years. A large number of case reports or small series favor the use of heparin.[178–187] Lifelong anticoagulation may have to be used in patients with abnormalities of coagulation parameters.[188,189]

Barnett and Hyland expressed reservations about the use of anticoagulation in sagittal sinus thrombosis.[190] Geittelfinger and Kokmen[191] advised against its use because two of their three heparin-treated patients died. One of those two patients had paroxysmal nocturnal hemoglobinuria, a situation in which heparin is contraindicated[182,192]; the other patient had also been treated with urokinase and had thrombocytopenia. Heparin can cause thrombosis in heparin-induced thrombocytopenia, which therefore is a contraindication for its use.[193] Hereditary antithrombin III–deficient patients with thrombosis may need heparin in addition to purified antithrombin III or fresh frozen plasma infusion.[194]

de Bruijn et al.[195] published the second randomized, placebo-controlled trial to evaluate the use of anticoagulation in CVT patients. Sixty patients were given either body-weight adjusted subcutaneous nadroparin, low-molecular-weight heparin, or placebo. Both arms were well matched except for a slightly higher number of pretreatment infarcts and hemorrhages in the nadroparin group. There was a marginally better outcome in the treatment group, but it was not statistically significant. The risk of hemorrhage was not increased in the treatment group. It is unclear why the results of this trial are different from the report by Einhäupl et al.[175] The study design was somewhat different, but it should not have affected the outcome to such an extent. The other difference between the two studies was that subcutaneous low-molecular-weight heparin was used instead of intravenous unfractionated heparin. de Bruijn et al. suggest another trial with at least 300 patients.

With the advent of better endovascular techniques, there have been more attempts to lyse venous clots locally and, at the same time, keep the patient anticoagulated to prevent propagation of residual thrombus. Experience with fibrinolytic agents consists of case reports and small series. Urokinase and, less frequently, streptokinase were infused locally, generally with good outcome.[196–198] In fact, a retrospective review of 49 cases of deep venous thrombosis treated with heparin or local thrombolytics with heparin revealed a mortality of 48% for untreated patients versus 13% for treated patients. There have been several reports in the literature of infusing recombinant tissue plasminogen activator.[199,200] Frey et al.[199] treated 12 patients by injecting recombinant tissue plasminogen activator via a microcatheter rostrally from the thrombus and pulling the catheter gradually through. The patients also received heparin. Complete blood flow was restored in six patients, incomplete flow in three patients, and none in the remaining three patients. Seven of the first two groups recovered; all patients were functionally independent at 6 months. The two patients who had an obvious hemorrhagic infarct before treatment experienced worsening of the hemorrhage, which shows that fibrinolysis increases the risk of parenchymal hemorrhage in higher-risk patients. Hemorrhage had been reported in a case by Rousseaux et al.,[181] and Geittelfinger and Kokmen,[191] who advised against the use of fibrinolytics.

Other methods of thrombolysis are in an experimental phase. Chow et al.[201] reported successful rheolytic thrombectomy combined with intra-arterial thrombolysis in two cases. They used a mechanical thrombectomy catheter (AngioJet), which breaks up the clot by vacuum and aspirates the debris. This device seems to be useful for the sinuses, but it is too stiff for the cerebral veins or the vein of Galen.

Surgical thrombus extraction is rarely attempted because of the friability of the swollen brain. At times it has been attempted during mastoidectomy.[202] Sindou et al.[203] report successful revascularization by bypassing a thrombosed transverse sinus to the superficial jugular vein, acutely reducing ICP.

In summary, CVT is not always easily diagnosed because of the nonspecific symptoms. In rare cases of local infection, antibiotics are required; otherwise, the currently preferred treatment is anticoagulation, and, in the future, possibly thrombolysis.

Conclusion

Appropriate and effective stroke therapy depends on knowledge about the pathogenesis and pathophysiology of stroke formation. This knowledge is difficult to obtain for unusual strokes. Great progress has been made in some of these unusual strokes, but because they are rare, clinicians continue to depend on case reports, small series, and multicenter studies to determine the appropriate therapy.

References

1. Waters WE, O'Connor PJ. Prevalence of migraine. J Neurol Neurosurg Psychiatry 1975;38:613–616.
2. Linet MS, Stewart WF. Migraine headache: epidemiological perspectives. Epidemiol Rev 1984;6:107–139.
3. Lipton RB, Stewart WF. Migraine in the United States: a review of epidemiology and health care use. Neurology 1993;43(Suppl 3):S6–S10.
4. Headache Classification Committee of the International Headache Society. Classification and diagnostic criteria for headache disorders, cranial neuralgias, and facial pain. Cephalalgia 1988;8:1–97.
5. Welch KMA, Levine SR. Migraine-related stroke in the context of the International Headache Society Classification of Head Pain. Arch Neurol 1990;47:458–462.
6. Featherstone HJ. Clinical features of stroke in migraine: a review. Headache 1986;26:128–133.
7. Rothrock J, North J, Madden K, et al. Migraine and migrainous stroke: risk factors and prognosis. Neurology 1993;43:2473–2476.
8. Carolei A, Marini C, De Matteis G. History of migraine and risk of cerebral ischemia in young adults. The Italian National Research Council Study Group on Stroke in the Young. Lancet 1996;347:1503–1506.
9. Tsourio C, Tehindrazanarivelo A, Iglesias S, et al. Case control study of migraine and risk of ischemic stroke in young women. BMJ 1995;310:830–833.
10. Iglesias S, Visy JM, Hubert JB, et al. Migraine as a risk factor for ischemic stroke: a case-control study. Stroke 1993;24(abstract):171.
11. Bogousslavsky FR, VanMelle G, Payot M, Uske A. Migraine stroke. Neurology 1988;38:223–227.
12. Del Sette M, Angeli S, Leandri M, et al. Migraine with aura and right-to-left shunt on transcranial Doppler: a case-control study. Cerebrovasc Dis 1998;8:327–330.
13. Anzola GP, Magoni M, Guindani M, et al. Potential source of cerebral embolism in migraine with aura: a transcranial Doppler study. Neurology 1999;52:1622–1625.
14. Desmond DW, Moroney JT, Lynch T, et al. The natural history of CADASIL: a pooled analysis of previously published cases. Stroke 1999;30:1230–1233.
15. Kalimo H, Viitanen M, Amberla K, et al. CADASIL: hereditary disease of arteries causing brain infarcts and dementia. Neuropathol Appl Neurobiol 1999;25:257–265.
16. Joutel A, Corpechot C, Ducros A, et al. Notch3 mutations in cerebral autosomal dominant arteriopathy with subcortical infarcts and leukoencephalopathy (CADASIL), a mendelian condition causing stroke and vascular dementia. Ann N Y Acad Sci 1997;826:213–217.
17. Andermann F, Lugaresi E, Dvorkin GS, Montagna P. The syndrome of prolonged classical migraine, epilepsia partialis continua, and repeated strokes: a clinically characteristic disorder probably due to mitochondrial encephalopathy. Funct Neurol 1986;1:481–486.
18. Hirano M, Ricci E, Koenigsberger MR, et al. MELAS: an original case and clinical criteria for diagnosis. Neuromuscular Disord 1992;2:125–135.
19. Lance JW. Current concepts of migraine pathogenesis. Neurology 1993;43(Suppl 3):S11–S15.
20. Shuaib A. Stroke from other etiologies masquerading as migraine-stroke. Stroke 1991;22:1068–1074.
21. Olesen J, Friberg L, Olesen TS, et al. Ischemia-induced (symptomatic) migraine attacks may be more frequent than migraine-induced ischemic insults. Brain 1993;116:187–202.
22. Solomon S, Lipton RB, Harris PY. Arterial stenosis in migraine: spasm or arteriopathy. Headache 1990;30:52–61.
23. Rothrock JF, Walicke P, Swenson MR. Migrainous stroke. Arch Neurol 1988;45:63–67.

24. Bardwell A, Trott JA. Stroke in migraine as a consequence of propranolol. Headache 1987;27:381–383.

25. Prendes JL. Considerations on the use of propranolol in complicated migraine. Headache 1980;20:93–95.

26. Gilbert GJ. An occurrence of complicated migraine during propranolol therapy. Headache 1982;22:81–83.

27. Welch KMA. Migraine: a biobehavioral disorder. Arch Neurol 1987;44:323–327.

28. Meyer JS, Okamoto S, Sari A, et al. Effects of beta-adrenergic blockade on cerebral autoregulation and chemical vasomotor control in patients with stroke. Stroke 1974;5: 167–179.

29. Aoyagi M, Desmukh VD, Meyer JS, et al. Effect of beta-adrenergic blockade with propranolol on cerebral blood flow, autoregulation, and CO_2 responsiveness. Stroke 1976;7:292–295.

30. Ganji S, Williams W, Furlow J. Bilateral occipital lobe infarction in acute migraine: clinical, neurophysiological, and neuroradiological study. Headache 1992;32: 360–365.

31. Bernsen HJ, Van de Vlasakker C, Verhagen WI, Prick MJ. Basilar artery migraine stroke. Headache 1990;30: 142–144.

32. Hess DC. Stroke associated with antiphospholipid antibodies. Stroke 1992;23(Suppl I):I23–I28.

33. Levine SR, Deegan MJ, Futrell N, Welch KM. Cerebrovascular and neurologic disease associated with antiphospholipid antibodies: 48 cases. Neurology 1990; 40:1181–1189.

34. Clinical and laboratory findings in patients with antiphospholipid antibodies and cerebral ischemia. The Antiphospholipid Antibodies in Stroke Study Group. Stroke 1990;21:1268–1273.

35. Briley DP, Coull BM, Goodnight SH. Neurological disease associated with antiphospholipid antibodies. Ann Neurol 1989;25:221–227.

36. Ascherson RA, Khamashta MA, Gil A, et al. Cerebrovascular disease and antiphospholipid antibodies in systemic lupus erythematosus, lupus-like disease, and the primary antiphospholipid syndrome. Am J Med 1989;86:391–399.

37. Harris EN, Gharavi AE, Asherson RA, et al. Cerebral infarction in systemic lupus: association with anticardiolipin antibodies. Clin Exp Rheumatol 1984;2:47–51.

38. Derksen RHWM, Bouma BN, Kater L. The association between the lupus anticoagulant and cerebral infarction in systemic lupus erythematosus. Scand J Rheumatol 1986; 15:179–184.

39. Anticardiolipin antibodies are an independent risk factor for first ischemic stroke. The Antiphospholipid Antibodies in Stroke Study (APASS) Group. Neurology 1993;43: 2069–2073.

40. Mackworth-Young CG, Loizou S, Walport MJ. Primary antiphospholipid syndrome: features of patients with raised anticardiolipin antibodies and no other disorder. Ann Rheum Dis 1989;48:362–367.

41. Asherson RA, Khamashta MA, Ordi-Ros J, et al. The "primary" antiphospholipid syndrome: major clinical and serological features. Medicine (Baltimore) 1989;68: 366–374.

42. Alarcón-Segovia D, Pérez-Vásquez ME, Villa AR, et al. Preliminary classification criteria for the antiphospholipid syndrome within systemic lupus erythematosus. Semin Arthritis Rheum 1992;21:275–286.

43. Harris EN, Gharavi AE, Tincani A, et al. Affinity purified anticardiolipin and anti-DNA antibodies. J Clin Lab Immunol 1985;17:155–162.

44. Gharavi AE, Harris EN, Asherson RA, Hughes GRV. Anticardiolipin antibodies: isotype distribution and phospholipid specificity. Ann Rheum Dis 1987;46:1–8.

45. Toschi V, Motta A, Castelli C, et al. Prevalence and clinical significance of antiphospholipid antibodies to noncardiolipin antigens in systemic lupus erythematosus. Haemostasis 1993;23:275–283.

46. Toschi V, Motta A, Castelli C, et al. High prevalence of antiphosphatidylinositol antibodies in young patients with cerebral ischemia of undetermined cause. Stroke 1998; 29:1759–1764.

47. Tuhrim S, Rand JH, Wu X, et al. Antiphosphatidyl serine antibodies are independently associated with ischemic stroke. Neurology 1999;53:1523–1527.

48. Coull BM, Kevine SR, Brey RL. The role of antiphospholipid antibodies in stroke. Neuro Clin 1992;10:125–141.

49. Feldmann E, Levine SR. Cerebrovascular disease with antiphospholipid antibodies: immune mechanisms, significance, and therapeutic options. Ann Neurol 1995;37 (Suppl 1):S114–S130.

50. Ginsburg KS, Liang MH, Newcomer L, et al. Anticardiolipin antibodies and the risk for ischemic stroke and venous thrombosis. Ann Intern Med 1992;117:997–1002.

51. Harris EN, Gharavi AE, Loizou S, et al. Cross-reactivity of antiphospholipid antibodies. J Clin Lab Immunol 1985;16:1–6.

52. Loizou S, Mackworth-Young CG, Cofiner C, et al. Heterogeneity of binding reactivity to different phospholipids of antibodies from patients with systemic lupus erythematosus (SLE) and with syphilis. Clin Exp Immunol 1990; 80:171–176.

53. Lafer EM, Rauch J, Andrzejewski C Jr, et al. Polyspecific monoclonal lupus autoantibodies reactive with both polynucleotides and phospholipids. J Exp Med 1981;153: 897–909.

54. Khamashta MA, Harris EN, Gharavi AE, et al. Immune mediated mechanism for thrombosis: antiphospholipid antibody binding to platelet membranes. Ann Rheum Dis 1988;47:849–854.

55. Freyssinet JM, Cazenave JP. Lupus-like anticoagulants, modulation of the protein C pathway, and thrombosis. Thromb Haemost 1987;58:679–681.

56. Cariou R, Tobelem G, Belluci S. Effect of lupus anticoagulant on antithrombogenic properties of endothelial cells: inhibition of thrombomodulin-dependent protein C activation. Thromb Haemost 1988;60:54–58.

57. Amer L, Kisiel W, Searles RP, Williams RC Jr. Impairment of the protein C anticoagulant pathway in a patient with systemic lupus erythematosus, anticardiolipin antibodies and thrombosis. Thromb Res 1990;57:247–258.

58. Bevers EM, Galli M, Barue T, et al. Lupus anticoagulant IgGs are not directed to phospholipids only, but to a com-

plex of lipid-bound human prothrombin. Thromb Haemost 1991;66:629–632.

59. Alarcon-Segovia D, Cabral AR. Functional and immunochemical heterogeneity of antiphospholipid antibodies: a classification. J Rheumatol 1992;19:1166–1169.

60. McNeil HP, Simpson RJ, Chesterman CN, Krilis SA. Antiphospholipid antibodies are directed against a complex antigen that includes lipid-binding inhibitor of coagulation: beta 2-glycoprotein I (apolipoprotein H). Proc Natl Acad Sci U S A 1990;87:4120–4124.

61. Gharavi AE. Antiphospholipid cofactor. Stroke 1992;23 (Suppl I):7–10.

62. Nimpf J, Bevers EM, Bumams PH, et al. Prothrombinase activity of human platelet is inhibited by beta 2-glycoprotein I. Biochem Biophys Acta 1986;884:142–149.

63. Nimpf J, Wurm H, Kostner GM. Beta 2-glycoprotein I (apoH) inhibits the release reaction of human platelets during ADP-induced aggregation. Atherosclerosis 1987; 63:109–114.

64. Ford SE, Lillicrap DP, Brunet D, Ford P. Thrombotic endocarditis and lupus anticoagulant: a pathogenic possibility for idiopathic "rheumatic type" valvular heart disease. Arch Pathol Lab Med 1989;113:350–353.

65. Asherson RA, Lubbe WF. Cerebral and valve lesions in SLE: association with antiphospholipid antibodies. J Rheum 1988;15:539–541.

66. Anticardiolipin antibodies and the risk of recurrent thrombo-occlusive events and death. The Antiphospholipid Antibodies and Stroke Study (APASS) Group. Neurology 1997;48:91–94.

67. D'Olhaberriague, Levine SR, Salowich-Palm T, et al. Specificity, isotype, and titer distribution of anticardiolipin antibodies in CNS diseases. Neurology 1998;51:1376–1380.

68. Finazzi G, Brancaccio V, Moia M, et al. Natural history and risk factors for thrombosis in 360 patients with antiphospholipid antibodies: a four-year prospective study from the Italian registry. Am J Med 1996;100:530–536.

69. Fields RA, Toubbeh H, Searles RP, Bankhurst AD. The prevalence of anticardiolipin antibodies in a healthy elderly population and its association with antinuclear antibodies. J Rheumatol 1989:16:623–625.

70. Tanne D, D'Olhaberriague L, Schulz LR, et al. Anticardiolipin antibodies and their associations with cerebrovascular risk factors. Neurology 1999;52:1368–1373.

71. Babikian VL, Levine SR. Therapeutic considerations for stroke patients with antiphospholipid antibodies. Stroke 1992;23(Suppl I):133–137.

72. Levine SR, Welch KMA. Cerebrovascular ischemia associated with lupus anticoagulant. Stroke 1987;18:257–263.

73. Brey RL, Hart RG, Sherman DG, Tegeler CH. Antiphospholipid antibodies and cerebral ischemia in young people. Neurology 1990;40:1190–1196.

74. Montalbán J, Codina A, Ordi J, et al. Antiphospholipid antibodies in cerebral ischemia. Stroke 1991; 22:750–753.

75. Nencini P, Baruffi MC, Abbate R, et al. Lupus anticoagulant and anticardiolipin antibodies in young adults with cerebral ischemia. Stroke 1992;23:189–193.

76. Huong DLT, Wechsler B, Edelman P, et al. Postpartum cerebral infarction associated with aspirin withdrawal in the antiphospholipid antibody syndrome. J Rheumatol 1993;20:1229–1232.

77. Digre KB, Durcan FJ, Branch DW, et al. Amaurosis fugax associated with antiphospholipid antibodies. Ann Neurol 1989;25:228–232.

78. Rosove MH, Brewer PM. Antiphospholipid thrombosis: clinical course after the first thrombotic event in 70 patients. Ann Intern Med 1992;117:303–308.

79. Recurrent thromboembolic and stroke risk in patients with neurological events and antiphospholipid antibodies. The Antiphospholipid Antibodies and Stroke Study (APASS) Group. Ann Neurol 1990;28:226.

80. Asherson RA, Gibson DG, Evans DW, et al. Diagnostic and therapeutic problems in two patients with antiphospholipid antibodies, heart valve lesions, and transient ischaemic attacks. Ann Rheum Dis 1988;47:947–953.

81. Landi G, Calloni MV, Sabbadini MG, et al. Recurrent ischemic attacks in two young adults with lupus anticoagulant. Stroke 1983;14:377–379.

82. McHugh NJ, Maymo J, Skinner RP, et al. Anticardiolipin antibodies, livedo reticularis, and major cerebrovascular and renal disease in systemic lupus erythematosus. Ann Rheum Dis 1988;47:110–115.

83. Derksen RH, Hasselaar P, Blokzijl L, deGroot PG. Lack of efficacy of plasma-exchange in removing antiphospholipid antibodies (letter). Lancet 1987;2:222.

84. Ingram SB, Goodnight SH, Bennett RM. An unusual syndrome of devastating noninflammatory vasculopathy associated with anticardiolipin antibodies: report of two cases. Arthritis Rheum 1987;30:1167–1172.

85. Perez MC, Wilson WA, Scopelitis E. Cyclophosphamide use in a young woman with antiphospholipid antibodies and recurrent cerebrovascular accident. South Med J 1989;82:1421–1424.

86. Case Record 42-1987. N Engl J Med 1987;317:1008–1020.

87. Wapner RJ, Cowchock FS, Shapiro SS. Successful treatment in two women with antiphospholipid antibodies and refractory pregnancy losses with intravenous immunoglobulin infusions. Am J Obstet Gynecol 1989;161:1271–1272.

88. Parke A, Maier D, Wilson D, et al. Intravenous gamma-globulin, antiphospholipid antibodies, and pregnancy. Ann Intern Med 1989;110:495–496.

89. Barbui T, Finazzi G, Falanga A, Corelazzo S. Intravenous gamma-globulin, antiphospholipid antibodies, and thrombocytopenia (letter). Lancet 1988;2:969.

90. Hagen PT, Scholz DG, Edwards WD. Incidence and size of patent foramen ovale during the first 10 decades of life: an autopsy study of 965 normal hearts. Mayo Clin Proc 1984;59:17–20.

91. Meissner I, Whisnant JP, Khandheria BK, et al. Prevalence of potential risk factors for stroke assessed by transesophageal echocardiography and carotid ultrasonography: the SPARC study. Stroke Prevention: Assessment of Risk in a Community. Mayo Clin Proc 1999;74:862–869.

92. Lechat PH, Mas JL, Lascault G, et al. Prevalence of patent foramen ovale in patients with stroke. N Engl J Med 1988;318:1148–1152.

93. Webster MWI, Smith HJ, Sharpe DN, et al. Patent foramen ovale in young stroke patients. Lancet 1988;2:11–12.

94. Ranoux D, Cohen A, Cabanes L, et al. Patent foramen ovale: is stroke due to paradoxical embolism? Stroke 1993;24:31–34.

95. Itoh T, Matsumoto M, Handa N, et al. Paradoxical embolism as a cause of ischemic stroke of uncertain etiology: a transcranial Doppler sonographic study. Stroke 1994;25: 771–775.

96. Di Tullio M, Sacco RL, Gopal A, et al. Patent foramen ovale as a risk factor for cryptogenic stroke. Ann Intern Med 1992;117:461–465.

97. deBelder MA, Tourikis L, Leech G, Camm AJ. Risk of patent foramen ovale for thromboembolic events in all age groups. Am J Cardiol 1992;69:1316–1320.

98. Schneider B, Hanrath P, Vogel P, Meinertz T. Improved morphologic characterization of atrial septal aneurysm by transesophageal echocardiography: relation to cerebrovascular events. Am J Cardiol 1990;16:1000–1009.

99. Barbosa MM, Pena JL, Motta MM, Fortes PR. Aneurysms of the atrial septum diagnosed by echocardiography and their associated cardiac abnormalities. Int J Cardiol 1990; 29:71–79.

100. Homma S, Di Tullio MR, Sacco RL, et al. Characteristics of patent foramen ovale associated with cryptogenic stroke. Stroke 1994;25:582–586.

101. Hanna JP, Sun JP, Furlan AJ, et al. Patent foramen ovale and brain infarct: echocardiographic predictors, recurrence, and prevention. Stroke 1994;25:782–786.

102. Agmon Y, Khandheria BK, Meissner I, et al. Frequency of atrial septal aneurysms in patients with cerebral ischemic events. Circulation 1999;99:1942–1944.

103. Mas JL, Zuber M. Recurrent cerebrovascular events in patients with patent foramen ovale, atrial septal aneurysm, or both and cryptogenic stroke or transient ischemic attack. French Study Group on Patent Foramen Ovale and Atrial Septal Aneurysm. Am Heart J 1995;130:1083–1088.

104. Steiner MM, Di Tullio MR, Rundek T, et al. Patent foramen ovale size and embolic brain imaging findings among patients with ischemic stroke. Stroke 1998;29:944–948.

105. Hausmann D, Mugge A, Daniel WG. Identification of patent foramen ovale permitting paradoxical embolism. J Am Coll Cardiol 1995;26:1030–1038.

106. Siebenlist D, Gattenlöhner W. Transit-thrombus im offenen foramen ovale mit pulmonaler und paradoxer embolisation. Dtsch Med Wochenschr 1993;118:1105–1109.

107. Silverman ME. Images in clinical medicine: paradoxical embolus. N Engl J Med 1993;329:930.

108. Meister SG, Grossman W, Dexter L, Dalen JE. Paradoxical embolism: diagnosis during life. Am J Med 1972;53: 292–298.

109. Comess KA, DeRook FA, Beach KW, et al. Transesophageal echocardiography and carotid ultrasound in patients with cerebral ischemia: prevalence of findings and recurrent stroke risk. J Am Coll Cardiol 1994;23:1598–1603.

110. Bogousslavsky J, Garazi S, Jeanrenaud X. Stroke recurrence in patients with patent foramen ovale: the Lausanne study. Lausanne Stroke with Paradoxical Embolism Study Group. Neurology 1996;46:1301–1305.

111. Nellessen U, Daniel WG, Matheis G, et al. Impending paradoxical embolism from atrial thrombus: correct diagnosis by transesophageal echocardiography and prevent by surgery. J Am Coll Cardiol 1985;5:1002–1004.

112. Quinn TJ, Plehn JF, Liebsen PR. Echocardiographic diagnosis of mobile right atrial thrombus: early recognition and treatment. Am Heart J 1984;108:1548–1550.

113. Schauer N, Kienpointner G, Scharfetter M, Stühlinger W. Echokardiographischer nachweis und operative entfernung eines flottierenden thrombus im rechten vorhof. Intensivmed 1986;23:366–368.

114. Müller C, Axthelm E-H. Thombolyse eines rechtsatrialen transit-thrombus. Dtsch Med Wochenschr 1992;117:1578.

115. Rosenow EC 3d, Osmundson PJ, Brown ML. Pulmonary embolism. Mayo Clin Proc 1981;56:161–178.

116. Chambers J. Should percutaneous devices be used to close a patent foramen ovale after cerebral infarction or TIA? Heart 1999;82:537–538.

117. Cardiogenic brain embolism: the second report of the Cerebral Embolism Task Force. Cerebral Embolism Task Force. Arch Neurol 1989;46:727–743.

118. Jeanrenaud X, Kappenberger L. Patent foramen ovale and stroke of unknown origin. Cerebrovasc Dis 1991;1:184–192.

119. Jones RJ Jr, Caplan LR, Come PC, et al. Cerebral emboli of paradoxical origin. Ann Neurol 1983;13:314–319.

120. Cheng TO. Paradoxical embolism: a diagnostic challenge and its detection during life. Circulation 1976;53:565–568.

121. Bridges ND, Perry SB, Keane JF, et al. Preoperative transcatheter closure of congenital muscular ventricular septal defects. N Engl J Med 1991;324:1312–1317.

122. Bridges ND, Hellenbrand W, Latson L, et al. Transcatheter closure of patent foramen ovale after presumed paradoxical embolism. Circulation 1992;86:1902–1908.

123. Nendaz MR, Sarasin FP, Junod AF, Bogousslavsky J. Preventing stroke recurrence in patients with patent foramen ovale: antithrombotic therapy, foramen closure, or therapeutic abstention? A decision analytic perspective. Am Heart J 1998;135:532–541.

124. Devuyst G, Paciaroni M, Bogousslavsky J. Secondary stroke prevention: a European trial. Cerebrovasc Dis 1999;9(Suppl 13):29–36.

125. Sturzenegger M, Huber P. Cranial nerve palsies in spontaneous carotid artery dissection. J Neurol Neurosurg Psychiatry 1993;56:1191–1199.

126. Ast G, Woimant F, Georges B, et al. Spontaneous dissection of the internal carotid artery in 68 patients. Eur J Med 1993;2:466–472.

127. Mokri B, Sundt TM Jr, Houser OW, Piepgras DG. Spontaneous dissection of the cervical internal carotid artery. Ann Neurol 1986;19:126–138.

128. Hart RG, Easton JD. Dissections of cervical and cerebral arteries. Neurol Clin 1983;1:155–182.

129. Mokri B, Houser OW, Sandok BA, Piepgras DG. Spontaneous dissections of the vertebral arteries. Neurology 1988;38:880–885.

130. Chiras J, Marciano S, Vega-Molina J, et al. Spontaneous dissecting aneurysm of the extracranial vertebral artery: 20 cases. Neuroradiology 1985;27:327–333.

131. Herr RD, Call G, Banks D. Vertebral artery dissection from neck flexion during paroxysmal coughing. Ann Emerg Med 1992;21:88–91.

132. Jentzer A. Dissecting aneurysm of the left ICA. Angiology 1954;5:232–234.

133. Caplan LR, Zarins CK, Hemmati M. Spontaneous dissection of the extracranial vertebral arteries. Stroke 1985;16: 1030–1038.

134. Anderson RM, Schechter MM. A case of spontaneous dissecting aneurysm of the internal carotid artery. J Neurol Neurosurg Psychiatry 1959;22:195–201.

135. Traflet RF, Barbaria AR, Bell RD, et al. Vertebral artery dissection after rapid head turning. AJNR Am J Neuroradiol 1989;10:650–651.

136. Tramo MJ, Hianline B, Petito F, et al. Vertebral artery injury and cerebellar stroke while swimming: case report. Stroke 1985;6:1039–1042.

137. Pryse-Phillips W. Infarction of the medulla and cervical cord after fitness exercises. Stroke 1989;20:292–294.

138. Bogousslavsky J, Despland PA, Regli F. Spontaneous carotid dissection with acute stroke. Arch Neurol 1987;44: 137–140.

139. Anglejan-Chatillon J, Ribeiro V, Mas JL, Bousser MG. Dissections Carotidiennes Extracrâniennes Spontanées Chez L'adulte: 47 Cas. In Indications et Résultats de la Chirurgie Carotidienne. Actualités de Chirurgie Vasculaire. Ed. AERCV 1988;245–252.

140. Mas JL, Bousser MG, Hasboun D, Laplane D. Extracranial vertebral artery dissections: a review of 13 cases. Stroke 1987;18:1037–1047.

141. Greiner AL. Spontaneous dissecting aneurysms of the cervical internal carotid artery. Stroke 1976;7(abstract):6.

142. Sellier N, Chiras J, Benhamou M, Boriers J. Spontaneous dissection of the internal carotid artery. Clinical, radiologic, and evolutive aspects. Apropos of 46 cases. J Neuroradiol 1983;10:243–259.

143. Ramsay TL, Mosquera VT. Dissecting aneurysm of the middle cerebral artery. Ohio State Med J 1948;44:168–170.

144. Thapedi IM, Ashenhurst EM, Rozdilsky B. Spontaneous dissecting aneurysm of the internal carotid artery in the neck. Arch Neurol 1970;23:549–554.

145. Schievink WI, Limburg M, Oorthuys JW, et al. Cerebrovascular disease in Ehlers-Danlos syndrome type IV. Stroke 1990;21:626–632.

146. Austin MG, Schaeffer RF. Marfan's syndrome with unusual blood vessel manifestations. Arch Pathol 1957;64:205–209.

147. Friedman AH, Drake CG. Subarachnoid hemorrhage from intracranial dissecting aneurysm. J Neurosurg 1984;60: 325–334.

148. Wilkinson IM. The vertebral artery: extracranial and intracranial structure. Arch Neurol 1972;27:392–396.

149. Fang H. A Comparison of Blood Vessels of the Brain and Peripheral Blood Vessels. In B Wright, CH Millikan (eds), Cerebral Vascular Diseases. New York: Grune & Stratton, 1958;17–22.

150. Saver JL, Easton JD, Hart RG. Dissections and Trauma of Cervicocerebral Arteries. In HJM Barnett, JP Mohr, BM Stein, FM Yatsu (eds), Stroke: Pathophysiology, Diagnosis, and Management (2nd ed). New York: Churchill Livingstone, 1992;671–688.

151. Kitanaka C, Tanaka J, Kuwahara M, Teraoka A. Magnetic resonance imaging study of intracranial vertebrobasilar artery dissections. Stroke 1994;25:571–575.

152. Zuber M, Meary E, Meder JF, Mas JL. Magnetic resonance imaging and dynamic CT scan in cervical artery dissections. Stroke 1994;25:576–581.

153. McCormick GF, Halbach VV. Recurrent ischemic events in two patients with painless vertebral artery dissection. Stroke 1993;24:598–602.

154. Levy C, Laissy JP, Raveau V, et al. Carotid and vertebral artery dissections: three-dimensional time-of-flight MR angiography and MR imaging versus conventional angiography. Radiology 1994;190:97–103.

155. Müllges W, Ringelstein EB, Leibold M. Non-invasive diagnosis of internal carotid artery dissections. J Neurol Neurosurg Psychiatry 1992;55:98–104.

156. Steiger HJ. Zur Behandlung der traumatischen Karotisdissektion. Neurochirugie 1988;31:128–133.

157. Landre E, Roux FX, Cioloca C. Spontaneous dissection of the extracranial internal carotid artery: therapeutic aspects. Presse Med 1987;16:1273–1276.

158. Pozzati E, Padovani R, Fabrizi A, et al. Benign arterial dissections of the posterior circulation. J Neurosurg 1991;75:69–72.

159. Youl BD, Coutellier A, Dubois B, et al. Three cases of spontaneous extracranial vertebral artery dissection. Stroke 1990; 21:618–625.

160. Young CA, Chadwick DW, Humphrey PR. Extracranial vertebral artery dissection following tonic clonic seizure. J Neurol Neurosurg Psychiatry 1991;54:365–366.

161. Hugenholtz H, Pokrupa R, Montpetit VJA, et al. Spontaneous dissecting aneurysm of the extracranial vertebral artery. Neurosurgery 1982;10:96–100.

162. Hodge CJ Jr, Lee SH. Spontaneous dissecting cervical carotid artery aneurysm. Neurosurgery 1982;10:93–95.

163. Kaplan SS, Ogilvy CS, Gonzalez R, et al. Extracranial vertebral artery pseudoaneurysm presenting as subarachnoid hemorrhage. Stroke 1993;24:1397–1399.

164. Ameri A, Bousser M-G. Cerebral venous thrombosis. Neurol Clin 1992;10:87–111.

165. Frerichs KU, Deckert M, Kempski O, et al. Cerebral sinus and venous thrombosis in rats induces long-term deficits in brain function and morphology—evidence for a cytotoxic genesis. J Cereb Blood Flow Metab 1994;14:289–300.

166. Bousser M-G, Chiras J, Bories J, Castaigne P. Cerebral venous thrombosis: a review of 38 cases. Stroke 1985; 16:199–213.

167. Einhäupl K, Villringer A, Haberl RL, et al. Clinical Spectrum of Sinus Venous Thrombosis. In K Einhäupl, O Kempski, A Baethmann (eds), Cerebral Sinus Thrombosis—Experimental and Clinical Aspects. New York: Plenum, 1990;275–279.

168. Sato S, Miyahara Y, Dohmoto Y, et al. Cerebral Microcirculation in Experimental Sagittal Sinus Occlusion in Dogs. In LM Auer, F Loew (eds), The Cerebral Veins. New York: Springer, 1983;111–117.

169. Smith AS, Cornblath WT, Deveikis JP. Local thrombolytic therapy in deep cerebral venous thrombosis. Neurology 1997;48:1613–1619.

170. Crawford SC, Digre KB, Palmer CA, et al. Thrombosis of the deep venous drainage of the brain in adults. Analysis of seven cases with review of the literature. Arch Neurol 1995;52:1101–1108.

171. Schutta HS, Williams EC, Baranski BG, Sutula TP. Cerebral venous thrombosis with plasminogen deficiency. Stroke 1991;22:401–405.

172. Carroll JD, Leak D, Lee HA. Cerebral thrombophlebitis in pregnancy and the puerperium. QJM 1966;139:347–367.

173. Cantú C, Barinagarrementeria F. Cerebral venous thrombosis associated with pregnancy and puerperium: review of 67 cases. Stroke 1993;24:1880–1884.

174. Singh B. The management of lateral sinus thrombosis. J Laryngol Otol 1993;107:803–808.

175. Einhäupl KM, Villringer A, Meister W, et al. Heparin treatment in sinus venous thrombosis. Lancet 1991;338:597–600.

176. Isensee CH, Reul J, Thron A. Magnetic resonance imaging of thrombosed dural sinuses. Stroke 1994;25:29–34.

177. Krayenbühl HA. Cerebral venous and sinus thrombosis. Clin Neurosurg 1967;14:1–24.

178. Fairburn B. Intracranial venous thrombosis complicating oral contraception: treatment by anticoagulant drugs. BMJ 1973;2:647.

179. Kaplan JM, Biller J, Adams HP Jr. Outcome in nonseptic spontaneous superior sagittal sinus thrombosis in adults: a 14-year experience. Cerebrovasc Dis 1991;1:231–234.

180. Buchanan DS, Brazinsky JH. Dural sinus and cerebral venous thrombosis: incidence in young women receiving oral contraceptives. Arch Neurol 1970;22:440–444.

181. Rousseaux P, Bernard MH, Scherpereel B, Guyot JF. Thrombose des sinus veineux intra-craniens (à propos de 22 cas). Neurochirurgie 1978;24:197–203.

182. Al-Hakim M, Katirji MB, Osorio I, Weisman R. Cerebral venous thrombosis in paroxysmal nocturnal hemoglobinuria: report of two cases. Neurology 1993;43:742–746.

183. Thron A, Wessel K, Linden D, et al. Superior sagittal sinus thrombosis: neuroradiological evaluation and clinical findings. J Neurol 1986;233:283–288.

184. Mattes W, Dörstelmann D. Hirnvenen-und sinusthrombose: diagnose und verlaufskontrolle der antikoagulantientherapic durch computertomographie. Dtsch Med Wochenschr 1981;106:744–747.

185. Halpern JP, Morris JGL, Driscoll GL. Anticoagulants and cerebral venous thrombosis. Aust N Z J Med 1984;14:643–648.

186. Jaillard AS, Hommel M, Mallaret M. Venous sinus thrombosis associated with androgens in a healthy young man. Stroke 1994;25:212–213.

187. Higashida RT, Helmer E, Halbach VV, Hieshima GB. Direct thrombolytic therapy for superior sagittal sinus thrombosis. AJNR Am J Neuroradiol 1989;10:S4–S6.

188. Rich C, Gill J, Wernick S, Konkol RJ. An unusual cause of cerebral venous thrombosis in a four-year-old child. Stroke 1993;24:603–605.

189. Cros D, Comp PC, Beltran G, Gum G. Superior sagittal sinus thrombosis in a patient with protein S deficiency. Stroke 1990;21:633–636.

190. Barnett HJ, Hyland HH. Non-infective intracranial venous thrombosis. Brain 1953;76:36–49.

191. Geittelfinger DM, Kokmen E. Superior sagittal sinus thrombosis. Arch Neurol 1977;34:2–6.

192. Rosse WF. Treatment of paroxysmal nocturnal hemoglobinuria. Blood 1982;60:20–23.

193. Kyritsis AP, Williams EC, Schutta HS. Cerebral venous thrombosis due to heparin-induced thrombocytopenia. Stroke 1990;21:1503–1505.

194. Tuite P, Ahmad F, Grant I, et al. Cerebral vein thrombosis due to hereditary antithrombin III deficiency. Can J Neurol Sci 1993;20:158–161.

195. de Bruijn SF, Stam J. Randomized, placebo-controlled trial of anticoagulant treatment with low-molecular-weight heparin for cerebral sinus thrombosis. The Cerebral Venous Sinus Thrombosis Study Group. Stroke 1999; 30:484–488.

196. Tsai FY, Higashida RT, Matovich V, Alfieri K. Acute thrombosis of the intracranial dural sinus: direct thrombolytic treatment. AJNR Am J Neuroradiol 1992;13:1137–1141.

197. Horowitz M, Purdy P, Unwin H, et al. Treatment of dural sinus thrombosis using selective catheterization and urokinase. Ann Neurol 1995;38:58–67.

198. Rael JR, Orrison WW, Baldwin N, Sell J. Direct thrombolysis of superior sagittal sinus thrombosis treated by direct endovascular thrombolysis. Surg Neurol 1997;48:261–266.

199. Frey JL, Muro GJ, McDougall CG, et al. Cerebral venous thrombosis: combined intrathrombus rtPA and intravenous heparin. Stroke 1999;30:489–494.

200. Kim SY, Suh JH. Direct endovascular thrombolytic therapy for dural sinus thrombosis: infusion of alteplase. AJNR Am J Neuroradiol 1997;18:639–645.

201. Chow K, Gobin P, Saver J, et al. Endovascular treatment of dural sinus thrombosis with rheolytic thrombectomy and intra-arterial thrombolysis. Stroke 2000; 31:1420–1425.

202. O'Connell JE. Lateral sinus thrombosis: a problem still with us. J Laryngol Otol 1990;104:949–951.

203. Sindou M, Mercier P, Bokor J, Brunon J. Bilateral thrombosis of the transverse sinuses: microsurgical revascularization with venous bypass. Surg Neurol 1980; 13:215–220.

Chapter 21
Restorative Therapy

Larry Bruce Goldstein

Despite the important advances in prevention and acute management of stroke reviewed in other chapters of this book, it is recognized that prevention is not universally effective and that the available acute intervention (recombinant tissue-type plasminogen activator) is appropriate for only a small minority of stroke patients. Of patients who survive the acute phase, approximately 50% are alive after 7 years.[1] It is estimated that there are more than 4 million Americans who have had a stroke. Approximately 10% of these patients return to work without disability, 40% have mild disabilities, 40% are severely disabled, and 10% require long-term institutional care.[2] The greatest portion of the country's $40 billion stroke-related annual expenditures is directed toward poststroke rehabilitation and long-term care. Nursing home costs account for more than 50% of the lifetime costs associated with stroke.[3,4] Therefore, developing effective treatments aimed at the poststroke recovery period is of critical importance from medical, social, and economic perspectives.

The major goals of interventions during the poststroke recovery period are (1) to implement secondary prevention strategies to reduce the risk of recurrent stroke (discussed in Chapters 1 and 9), (2) to avoid and manage stroke-related complications (Chapters 13 and 14), and (3) to maximize functional recovery (and optimize compensation for residual deficits in patients with incomplete recovery) (Chapter 17). This chapter focuses on data regarding factors that may influence recovery after stroke, including new and experimental approaches.

Assessing Stroke-Related Outcomes: Levels of Measurement

The impact of any intervention first requires a uniform method of evaluating and comparing outcomes. The functional impact of stroke may be considered at several levels.[5,6] The World Health Organization scheme refers to stroke-related deficits at the levels of impairment, disability, and handicap. *Impairment* refers to specific physiologic functions, such as language, spatial perception, sensation, strength, and coordination. *Disability* is the result of physiologic impairments and is reflected in specific activities (i.e., activities of daily living, such as bathing, walking, and dressing). *Handicap* results from impairments and disabilities and refers to loss of function at a societal level (i.e., loss of employment). Handicap can be conceptualized as the interaction between disability and the surrounding environment.

It is important to recognize that progress at the impairment level may not be mirrored by improvement in disabilities and handicaps, and that diminished disability and handicap may not reflect decreased impairment. For example, limb paresis may improve after stroke, but the patient may still be unable to walk without assistance (disability) or return to work (handicap). A patient with an upper limb amputation (fixed impairment) may learn to use a prosthesis and the remaining arm to dress (improved disability) and provide childcare (reduction of handicap). Therefore, in considering the impact of experimental and clinical interventions aimed at improving poststroke "functional" recovery, the level of function must be clearly understood. This distinction is also important when assessing the impact of poststroke treatment paradigms.

A variety of different clinical instruments have been developed to measure stroke-related deficits and recovery at each of the three principal functional levels. The National Institutes of Health Stroke Scale (NIHSS) is both reliable and valid and has become the standard stroke impairment scale for use in clinical studies in the United States.[7–10] Reliability can be further improved through the use of standardized video training.[11,12] The European Stroke Scale is similar to the NIHSS and is also reliable and partially validated.[13] The Canadian Neurological Scale is simpler and more rapidly performed, but does not capture many stroke-related impairments.[14,15] However, it has been validated for use retrospectively based on information available in medical records.[16] Scales to measure specific types of impairments, such as the Fugl-Meyer Assessment (motor) and the Berg Balance Scale (balance), have also been developed and validated in stroke patients.[17]

Disability is commonly measured with the Barthel Index (BI).[18,19] Pivotal scores have been established that correspond to severe dependence (score <40) and assisted independence (score >60).[19] Despite being widely used, the BI has significant limitations, including a low-ceiling effect.[20] As a result, some patients with significant stroke-related functional limitations may not have deficits measurable with the BI. The Functional Independence Measure is another valid, reliable, and widely used measure of disability.[21,22] The Functional Independence Measure is popular in the rehabilitation community for monitoring functional improvements in disability through the course of rehabilitation therapy. Instrumental activity of daily living scales attempt to bridge the gap between disability and handicap.[23] These scales attempt to measure the patient's ability to live independently in the home, capturing certain core activities, such as domestic chores, household management, outdoor activities, and transportation. None of the instrumental activity of daily living scales has been fully validated, and reliability has not been fully established.

The Rankin Scale has been used as a measure of stroke-related handicap in many interventional trials.[24] However, the Rankin Scale is a global func-tional health index emphasizing physical disability.[25] The scale may be reliably applied, and because it is weighted towards physical function, the results correlate closely with scores on the BI.[26–28] The Craig Handicap Assessment and Reporting Technique was specifically designed to assess handicap and may prove applicable to stroke patients.[29]

In addition to these physically based measures, it is becoming increasingly important to assess patients' quality of life. Issues related to proxy responses, reliability, and validity in this setting have generally not been systematically evaluated in a prospective study, although relevant data are becoming available.[30–32] Because many of the measures are lengthy, issues related to feasibility in patients recovering from acute stroke also should be assessed. The Sickness Impact Profile (SIP), Health Utilities Index, and EuroQol have been used in the evaluation of stroke patients.[31–34] The physical subscore of the SIP correlates with stroke-related impairments as measured with the NIHSS and Canadian Neurological Scale, but the psychosocial subscore does not correlate as well.[27] Disability scores measured with the BI and handicap scores measured with the Rankin Scale explain only 33% of the variance in SIP scores.[35]

Another stroke outcome scale has been developed that is reliable, valid, and sensitive to change.[36] The Stroke Impact Scale is dependent on patient report, and cannot be obtained in the hyperacute setting. Because it requires patient report, it cannot be obtained from patients with significant language or cognitive impairments. Further study is required to determine the reliability and validity of surrogate-completed assessments.

The World Health Organization is in the process of revising its classification scheme for functional disability.[37] The International Classification of Functioning and Disability-2 organizes information into three dimensions: (1) *Body dimension* (corresponding to impairment) refers to the structure and function of body systems, (2) *activities dimension* (corresponding to disability) refers to the complete range of activities performed by an individual, and (3) *participation dimension* (corresponding to handicap) classifies areas of life in which an individual is involved, has access to, or has societal opportunities or barriers. These dimensions of function may be used in describing stroke-related deficits in the future.

Health Care System Level Factors: Effects of Setting of Rehabilitative Care on Poststroke Recovery

General Setting of Care

More than 70% of stroke survivors receive either postacute institutional or ambulatory rehabilitation care during the first 6 months after stroke.[4] These services are provided in a variety of settings that could affect stroke-related outcomes.[38] In the United States, nearly one-third of rehabilitation services during the first 6 months after stroke are provided in rehabilitation hospitals, approximately 25% in skilled nursing facilities, 16% in acute care hospitals, and 11% through home health agencies.[4] Ideally, the optimal setting of care should be influenced by a variety of factors, including the patient's deficits, capacity to participate in rehabilitative therapy, and potential home support.[38] However, there are wide variations across the country in the use of specific rehabilitation services.[4] For example, the percentage of stroke survivors admitted to a rehabilitation hospital varies from 10% in Tampa-St. Petersburg, Florida, to 31% in Houston, Texas. Use of skilled nursing facilities varies from 14% in Newark, New Jersey, to 41% in Minneapolis-St. Paul, Minnesota. The percentage of stroke patients receiving home health services varies from 19% in the Minneapolis-St. Paul area to 57% in Miami, Florida. There are also large differences between urban and rural areas. Stroke patients living in rural areas are 25% less likely to be admitted to a rehabilitation hospital, 10% less likely to receive home health services, and 41% less likely to receive rehabilitation services from independent providers than stroke patients residing in urban areas.[4] Therefore, the location where a patient resides may be equally, if not more, important than clinical and social factors in determining the setting of rehabilitative care that is offered.

Despite its potential clinical and economic importance, well-controlled outcome data addressing differences based on rehabilitation settings are generally lacking. In one study conducted in Norway, 251 stroke patients initially treated in an acute care hospital were randomized to receive subacute rehabilitation in a hospital rehabilitation unit or routine care offered through community health services.[39] Although there were no differences in mortality after 7 months or health-related quality of life, significantly fewer patients treated in inpatient units were dependent in their activities of daily living. However, 30% of community-treated patients received no organized rehabilitative services. Furthermore, it is not certain whether the differences in outcome were related to the intensity of rehabilitation or the setting in which the rehabilitation was provided. Two prospective studies comparing care in a rehabilitation hospital with that provided in nursing homes indicated better functional outcomes for stroke patients cared for in the rehabilitation hospital setting.[40,41]

Specialized Stroke Rehabilitation Units

The purpose of specialized stroke rehabilitation units is to bring together a team of dedicated experts to provide a tailored, organized, intensive rehabilitative program aimed at optimizing poststroke recovery. The benefit of such programs has been the subject of debate.[42] Observational studies suggested little benefit from a dedicated stroke rehabilitation unit. For example, conventional rehabilitation in general medical wards was compared to comprehensive rehabilitation in geriatric/rehabilitation units in a study conducted in Australia.[43] Care in a dedicated rehabilitation unit was 35% less efficient (i.e., was associated with longer hospital stays) and did not improve discharge scores, accelerate the process of rehabilitation, or decrease the demand for extended care beds after controlling for potential confounding variables. However, several randomized trials of stroke rehabilitation unit care have been completed. Although not every trial demonstrated a positive effect, meta-analyses of randomized trials of organized stroke units (including rehabilitation units) showed a reduction in mortality and improved functional outcome when compared to traditional care.[44,45] Characteristics differentiating organized stroke rehabilitation from traditional care included the presence of a coordinated, multidisciplinary rehabilitation team, staff education and training in stroke, specialization of the medical and surgical staff, and the availability of a geographically distinct ward.[46] In summary, although these data suggest that the provision of organized rehabilitative services has a positive influence on outcomes, the specific features of care that lead to these improvements have not been elucidated.

Patient Level Factors: Effects on Poststroke Recovery

Although some individuals may continue to recover over a period of years,[47] the greatest amount of spontaneous recovery after stroke occurs over the first month.[48–53] Functional improvements tend to be limited after the first 3–6 months.[54] The strongest predictor of the extent of eventual recovery is the severity of the initial neurologic deficit.[48,55–57] Reflecting these observations, the probability of being able to walk 150 ft without assistance after a hemispheric stroke is strongly related to whether the patient has a motor deficit alone, motor and somatic sensory deficits, or combined motor, somatic sensory, and visual field deficits.[58]

A variety of other factors may affect the degree of recovery after stroke. Older individuals tend to have poorer recoveries than younger patients.[59–62] Blacks tend to have greater residual physical deficits after stroke than whites.[63,64] The location of the brain lesion resulting in a specific clinical deficit and the presence of prior lesions are also critical. For example, language recovery in patients with intermediate-sized lesions depends largely on lesion location.[65] The importance of lesion location was also demonstrated in a study in which infarct size and location were determined by brain computed tomography or cerebral angiography and correlated with poststroke motor deficits.[66] The site of the lesion (subcortical vs. cortical) correlated with ultimate recovery, but the size of the lesion did not. Nutritional status, prelesion experience, and postlesion training are also relevant to recovery.[67] Grafman and coworkers[68] investigated the relationships of preinjury intelligence or education, brain-tissue volume loss, and lesion location on the persistence of cognitive deficits after penetrating brain injuries. Preinjury intelligence and education were more important predictors of postinjury performance than other variables. Other potentially important covariates that can have an important impact on recovery after stroke include comorbid neurologic[62] (e.g., cognitive, motor, perceptual) and non-neurologic (e.g., limb amputation, severe arthritis, refractory congestive heart failure) conditions, the presence of

mood disorders,[69,70] and the relative availability of social support mechanisms.[57,71–73]

Facilitation of Recovery: Standard Physiotherapy

Interventions aimed at facilitating poststroke recovery must demonstrate an improvement compared to the "spontaneous" recovery that occurs, in varying degrees, in most stroke patients. The various techniques of physical therapy form the cornerstone of these interventions and are intended to augment normal compensatory strategies[74] or specifically improve lost functions.[75–78]

The standard physiotherapeutic approaches include neurofacilitatory methods using sensory stimulation, exercises that include a progression from assistive to active and resistive modes, and techniques to normalize tone.[79] The methods used by physical therapists to achieve these goals are varied and, in some cases, conflicting. Some approaches discourage excessive effort because of concern that it increases abnormal tone. Other approaches encourage maximal effort to facilitate movement. Because treatment effects are relatively small and the trials have been underpowered,[80] conclusive data supporting the efficacy of specific interventions as compared to each other or to spontaneous recovery are lacking.[79]

Timing and Intensity of Therapy

Early physiotherapeutic intervention may reduce the length of hospital stay and improve functional outcome after stroke.[81] In part, this may be true because early mobilization helps to reduce the incidence of some of the medical complications of stroke, such as deep vein thrombosis, pressure ulcers, and contractures. However, some experimental studies suggest that aggressive early intervention should be considered carefully. These laboratory studies show that intense use of a paretic limb soon after stroke may significantly increase the volume of infarcted brain.[82,83]

Intensive rehabilitation generally begins after the hyperacute stage of stroke. An early randomized trial studying the impact of therapy intensity had methodologic limitations but found that those treated with intensive therapy were less dependent after 3 months, despite being more dependent initially.[84] A subsequent single-blind, randomized trial found that an enhanced physiotherapeutic regimen resulted in a small but statistically significant improvement in arm strength, range, and speed of movement 6 months after stroke.[85] However, these benefits at the level of impairment were not reflected in a reduction in disability as measured by the BI. Another trial compared standard arm physiotherapy with a more intensive regimen in which patients were given an additional 10 hours of therapy over 5 weeks.[86] There was no effect of the additional treatment as measured by a variety of scales at 3 weeks or 6 months after stroke. A program that added arm sensorimotor stimulation to standard therapy resulted in an improvement in motor impairment but had no effect on disability after 6 weeks.[87] Another study compared functional recovery in three groups of patients: a rehabilitation program focused on arm or leg retraining versus a control program in which the paretic limb was transiently immobilized.[88] All patients otherwise underwent standard physiotherapy. Patients who had leg retraining had better outcomes after 20 weeks compared to the controls, and there was an improvement in dexterity in the arm with treatment. However, it is unclear whether the benefits would have been similar if the controls were not immobilized. Taken together, these studies suggest that there may be some benefit to increasing the intensity of arm physiotherapy, but the benefit tends to be small and leads to limited functional improvement. More intensive regimens may result in greater gains in leg function, but the data remain inconclusive.

New and Experimental Approaches

Adjunctive Therapies

The potential impacts of a variety of adjunctive treatments, including electrical stimulation and biofeedback training, on poststroke recovery have been investigated. A meta-analysis of four studies on the effects of electrical stimulation applied to nerves or paretic muscles suggests that the treatment may lead to an overall improvement in strength, but there is no clear evidence that this results in enhanced functional recovery.[89] Data

regarding the impact of biofeedback training are conflicting. One meta-analysis supported an improvement in motor function with biofeedback,[90] whereas a second concluded that biofeedback was of no benefit.[91] These disparate results may have occurred because the specific biofeedback techniques, duration of treatment, and other factors varied among the individual studies.

Novel Physiotherapeutic Approaches

Experimental studies suggest that the nature of postlesion experience may affect recovery after brain injury. A variety of approaches to poststroke physiotherapy are being investigated to determine whether they may lead to greater improvements in functional recovery as compared to more traditional methods.

Repetitive Training. A repetitive training paradigm focused on hand function was found to improve basic movements and manual dexterity in comparison to standard physiotherapy.[92] However, the duration of the benefit after therapy was discontinued, and the impact on overall disability and quality of life was not assessed.

Robot-Assisted Therapy. Robot-assisted therapy provides an automated method of repetitive training. The patient actively or passively interacts with a robotic arm that delivers a precise degree of force, velocity, duration, and repetition of movement in a stereotyped pattern.[93] A randomized study of 20 paretic stroke patients found no significant improvement in disability, motor power, or arm pain with robotic training of the upper extremity, but some improvement in accuracy of proximal arm movements.[94] Twelve of the patients were re-evaluated 3 years later.[95] Those who had received robot training continued to have significantly less motor impairments. A larger study with long-term follow-up is required to determine the clinical value of this approach.

Supported Treadmill Training. Supported treadmill training allows nonambulatory patients to practice patterned walking movements (i.e., repetitive task-specific training). This approach was first assessed in seven nonambulatory stroke patients in a crossover design study.[96] Patients were first treated with supported treadmill training, then crossed over to standard physiotherapy, and then crossed back to treadmill training. There were significant improvements in functional ambulation and walking velocity during the periods of treadmill training, with the patients being able to ambulate by the end of the study. This was followed by a trial in which body-weight–supported treadmill training was compared to treadmill training without body-weight support in 100 gait-impaired stroke patients.[97] Those in the body-weight support group had significant improvements in functional balance, voluntary movement and mobility, walking speed, and endurance at the end of the 6-week training period. Significant benefits in voluntary movement and mobility and walking speed were still evident 3 months after the completion of training.

Forced Use. Forced use (constraint-induced movement) therapy is based on laboratory observations that indicate animals with paretic limbs can regain function if the normal limb is restrained, "forcing" the use of the paretic limb.[98] In a study of 16 stroke and five traumatic brain injury patients with some volitional hand movement more than 1 year after injury, restraining the noninvolved hand for 2 weeks led to significant improvements in the performance of timed tasks.[99] This effect was replicated in a case series of patients with stable deficits more than 1 year after stroke[100] and further supported by an initial randomized study.[101]

Potential Pharmacotherapeutic Approaches. Laboratory studies clearly show that drugs influencing the activity of specific central neurotransmitters can modulate the recovery process.[102] These data suggest that pharmacotherapy to enhance recovery of lost function may be possible and that some commonly prescribed medications used for the treatment of coincident medical conditions in recovering stroke patients may be harmful.

Amphetamine. Several anecdotal reports and small controlled studies suggest that treatment with amphetamine may enhance functional recovery after focal brain injury under certain conditions. These studies vary significantly with regard to patient populations, dosing regimens, and the timing of the interventions. In one study, eight patients with stable motor deficits were randomized to receive either a single dose of amphetamine or placebo within 10 days of ischemic stroke.[103] Within 3 hours of drug administration, all of the patients underwent intensive physical therapy (i.e., drug administration was coupled with task-specific experience). The next day, the amphetamine-treated group showed a significant improvement in motor performance, whereas there was little change in the placebo-treated group. This study was limited because only a small group of highly selected patients was included and only short-term effects were measured. Furthermore, only two of the four amphetamine-treated patients had a "dramatic" motor improvement (the intervention had a variable effect even in this highly selected group).

A second double-blind, placebo-controlled trial included five amphetamine-treated and five placebo-treated patients.[104] Drug or placebo was given once every 4 days for 10 sessions beginning 15–30 days after stroke. Each dose was given in tight conjunction with a session of intensive physical therapy. Evaluations performed 1 week and 1 year after the last dose found amphetamine-treated patients had significantly greater improvements in motor scores compared to placebo-treated patients.

A third double-blind, placebo-controlled trial included 12 patients given 10 mg of amphetamine daily for 14 days followed by 5 mg for 3 days and 12 placebo-treated patients.[105] Interventions began more than 1 month after stroke, and the administration of the drug/placebo was not tightly linked with physical therapy sessions. This study was negative, but varied in several significant ways from the previous trial, including a different dosing regimen, a longer delay between stroke and treatment, and a lack of a tightly coupled drug-physical therapy regimen. Laboratory animal studies suggest that these differences may be critical.

In addition to poststroke motor recovery, speech pathologists have begun to study the effects of amphetamine on language recovery in aphasic stroke patients.[106,107] In one study,[107] six aphasic patients had language function rated with the Porch Index of Communicative Ability 10–30 days after stroke. Language scores at 6 months were predicted for each patient based on this initial evaluation. All patients were then given 10 mg of d-amphetamine followed by speech therapy every 4 days for 10 sessions. The patients' actual language scores after 3 months were then compared with their 6-month predicted scores. Most patients achieved or exceeded this 6-month prediction by the 3-month assessment.

In summary, there are encouraging data suggesting that treatment with amphetamine may facilitate poststroke recovery. However, only a few patients have been studied prospectively, one of three studies was negative, and a second did not include clinically meaningful outcomes. Therefore, use of amphetamine to facilitate poststroke recovery should be viewed as experimental pending the completion of well-designed, multicenter clinical trials.

Methylphenidate. Methylphenidate, another sympathomimetic drug, has also been used in attempts to improve postbrain injury rehabilitation outcome, particularly in depressed patients who are not optimally participating in physical therapy.[108–112] The effect of treatment with methylphenidate on stroke-related disability has been studied in a small placebo-controlled trial.[113] As a group, the methylphenidate-treated patients had less severe motor deficits at the start of the study. Although methylphenidate is safe to administer to stroke patients, there were similar improvements in motor function based on the Fugl-Meyer Assessment motor scores when methylphenidate and placebo-treated patients were compared. Experimental studies suggest a complex relationship between methylphenidate dose and training,[114] which should be systematically explored in a large number of patients to determine whether a specific regimen might be associated with a clinically meaningful benefit.

Tricyclic Antidepressants. Clinical depression is associated with impaired recovery after stroke in humans.[115] Tricyclic antidepressants are commonly used to treat mood disorders in stroke patients. Trazodone, a drug that impairs recovery from hemiplegia in the rat, was found to improve outcome as measured with the BI in depressed stroke patients.[70] Other clinical studies have found a beneficial effect of the serotonin reuptake blocker fluoxetine[116] and no significant effect of the norepinephrine reuptake blockers maprotiline[116] and nortriptyline.[117] Further study is required to verify these preliminary studies and to determine the generalizability of the effect.

Other Drugs. Preliminary studies indicated that the administration of bromocriptine improved flu-

ency in certain aphasics.[118–120] However, two small controlled studies were negative.[121,122] These disappointing results may have been due to a variety of factors. Both controlled trials included patients long after stroke onset and one included several patients with traumatic brain injury.

Potential Detrimental Drug Effects

Laboratory studies also suggest that some drugs may interfere with recovery. Clinical studies have been limited because they can only be carried out based on retrospective analyses. Anecdotal reports indicate that treatment with haloperidol[123,124] and certain antihypertensives[125] may slow or block language recovery in aphasic stroke patients. A retrospective study specifically tested the hypothesis that drugs that are harmful during recovery in laboratory animals (e.g., the antihypertensives clonidine and prazosin, neuroleptics, benzodiazepines, phenytoin, and phenobarbital) would interfere with motor recovery in humans.[64] Patients who received one or a combination of the hypothesized "detrimental" drugs at the time of stroke or during subsequent hospitalization had significantly slower motor recoveries than a comparable group of patients who did not receive any of these drugs. Multivariate analysis indicated a significant effect of "drug group" after correcting for the contributions of other variables, including the initial severity of the deficit. The deleterious effect of these same drugs on motor recovery was also found in a separate cohort of patients with anterior circulation ischemic stroke.[126] These patients were control subjects in a prospective acute interventional stroke trial.[127] Nearly 40% of the control patients enrolled in this study received one or a combination of drugs hypothesized to impair recovery after stroke. As with the previous study, stepwise regression models indicate that those receiving potentially detrimental drugs had poorer motor recoveries independent of the degree of the initial motor impairment, comorbid conditions, and other patient characteristics. However, because both of the studies involved retrospective analyses, it cannot be certain that the reason for the administration of a given drug, rather than the drug itself, influenced recovery. These studies did not permit an analysis of the impact of specific "detrimental" drugs, nor did they permit analyses of dose or timing effects. Whenever possible, however, these drugs should be avoided during the poststroke recovery period. These potential drug effects should also be considered in the design of interventional acute stroke trials because a relatively small clinical benefit of a new experimental drug could be obscured by detrimental effects of others drugs given to treat coincident medical problems.

Other Novel Approaches

Several additional new approaches to improve poststroke recovery are beginning to be explored and could be topics of separate reviews. These include the use of growth factors to facilitate recovery and the possibility of transplanting neural tissue into the damaged brain.

A variety of polypeptide growth factors have been identified that may influence recovery after brain injury.[128–130] These have been classified as neurotrophic (promoting neuronal survival or outgrowth, or both), gliotrophic (supporting glial proliferation and survival), and angiogenic (promoting capillary proliferation) growth factors.[129] Nerve growth factor (NGF) is an example of a neurotrophic factor. Intraventricular infusion of NGF improved behavioral performance on spatial learning tasks in rats with localized brain lesions.[131–133] Much emphasis has been placed on the role of basic fibroblast growth factor (bFGF), which is expressed at the site of focal brain injury.[134] Blockade of bFGF retards recovery from motor cortex injury in rats.[135]

Intracisternal administration of bFGF enhances functional recovery after focal cerebral infarction in rats,[136] an effect blocked by intracisternal antisense oligonucleotide to growth protein-43.[137] The latter finding suggests that bFGF may act by enhancing axonal sprouting in uninjured brain.

Transplantation of non-neural and neural tissue into injured brain offers another potential mode of therapy to enhance poststroke recovery. For example, in one experiment, adult cats that received adrenal medullary autografts onto the floor of a cortical wound 21 days after a frontal cortical lesion had a significant and enduring improvement of locomotor ability.[138] Fetal neocortex can become functionally integrated into the area of brain damaged by infarction in adult rats.[139,140] These types of transplants can lead to improved behavioral outcomes.[141,142]

There appears to be a complex relationship between the viability of transplanted tissue and the behavioral experience of the animal after the graft is placed,[142–145] however, and the mechanism(s) of any behavioral effects remains uncertain.[130] The use of fetal transplants is clearly problematic from the standpoint of human disease. The use of a variety of different types of progenitor cells in transplantation studies is being explored,[146] and at least one human stroke patient has received transformed, fully differentiated neurons made from a teratocarcinoma cell line.[147]

Conclusion

Although advances in treatments directed at the poststroke recovery period have lagged behind preventive and acute therapies, they offer the possibility of entirely new avenues of therapy. Properly timed, specific, intensive physiotherapeutic intervention holds the potential to enhance recovery in comparison to standard approaches. Drugs that may impair recovery can be avoided based on available information, and pharmacotherapy to enhance poststroke recovery should be rigorously tested over the next few years. These approaches may be combined with the use of specific growth factor or transplants, or both, to improve the outcome of patients who would otherwise be disabled by stroke.

References

1. Dombovy ML, Sandok BA, Basford JR. Rehabilitation for stroke: a review. Stroke 1986;17:363–369.
2. Heyman A, Leviton A, Millikan CH, et al. Transient focal cerebral ischemia: epidemiological and clinical aspects. Stroke 1974;5:277–287.
3. Taylor TN, Davis PH, Torner JC, et al. Lifetime cost of stroke in the United States. Stroke 1996;27:1459–1466.
4. Lee AJ, Huber J, Stason WB. Poststroke rehabilitation in older Americans. The Medicare experience. Med Care 1996;34:811–825.
5. International Classification of Impairments, Disabilities, and Handicaps. Geneva: World Health Organization, 1980.
6. Granger CV, Gresham GE. International Classification of Impairments, Disabilities, and Handicaps (ICIDH) as a conceptual basis for stroke outcome research. Stroke 1990;21(Suppl II):66–67.
7. Brott T, Adams HP Jr, Olinger CP, et al. Measurements of acute cerebral infarction: a clinical examination scale. Stroke 1989;20:864–870.

8. Goldstein LB, Bertels C, Davis JN. Interrater reliability of the NIH Stroke Scale. Arch Neurol 1989;46:660–662.

9. Goldstein LB, Samsa GP. Extension of the reliability of the NIH Stoke Scale to non-neurologists. Stroke 1997; 28(abstract):236.

10. Wityk RJ, Pessin MS, Kaplan RF, Caplan LR. Serial assessment of acute stroke using the NIH Stroke Scale. Stroke 1994;25:362–365.

11. Lyden P, Brott T, Tilley B, et al. Improved reliability of the NIH Stroke Scale using video training. NINDS TPA Stroke Study Group. Stroke 1994;25:2220–2226.

12. Albanese MA, Clarke WR, Adams HP Jr, Woolson RF. Ensuring reliability of outcome measures in multicenter clinical trials of treatments for acute ischemic stroke. The program developed for the Trial of ORG 10172 in Acute Stroke Treatment (TOAST). Stroke 1994;25:1746–1751.

13. Hantson L, De Weerdt W, De Keyser J, et al. The European Stroke Scale. Stroke 1994;25:2215–2219.

14. Cote R, Battista RN, Wolfson C, et al. The Canadian Neurological Scale: validation and reliability assessment. Neurology 1989;39:638–643.

15. Cote R, Hachinski VC, Shurvell BL, et al. The Canadian Neurological Scale: a preliminary study in acute stroke. Stroke 1986;17:731–737.

16. Goldstein LB, Chilukuri V. Retrospective assessment of initial stroke severity with the Canadian Neurological Scale. Stroke 1997;48:1181–1184.

17. Post-Stroke Rehabilitation Guidelines Panel. Post-Stroke Rehabilitation. Rockville, MD: Agency for Health Care Policy Research, 1995.

18. Mahoney FI, Barthel DW. Functional evaluation: the Barthel Index. Md Med J 1965;14:61–65.

19. Granger CV, Dewis LS, Peters NC, et al. Stroke rehabilitation: analysis of repeated Barthel Index measures. Arch Phys Med Rehabil 1979;60:14–17.

20. Duncan PW, Samsa GP, Weinberger M, et al. Health status of individuals with mild stroke. Stroke 1997;28:740–745.

21. Data Management Service of the Uniform Data System for Medical Rehabilitation. Guide for the Use of the Uniform Data Set for Medical Rehabilitation. Buffalo, NY: Research Foundation—State University of New York, 1990.

22. Segal ME, Schall RR. Determining functional/health status and its relation to disability in stroke survivors. Stroke 1994;25:2391–2397.

23. Chong DK. Measurement of instrumental activities of daily living in stroke. Stroke 1995;26:1119–1122.

24. Rankin J. Cerebral vascular accidents in patients over the age of 60: II. Prognosis. Scott Med J 1957;2:200–215.

25. De Haan R, Limburg M, Bossuyt P, et al. The clinical meaning of Rankin "handicap" grades after stroke. Stroke 1995;26:2027–2030.

26. Wolfe CD, Taub NA, Woodrow EJ, Burney PG. Assessment of scales of disability and handicap for stroke patients. Stroke 1991;22:1242–1244.

27. De Haan R, Horn J, Limburg M, et al. A comparison of five stroke scales with measures of disability, handicap, and quality of life. Stroke 1993;24:1178–1181.

28. Burn JP. Reliability of the modified Rankin Scale. Stroke 1992;23:438.

29. Whiteneck GG, Charlifue SW, Gerhart KA, et al. Quantifying handicap: a new measure of long-term rehabilitation outcomes. Arch Phys Med Rehabil 1992;73:519–525.

30. De Haan R, Aaronson N, Limburg M, et al. Measuring quality of life in stroke. Stroke 1993;24:320–327.

31. Mathias SD, Bates MM, Pasta DJ, et al. Use of the Health Utilities Index with stroke patients and their caregivers. Stroke 1997;28:1888–1894.

32. Dorman P, Slattery J, Farrell B, et al. Qualitative comparison of the reliability of health status assessments with the EuroQol and SF-36 questionnaires after stroke. United Kingdom Collaborators in the International Stroke Trial. Stroke 1998;29:63–68.

33. Bergner M, Bobbitt RA, Carter WB, Gilson BS. The Sickness Impact Profile: development and final revision of a health status measure. Med Care 1981;19:787–805.

34. Rothman ML, Hedrick S, Inui T. The Sickness Impact Profile as a measure of the health status of noncognitively impaired nursing home residents. Med Care 1989;27: S157–S167.

35. De Haan R, Limburg M. The relationship between impairment and functional health scales in the outcome of stroke. Cerebrovasc Dis 1994;4(Suppl 2):19–23.

36. Duncan PW, Lai SM, Johnson D, et al. The Stroke Impact Scale Version 2.0. Evaluation, reliability, validity, and sensitivity to change. Stroke 1999;30:2131–2140.

37. World Health Organization. International Classification of Functioning and Disability. www.who.int/icidh.

38. Feigenson JS. Stroke rehabilitation. Outcome studies and guidelines for alternate levels of care. Stroke 1981;12: 372–375.

39. Ronning OM, Guldvog B. Outcome of subacute stroke rehabilitation: a randomized controlled trial. Stroke 1998; 29:779–784.

40. Kane RL, Chen Q, Blewett LA, Sangl J. Do rehabilitative nursing homes improve the outcomes of care? J Am Geriatr Soc 1996;44:545–554.

41. Kramer AM, Steiner JF, Schlenker RE, et al. Outcomes and costs after hip fracture and stroke: a comparison of rehabilitation settings. JAMA 1997;277:396–404.

42. Reding MJ, McDowell FH. Focused stroke rehabilitation programs improve outcome. Arch Neurol 1989;46:700–701.

43. Shah S, Vanclay F, Cooper B. Stroke rehabilitation—who benefits? A comparison of medical wards and rehabilitation units. Restor Neurol Neurosci 1992;4:401–410.

44. Langhorne P, Wiliams BO, Gilchrist W, Howie K. Do stroke units save lives? Lancet 1993;342:395–398.

45. Ottenbacher KJ, Jannell S. The results of clinical trials in stroke rehabilitation research. Arch Neurol 1993;50:37–44.

46. Collaborative systematic review of the randomised trials of organised inpatient (stroke unit) care after stroke. Stroke Unit Trialists' Collaboration. BMJ 1997;314:1151–1159.

47. Bach y Rita P. Central nervous system lesions: sprouting and unmasking in rehabilitation. Arch Phys Med Rehabil 1981;62:413–417.

48. Duncan PW, Goldstein LB, Matchar D, et al. Measurement of motor recovery after stroke. Outcome assessment and sample size requirements. Stroke 1992;23:1084–1089.

49. Newman M. The process of recovery after stroke. Stroke 1972;3:702–710.

50. Wade DT, Langton HR, Wood VA, et al. The hemiplegic arm after stroke: measurement and recovery. J Neurol Neurosurg Psychiatry 1983;46:521–524.

51. Loewen SC, Anderson BA. Predictors of stroke outcome using objective measurement scales. Stroke 1990;21:78–81.

52. Wade DT, Wood VA, Hewer RL. Recovery after stroke: the first three months. J Neurol Neurosurg Psychiatry 1985;48:7–13.

53. Kinsella G, Ford B. Acute recovery patterns in stroke patients. Med J Aust 1980;2:662–666.

54. Skilbeck CE, Wade DT, Hewer RL, Wood VA. Recovery after stroke. J Neurol Neurosurg Psychiatry 1983;46:5–8.

55. Jongbloed L. Prediction of function after stroke: a critical review. Stroke 1986;17:765–776.

56. Heinemann AW, Roth EJ, Cichowski K, Betts HB. Multivariate analysis of improvement and outcome following stroke rehabilitation. Arch Neurol 1989;44:1167–1172.

57. Lincoln NB, Blackburn M, Ellis S, et al. An investigation of factors affecting progress of patients on a stroke unit. J Neurol Neurosurg Psychiatry 1989;52:493–496.

58. Reding MJ, Potes E. Rehabilitation outcome following initial unilateral hemispheric stroke. Life table analysis approach. Stroke 1988;19:1354–1358.

59. Granger CV, Hamilton BB, Fiedler RC. Discharge outcome after stroke rehabilitation. Stroke 1992;23:978–982.

60. Kotila M, Waltimo O, Niemi M, et al. The profile of recovery from stroke and factors influencing outcome. Stroke 1984;15:1039–1044.

61. Lindmark B, Hamrin E. Evaluation of functional capacity after stroke as a basis for active intervention. Scand J Rehab Med 1988;20:103–109.

62. Novack TA, Haban G, Graham K, Satterfield WT. Prediction of stroke rehabilitation outcome from psychologic screening. Arch Phys Med Rehabil 1987;68:729–734.

63. Horner RD, Matchar DB, Divine GW, Feussner JR. Racial variations in ischemic stroke-related physical and functional impairments. Stroke 1991;22:1497–1501.

64. Goldstein LB, Matchar DB, Morgenlander JC, Davis JN. Influence of drugs on the recovery of sensorimotor function after stroke. J Neuro Rehab 1990;4:137–144.

65. Knopman DS, Selnes OA, Niccum N. A longitudinal study of speech fluency in aphasia: CT correlates of recovery and persistent nonfluency. Neurology 1983;33:1170–1178.

66. Lundgren J, Flodstrom K, Sjogren K, et al. Site of brain lesion and functional capacity in recovered hemiplegics. Scand J Rehab Med 1982;14:141–143.

67. Finger S, Stein DG. Brain Damage and Recovery. New York: Academic Press, 1982.

68. Grafman J, Salazar A, Weingartner H. The relationship of brain-tissue loss volume and lesion location to cognitive deficit. J Neurosci 1986;6:301–307.

69. Finklestein S, Benowitz LI, Baldessarini RJ, et al. Mood, vegetative disturbance, and dexamethasone suppression test after stroke. Ann Neurol 1982;12:463–467.

70. Reding MJ, Orto LA, Winter SW, et al. Antidepressant therapy after stroke. A double-blind trial. Arch Neurol 1986;43:763–765.

71. Shah S, Vanclay F, Cooper B. Predicting discharge status at commencement of stroke rehabilitation. Stroke 1989; 20:766–769.

72. Vogt TM, Mullooly JP, Ernst D, et al. Social networks as predictors of ischemic heart disease, cancer, stroke, and hypertension: incidence, survival, and mortality. J Clin Epidemiol 1992;45:659–666.

73. Glass TA, Matchar DB, Belyea M, Feussner JR. Impact of social support on outcome in first stroke. Stroke 1993;24: 64–70.

74. Wescott EJ. Traditional exercise regimens for the hemiplegic patient. Am J Phys Med 1967;46:1012–1023.

75. Bobath B. Adult Hemiplegia: Evaluation and Treatment. London: Heinemann, 1984.

76. Brunnstrom S. Movement Therapy in Hemiplegia: A Neurophysiological Approach. New York: Harper & Row, 1970.

77. Wolf SL, Binder-MacLeod SA. Electromyographic biofeedback applications to the hemiplegic patient. Phys Ther 1983;63:1393–1403.

78. Basmajian JV, Gowland CA, Finlayson AJ, et al. Stroke treatment: comparison of integrated behavioral-physical therapy vs traditional physical therapy programs. Arch Phys Med Rehabil 1987;68:267–272.

79. Duncan PW. Synthesis of intervention trials to improve motor recovery following stroke. Top Stroke Rehabil 1997;3:1–20.

80. Matyas TA, Ottenbacher KJ. Confounds of insensitivity and blind luck: statistical conclusion validity in stroke rehabilitation clinical trials. Arch Phys Med Rehabil 1993; 74:559–565.

81. Hayes SH, Carroll SR. Early intervention care in the acute stroke patient. Arch Phys Med Rehabil 1986;67:319–321.

82. Kozlowski DA, James DC, Schallert T. Use-dependent exaggeration of neuronal injury after unilateral sensorimotor cortex lesions. J Neurosci 1996;16:4776–4786.

83. Humm JL, Kozlowski DA, James DC, et al. Use-dependent exacerbation of brain damage occurs during an early postlesion vulnerable period. Brain Res 1998;783:286–292.

84. Sivenius J, Pyorala K, Heinonen OP, et al. The significance of intensity of rehabilitation of stroke: a controlled trial. Stroke 1985;16:928–931.

85. Sunderland A, Tinson DJ, Bradley EL, et al. Enhanced physical therapy improves recovery of arm function after stroke. A randomised controlled trial. J Neurol Neurosurg Psychiatry 1992;55:530–535.

86. Lincoln NB, Parry RH, Vass CD. Randomized, controlled trial to evaluate increased intensity of physiotherapy treatment of arm function after stroke. Stroke 1999;30:573–579.

87. Bornstein NM, Bova IY, Korczyn AD. Infections as triggering factors for ischemic stroke. Neurology 1997;49 (Suppl 4):S45–S46.

88. Kwakkel G, Wagenaar RC, Twisk JWR, et al. Intensity of leg and arm training after primary middle-cerebral artery stroke: a randomised trial. Lancet 1999;354:191–196.

89. Glanz M, Klawansky S, Stason W, et al. Functional electrical stimulation in post-stroke rehabilitation: a meta-analysis of randomized controlled trials. In Center for Health Economics Research: Post-stroke Rehabilitation Guideline Technical Report. Boston: Harvard School of Public Health, 1995.

90. Schlennbaker RE, Mainous AG. Electromyographic biofeedback for neuromuscular reeducation in the hemiplegic stroke patient: a meta-analysis. Arch Phys Med Rehabil 1993;74:1301–1304.

91. Glanz M, Klawansky S, Stason W, et al. Biofeedback therapy in poststroke rehabilitation: a meta-analysis of randomized controlled trials. Arch Phys Med Rehabil 1995; 76:508–515.

92. Butefisch C, Hummelsheim H, Denzler P, Mauritz K-H. Repetitive training of isolated movements improves the outcome of motor rehabilitation of the centrally paretic hand. J Neurol Sci 1995;130:59–68.

93. Aisen ML, Krebs HI, Hogan N, et al. The effect of robot-assisted therapy and rehabilitative training on motor recovery following stroke. Arch Neurol 1997;54:443–446.

94. Wijdicks EF, St Louis E. Clinical profiles predictive of outcome in pontine hemorrhage. Neurology 1997;49: 1342–1346.

95. Volpe BT, Krebs HI, Hogan N, et al. Robot training enhanced motor outcome in patients with stroke maintained over 3 years. Neurology 1999;53:1874–1876.

96. Hesse S, Bertelt C, Jahnke MT, et al. Treadmill training with partial body weight support compared with physiotherapy in nonambulatory hemiparetic patients. Stroke 1995;26:976–981.

97. Visintin M, Barbeau H, Korner-Bitensky N, Mayo NE. A new approach to retrain gait in stroke patients through body weight support and treadmill stimulation. Stroke 1998;29:1122–1128.

98. Taub E, Crago JE, Burgio LD, et al. An operant approach to rehabilitation medicine: overcoming learned nonuse by shaping. J Exp Anal Behav 1994;61:281–293.

99. Wolf SL, Lecraw DE, Barton LA, Jann BB. Forced use of hemiplegic upper extremities to reverse the effect of learned nonuse among chronic stroke and head-injured patients. Exp Neurol 1989;104:125–132.

100. Miltner WH, Bauder H, Sommer M, et al. Effects of constraint-induced movement therapy on patients with chronic motor deficits after stroke: a replication. Stroke 1999;30:586–592.

101. Taub E, Miller NE, Novack TA, et al. Technique to improve chronic motor deficit after stroke. Arch Phys Med Rehabil 1993;74:347–354.

102. Goldstein LB. Potential Impact of Drugs on Poststroke Motor Recovery. In LB Goldstein (ed), Restorative Neurology. Advances in Pharmacotherapy for Recovery After Stroke. Armonk, NY: Futura Publishing Company, 1998; 241–256.

103. Crisostomo EA, Duncan PW, Propst MA, et al. Evidence that amphetamine with physical therapy promotes recovery of motor function in stroke patients. Ann Neurol 1988; 23:94–97.

104. Walker-Batson D, Smith P, Curtis S, et al. Amphetamine paired with physical therapy accelerates motor recovery after stroke. Further evidence. Stroke 1995;26:2254–2259.

105. Reding MJ, Solomon B, Borucki SJ. Effect of dextroamphetamine on motor recovery after stroke. Neurology 1995;45(Suppl 4)(abstract):A222.

106. Homan R, Panksepp J, Mcsweeny J, et al. d-amphetamine effects on language and motor behaviors in a chronic stroke patient. Soc Neurosci Abstr 1990;16:439.

107. Walker-Batson D, Unwin H, Curtis S, et al. Use of amphetamine in the treatment of aphasia. Restor Neurol Neurosci 1992;4:47–50.

108. Johnson ML, Roberts MD, Ross AR, Witten CM. Methylphenidate in stroke patients with depression. Am J Phys Med Rehabil 1992;71:239–241.

109. Lazarus LW, Moberg PJ, Langsley PR, Lingam VR. Methylphenidate and nortriptyline in the treatment of poststroke depression: a retrospective comparison. Arch Phys Med Rehabil 1994;75:403–406.

110. Lazarus LW, Winemiller DR, Lingam VR, et al. Efficacy and side effects of methylphenidate for poststroke depression. J Clin Psychiatry 1992;53:447–449.

111. Rosenberg PB, Ahmed I, Hurwitz S. Methylphenidate in depressed medically ill patients. J Clin Psychiatry 1991; 52:263–267.

112. Larsson M, Ervik M, Lundborg P, et al. Comparison between methylphenidate and placebo as adjuvant in care and rehabilitation of geriatric patients. Compr Gerontol 1988;2:53–59.

113. Grade C, Redford B, Chrostowski J, et al. Methylphenidate in early poststroke recovery: a double-blind, placebo-controlled study. Arch Phys Med Rehabil 1998;79:1047–1050.

114. Kline AE, Chen MJ, Tso-Olivas DY, Feeney DM. Methylphenidate treatment following ablation-induced hemiplegia in rat: experience during drug action alters effects on recovery of function. Pharmacol Biochem Behav 1994; 48:773–779.

115. Morris PL, Raphael B, Robinson RG. Clinical depression is associated with impaired recovery from stroke. Med J Aust 1992;157:239–242.

116. Dam M, Tonin P, De Boni A, et al. Effects of fluoxetine and maprotiline on functional recovery in poststroke hemiplegic patients undergoing rehabilitation therapy. Stroke 1996;27:1211–1214.

117. Lipsey JR, Pearlson GD, Robinson RG, et al. Nortriptyline treatment of post-stroke depression: a double-blind study. Lancet 1984;1:297–300.

118. Albert ML, Bachman DL, Morgan A, Helm-Estabrooks N. Pharmacotherapy for aphasia. Neurology 1988;38:877–879.

119. Bachman DL, Morgan A. The role of pharmacotherapy in the treatment of aphasia. Aphasiology 1988;3–4:225–228.

120. Sabe L, Leiguarda R, Starkstein SE. An open-label trial of bromocriptine in nonfluent aphasia. Neurology 1992;42: 1637–1638.

121. Gupta SR, Mlcoch AG, Scolaro C, Moritz T. Bromocriptine treatment of nonfluent aphasia. Neurology 1995;45: 2170–2173.

122. Sabe L, Salvarezza F, Cuerva AG, et al. A randomized, double-blind, placebo-controlled study of bromocriptine in nonfluent aphasia. Neurology 1995;45:2272–2274.

123. Porch B, Wyckes J, Feeney DM. Haloperidol, thiazides, and some antihypertensives slow recovery from aphasia. Soc Neurosci Abstr 1985;11(abstract):52.

124. Feeney DM, Sutton RL. Pharmacotherapy for recovery of function after brain injury. Crit Rev Neurobiol 1987;3: 135–197.

125. Porch BE, Feeney DM. Effects of antihypertensive drugs on recovery from aphasia. Clin Aphasiology 1986;16: 309–314.

126. Goldstein LB. Common drugs may influence motor recovery after stroke. The Sygen in Acute Stroke Study Investigators. Neurology 1995;45:865–871.

127. Ganglioside GM1 in acute ischemic stroke. The SASS trial. Stroke 1994;25:1141–1148.

128. Lipton SA. Growth factors for neuronal survival and process regeneration. Implications for the mammalian central nervous system. Arch Neurol 1989;46:1241–1248.

129. Kawamata T, Speliotes EK, Finklestein SP. The role of polypeptide growth factors in recovery from stroke. Adv Neurol 1997;73:377–382.

130. Johansson BB. Neurotrophic Factors and Transplants. In Restorative Neurology: Advances in Pharmacotherapy for Recovery after Stroke. Armonk, NY: Futura Publishing Company, 1998;141–166.

131. Mandel RJ, Gage FH, Thal LJ. Spatial learning in rats: correlation with cortical choline acetyltransferase and improvement with NGF following NBM damage. Exp Neurol 1989;104:208–217.

132. Pallage V, Orenstein D, Will B. Nerve growth factor and septal grafts: a study of behavioral recovery following partial damage to the septum in rats. Behav Brain Res 1992;47:1–12.

133. Dekker AJ, Gage FH, Thal LJ. Delayed treatment with nerve growth factor improves acquisition of a spatial task in rats with lesions of the nucleus basalis magnocellularis: evaluation of the involvement of different neurotransmitter systems. Neuroscience 1992;48:111–119.

134. Finklestein SP, Apostslides PJ, Caday CG, et al. Increased basic fibroblast growth factor (bFGF) immunoreactivity at the site of focal brain wounds. Brain Res 1988;460:253–259.

135. Rowntree S, Kolb B. Blockade of basic fibroblast growth factor retards recovery from motor cortex injury in rats. Eur J Neurosci 1997;9:2432–2442.

136. Kawamata T, Dietrich WD, Schallert T, et al. Intracisternal basic fibroblast growth factor enhances functional recovery and up-regulates the expression of a molecular marker of neuronal sprouting following focal cerebral infarction. Proc Natl Acad Sci U S A 1997;94:8179–8184.

137. Kawamata T, Ren J, Cha JH, Finklestein SP. Intracisternal antisense oligonucleotide to growth associated protein-43 blocks the recovery-promoting effects of basic fibroblast growth factor after focal stroke. Exp Neurol 1999;158:89–96.

138. Sutton RL, Hovda DA, Feeney DM. Intracerebral chromaffin cell autografts accelerate functional recovery in adult cats unilateral frontal cortex ablation. Brain Dysfunct 1989;2:201–210.

139. Grabowski M, Brundin P, Johansson BB. Functional integration of cortical grafts placed in brain infarcts of rats. Ann Neurol 1993;34:362–368.

140. Tillotson GL, Schulz MK, Hogan TP, Castro AJ. Analysis of neocortical grafts placed into focal ischemic lesions in adult rats. Neurosci Lett 1995;201:69–72.

141. Plumet J, Ebrahimi A, Guitet J, Roger M. Partial recovery of skilled forelimb reaching after transplantation of fetal cortical tissue in adult rats with motor cortex lesion: anatomical and functional aspects. Restor Neurol Neurosci 1993;6:9–27.

142. Mattsson B, Sorensen JC, Zimmer J, Johansson BB. Neural grafting to experimental neocortical infarcts improves behavioral outcome and reduces thalamic atrophy in rats housed in enriched but not in standard environments. Stroke 1997;28:1225–1231.

143. Bragin AG, Vinogradova OS, Stafekhina VS. Sensory deprivation prevents integration of neocortical grafts with the host brain. Restor Neurol Neurosci 1992;4:279–283.

144. Christie MA, Dalrymple-Alford JC. Behavioural consequences of frontal cortex grafts and enriched environments after sensorimotor cortex lesions. J Neural Transplant Plast 1995;5:199–210.

145. Grabowski M, Sorensen JC, Mattsson B, et al. Influence of an enriched environment and cortical grafting on functional outcome in brain infarcts of adult rats. Exper Neurol 1995;133:96–102.

146. Gage FH, Coates PW, Palmer TD, et al. Survival and differentiation of adult neuronal progenitor cells transplanted to the adult brain. Proc Natl Acad Sci U S A 1995;92:11879–11883.

147. Bonn D. First cell transplant aimed to reverse stroke damage. Lancet 1998;352:119.

Chapter 22

Management of Poststroke Neurobehavioral Disturbances

James Paskavitz

Virtually any symptom of cognitive or behavioral dysfunction can occur as a result of stroke. On rare occasions, these symptoms are the only manifestation of the stroke. More often, other prominent physical symptoms and signs overshadow the cognitive or behavioral symptoms. This makes it difficult for the clinician to determine the extent of neurobehavioral dysfunction. For instance, unilateral apraxia cannot be appreciated with a concomitant hemiplegia. Mild aphasia may not be appreciated if there is a severe dysarthria. As recovery from physical deficits occurs, these neurobehavioral deficits may become more apparent and may interfere with the patient's ability to function independently.

Acute occlusive vascular events may cause the most dramatic presentations, but the neurobehavioral consequences are at least additive for gradually progressive small vessel ischemic events or the accumulation of multiple discrete ischemic events. Therefore, multiple neurobehavioral syndromes (i.e., aphasia and apraxia) may be present in a single patient to the degree that they may be demented. Poststroke dementia as a single diagnosis is not discussed here.

In this chapter, specific neurobehavioral syndromes from discrete lesions are discussed. The discussion is limited to syndromes that significantly affect the patient's ability to function in daily life, and many interesting neurobehavioral diagnoses are not addressed. This chapter includes the syndromes of confusional states, neglect, aphasia, amnesia, abulia, apraxia, depression, mania, hallucinations,

and delusions. Methods for examining the patient to diagnose these syndromes go beyond the scope of this chapter, but an attempt is made to define and localize these syndromes, with attention to prognosis and treatment. Much of the literature on treatment of neurobehavioral disorders is anecdotal or lacks vigorous study design; therefore, many of the therapeutic interventions remain unproven.

Confusional States

The development of a confusional state is usually seen in right middle or posterior cerebral artery infarctions[1–4] or multifocal bihemispheric events (i.e., multiple emboli or global hypoperfusion). In a confusional state, level of arousal typically is normal with impaired or fluctuating attention. These patients therefore have memory disturbances and word-finding and comprehension problems and are usually disoriented and unable to engage in high-level cognitive tasks. Right middle cerebral artery infarctions causing confusion usually mature with time into a neglect syndrome (see subsequent discussion of neglect). Bihemispheric events from multiple emboli or global hypoperfusion tend to have more permanent confusional states. Likewise, posterior cerebral artery infarcts have long-lasting effects, presumably due to diencephalic injury in either hemisphere.

Recovery from inattention due to stroke has not been well studied. Neurorehabilitation is unlikely to be helpful because the impaired attention of patients makes them unable to cooperate. No pharmacologic interventions have been established. If agitation and combativeness accompany the confusional state, low-dose neuroleptics may provide some symptomatic improvement.

Neglect

Unilateral neglect is a common neurologic deficit after strokes in the nondominant hemisphere, although transient neglect can be seen in dominant hemispheric strokes. Unilateral neglect is therefore almost always left-sided. Also called *hemi-inattention*, left neglect can be subtle and modality-specific (i.e., visual, somatosensory, or auditory) or dense and disabling if it involves multiple brain modalities, including sensory and motor. Neglect may also encompass impaired appreciation of personal and extrapersonal space.[5]

Left neglect is most commonly seen in patients who have experienced right parietal stroke, typically in the inferior parietal cortex. It can also be seen in patients with right thalamic strokes and white matter infarcts in the parietal lobe. Frontal and cingulate cortical infarcts, as well as midbrain and basal ganglia strokes, are more rare causes of neglect. The severity of neglect usually reflects the size of the stroke.[5,6]

Anosognosia (lack of knowledge of one's deficit) may compound the neglect syndrome. Patients who are unable to appreciate left hemispace may not appreciate their own left-sided paralysis and are at risk for injuries should they try to walk. Anosognosia is not specifically localized to the right hemisphere but is usually present if left neglect is severe.[7]

Recovery from left neglect depends on how dense the neglect is and is related to stroke size. Improvements are seen most rapidly in the first week after stroke. Impairments continue to decrease for up to 4 months thereafter. If no improvement has occurred after 2 months, however, it is unlikely that any recovery will occur.[8] Overall, the presence of neglect confers a poor prognosis for functional recovery of activities of daily living.[6]

Treatment of neglect is an attempt to improve the patient's function beyond the level expected in spontaneous recovery. Most pharmacologic or rehabilitation treatment approaches are only somewhat successful or have not been demonstrated to show generalized, sustained effectiveness.[6,9] Often, the reported improvements for the interventions only reflect improvement on specific tests and do not generalize to overall functional improvement.[5] For instance, Fresnel prism spectacles displace images from the impaired or neglected visual field toward the center and functioning visual field. Patients with left hemianopia or left neglect, or both, showed improvements with Fresnel prisms on a visuoperceptual task but did not improve in activities of daily living.[10]

Other manipulations of visual fields have shown some positive results as well. A small study showed that patients with left neglect had initial improvement in function when the right hemifield of each eye was covered with a patch, forcing patients to attend to left space.[11] Another small study used sunglasses that were shaded on the right half of each lens in patients with left neglect and showed mixed improvements on line bisection, line cancellation, and copying tasks.[12]

Behavioral strategies that involve repetitive training tasks have been shown to variably improve neglect. Patients with neglect who frequently repeated tasks for scanning visual space and becoming aware of personal and extrapersonal space and perceptual organization in a rehabilitation setting showed some improvement in both scanning visual space[13] and somatosensory personal and extrapersonal space perception.[14] Another study confirmed these short-term improvements but found that the benefit did not persist.[15]

External stimulation of the right hemisphere has shown variable results in improving neglect during specific tasks but has not been found to be generalizable.[6] Auditory cueing while a patient is trying to bisect a line, visual stimulation of left hemispace with flashing lights during a line bisection task, and patching the right eye while visually stimulating the left visual field all improve neglect during the task.[16–18] Listening to background music during a task may also improve neglect because of proposed activation of the right hemisphere.[19]

Other approaches involving external stimuli with actual sensory or conceptual feedback may improve task-specific neglect. For instance, visual neglect has been shown to improve with proprioceptive feedback in a study in which subjects were told to pick up a metal rod by holding it in the middle. When subjects picked up the rod to the right of center, the proprioceptive perception of weight imbalance allowed them to correct their mistaken visual perception of center.[20] In a similar approach, patients with neglect mistakenly point to the right of center when asked to find the center of a balancing-lever apparatus. When asked to place an object on the center of the lever to achieve balance and prevent the object from tilting the lever and falling, patients with neglect tended to place the object closer to the center than the spot where they originally pointed.[21] This suggests that anticipating the consequences of an action may improve neglect. Although these benefits were task-specific, a randomized controlled trial using a trunk-rotation and scanning paradigm showed improvement in tests of neglect that generalized to activities of daily living among patients who had neglect for less than 3 months. This technique also resulted in improvement among neglect patients with symptoms longer than 6 months in duration.[22] This improvement may have been due to the appreciation of the incongruity between the proprioceptive feedback with trunk rotation and visual perception during scanning, with the appropriate response requiring integration of both modalities.

Vestibular stimulation is another approach to treating neglect with external sensory stimulation techniques that has shown task-specific improvement. Stimulating the external auditory canal on the neglected side with cold water makes the patient's eyes move toward the left (cold water caloric reflex) and improves midline pointing and cancellation and counting tasks.[23] Caloric stimulation has been shown to improve neglect even in patients with closed eyes,[24] and it helps patients appreciate their left-sided paralysis, suggesting improved anosognosia.[24,25] However, this improvement in neglect and anosognosia appears only during stimulation and, therefore, is not of practical significance.

Pharmacologic intervention for neglect has not been studied extensively. In two studies, dopamine agonist therapy improved neglect. One study involved two patients who improved with bromocriptine for 1 month,[26] whereas the other used apomorphine in four patients compared with a placebo in those same four patients.[27] Other medicines thought to have effects on arousal and, therefore, potentially improve attention, such as cholinergic medications and stimulants, have not been studied thus far.

Aphasia

Language disturbances have been well studied in patients after stroke and occur in approximately 33% of patients who survive an acute stroke, with 20% of the remaining survivors being phasic at 6 months.[8] Language dysfunction includes problems with both spoken and written language. Deficits in spoken language (*aphasia*) are a more significant determinant of functional recovery than deficits in written language (*alexia*, *agraphia*) because social interactions and activities are more speech-based. The severity of the language deficit usually reflects the size of the stroke.

Aphasia typically results from dominant hemisphere strokes. The nondominant hemisphere contributes prosody and inflection to speech. Aphasic syndromes are generally divided into *global*, *fluent*, or *nonfluent* aphasias. Most acute aphasias are global, but mature into either nonfluent or fluent aphasias depending on the location of the stroke. In fluent aphasia, the stroke is usually posterior to the central sulcus or inferior to the sylvian fissure, or both. Nonfluent aphasias arise from lesions in the frontal lobe. Aphasia can also result from strokes in the left caudate or thalamic nuclei.

Nonfluent aphasias demonstrate effortful speech with grammatic errors and few spontaneous words, but comprehension is usually intact. In fluent aphasia, speech is spontaneous and effortless, but is usually nonsensical with impaired comprehension. Milder fluent aphasia may be manifest as neologisms and paraphasic errors with only mildly impaired comprehension. Naming problems and impaired repetition of speech help further clarify aphasia subtypes and reflect anatomic localization. For instance, anomic aphasia occurs exclusively in left temporal lobe lesions, but all aphasia subtypes show impaired naming.[7] Delineation of aphasia subtypes goes beyond the scope of this chapter.

Recovery from aphasia also reflects the location and severity of the stroke. Pure anomic aphasia has the best prognosis, given the relatively small lesion size sufficient to cause this type of deficit. Severe fluent aphasias with impaired comprehension usually have significant comprehension deficits that persist. Nonfluent aphasias also remain nonfluent to a similar relative extent. Recovery is fastest 1–3 months poststroke, with less recovery thereafter, although comprehension deficits can improve for up to a year after stroke onset.[8,28]

Strategically localized strokes in combination, even if small in size, can be as devastating to language function as large strokes. For example, discrete white matter lesions adjacent to the head of the caudate and anterior corpus callosum, combined with lesions in the periventricular white matter that extend to motor and sensory cortical regions for the mouth, are associated with poor recovery of spontaneous speech in severe nonfluent aphasia, much like large hemispheric infarction.[29] In global aphasia, recovery of language comprehension is worse for cortical lesions involving posterior superior temporal gyrus than large white matter lesions in the same region.[30]

Treatment for aphasia has included rehabilitation and pharmacologic approaches but has been inconclusive regarding efficacy and outcomes, largely due to problems related to study design and inclusion of heterogeneous aphasia subtypes. Many theoretical models guide the structure of rehabilitation from behavioral stimulus-response-reinforcement paradigms to cognitive psychological paradigms. Despite the variety of approaches and study designs, meta-analysis of rehabilitation versus spontaneous recovery seems to favor treatment.[9] Pharmacotherapy for aphasia has not been shown to work in most cases; however, anecdotal cases of improvement with bromocriptine and amphetamine have been reported and critiqued.[31]

The only rehabilitation approach for aphasia that has been endorsed by the American Academy of Neurology is melodic intonation therapy (MIT). MIT is a technique that attempts to use the right hemisphere to improve fluency in nonfluent aphasias. Teaching patients to sing and modulate tone and prosody instead of speaking in a monotone accounts for the improved fluency. The improvement in fluency is not present unless melodic intonation is being performed. It was initially thought that MIT activates the right hemisphere to override the left hemisphere deficit; however, one positron emission tomography study showed that MIT actually enhances left hemisphere language areas and decreases activity in right hemisphere language areas.[32]

Other therapy approaches attempt to help patients adjust to and compensate for their language dysfunction. Some strategies try to reteach the rules of language, whereas others attempt to teach nonverbal strategies of communication, including sign language (which uses symbolic hand representations to convey information) and gestural techniques. Other therapies use icons (or pictures) to convey information, either with stacks of cards or computer images with visual representations of information to be shown by the aphasic patient and structured in a way as to convey that information in a "conversation." Choosing the therapy appropriate for an individual patient cannot be based on good outcomes data because there is no consistently good method; instead, therapy should be tailored to the abilities of the patient. For instance, a mild nonfluent aphasic patient may experience some improvement with MIT, such that functional communication may improve, whereas a patient with severe global aphasia would probably need an iconic representational approach to both understand and communicate.

Amnesia

Memory disorders resulting from acute stroke are rare in isolation and may be difficult to detect if there is prominent language or visuospatial dysfunction, or both. Memory deficits are common in more chronic, slowly progressive cerebrovascular diseases. *Antegrade amnesia* is the term used to describe memory acquisition deficits and must be distinguished from attentional disturbances. There are many kinds of memory subtypes, such as declarative and procedural, episodic and implicit, with these subtypes having overlapping features. Despite the overlap, it seems that hemispheric laterality plays a role in determining the type of information that cannot be remembered.[7,8] Left hemisphere events usually cause impairment in learning linguistic information, whereas right hemisphere events impair learning of visuospatial information.

Medial temporal lobe infarction involving the hippocampus or adjacent structures, or both, can cause global amnesia if there is bilateral involvement. Similarly, bilateral basal ganglia infarcts can cause global amnesia, as can thalamic infarctions. Basal forebrain infarcts are rarely due to vascular occlusion in vivo but can occur as a result of clipping unruptured anterior communicating artery aneurysms with consequent severe global amnesia.[33]

There are no pharmacologic treatments for amnesia. Rehabilitation does not improve memory deficits but should be viewed as an attempt to compensate for lost function or maximize residual function.[8,34] Memory diaries, calendars, alarms, and so forth may all work as cues, but patients must learn how to use them and respond to them. Patients with explicit memory deficits can learn implicitly, so repetitive procedural training may create patterns of behavior conducive to environmental cues (i.e., putting the memory diary with daily schedule next to the alarm so the patient has it in hand when waking in the morning).

Abulia

Abulia refers to signs of apathy and decreased initiative. Patients with abulia may have completely intact cognitive function but make no attempt to interact with their environment. If it is severe enough, they may have no spontaneous activity or reaction to uncomfortable environmental circumstances. They may be incontinent of stool or urine because they do not respond to the urge to go to the bathroom and may not change their clothing after soiling themselves. They may not groom, change clothes, prepare meals, or show any social interests. Injury to medial frontal cortex from anterior cerebral artery infarctions causes abulia. If bilateral infarction of the cingulate gyrus occurs, patients may have no spontaneous speech or body movements (akinetic mutism). Abulia can occur in depression and dementing illnesses as well, but other neurologic features are not usually present. Stimulants, such as methylphenidate and amphetamine, and dopaminergic agents, such as levodopa, amantadine, and bromocriptine, have been used to treat abulia with anecdotal success. No trials have been randomized and controlled and no reports are restricted to poststroke abulia.[35]

Disinhibition

The opposite of abulia would be disinhibition, which can manifest itself in a variety of ways ranging from aggression to inappropriate behaviors and impulsivity. Aggression can be spontaneous or reactive in poststroke behavioral dysfunction, but it is unlikely to be premeditated. Emotional disinhibition may be exemplified by inappropriate laughter or tearfulness (pseudobulbar affect), irritability, and labile mood. Impulsivity can be manifested as inappropriate responses to circumstances whereby the patient misjudged or did not consider the consequences of his or her action. They may say insulting things without the intention of insulting or may behave in a way that causes physical harm to themselves due to the misjudgment. The combination of impulsivity and aggressiveness may be difficult to manage. Damage to inferior frontal lobes seems to lead to disinhibition and can be seen in infarcts of anterior cerebral artery branches.

As in other stroke syndromes, recovery levels off in a few months, but management of disinhibition is difficult. Often, these patients need to live in structured and socially isolating environments. Sometimes their behavior is bad enough that they should be institutionalized. Behavioral programs, whether at home or in an institution, revolve around external control of behavior outputs. Family or health care staff often need to cue and defuse situations, which requires significant attention and effort. Reward- and punishment-based behavioral paradigms are sometimes helpful but can be difficult to implement, especially if the patient is not institutionalized.

Pharmacologic management of disinhibition after stroke is not well studied. Aggression is one manifestation of disinhibition that usually requires pharmacologic management. Lithium and beta blockers have been used in poststroke aggression.[7] Other medications that may be helpful include mood stabilizers such as carbamazepine or valproic acid. Benzodiazepines and neuroleptics are the last choice; their use depends on how aggressive the patient is because they induce more of a sedative effect, acting as a chemical restraint, and may retard stroke recovery.[35] The lowest possible dose of any medicine should be used to avoid sedation or other side effects, such as depression with beta blockers.

Apraxia

Apraxia is an intentional disorder in which patients are unable to execute purposeful motor behavioral pantomimes, either spontaneously, to command, or even imitation. There are many different kinds of apraxia, but ideomotor apraxia is the most common manifestation of stroke-induced apraxia and seems to localize to lesions of the dominant hemisphere supplementary motor area, corpus callosum, inferior parietal lobe, or basal ganglia and adjacent subcortical white matter. Ideomotor apraxia consists of errors in the production of movements, either by spatial or temporal misjudgment, but the intention of the motor behavior can usually be appreciated.[36] Using an object or imitating a behavior that someone else is performing may produce better results than pantomiming to command. Because of the localization of apraxia to the dominant hemisphere, this deficit may be obscured by or confused with language comprehension deficits, especially in large hemispheric lesions.

For some reason, recovery from apraxia is more promising than other behavioral stroke syndromes. Fifty percent of patients with apraxia recover at 5 months and another 25% recover as late as 3 years after stroke. Prognosis is somewhat worse if the parietal lobe is involved. There are no substantiated rehabilitation or pharmacologic treatments for apraxia.[8] Because they are usually somewhat improved when imitating a behavior or using an implement to guide behavior, patients may be able to function with a milder deficit than is demonstrable by pantomiming.

Depression

Depression is a common consequence of stroke—occurring after approximately one-third to one-half of strokes—and is more common than apraxia, amnesia, and aphasia.[8] There is a debate about whether depression is caused by the stroke or in reaction to the deficits appreciated by the patient. It was thought that depression was more common after left-sided strokes, but it may be that right hemisphere strokes resulting in neglect and anosognosia made it difficult to make depression detectable. Left-sided strokes may result in more severe depression.[8] Left frontal pole, left or right thalamus, left caudate, and right or left parietal lesions have all been thought to contribute to acute depression or dysthymia,[7,35] but long-term follow-up shows lesion location to be a more ambiguous variable.[37–39] Depression can affect participation performance and outcome of rehabilitation. Patients may decline in function, and their poststroke physical and cognitive deficits may appear worse than they would be had they not been depressed.[8,9,40]

Despite the abundance of antidepressant medications and the frequency of poststroke depression, few good clinical studies exist to corroborate their usefulness. The few randomized, double-blind, placebo-controlled trials that have been done all involved relatively small numbers of patients; however, they did show benefits from antidepressants. Trazodone was shown to be effective in depressed poststroke patients who had a positive dexamethasone suppression test.[41] Nortriptyline was found to have a dramatic effect on poststroke depression in another small study, with a 100% response rate to treatment and a 0% response rate to placebo. There was a one-third dropout rate for both placebo and treatment groups. Both the response rate and dropout rate may reflect some of the methodologic flaws in this study.[42] A study of citalopram, a selective serotonin reuptake inhibitor, showed a two-thirds response rate to treatment versus a 15% response rate to placebo, with 25% of the treated patients and 5% of the placebo patients withdrawing from the study due to side effects.[43] Prospective and retrospective open-label studies using methylphenidate also have found benefit with this medicine in a small number of patients.[35]

Given the potential outcome effect of untreated depression and the suggestive evidence of treatment efficacy, it is worth risking side effects to treat depression in stroke patients. The lower side effect profile of selective serotonin reuptake inhibitors makes them the best choice, and low doses should be the rule with titration upward based on effect. Because stroke patients tend to be elderly and medication side effects are more frequent in elderly populations, it is best to give patients up to 2 weeks of a low-dose medicine before increasing it, as beneficial effects may take up to 2 weeks to appear.

Mania

Mania after stroke is rare and seems to occur with infarctions in the right hemisphere. Lesions in the right caudate, right thalamus, and combinations of lesions in the right caudate, basolateral frontal, and inferior temporal cortex have resulted in secondary manic-depression.[44] Pure mania can be caused by right hemisphere caudate, thalamic, occipitotemporal, and combinations of caudate and temporal lobe infarcts,[44,45] but left hemisphere events have also been reported.[46] A family history of mania seems to be a risk factor for secondary mania in some cases,[7] and the cerebrovascular event may unmask the predisposition.

No clinical studies have been conducted to test the efficacy of pharmacotherapy in pure poststroke mania, but anecdotal use of lithium has suggested beneficial effects.[45,47] Other mood stabilizing agents, such as valproic acid and carbamazepine, have yielded encouraging results in small trials of patients with secondary mania.[35] The clinical course of untreated secondary mania may be self-limited,[45] suggesting the need to reassess continuation of treatment if initiated.

Hallucinations and Delusions

Poststroke hallucinations have a variety of presentations, from simple visual, auditory, or sensory illusions to complex visual or auditory phenomena that are difficult to distinguish from reality. Generally speaking, the quality of the hallucination reflects the area of brain that is affected. For instance, spots of light or color called *positive spontaneous visual phenomena* or *release hallucinations* may be present in or around the blind visual field of patients with infarctions in the primary visual cortex.[48–50] Stroke involving areas of higher order visual integration may result in visual distortions or more complex hallucinations.[50] *Peduncular hallucinations* are well-formed visual hallucinations that may occur in brain stem strokes, in which the patient knows what he or she is perceiving is not real.

Hallucinations in which patients cannot distinguish between their perceptions and reality, and are therefore psychotic, tend to occur after right hemisphere strokes but are not more localizable. Psychotic visual hallucinations are more common than auditory hallucinations after stroke, and patients may have associated delusions that are organized and paranoid.[51]

Delusions are beliefs that are not grounded in reality and thus are psychotic. Delusions without hallucinations occur more frequently in right hemisphere strokes but can occur in left hemisphere events as well.[35,52,53] There are no consistent lesion locations associated with delusions. Paranoia can be present in fluent aphasia from left hemisphere strokes but is more likely a combination of anosognosia and impaired comprehension than a delusion. Patients experiencing paranoia become suspicious when people do not respond to them in a manner they believe would be appropriate to the conversation because the patients do not realize that they are delusional.

Pharmacologic treatment should be reserved for patients who are significantly disturbed by their hallucinations. For instance, peduncular hallucinations can be extremely well formed, but if the patient knows that they are not real and is not acting on them there is little need to subject the patient to the side effects of a medicine. Psychotic hallucinations and delusions should always be treated. There are no clinical studies to corroborate the effectiveness of neuroleptics in poststroke hallucinations or delusions, but anecdotal communications suggest they work.[52,53] Newer antipsychotic medications, such as risperidone, clozapine, and olanzapine, are probably the best initial treatment choices because they have better side-effect profiles than older antipsychotic agents.

Conclusion

Strokes cause a variety of neurobehavioral syndromes. Combinations of multiple syndromes can result in severe functional disability and dementia, but the few syndromes described in this chapter can occur from single ischemic events. Although rehabilitation can help improve function in patients with neglect, aphasia, amnesia, and, possibly, apraxia, it does not improve overall brain recovery from stroke. Pharmacologic interventions have not been shown to improve these syndromes. Conversely, pharmacologic interventions may help with poststroke disinhibition, abulia, depression, mania, hallucinations, and delusions, whereas rehabilitation is less likely to improve functionality. More controlled clinical trials with strict inclusion criteria and homogeneous neurobehavioral syndromes may help clarify the efficacy of drug or rehabilitation approaches in helping these patients.

References

1. Mesulam MM, Waxman SG, Geschwind N, Sabin TD. Acute confusional states with right middle cerebral artery infarctions. J Neurol Neurosurg Psychiatry 1976;3:84–89.
2. Mori E, Yamadori A. Acute confusional state and acute agitated delirium, occurrence after infarction of the right middle cerebral artery. Arch Neurol 1987;44:1139–1143.

3. Devinsky O, Bear D, Volpe BT. Confusional states following posterior cerebral artery infarction. Arch Neurol 1988; 45:160–163.

4. Nicolai A, Lazzarino LG. Acute confusional states secondary to infarctions in the territory at the posterior cerebral artery in elderly patients. Ital J Neurol Sci 1994;15: 91–96.

5. Heilman KM, Watson RT, Valenstein E. Neglect: Clinical and Anatomic Aspects. In Feinberg and Farah (eds), Behavioral Neurology and Neuropsychology. New York: McGraw-Hill, 1997;309–317.

6. Chatterjee A, Mennemeier M. Diagnosis and Treatment of Spatial Neglect. In RB Lazar (ed), Principles of Neurologic Rehabilitation. New York: McGraw-Hill, 1998;567–612.

7. Absher JR, Toole JF. Neurobehavioral Features of Cerebrovascular Disease. In BS Fogel, RB Schiffer, SM Rao (eds), Neuropsychiatry. Baltimore: Williams & Wilkins, 1996;895–912.

8. Alexander MP. Medical, Neurologic, and Functional Outcome of Stroke Survivors. In VM Mills, JW Cassidy, DI Katz (eds), Neurologic Rehabilitation. Oxford, UK: Blackwell, 1997;29–57.

9. U.S. Department of Health and Human Services. Post-Stroke Rehabilitation: Clinical Practice Guidelines. Number 16. Washington, D.C.: 1995;85–142.

10. Rossi PW, Kheyfets S, Reding MJ. Fresnel prisms improve visual perception in stroke patients with homonymous hemianopia or unilateral neglect. Neurology 1990;40: 1597–1599.

11. Beis JM, Andre JM, Baumgarten A, Challier B. Eye patching in unilateral spatial neglect; efficacy of two methods. Arch Phys Med Rehab 1999;80:71–76.

12. Arai T, Ohi H, Sasuki H, et al. Hemispatial sunglasses: effect on unilateral spatial neglect. Arch Phys Med Rehab 1997;78:230–232.

13. Weinberg M, Diller L, Gordon WA, et al. Visual scanning training effects on reading-related tasks in acquired right brain damage. Arch Phys Med Rehab 1977;58:479–486.

14. Weinberg M, Diller L, Gordon WA, et al. Training sensory awareness and spatial organization in people with right brain damage. Arch Phys Med Rehab 1979;60:491–496.

15. Gordon WA, Hibbard MR, Egelko S, et al. Perceptual remediation in patients with right brain damage: a comprehensive program. Arch Phys Med Rehab 1985;66:353–359.

16. Riddoch MJ, Humphreys GW. The effect of cueing on unilateral neglect. Neuropsychologia 1983;21:589–599.

17. Butter CM, Kirsch NL, Reeves G. The effect of dynamic stimuli on unilateral spatial neglect following right hemisphere lesions. Rest Neurol Neurosci 1990;2:39–46.

18. Butter CM, Kirsch NL. Combined and separate effects of eye patching and visual stimulation on unilateral neglect following stroke. Arch Phys Med Rehab 1992;73:1133–1139.

19. Hommel M, Peres B, Pollack P, et al. Effects of passive tactile and auditory stimuli on left visual neglect. Arch Neurol 1990;47:573–576.

20. Robertson IH, Nico D, Hood BM. Believing what you feel: using proprioceptive feedback to reduce unilateral neglect. Neuropsychology 1997;11:53–58.

21. Robertson IH, Nico D, Hood BM. The intention to act improves unilateral left neglect: two demonstrations. Neuroreport 1995;7:246–248.

22. Wiart L, Lome AB, Debelleix X, et al. Unilateral neglect syndrome rehabilitation by trunk rotation and scanning retraining. Arch Phys Med Rehab 1997;78:424–429.

23. Rubens A. Caloric stimulation and unilateral neglect. Neurology 1985;35:1019–1024.

24. Cappa S, Sterzi R, Vallar G, Bisiach E. Remission of hemineglect and anosognosia during vestibular stimulation. Neuropsychologia 1987;25:775–782.

25. Geminiani G, Bottini G. Mental representations and temporary recovery from unilateral neglect after vestibular stimulation. J Neurol Neurosurg Psychiatry 1991;55:332–333.

26. Fleet WS, Valenstein E, Watson RT, Heilman KM. Dopamine agonist therapy for neglect in humans. Neurology 1987;37:1765–1770.

27. Geminiani G, Bottini G, Stenzi R. Dopamine stimulation in unilateral neglect. J Neurol Neurosurg Psychiatry 1998; 65:344–347.

28. Kertesz A. Recovery of Aphasia. In Feinberg and Farah (eds), Behavioral Neurology and Neuropsychology. New York: McGraw-Hill, 1997;167–182.

29. Naeser MA, Palumbo CL, Helm-Estabrooks N, et al. Severe nonfluency in aphasia. Role of medical subcallosal fasciculus plus other white matter pathways in recovery of spontaneous speech. Brain 1989;112(Pt 1):1–38.

30. Naeser MA, Gaddie A, Palumbo CL, Stiassmy-Eder D. Late recovery of auditory comprehension in global aphasia. Improved recovery observed with subcortical temporal isthmus lesion versus Wernicke's cortical area lesion. Arch Neurol 1990;47:425–432.

31. Small SL. Aphasia Rehabilitation. In RB Lazar (ed), Principles of Neurologic Rehabilitation. New York: McGraw-Hill, 1998;517–551.

32. Belin P, Van Eeckhout P, Zilbovicius M, et al. Recovery from nonfluent aphasia after melodic intonation therapy: a PET study. Neurology 1996;47:1504–1511.

33. Abe K, Inokawa M, Kashiwagi A, Yanagihara T. Amnesia after a discrete basal forebrain lesion. J Neurol Neurosurg Psychiatry 1998;65:126–130.

34. Glisky EL. Rehabilitation of Memory Dysfunction. In Feinberg and Farah (eds), Behavioral Neurology and Neuropsychology. New York: McGraw-Hill, 1997;491–495.

35. Gaviria M, Furmaga K. Clinical Aspects and Treatment of Neuropsychiatric Disturbances in Patients with Chronic Neurologic Disorders. In RB Lazar (ed), Principles of Neurologic Rehabilitation. New York: McGraw-Hill, 1998;553–563.

36. Heilman KM, et al. Disorders of Skilled Limb Movements: Limb Apraxia. In Feinberg and Farah (eds), Behavioral Neurology and Neuropsychology. New York: McGraw-Hill, 1997;227–236.

37. Kauhanen M, Korpelainen JT, Hiltunen P, et al. Poststroke depression correlates with cognitive impairment and neurologic deficits. Stroke 1999;30:1875–1880.

38. Shimoda K, Robinson RG. The relationship between poststroke depression and lesion location in long-term follow-up. Biol Psychiatry 1999;45:187–192.

39. Singh A, Herrmann N, Black SE. The importance of lesion location in poststroke depression: a critical review. Can J Psychiatry 1998;43:921–927.

40. Paolucci S, Antonucci G, Pratesi L, et al. Poststroke depression and its role in rehabilitation of inpatients. Arch Phys Med Rehabil 1999;80:985–990.

41. Reding MJ, Orto LA, Winter SW, et al. Antidepressant therapy after stroke. A double-blind trial. Arch Neurol 1986;43:763–765.

42. Lipsey JR, Robinson RG, Pearlson GD, et al. Nortriptyline treatment of post-stroke depression: a double-blind study. Lancet 1984;1:297–300.

43. Andersen G, Vestergaard K, Lauritzen L, et al. Effective treatment of poststroke depression with selective serotonin reuptake inhibitor citalopram. Stroke 1994,25:1099–1104.

44. Starkstein SE, Fedoroff P, Berthier ML, Robinson RG. Manic-depressive and pre-manic states after brain lesions. Biol Psychiatry 1991;29:149–158.

45. Cummings JL, Meadey MF. Secondary mania with focal cerebrovascular lesions. Am J Psychiatry 1984;141:1084–1087.

46. Fenn D, George K. Post-stroke mania late in life involving the left hemisphere. Aust N Z J Psychiatry 1999;33:598–600.

47. Rosenbaum AH, Barrn MJ. Positive therapeutic response to lithium in hypomania secondary to organic brain syndrome. Am J Psychiatry 1975;132:1072–1073.

48. Vaphiades MS, Celesia GG, Brigell MG. Positive spontaneous visual phenomena limited to the hemiscopic field in lesions of central visual pathways. Neurology 1996;47:408–417.

49. Anderson SW, Rizzo M. Hallucinations following occipital lobe damage: the pathological activation of visual representations. J Clin Exp Neuropsychol 1994;16:652–663.

50. Brust JC, Behrons MM. Release hallucinations as the major symptom of posterior cerebral artery occlusion. Ann Neurol 1977;2:432–436.

51. Price BH, Mesulam M. Psychiatric manifestations or right hemisphere infarctions. J Nerv Ment Dis 1985;173:610–614.

52. Levine DN, Grek A. The anatomic basis of delusions after right cerebral infarction. Neurology 1984;34:577–582.

53. Gorman DG, Cummings JL. Organic delusional syndrome. Sem Neurol 1990;10:229–238.

Index